CW00696331

1 MONTH OF
FREE
READING

at

www.ForgottenBooks.com

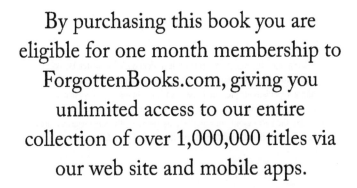

By purchasing this book you are eligible for one month membership to ForgottenBooks.com, giving you unlimited access to our entire collection of over 1,000,000 titles via our web site and mobile apps.

To claim your free month visit:
www.forgottenbooks.com/free678891

ISBN 978-0-483-37412-6
PIBN 10678891

Official Journal Ohio State Eclectic Medical Association.

JANUARY, 1908.

SIXTY-EIGHTH YEAR. VOL. LXVIII, No. 1.

The
Eclectic Medical
Journal

Edited by

JOHN KING SCUDDER, A. M., M. D.

Assisted by the Faculty of the Eclectic Medical Institute

A MONTHLY JOURNAL OF ECLECTIC MEDICINE AND SURGERY
strongly advocating a re-study of Practice and Materia Medica
along the lines of the well-known doctrines of Specific
Medication and Specific Diagnosis.

ἐκλέγω

Published by
THE SCUDDER BROTHERS COMPANY, 1009 Plum Street, Cincinnati, Ohio.

SUBSCRIPTION PRICE, TWO DOLLARS A YEAR, IN ADVANCE
SINGLE NUMBERS, 20 CENTS

Table of Contents, Page 1.

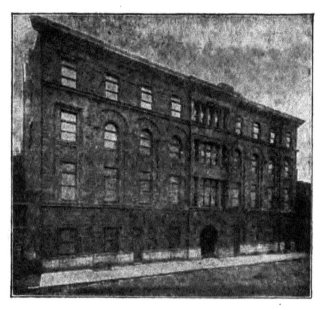

THE

ECLECTIC MEDICAL JOURNAL

EDITED BY

JOHN K. SCUDDER, A.M., M.D.,

ASSISTED BY THE FACULTY OF THE ECLECTIC MEDICAL INSTITUTE,
CINCINNATI, OHIO.

JANUARY TO DECEMBER, 1908.
VOLUME LXVIII.

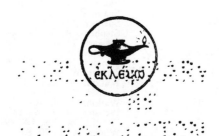

PUBLISHED BY
The Scudder Brothers Co., Medical Publishers,
1009 PLUM STREET, CINCINNATI, OHIO.
1908.

INDEX TO AUTHORS.

INDEX.

INDEX.

THE ECLECTIC MEDICAL JOURNAL

ESTABLISHED 1836.

VOL. LXVIII.   CINCINNATI, JANUARY, 1908.   No. 1.

BIOGRAPHICAL SKETCHES.*

WOOSTER BEACH, M.D.

By HARVEY WICKES FELTER, M.D.,
CINCINNATI.

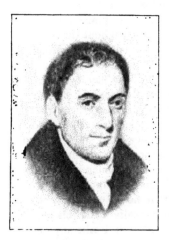

WOOSTER BEACH, M. D.

Wooster Beach, M.D., the "Founder of Eclecticism," was born at Trumbull, Conn., in 1794, and died in 1868. He was connected with the Woosters of Connecticut — one of whom, General David Wooster, served with distinction in the Revolutionary War, losing his life for his country. Early in life Dr. Beach showed a strong leaning toward education, which finally shaped itself into an ardent passion for research, particularly in the fields of theology and medicine. A strong distrust and antipathy to the current medical practice of his day marks his entrance into a subsequently eminent career. He pursued eagerly all the adverse criticisms upon medicine, such as were frequently indulged in by the leaders of medical thought, among whom may be mentioned the celebrated Dr. Benjamin Rush, of Philadelphia. He paid particular attention to the results of heroic medication, and was appalled by the sights that he beheld in the recognized regular practice of medicine. Says he, in that rare publication, "The Rise, Progress, and Present State of the New York Medical Institution and Reformed Medical Society of the United States," published by him in 1830:

---

* Reprinted from the "History of the Eclectic Medical Institute," 1902.

"With such facts staring me in the face, my soul was filled with indignation at these instru ments of cruelty and misery, administered under the specious pretext of removing disease. These sentiments ' grew with my growth and strengthened with my strength.' Constant observation confirmed me in the truth of these things, and I felt a deep solicitude to effect a reformation; but how to do this I knew not. I had no idea that there was a single individual in existence who practiced medicine on different principles, until one day I accidentally saw a medical preparation brought from a distance by a relative, which had cured him of a critical complaint. Upon further inquiry respecting its origin, I was informed that it had been given by a celebrated physician, of the name of Tidd,' residing in a seeluded part of New Jersey. He informed me that he was an aged man, ·very noted, and remarkably skillful in the cure of various diseases. From that hour a hope sprang up in my mind that I should be enabled to obtain a knowledge of his practice, and it was not long before Providence called me near his residence. I then found the ' half had not been told me.' His praise was in the mouth of almost every one, and his fame was throughout the country. One would show me a scar of some great cure which he had performed, while others would relate cases where his skill had been tested and demonstrated. I therefore had an increasing desire to pay a visit to this physician, that I might learn his practice for the good of my fellow-men. I accordingly commenced my journey. After I had traveled about thirty miles, I arrived at his residence; and instead of finding a dashing, popular man, I found his appearance plain and even ordinary. I made known my business, and expressed a great desire to obtain a knowledge of his practice. The old gentleman was not disposed to receive me as a student—he had repeated applications from physicians and others, but he observed that he did not think it was right to make his practice known.[2] He sarcastically made this expression to me: ' Doctors wish to be gentlemen, but if I take any one to learn, I want another hog like myself to root around the mountains in search of medicines; they wish to be gentlemen, but they ought to be the servants of all men.' . . . Notwithstanding my urgent solicitations, however, I could not persuade him to receive me as a student, and I was obliged to return home disappointed. But the same anxiety continued; and I felt, respecting medicine, something as the Apostle Paul is represented to have felt respecting religion, when he said, 'A dispensation of the gospel is committed unto me, and woe be unto me if I preach not the gospel.' "

1 Dr. Jacob Tidd, of Amwell, Hunterdon County, New York.
2 Had he done so in his day, he would have had his means of livelihood taken from him.

Another journey was made, and again was Beach repulsed, but not hopeless. He further relates:

"After teaching school awhile, I turned my attention to mercantile pursuits. But this appeared not to be the sphere in which Providence designed that I should move. A series of misfortunes attended all my pursuits. But it is remarkable that, in whatever business I was engaged, I never ceased praying the Almighty that he would yet enable me to learn this practice, which I so much desired, and, like the importunate widow, continued my intercessions for the space of six or seven years, and during most of which period I was several hundred miles from the doctor's residence. But a well-directed train of events finally brought me to Philadelphia, and I concluded once more to pay a visit to the old doctor. I went, and it happened (but I will not say happened, for it was providential) just at the time when a grandson of his had emigated to the western country, and left him without assistance. When I again made my errand known, he appeared pleased, and gave me encouragement. I informed him that I came with a determination of staying, and did not mean to leave his house till I learned his knowledge of the healing art. He finally gave his consent, provided I could obtain that of his family; and, after much hesitation, fearing I should make known the practice to their injury, they agreed to receive me. I remained with him a sufficient length of time to learn his practice, when he departed this life at the age of seventy-four years. . . . I then succeeded him for some time, until I was called to this city (New York) to treat some difficult cases, which, having cured, I was introduced into practice. Having located myself here, I attended a course of lectures in the University of the State of New York during the time Drs. Post, Hosack, Mott, and others, were professors. I concluded this was best, were it only to detect the errors of the modern practice; and subsequently I obtained a *diploma*, according to the law of the State, which, should any wish to peruse, they will find it recorded in the County Clerk's Office, in the City Hall, New York. And to refute calumny, I will here subjoin the recommendation of the Censors to the President of the Medical Society, viz.: ' We certify that we have examined Dr. W. Beach, that he has produced to us sufficient vouchers that he has studied the practice of Physic and Surgery the term required by law; that he possesses a good moral character, and that he has sustained an examination before us which does him honor; and we cheerfully recommend him to the President of the Medical Society for a diploma to practice Physic and Surgery.' "

Dr. Beach at once began his active career. He learned much from a Dr. Ferris, and other botanic physicians, and, in fact, from any source which promised a reform in medicine. It was about the year 1825 when he located in New York, at 93 Eldridge Street. He practiced with marked success, instructed private students, and dispensed medicines. He now conceived a plan for a clinical institution and a medical school, and accordingly opened, in 1827, the United States Infirmary, and in 1829, the Reformed Medical Academy, which, in 1830, became the Reformed Medical College. Among those connected with this school, either as students, and some as teachers, were Drs. T. V. Morrow, I. G. Jones, John King, John J. Steele, and one afterward a distinguished surgeon of New York City, Dr. James R. Wood, for many years a leader of medical opinion in his city, and one who had a very flattering opinion of Dr. Beach, characterizing him as one of the "really great men of his day." In 1829 a pioneer national society was formed, known as the Reformed Medical Society of the United States. Of this, Dr. Beach was elected (November 29, 1829) President. From this society was sent out, on May 3, 1830, a circular of resolutions, which culminated in locating the Reformed Medical College of Ohio, at Worthington, Ohio. In 1832 he distinguished himself in New York City by his success over his competitors in the treatment of Asiatic cholera, he having been assigned to treat the out-door poor of the Tenth Ward. Dr. Beach subsequently became much interested in religious controversies, and published papers and magazines in support of his views, among them the *Battle-Axe*, the *Ishmaelite*, the *Medical Reformer*, and the *Telescope*, a weekly journal on religious, social and medical topics. Upon the establishment of the Eclectic Medical Institute, Dr. Beach was added to the faculty in December, 1845, as Professor of Clinical Surgery and Medicine, holding his position for one session, when he was made an Emeritus Professor, and later was dropped from the faculty, not being altogether acceptable to Professor Buchanan and his associates. He also lectured one term at the Central Medical College of New York. In 1855 he was made President of the National Eclectic Medical Association. Since that period there seems to have been a coldness between Beach and the other teachers of Reformed and Eclectic Medicine. About the latter part of 1855, Dr. Beach began a two years' tour of inspection of the hospitals, public and private, of Europe, in order to collect new material for a revised edition of his practice. Dr. Beach was a voluminous writer. Besides his professional labors and editorial work, he published, in 1833, the first great work on Reformed Medicine,' his three-volume compilation, "The American Practice of Medicine," which at once became the standard work on practice among the reform-

---

1 Not botanic. Dr. Elisha Smith published in 1830 the *Botanic Physician*, and Thompson had preceded him.

ers, and received gold medals and other distinctions from foreign poten-
tates and distinguished European physicians. It was afterward condensed into one volume, and had a large sale, and contributed greatly
to the popularity of the reform movement. In 1850 a new edition of
his larger work was published, being embellished with the engravings
of medicinal plants from Rafinesque's " Medical. Botany.'" This edition, however, proved a pecuniary loss to him. He also prepared a
" Medical Dictionary," a work on " Midwifery," with elegant plates,
and a " Human Physiology." On account of his excellent works he
was made a member of several European medical societies. Shortly
after his connection with the Institute a heavy blow fell upon him in
the loss of a favorite son, by drowning, in the East River. This son,
he had hoped, would continue his reform movement. From that time
on his life was saddened. Though he traveled from point to point,
and instructed students, and delivered lectures from time to time, and
even purchased a large and expensive anatomical museum in Paris,
with a view of founding a great medical institution, his life's work
had been accomplished, and he keenly felt his inability to carry out
his designs. For years after he suffered from mental despondency, and
died in 1868. Dr. Beach married Miss Eliza DeGrove in 1823, by
whom he had seven children. Two of his sons became practitioners of
medicine of the dominant school. Dr. Beach was tall, heavy-boned, and
of dark complexion. He cared little for the conventionalities of life,
and possessed poor financial ability. Dr. Horatio Firth says of him:

" Dr. Wooster Beach was, in many respects, a remarkable man.
He was ' brimful ' of restless enthusiasm. He labored as one having
faith in the purity of his mission. His devotion to the cause of medical reform was without a parallel in the history of medicine. He considered no sacrifice too great, no labor too hard, if he could only thereby
advance the interests of medical reform. Although Dr. Beach possessed but limited capacity as a lecturer, and was not in reality a highly
educated man, he was, nevertheless, one of the greatest compilers and
collectors of medical experiences that the reformed practice has ever
known. His intimate knowledge of the nature of disease and of the
action of remedies, and his skillful plan of treating all diseases, were
appreciated by his patients, and even acknowledged by his enemies."
Notwithstanding all that he did, he " was one of the poorest of finan-
ciers. He was ever writing and publishing books, periodicals and
papers; but shrewd and designing men were ever on his path to pocket
the proceeds of his labor. He collected great museums, but never realized any pecuniary advantage therefrom. He organized societies, colleges and infirmaries. He labored with untiring zeal to relieve the
distressed, the sick and the poor. He visited various parts of the country as consulting physician, and to the pursuits of his profession he
gave untiring diligence; but for all this ceaseless labor he scarcely
received money enough to secure him a livelihood."

DISEASES OF THE UTERUS.*

BY A. F. STEPHENS, M.D.,
ST. LOUIS, MO.

Normally the uterus lies, or is suspended, in the pelvis, with its anterior surface in contact with the urinary bladder, its fundus looking towards the umbilicus, the cervix pointing backwards towardr the hollow of the sacrum, its long axis practically at right angle with the axis of the vaginal canal. It is so adjusted and suspended in the

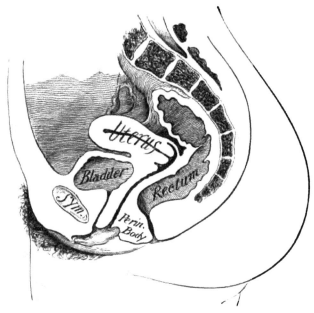

FIG. 8.—Median sagittal section of the normal female pelvis. (Penrose.)

pelvis that ordinary movements of the body do not affect it, hence no injury or discomfort results from any position the woman may assume.

The normal non-gravid uterus of the adult woman is about three inches in length, two inches in breadth at its broadest part, and one inch in thickness. It varies according to the age of the subject, being quite small before the age of puberty, and again in old age from atrophy. In women who have borne children it does not return to the size it was before child-birth, but remains somewhat larger. However, its size should not exceed an ounce and a half to two ounces in

* A portion of Chapter VIII of Professor Stephens' new book on "Medical Gynecology," 12 mo. of 428 pp. Cloth, $3.00.

weight. At the end of gestation its weight is from a pound and a half to three pounds. It decreases rapidly to its normal size and weight after the termination of pregnancy.

The uterus is arbitrarily divided into a fundus, a body and a neck. It is a hollow organ, and the entrance to its cavity is through the os uteri and cervical canal. The entrance is guarded by circular bands of muscular fibres, which exert considerable strength, especially at the internal os, or constriction at the upper extremity of the cervical canal.

The fundus of the uterus is that portion of the organ which rises above the insertion of the Fallopian tubes. It is directed upwards and forwards, and is covered by the peritoneum. The body is that portion below the insertion of the tubes, and extends to the constriction, which marks the beginning of the cervix or neck. The boundary between the fundus and body is unmarked and entirely arbitrary. In fact, there is no valid reason for the division. For all practical purposes the division of the organ into a body and a neck would be sufficient.

The uterus is situated in the pelvis between the urinary bladder and the rectum, being united to these organs by folds of the peritoneum, which are reflected from its body both anteriorly and posteriorly, and which are termed the anterior and posterior ligaments of the uterus. By like reflections of the peritoneal covering laterally the broad ligaments are formed. Within the folds of the broad ligaments are contained the Fallopion tubes, ovaries, and their ligaments, the round ligaments, and the nutrient vessels and nerves.

The cavity of the uterus is small, triangular, flattened from before backwards, with its base directed upwards and its walls closely approximated. At each upper angle is a funnel-shaped cavity, at the bottom of which are the orifices of the Fallopian tubes. At the inferior angle is the constricted opening, or ostium internum, which leads to the canal of the cervix. This canal is cylindrical, broadest at the middle, and ends at the ostium externum, which communicates with the vaginal canal.

The cervix uteri is from an inch to an inch and a quarter in length normally, a portion of which extends into the vaginal canal, and can be felt by the examining finger in the vagina and may be seen by the aid of a speculum. At the termination of the cervix is the external os, or mouth of the uterus. This opening into the vagina is small, circular in women who have never borne children, and appears as a simple indentation in the lower end of the cervix. After the woman has given birth to a child the os is much larger, and usually fissured laterally, which divides the cervix into an anterior and posterior lip.

This lateral laceration of the cervix by child-birth, while it results in nearly all cases, yet it is possible for a woman to give birth to a child and not destroy the circular shape of the os. The healthy cervix is smooth, firm, and elastic to the touch, and of a pale rose color. Sensibility is deficient, no pain being felt on pressure. Decided variations from the above are evidences of disease.

Appendages.—The uterine appendages are the *Fallopian tubes, ovaries* and their *ligaments,* and the *round ligaments.*

The Fallopian tubes and ovaries are very frequently the seat of disease.

Fallopian Tubes.—The Fallopian tubes are two in number, one on either side of the uterus, and situated in the free margin of the broad ligament. They are ducts which convey the ova from the ovaries to the uterus. They are about four inches in length, extending from the uterus to the ovaries. Their canals are very minute, the entrance to them at the superior angles of the uterine cavity scarcely admitting an instrument the size of a bristle.

Ovaries.—The ovaries, which are analogous to the testes in the male, are two in number. They are elongated, oval-shaped bodies flattened from above downwards, and situated, one on either side of the uterus, in the posterior portion of the broad ligaments. They are connected with the uterus by ligaments, and to the fimbriated extremity of the Fallopian tubes by a sort of cord. Normally they are whitish in color, about an inch and a half in length, three-fourths of an inch in breadth, and about a third of an inch in thickness. Their anterior surfaces are attached to the broad ligaments, their posterior surfaces being free. They are invested by a peritoneal covering, except at the attached border.

DISEASES OF THE BODY OF THE UTERUS.

DISPLACEMENTS.—The uterus may be displaced as a whole, as in prolapse; or it may simply change its relative position, as is seen in version; or it may change its shape, as in the different flexions.

The various displacements are known as *versions, flexions,* and *prolapses.*

A *retroversion* is that in which the uterus turns on its transverse axis, so that the intra-abdominal pressure lies upon its anterior wall instead of the posterior, as in the normal state.

A *retroflexion* is one in which the uterus is bent upon itself, the body being bent backwards towards the hollow of the sacrum.

Anteversion is normal to the uterus, but the position is sometimes exaggerated, when it becomes abnormal.

A *prolapse* is that condition wherein the uterus descends along the vaginal canal downwards. The prolapse may reach an extreme degree, the uterus descending until it emerges from the vulva. As a rule the prolapse is only partial, the organ remaining in the vagina, but lower in the pelvis than normal.

ANTEFLEXION.—While a slight anteflexion is the normal position of the uterus, and is therefore of no pathological significance, an exaggerated anteflexion may be the cause of dysmenorrhea, endometritis, or sterility. The disease is most frequently met with in women who have never borne children.

Etiology.—Anteflexion in women who have borne children has its origin from the puerperal state. The uterus may be flexed in a forward direction by ligamentous contraction, and pressure of the adominal viscera upon the body has a tendency to increase it.

The cause of anteflexion in women who have not borne children is not well established, but seems to be an increase of the normal anteflexion of childhood, which may be due to accident or congestion of the organ.

Symptoms.—A frequent symptom of anteflexion is menstrual pain. Pain is due to the obstruction in the cervical canal, because of the bending of the body of the uterus upon the cervix and the consequent endometritis brought on by the unrelieved congestion of the endometrium.

Sterility is another frequent consequence of anteflexion, which is due to structural changes in the uterine mucous membrane as a result of chronic endometritis.

Anteflexion, by interfering with the normal circulation, causes passive congestion and chronic edometritis. This gives rise to excessive secretion of mucus, which escapes from the uterus as a leucorrhea. This discharge is whitish in color and more or less profuse in amount, dependent upon the degree of congestion. It is most abundant just before and after a menstrual period.

Diagnosis.—Anteflexion may be detected by digital examination. A finger is introduced into the vagina, with which the anterior surface of the uterus is traced while pressing the organ downward, with the points of the fingers placed on the abdomen directly above the symphysis pubis. The uterus can be easily palpated between the two hands, unless the patient is extremely fat and has very thick abdominal walls. Being familiar with the normal curve of the uterus, one can easily recognize an exaggerated anteflexion.

Additional evidence may be had by the passage of a uterine sound, which will meet with obstruction at the entrance to the uterine cavity, and will require a short curve at the end of the sound before it can be passed into the uterine cavity.

Prognosis.—Anteflexion occurring in a normal sized uterus is readily curable. When associated with an infantile uterus it is probably incurable.

Treatment.—The treatment for anteflexion is operative by dilatation. The operation should be done about ten days after menstruation. If there is a chronic endometritis, curetment should also be done.

RETROVERSION.—Retroversion is that position of the uterus assumed when the organ is tilted upon its transverse axis, with its fundus looking backward, the cervix pointing forward towards the bladder, while the natural curve of the canal remains unchanged.

Retroversion is the most frequent displacement of the uterus, and is found oftenest in women who have borne children.

Etiology.—Posterior displacements are due to relaxation of the pelvic tissues; lacerations of the pelvic floor; abnormally large pelvis;

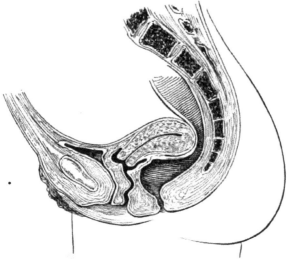

FIG. 11.—Retroversion of the Uterus.   (Penrose.)

increased weight of the uterus, due to subinvolution following labor or miscarriage; sudden or extreme muscular effort, as in lifting or straining; tight lacing and weakening of the pelvic tissues from general debility or exhaustion.

Symptoms.—The symptoms are backache, pain and weight, with a sensation of dragging in the pelvis; pain extending to the hips and down the thighs; a sensation of fullness in the rectum and constipation; irregular menstruation, usually in the form of menorrhagia, which is due to the congestion caused by displacement. Pain in the top of the head is often complained of, as well as pain in the occiput.

The patient finally becomes neurasthenic if the displacement is not overcome. Milder reflex neuroses precede general neurasthenia, such as gastric and intestinal disturbances. The disease eventually causes a lack of energy, the patient complains of being tired on the least exertion, and even moderate exercise increases her suffering.

Diagnosis.—The group of symptoms above outlined will suggest disease of the pelvic organs, when an examination should be made. On making a digital examination the cervix will be found pointing towards the bladder, instead of backwards in the direction of the hollow of the sacrum. With the fingers of the free hand pressing downward from above the symphysis pubis, the fundus of the retroverted uterus cannot be felt anteriorly as it should be if in the normal state, but will be found lying in the hollow of the sacrum. If the vaginal finger is carried backwards and upwards to the posterior cul-de-sac and pressure made in an upward and forward direction, the fundus can be brought under the fingers of the hand on the abdomen. If a finger is then passed into the rectum, the position of the uterus may be very readily determined and the diagnosis confirmed.

Retroversion is differentiated from retroflexion by the fact that in the former the normal curve remains unchanged, while in retroflexion the concavity of the curve is reversed.

Finally, a uterine sound carried through the canal to the fundus will follow the direction of the retroverted organ, passing upwards and backwards towards the hollow of the sacrum, instead of upwards and forwards, as in the normal position.

Prognosis.—The danger to life need not be considered, except that the displacement, by its debilitating effects upon the general health, renders the patient less able to resist other diseases to which she may be liable, thus proving serious. Unless the displacement is corrected, it may result in permanent invalidism.

Treatment.—In cases of recent displacement the tissues have not undergone changes which make it almost impossible to correct without resorting to operative measures, and the treatment by other methods may be undertaken with the assurance of success. However, the longer the lesion has existed, the less likely are we to meet with success and the longer will the treatment have to be continued to attain it. In recent cases, however, the treatment will have to be continued for several months, and in some cases longer, in order to gain the desired end. It requires a long time in many cases to bring the tissues back to their normal condition and strength.

The treatment will include the removal of the cause, replacement of the uterus in its normal position and maintaining it there, reducing the organ to its normal size if enlarged, stimulating and strengthening the holding structures, constitutional treatment, and hygiene. The latter will include the right kind of clothing, proper exercise, bathing and massage.

Whatever existing cause is found must be first removed. It may be a laceration of the pelvic floor or cervix, endometritis or subinvolution; whatever it may be must be relieved before we can hope to replace a retroverted uterus to its normal position and retain it there.

Having removed all causes of displacement, the next step in the treatment is to replace the uterus in its normal position and maintain it in that position.

The knee-chest position is the best attitude for the patient to assume during the replacement of a retroverted uterus. In this position we are assisted by the force of gravity, the fuudus dropping back into place by its own weight. The air-pressure within the distended vagina also aids in pushing the organ into its proper position. The proceeding is as follows: The patient having been placed in the knee-chest position, a Sims' speculum is introduced and the perineum retracted. If the uterus does not assume its normal position of itself, the anterior lip of the cervix is seized with a pair of bullet forceps and pulled downwards and backwards, thus allowing the fundus to clear the promontory of the sacrum and drop forward, where it normally belongs. If necessary a small ball of absorbent cotton may be grasped with dressing forceps, and being placed against the fundus a pushing force can be applied, which will aid in sending the fundus anteriorly, where it belongs.

The uterus having been placed in its proper position, the next thing is to keep it there. This is to be done by means of some contrivance which will hold the organ steady in the position in which we have placed it. For this purpose there have been many pessaries fashioned, the best of which is probably the Thomas hard rubber, or the Smith-Hodge. The instrument can be placed while the patient is in the knee-chest position, or she may lie upon her back. In inserting the pessary the labia are separated with the thumb and finger of the left hand, while the pessary is held by its anterior bar between the thumb and fingers of the right hand, and the posterior bar is made to enter between the separated labia, the bar being held in the transverse diameter of the vagina. It is pushed upwards, followiug the curve of the pelvis until it reaches a position against the anterior lip of the cervix. An index finger is now inserted under the anterior bar of the pessary and conducted upwards to the posterior bar, against which it rests and which it carries behind the cervix and high enough to sustain the uterus in the desired position. To remove the pessary the patient is to hook her finger behind the anterior bar and carefully pull it from the vagina.

Careful adjustment of the pessary is necessary to success, and the instrument must fit properly, hence it is always well to have a number of different sizes at hand, so that the proper size may be adjusted. If it is necessary to change the shape of a pessary, it may be coated with vaseline and held over the flame of an alcohol lamp until it becomes pliable, when it can be bent to any shape desired and allowed to cool. The pessary should not be too large, for if so it will in all probability interfere with the rectum or bladder, and thereby cause trouble. It is to be borne in mind that a pessary should cause no pain or discomfort while worn if it fits perfectly. Neglect of this precaution may, by producing excoriations about the vagina, cause the patient much suffering. After the pessary is properly adjusted the patient is to remain under the care of the physician, and the condition of the parts is to be examined every day or two for a week to see that the instrument remains in place, and that the uterus is held in its normal position without inconvenience to the woman. Afterwards it should be examined once a month. A new one should be substituted every few months, or as often as may be necessary, or whenever the pessary becomes defective. At any time the patient complains of pain or discomfort from the presence of the pessary she is to notify the physician of such pain or discomfort, when the cause of the trouble is to be sought for and removed. While wearing a pessary the vagina must be kept perfectly clean. This is to be done by using the plain hot water douche once or twice a day.

The general health of the patient is to be carefully looked after and any wrong corrected. If constipation is present it is to be overcome, but all means to that end should be directed so as to avoid active catharsis. Proper food and drink, together with regular habits, will, as a rule, overcome the difficulty without having to resort to physic. Bathing, especially the cold sponge bath, followed by thorough rubbing dry with the hands, is recommended. By this method she gives the pelvic structures a massage that in time will strengthen them greatly by the increased circulation induced by the rubbing. At the same time it is a splendid exercise to all the muscles of the body. In addition, the various physical culture exercises practiced faithfully will do much good to bring about the desired physical well-being. Exercise in the open air is a necessity, and exercise to be beneficial should be accompanied by intelligent thought. In other words, to exercise properly one must have some object in view in doing so. Otherwise even a little exercise becomes tiresome and exhausting, rather than recuperative. Different methods will suggest themselves in different cases, and one must invent means to suit the different cases.

The clothing is to be worn with a view to comfort and the avoidance of constriction about the waist, or dragging and pressure upon abdomen, as all such will tend to force the uterus out of position, by crowding the abdominal viscera downward upon the pelvic organs.

We have a few remedies which we know exert a beneficial influence upon the pelvic organs, remedies which, acting upon these structures, give a better circulation and innervation, thereby strengthening them and aiding in the correction of any wrong which may be due to relaxation and congestion of the tissues. I will mention only a few.

Viburnum prunifolium is one of the most important uterine tonics we possess. It is indicated when dysmenorrheic symptoms are present. Macrotys is indicated by muscular pain in the back and dragging pains in the uterus. These symptoms are very often present in displacements. Belladonna is indicated in all forms of congestion in whatever part of the body it may be. The indications are capillary congestion, with deep, dull, aching pains in the loins and back, with a sense of fullness; dull, heavy headache and dizziness or drowsiness. Nux vomica will prove an aid to the treatment when the patient is debilitated and the tissues need a better innervation. These patients are apt to look sallow or pale; the tongue is broad and pale in color; the patient is weak and does not care to take exercise. The remedy will wake them up and give a better appetite and better digestion, which is bound to aid us in our effort to strengthen the tissues involved in the displacement.

Many other remedies might be mentioned, but after all it is impossible to give a treatment that will fit every case, as cases must necessarily differ as widely as do the patients, and one must meet the indications as they arise in each individual case.

In those cases which may be termed chronic, and when the displacement cannot be overcome and replacement sustained, operation becomes a necessity. Such operations have for their object either shortening of the round ligaments, or ventral suspension of the uterus.

KEY TO THE TESTING OF DRUG ACTION.

By F. J. PETERSEN, M.D.,
LOMPOC, CAL.

A subject that has caused much misunderstanding amongst practitioners in general and the various schools of medicine, is the physiological effect of drugs. A more thorough understanding of this subject would cause a better feeling and result in deeper investigations into a subject which is far from being well understood at the present time.

The true disciples of Hahnemann prove the action of a drug by giving potencies, generally the sixth to the thirtieth, three to four times a day to a healthy person, until the physiological effect becomes pronounced. He does not believe that the effect of physiological doses can serve him as a guide to its primary use. The fact of the matter is that many drugs can be tested by giving physiological doses; others can only be tested satisfactorily by Hahnemann's system of proving.

Where possible to test the action of a drug by physiological doses, it is more satisfactory in giving us the basic indication than the system of proving, as the latter is so broad in its symptomatology that it is not always easy to get the basic indications fully isolated. Minor indications are often misleading. Most of the old school physicians deny the possibility of testing the action of a drug by provings, and deny that there is any virtue in potencies. Still, they believe in serum therapy, which, in fact, is nothing but Homeopathy in a crude and cruel form; it is given in homeopathic doses.

Electricity is quite often used now for its primary effect. This does not mean a primary current, but it means that if the vibrations of a current are carried way up in the thousands a minute we begin to get the primary effect, which is more pronounced as the number of vibrations are increased in a minute. Still, the allopaths deny that there is any value in potencies.

We, as Eclectics, fully understand that there is virtue in medicine in various forms and strengths, and for that reason use drugs, no matter in what strength, if it will meet certain indications, and thus conform to our system of specific medication. Thus our school has formulated a system which deserves the good will of the public. However, in order to get the credit we deserve, our school of medicine must become better known, and there is only one way to do this, and that is to *come to the front* and *stay there*. Let the public know who we are, what advantages our system has, and show them what we can do. Our work speaks for itself; but what good does it do the Eclectic school of medicine if the public does not know the work is done by Eclectics? We must do missionary work, show the advantages of our system of medication, enlighten the public on the subject through the public press.

The necessity of just laws, such as will give equal rights and representation to all schools and special favors to none, must be impressed upon them through the public press. Thus the danger of a one-school medical trust will come home to the people, and, as a result, we can expect justice.

The public owes the Eclectic and Homeopathic schools a lasting gratitude for changing the old, obsolete way of medication. What would therapeutics be to-day without the *regular* Eclectic and *regular* Homeopathic materia medica and therapeutics? Let us impress this on the minds of the people through the public press, and we will eventually get our just dues.

To come back to our subject of physiological effects of drugs, we will say that, to a certain extent, both the test by physiological doses as well as by proving can be used. In some drugs the former is more desirable, and in some the latter can only be used.

To illustrate: Belladonna, gelsemium, glonoin, lobelia, jaborandi and many other drugs of a dual nature can be tested by both methods, as we get in both our basic symptoms. The physiological tests, however, do not apply to drugs which are markedly irritating to the gastro-intestinal tract, because the direct effect of contact is so irritating that its test cannot be carried far enough to give us all the basic symptoms of the physiological effects. Drugs in which immediate vomiting is produced simply through the direct irritation to mucous surfaces can be best tested by the system of provings for reasons given above. Bryonia is a drug which causes so much direct irritation to the gastro-intestinal tract by contact that it must be tested by provings. Ipecac is another drug that is best tested by provings. I could mention many others, but the above will give the reader an idea of what I mean.

Speaking about bryonia, we will say that this is a remedy of great value; and still the old school generally gives it credit for something it should never be used for, and that is a cholagogue cathartic. Its true medicinal value they do not seem to realize.

Those who have seen my scales in the March issue of the *Chicago Medical Times* and the *California Medical Journal*, will understand that Eclectics and Homeopaths use bryonia for its primary effect, the difference being that we, as Eclectics, at times come very near the border-line, where the primary blends into that of the secondary action. The secondary effect is too irritating to the gastro-intestinal tract, while in full physiological doses it is dangerous. Lloyd's specific bryonia, five drops to four ounces, is strong enough, and in some cases, especially where there is nausea and much irritation in the gastro-intestinal tract, bryonia 2x—say ten to twenty drops in four ounces of water—can be tolerated better.

The above, in a general way, will explain points which are so often disputed. Bear in mind, however, that what the Homeopaths call proving of a drug and our physiological tests, although vastly different in their application, are both practically physiological tests.

In the large doses we get almost immediate physiological effects, at least very soon, while in potencies it takes a long while to impress the system to such an extent as to get the physiological effect. The difference is, that if full physiological doses are given of some drugs that are very irritating to the gastro-intestinal tract or produce immediate vomiting, we fail to get all our basic symptoms, thus depriving us of some of our basic indications so necessary to know in applied therapeutics.

In summing up the whole subject of the successful study of drug action, it is necessary to consider the following, viz.:

1. That many drugs with a dual action can be proven by the physiological test.

2. That some drugs cannot be tested by the above method on account of pronounced irritating effect by direct contact, in such cases only giving us very few symptoms of the action of the drug, and we thus lose many of our guiding basic indications so important in the successful administration of the drug in the treatment of the sick.

3. That such drugs should be proven by giving them in potencies in the primary form for some time to healthy individuals, until physiological effects show themselves.

4. That, where possible, our best mode of testing the physiological effect is by physiological doses, as we generally get pronounced basic indications for its use in the primary form, without the many often misleading minor symptoms that appear in the provings with potencies.

5. That some drugs, even in tincture form, or fluid extracts, only develop the primary effect, not being strong enough for secondary or physiological effect. Such drugs, of course, cannot be tested by the physiological or proving test, clinical tests being the best in such cases.

6. Therefore, in order to be most successful and to get the leading basic indications, some drugs must be tested by physiological doses, and others by provings, as stated. Good judgment will enable the practitioner to differentiate.

7. That the physiological test, or mode of provings, are both based on pathology. Whether one or the other, in the tests we get functional or organic changes; these produce temporary symptoms, the leading symptoms of which serve us as a guide for the use of the drug in its primary form. In case of drugs with dual action, it will also serve us as a guide for its use in the secondary form.

8. This all teaches us that, in order to be most successful, drug action, pathology and diagnosis must be well understood.

9. That, once clear why some drugs must be tested by one method, others by another, and many by either one, a question will be cleared up which has been the cause of many disputes.

BLEEDING after coitus is sometimes the earliest sign of cancer of the cervix.—*American Journal of Surgery*.

SULPHUR—AND OTHER COMMENTS.

By J. S. NEIDERKORN, M.D.,
VERSAILLES, O.

If there is anything likely to agreeably entertain me it is the reading of an article written by some member of the allopathic fraternity "way up" about how we irregulars do business, and which insinuates about the propriety of being permitted to thrive as a scientific body, wondering why we should dare to legally exist, and why sectarian schools can't be gotten out of existence, should they refuse to die the natural death commonly ascribed to faddists.

Somehow or another some of these "higher luminaries" cannot refrain from giving vent to their ingrained prejudice, and in doing this an occasion of a gathering of medical men of their faith is selected in order to win applause and the false claim to a pretended distinction.

Their object is to ridicule those not in accordance with their therapeutic belief and to ingratiate themselves into the confidence of their disciples, particularly so in the case where the writer or speaker is reputed to be some specialist who is desirous of pulling work from the general field. These "higher luminaries" of the dominant school are so eager of posing as authorities and leaders in matters pertaining to medicine that in their anxiety they forget they are surrounded with therapeutic darkness which they can never hope to penetrate, and will not unless and until they adopt such therapeutic measures as are advocated by their much-hated sectarians; their therapeutic conceptions have been so blunted by their persistent inclinations to follow the "anti" toxin and serum crazes that they cannot be made to realize that their real medical knowledge is of mediocre quality, and really not worthy of any serious consideration. A redeeming feature is that there are many members in the rank and file of the regular fraternity who graciously and with confidence acknowledge the therapeutic exactness which we propound, and who ignore the proffered opinion of their political dignitaries.

They want us to believe, for instance, that arsenic is practically a panacea for disorders of the skin, and offer the advice of its universal adaptness to these lesions. That, they say, is science, for its physiological action has been proven in the laboratory; its action upon living tissue and organ and fluids of the body and manner of excretion from the body has been demonstrated. But when we say that sulphur is indicated in cases of obstinate cough with profuse expectoration, and where the skin has a tawny-sallow color, and this in the case where the patient really looks sick, then we are all wrong, because, in spite of the fact that clinical, bedside experience has times untold proven its worth under these circumstances, we are told that "every fact and observation in order to attain value must be interpreted in the light of science."

What do you think of that? Is it possible that bedside experience and clinical demonstrations are not of sufficient value to be classed as scientific information and conclusions? If I and others have proven that sulphur is curative in the conditions named, and my mind and eye are quick enough to catch these special features in the case soliciting medication, and without first stopping to give my patient a name for his affliction before I can select the remedy, is there any plausible reason why I should be condemned for failing to comply with the ancient and proverbial orthodox way of knowing of *what* my patient is suffering, and by *what* is meant a nosological term? Is my ridicule justified if I clearly give the indications for which a specific remedy is administered and a cure follows in a case where a half-dozen orthodox fellows vainly tried to relieve the patient? Can any specialist do more than cure his case, even though he fully understands of *what* his patient suffers? If I cure my case with sulphur, and state why I select that remedy, and further state that those conditions are met in every case, irrespective of its *name*, then it would seem that I have accomplished something definite. Can the laboratory test-tube or the guinea-pig experiment be as definite in its conclusion, provided you carry the experiment further and put it to a clinical test?

Many of us know that if a sick man has been under routine regular treatment for several years without any benefit to his health, he would look sick as a natural sequence, and there would not be any doubt but what he really is sick; and it probably would require sharp discrimination to differentiate the real sickness from the drug-induced derangement. Now, if such a case should apply for treatment and I were undecided of *what* he was suffering, to give nature a chance I would be justfied in prescribing a placebo until a future examination would disclose just where the real trouble is. If there are physicians who consider sulphur 3-x to be of no therapeutic value—a placebo— then such a prescription can do no harm in their estimation. Granting that such be the case, wherein have I erred? But there are many physicians who know that sulphur in the second or third or sixth decimal trituration, administered internally, has a decided effect upon the human economy; and there are capable physicians who insist that the higher the trituration of the remedy the deeper the effect. There isn't any questioning the fact that the effect of sulphur in the third decimal trituration given internally under certain conditions will give decidedly better therapeutical results than the remedy can if given in its crude state, or in the form in which it is ordinarily used. Any fair-minded physician, specialist included, can convince himself of the correctness of this statement if he will use the preparation in the form suggested, not indiscriminately, but in conditions as mentioned.

Sulphur is an alterative and a reconstructor, and is usually used in chronic constitutional ailments due to a general lack of tonicity of the body cells—disturbance of the electrical equilibrium, electro-tonus, if you please. From some reason nerve force has become exhausted, tissue metabolism cannot be carried on normally, for the reason that nutrition is impaired; there is a lack of tissue contractility and a consequently imperfect elimination of waste; capillary function is impaired, a toxemic condition—the product of body cells or that of micro-organisms—develops, the quality of the blood suffers, the opsonic index is lowered, and there is an abnormal discoloration of the skin. Excluding hepatic inefficiency, some organic disease or malignancy, a sallow color of the skin is the result of imperfect elimination —a tissue toxemia. Sulphur, in small doses, acts as a gentle stimulant to the organs of excretion and to the sebaceous glandular system; it counteracts cachectic constitutional conditions, favors nutrition, metabolism and elimination of worn-out tissues; modifies functions, is a reconstructive because it stimulates cell life, agitates nerve periphery and excites vaso-motor activity. The effect of small doses of sulphur, internally administered, is deep and long lasting, and it is the experience of those who observe that the more trituration the drug is subjected to, the more completely it is attenuated, the more effective is its action.

Given a case of chronic ailment, non-organic, where the patient has a non-elastic, tawny-colored skin, and where it is evident that he feels sick *and looks sick* (that physician who needs not consider the looks of his patient in order to decide upon his treatment of the case is either one of those lightning diagnosticians one reads or hears about but never meets, or he is so overwhelmingly full of theoretical knowledge that he is unconscious of his ignorance), I would think of sulphur as the remedy for him; and if in addition to that he has an obstinate cough and expectorates a muco-purulent sputum freely, he would certainly get sulphur, with the confident expectation of a satisfactory recovery to good health.

The functions of the skin and pulmonary organs are especially influenced by sulphur, if given in small doses. Excessive bronchial secretion, muco-purulent in character, is the result of impoverished, debilitated and relaxed bronchial mucous membrane, as well as constitutional debility, and these conditions are usually accompanied by an obstinate cough. If I have repeatedly demonstrated to my own satisfaction and to the gratification of my patients that sulphur will cure such conditions, and it does cure, then there will be no occasion to consult "authority;" my own observation and demonstration will be authority sufficient.

I can agree with the proposition that anything based on a reality will prosper, but, if based on a fad, it will go out of existence. The proof is the present sound, substantial and distinguished position the Eclectic materia medica now occupies in the medical world, and the present dilapidated condition of an almost obsolete allopathic materia medica, with its indefinite therapeutic propositions.

Uncertain therapeutic applications, "may be's," "mights" and "isms," are some of the causes of loss of confidence in medicine; whilst the definite and progressive spirit of Eclectic therapeutics has placed a goodly number of the higher luminaries of the dominant school on the defensive, and has caused various and vain efforts to either absorb or drive us out of existence.

The modern Eclectic materia medica is a scientific proposition, and since the practice of preventing, alleviating and curing human mental and physical infirmities medicinally is a science demonstrated systematically and skilfully, and since medicine has legal recognition, it would seem that we are conforming to the proposed requirements of those whose fervent desire is to rule or ruin. Incompetent to successfully execute the former and chagrined because of their inability to produce the latter, a few of the leaders resort to dramatic measures, hoping thereby to place us open to public ridicule and to regain lost prestige from their followers.

Eclectic physicians are familiar with the piratical practice of some of the distinguished scientific luminaries of appropriating specific therapeutic facts which did not emanate from the cranium of any regular chieftain, as well as with the adroitness of their method of concealing originality of the material they elect to purloin. Their simulation of scientific goodness to suffering humanity for the special purpose of attracting and winning approbation might be compared to the slightly orthographically modified axiom, "Let us prey."

THE MILK SUPPLY.*

By H. J. SHELLEY, M.D.,
MIDDLETOWN, N. Y.

I will try to tell you of some of the difficulties that exist in procuring pure milk, the more common sources of contamination about the farm, and the difficulties in removing the same. These deductions

* Read before First District Medical Society, October 28, 1907.

are the results of the inspection of the farms·and creameries that supply Middletown, N. Y.

In our milk ordinance and control of supply we have attempted clean milk in the macroscopic rather than the microscopic sense of the word. We have examined farm and dairies rather than the milk, believing that for all practical purposes we should remove the source of infection on the farm.

We know from experience that where we have dirty farms and dairies the bacterial count is high, and that as we clean up our source of supply the count will be correspondingly low. · To the average farmer an inspection of his dairy, with certain prescribed rules and regulations governing the production and distribution of milk, is as if one should challenge his vote at a presidential election. The effect is the same, whether the rule emanates from Greater New York or a smaller city. The right of the farmer is being violated, his sanctity wrested from him. He meets the inspector, at the best, in a sullen mood, and follows out the rules only when he confronts the alternative of having the sale of his milk stopped by the health authorities.

Much of this, strange as it may seem, is due to ignorance; for it is a common occurrence in some dirty, poorly-ventilated and illy-lighted barn to have the farmer tell you he produces the best of milk, his cows are graded stock, and that he feeds only the best of feed. Men of this stamp are honest in their belief that if they have graded stock they are producing pure milk. In this class, education (sometimes it has to be done with a hammer) is bringing about a betterment of conditions.

Though much has been accomplished throughout the country by the various boards of health, and by legislative enactments, the great work of education to be accomplished, both by beetle and wedge, and by diplomacy, is appalling.

The farmer has learned that the cow's foot in the pail and manure scooped out with an equally dirty hand is not looked upon favorably by health authorities; but to the great majority cleanliness further than to prevent this is a waste of time, and a finicky notion of some city fellow who does not know a cow from a bull.

There is some ground for this belief, for it is amusing to the farm-bred man to hear some of the ideas regarding milk advanced by the big dealers, to say nothing of the educated medical man or the theoretical health expert.

Brought up on a farm, having pulled teats in cow manure four to eight inches deep, practiced medicine in a farming country for nineteen years, I feel I can appreciate the subject from both the farmer and board of health standpoint.

With this introduction, we will explain how we are working for pure milk in Middletown. If we refer to self frequently it is not from egotism, but rather to show the obstacles and how they can be overcome in enforcing a milk ordinance.

In the city of Middletown, for a long period of years, efforts had been made to have a milk ordinance, and some form of milk inspection. This met with repeated opposition for three reasons : (1) On the part of the dealer, who did not want the source of his supply looked into ; (2) the public, which is always looking for a cheap milk, and feared that a milk law would cause the dealer to put up his price ; the third and last reason is like that of the Irishman who offered three reasons why he could not enter a poker game. The first was that he had no money ; the others his companions did not care to hear. One great reason was the Board of Health did not have money to go on with the work.

Early in the summer of 1906 the conditions were such that the Health Officer, Dr. Horner, and myself, in my rig, visited the most of the dairies that supplied the city with milk. This was purely a work of love, as is the inspection at the present time.

The existing conditions were brought before the local board ; the dealers and farmers were notified that the key-note of the board was to clean up and to keep clean. This brought abuse galore upon those who had visited the farms, as well as upon the local board.

Late in the fall of 1906 a milk ordinance was passed, and while it has many defects and needs to be changed, its enforcement is bringing about a better condition on the farm and purer milk to the consumer.

Our ordinance, briefly, requires the dealer to file an application, giving number of wagons, health of dairies, location of creamery, etc. With his application he files a statement signed by the farmer from whom he procures his milk, giving a description of his farm buildings, air-space, number of cows, and general information in regard to feed, water supply and health of family.

These applications are approved by the Board if they contain nothing radically wrong, and a license is granted for each wagon, the cost of which is $5.00 per wagon a year. Our dairy rules are printed on water-proof card muslin, and are issued to each farmer, who keeps a copy posted in his barn. They are as follows :

"RULES AND REGULATIONS.

"1. The room in which the cows are kept shall contain at least 500 cubic feet for each cow housed therein ; shall be well ventilated and lighted ; have a dry, well-drained floor, and be cleaned each day, the manure being removed at least twenty feet from the barn at each cleaning.

"2. The ceiling and side walls shall be whitewashed twice each year and be kept free from dust, cobwebs, and filth at all times.

"3. No swine shall be kept in the same room with the cows.

"4. No musty or dirty litter shall be used for bedding.

"5. The food and water given the cows shall be at all times pure and wholesome and subject to the approval of the Board of Health.

"6. All cows shall be free from stable filth and loose dust, and the milkers shall have clean hands and clothing at the time of milking.

"7. Milk shall be removed immediately after being drawn from each cow to a well-ventilated milk-room separate from the stable-room and there aërated and cooled before being placed in the cans.

"8. Milk must be strained through a cotton flannel or other equally efficient strainer, which shall be renewed as often as necessary. All strainers shall be cleansed and sterilized after each milking.

"9. All vessels having contained milk shall be washed clean and sterilized after each milking or using.

"10. Milk delivered in bottles shall be bottled in the milk-room at the dairy or creamery, and bottles shall be cleaned and sterilized at the dairy or creamery, even though having been washed by the customers, and no milk shall be sold dipped from cans and poured into other vessels.

"11. No milk bottles, tickets or other things shall be taken from a house while it is under quarantine for a contagious disease.

"12. No milk tickets shall be used by customers more than once.

"13. All wagons, sleighs or other vehicles from which milk is delivered shall be kept cleaned in a manner satisfactory to this board or its authorized agent.

"14. All wagons upon which milk is brought from the dairy or from which it is delivered to customers shall be kept covered to protect the milk from the rays of the sun, in a manner satisfactory to this board or its authorized agent."

(*Concluded next month.*)

BISMUTH SUBSALICYLATE.

BY P. A. DE OGNY, M.D.,
BENTON, KAS.

In looking over my list of anti-ferments I find none equal to bismuth salicylate. During the convalescence of all acute bowel troubles, when the food causes fermentation, distention and more or less distress, give your bismuth. In morning diarrhea, chronic diarrhea, diarrhea of tuberculosis, it will be found your best remedy. Given to the chronic dyspeptic it arrests fermentation, promotes a better digestion, and makes you a friend. Migraine the result of fermentation in the stomach and bowels is surely relieved by this remedy. It stops diarrhea, but does not constipate.

Indications.—Putrefactive fermentation of food, gastric or intestinal, associated with either constipation or diarrhea.

Dose.—Dr. jss to dr. iij to water oz. jv. Shake well. One teaspoonful every three hours.

Ohio State Eclectic Medical Association.
Proceedings Annual Meeting, 1907

W. N. MUNDY, M.D., EDITOR.

SECTION VIII.

OPHTHALMOLOGY, OTOLOGY AND LARYNGOLOGY.

KENT O. FOLTZ, M.D., PRESIDING.

MATERIA MEDICA OF THE EYE.

By KENT O. FOLTZ, M.D.,

CINCINNATI, O.

Local measures are usually well known, but a few local applications which are not often used, or are used indiscriminately, will be mentioned.

Ergot.—In subconjunctival congestion this is a valuable remedy. It does not give as good results in ordinary conjunctivitis, however. Lloyd's ergot, gtt. xx–dr. ss; solution boric acid, q.s. oz. ss. Sig. Two drops in the eye every two or three hours. The preparation of ergot should contain no alcohol, and should be kept in a cool place, as the dilution soon spoils.

Calendula.—The form employed is Lloyd's non-alcoholic fluid extract. This can be used either alone or combined with hydrastis. In conjunctivitis, especially with a tendency to muco-purulent or purulent secretions. The use of the hydrastis with calundula seems to increase its activity. There is a burning sensation when first introduced into the cul-de-sac, lasting for a few seconds, when a sensation of coolness follows, and the relief from the uncomfortable sensations prevalent in this form of conjunctivitis is very marked. The drug or its combination is used in the same proportions as the ergot.

Hamamelis.—The distilled hamamelis is used in those cases where the secretions are thin, watery and non-excoriating. It may be combined with other drugs, or simply use the hamamelis and solution boric acid, aa, q.s. The local use of this drug for catarrhal conditions elsewhere is worthy of study.

Internal remedies are so numerous I will mention only a few of those more frequently employed.

Calcium Sulphide (Hepar sulphur of the homeopathic pharmacy). —This is used in all cases when there is a tendency to pus formation, either within the eye, its tunics, or from the mucous surfaces. It may be carried to the point of saturation or not, as deemed advisable. In babies the lime water is used instead of the sulphide, and it is easier administered. The sulphide is given in doses ranging from 1-100 gr. to 1-5 gr.

Hamamelis.—As for the local use, the distilled is used. The thin, watery, non-excoriating secretion being the indication. Dose, dr. ss–ij, aqua q.s. oz. jv. Teaspoonful every two hours.

Liquor Potassii Arsenitis (Fowler's solution).—The indication for this drug is the thin, watery, excoriating secretion. Dose, gtt. x–xxx, aqua oz. jv. Teaspoonful every two or three hours.

Cimicifuga (Macrotys).—When the eye or the surrounding tissues have a bruised feeling, dose, gtt. x–xxv, aqua oz. jv. Teaspoonful every one to three hours.

Bryonia.—When motion of the eye or lids increases the pain. Dose, gtt. xv–xxv, aqua oz. jv. Teaspoonful every one or two hours. In supraorbital neuralgia, the combination of gelsemium with bryonia will usually afford relief in a short time. Bryonia gtt. xx, gelsemium, dr. ss, aqua q.s. oż. jv. Teaspoonful every hour until the pain is less severe, then every two or three hours as required.

Phytolacca.—In conjunctival conditions, where the mucous glands are distended with secretion. If the lymphatic glands of the face or neck are also affected, it is an additional indication. Dose, phytolacca dr. ss–j, aqua q.s. oz. jv. Teaspoonful every four hours.

Potassium Bichromate.—In conjunctivitis when the secretion is sticky, tough and tenacious. Not often required, but a valuable drug with this condition. Dose, 1-100 gr. every three hours. Tablets are preferred.

Rhus Tox.—When motion of eye or lids affords relief from pain or discomfort. The burning pain is less an indication than the relief obtained by motion. Dose, gtt. iij, aqua oz. jv. Teaspoonful every one or two hours.

Potassium Iodide.—Of most value in specific diseases, as syphilitic iritis or neuritis, although in interstitial keratitis, and occasionally in conjunctivitis complicated with the syphilitic taint, the drug will be required, usually in small doses. In iritis or neuritis, however, the drug should be administered in large doses, until iodism results, then just inside this effect until a cure is effected.

ALBUMINURIC RETINITIS.

BY J. P. HARBERT, M.D.,
BELLEFONTAINE, O.

Ocular manifestations of general disease are quite common, and are alike interesting to the general practitioner and specialist in medicine. Albuminuric retinitis, or renal retinitis, is one of the most characteristic of such manifestations. It is an inflammation of the retina accompanying diseased conditions of the kidneys characterized by the presence of albumin in the urine. It is frequently complicated with an inflammation of the intraocular end of the optic nerve, giving rise to the condition known as neuro-retinitis or papillo-retinitis.

Albuminuric retinitis is essentially a complication of the later forms of kidney disease, and sometimes the lastest. However, retinitis had been found in some of the acute forms of nephritis; as, for instance, following the exanthemata, in child birth, during pregnancy, in erysipelas and diphtheria. It is said to be a more frequent complication of chronic interstitial nephritis than any other form of renal disease. Authorities differ as to the frequency of retinitis in kidney disease, some placing it as high as 33 per cent., others as low as 7 per cent. Age seems to have little influence over the frequency of the disease, and it is found alike in the young as well as the aged.

It most always attacks both eyes, yet one may become affected long before its fellow, and it may be much more severe in one eye than the other. Very frequently the ocular affection will be the first intimation that the patient will have of any serious disease, and an oculist will be consulted on account of the failing vision. The opthalmoscopic examination will reveal the true nature of the disease, and while no two cases will be found exactly alike, there should be no trouble in making a correct diagnosis. The optic nerve head appears opaque, swollen and hyperemic, or actively inflamed, its edges in some cases not being visible; large, round, white massings are seen to surround the disc, and have been termed "snow banks," and are distinctive of albuminuric retinitis. The macula is often red, and is surrounded by white spots caused by degeneration of the exudates and retinal elements; later the spots coalesce into radiations like the spokes of a wheel with the macula at the centre, the radiations resembling the points of a star, and hence the name "stellate" or "macular figure." This is considered pathognomonic of the disease. In fact, the two conditions, viz., "snow banks" and "stellate macula," either partial or complete, would warrant a diagnosis of albuminuric retinitis until positively disproven by other factors. The arteries are usually thin, and may be traced only by whitish stripes; the veins are slightly tortuous and dark in color. Extravasations of the blood may be seen and may occur at any time during the course of the disease; these hemorrhages are usually in the nerve fiber layer of the retina and are therefore flame-shaped.

The visual disturbance is not always in proportion to the severity of the kidney disease.

The course of the disease varies; as a rule, the changes noted above persist, although undergoing some change, to the end. In rare cases the lesions may clear up or entirely disappear, as after pregnancy or where the general disease is benefited by treatment. The improvement in vision corresponds, as a rule, to the diminution in the retinal disease. In some cases the retina is damaged to such an extent that even though the exudates and hemorrhages are absorbed, little or no improvement in vision can occur. Betterment of vision without improvement of the primary or general disease, is of brief duration. Central vision will remain fairly good if the macula does not become markedly affected; it will be seriously damaged or destroyed if the macula is much involved. Peripheral vision usually remains good.

Prognosis.—So far as vision is concerned the prognosis is unfavorable, though some improvement may occur under suitable treatment.

The prognosis regarding life is very grave, and in almost all instances death must be expected in a few months, or years.

Retinitis appearing during the course of kidney diseases must indeed be considered a very grave indication. As a rule, the kidney disease has reached a stage from which recovery is impossible before the ocular disturbance occurs, and most cases will die within a few months to two years from the time of the retinal involvement.

Retinitis complicating albuminuria, occurring during pregnancy, is not nearly so serious, either in regard to vision or life, as in other varieties, restoration of useful vision and almost complete recovery from the retinal lesions as well as permanent recovery from the renal disease, not being uncommon.

Treatment.—So far as the ocular disturbance is concerned, the eyes should be protected with dark glasses, and all close work should be prohibited, together with any cleansing or soothing lotion that may be desired.

Internally, the treatment should be directed to the kidneys and to the underlying cause of the disease.

In nearly all cases developing albuminuric retinitis during pregnancy, premature labor should be induced. In some cases of albuminuria delivery should be expedited without reference to the retinal involvement, but when severe retinitis develops there should then no longer be any hesitancy in bringing the gestation to a close, and thus relieving the patient before such marked changes have occurred as to render restoration of useful vision impossible.

Report of a Case.—Mr. K., aged fifty, locomotive engineer, consulted me in October, 1902, on account of rapidly failing vision. He came into the office right from his engine, and was much concerned lest the railroad company should learn of his visit to me. He said that on the last few trips he had made that he had had to depend entirely on the fireman, as he was unable to see the signals. He was a strong, healthy looking man, and the disease had been so insidious that he was not aware of its presence until his vision became so much reduced that he was compelled to seek consultation.

Ophthalmoscopic examination revealed a fairly typical picture of renal retinitis in each eye, and an analysis of the urine confirmed the diagnosis. This patient made no improvement whatever, and died within six weeks after his first visit to my office.

ASTHENOPIA AND ASTIGMATIC ABSURDITIES.

BY A. RIGGS, M.D.,
CINCINNATI, O.

The terms asthenopia and astigmatism are used somewhat in a similar way by the novice. I do not think that there are any other two names in the oculist's nosology that are so frequently referred to, and probably no others so badly abused. These terms are often used by opticians as a "shrapnell bomb," a sure "hit," so to speak. In many localities the terms have been used so frequently that the glass-wearing people have learned to used them as a fad. For convenience, I will combine the two and treat them roughly as one. I will not try to elucidate upon the differential minute points, for they are to the average physician superfluous.

Asthenopia seems to be a disease of civilization, and America leads in producing the greatest number of cases; England, Germany and France come next in the production, as in the manner named. Our American compulsory and cramming methods of education are responsible for a large percentage of the cases in this country, while congenital anomalies of the eyes, local catarrhal troubles, debilitated constitutional conditions, hereditary weakness of the eye muscles, improper nourishment, bad hygiene, diseases of the genital, eliminative and digestive organs, irritation from smoke, gases, chemicals, dust, refractions of strong light, excessive use of the eyes, using the eyes on fine work by unsteady or flickering light, etc., are enumerated as causes.

The principal symptoms of asthenopia are photophobia, irritability, want of endurance of the ciliary muscles, with some conjunctival inflammation, pain in back of the eyes, headache, and neuralgia in the head, with dazzling vision. Acuteness of sight is usually perfect, and refraction almost, if not, normal. All symptoms are increased by various work; close application at reading or needlework aggravate the disease.

Astigmatism, in the majority of cases, has symptoms identical with those of asthenopia, with the exception that the acuteness of sight is always impaired. Astigmatism is largely an organic, and not a functional, affection. The usual causes are hypermetropia, deviations of the crystalline lens, defects of the cornea, etc. Otherwise, all that can be said about asthenopia may be applied to astigmatism.

Treatment of asthenopia should be along proper hygienic and dietetic lines. Glasses will not cure the disease, and it would be practicing a deception to lead our patients to believe anything to the contrary. The free bathing of the eyes with cold water and the application of weak astringent lotions are useful. Out-door exercise and resting of the eyes should be encouraged. The general health is to be carefully looked after, and any wrongs of the eliminative, digestive and generative organs should be corrected. Susceptible persons should not, under any conditions, use the eyes for reading or sewing in an unsteady, flickering light. Our school boards should pass rules prohibiting the use of glazed paper on which school books are printed. A paper with a dead finish should only be used.

Treatment for astigmatism would be the same, practically, as that for asthenopia, with the exceptions that the refraction and the state of the internal and external recti muscles should always be carefully tested, and any error corrected by lenses. Unless corneal astigmatism reaches a diopter with the rule or a quarter of a diopter against the rule, it would be useless to give such patients glasses, for they would be but a little better than placebo. In my judgment no one is ever better for glasses unless they see better with them, or are much more comfortable with them. Even when vision for distance is perfect with glasses I do not urge such patients to wear glasses except for the near.

It would be quite difficult for any physician who has not made the eyes a special study, to know just what errors in diagnosis are being made by the majority of unskilled opticians. When the average vender of glasses can find no other excuse for the placing of glasses before the eyes of the credulous, he invariably falls back onto one of the two mentioned ocular entities. I am too liberal minded to think that the optical profession has no conscience and is thinking only of the almighty dollar. I am more inclined to think that the principal reason for their fooling the people is due to their lack of knowledge of the pathological diseases of the organs of sight. It is impossible to conceive the number of people, especially children, that are being injured by the unnecessary wearing of lenses. It seems as though the spectacle venders would have the people believe that all the ills that man is heir to, no matter of what kind or nature, can be cured by naming the ailment asthenopia or astigmatism and by prescribing glasses. Their prescriptions, however, are not always scientifically (?) written, for more than one person has come under my observation who were wearing, or trying to wear, glasses they could not see through. I remember, òn one occasion, I was called to attend a woman with normal vision who was made a nervous wreck by her trying to wear a pair of prisms of 2° strength. On inquiry, she said an optician examined her eyes and told her that she had asthenopia, and sold her the mentioned lenses. She could not use the glasses on account of the drawing and blurring of the eyes, and upon several occasions she called upon the optician and stated her inability to wear the glasses, but all the satisfaction she received was for her to go right on wearing the glasses, and possibly she would get used to them bye and bye. It would not be hard for any physician to conceive the severe headaches and· nervous irritability that would result from the excessive eye-strain due to using prisms over normal sight.

The present indiscriminate prescribing of glasses for our children, as practiced by our public school corps—district physician, principal and teacher – is certainly laying a foundation for a coming generation with defective eyesight. I think that we, the medical fraternity, owe it to ourselves, as well as to posterity, that the present status of the promiscuous prescribing and encumbering of the eyes of our people with unnecessary glasses should be discouraged,

COMMON INJURIES OF THE EYE.

By A. S. McKITRICK, M. D.,
KENTON, O

Among the more common injuries of the eye are lodgment of particles of steel, particles from emery wheels, etc. A great many times these burn more or less in coming in contact with the·eye.

The first thing to do when a patient presents himself with an injured eye is to thoroughly examine it. Often there will be blepharospasm and the eyeball strongly turned up. Usually the eye can be opened easily, sufficiently to drop in a few drops of 4 per cent. solution of cocaine. Wait two or three minutes and then place the thumb of the left hand against the lower·border of the upper lid and let the finger rest against the forehead, and with the right hand on the lower lid. This increases the spasm. If you do not use much force, but wait patiently a minute or two the muscles will tire and relax and can be separated without difficulty. Drop in another drop of cocaine and wait and the eyeball will rotate downward and can be inspected. And here it may be necessary to use a double convex lens to focus the light. A little experience will enable you to hold the lids open and do this. The foreign substance is likely to be found in the cornea although the patient will tell you that it is under the upper lid. If not found, then turn the upper lid over the point of a lead pencil and inspect it. The foreign body should be carefully removed with a spud. If it has been in long enough, or if the injury has caused much inflammation, instill two drops of 4 per cent. solution of atropine. Order ice-cold compresses to the eye and it will be all right in a short time.

If the injury is more severe, causing penetration of the eyeball, it is not so simple. If the wound is in the cornea the aqueous humor escapes. The iris may be injured and prolapsed, in which case it should be either returned to its place or cut off and the remaining part returned. If the lens is injured it may become opaque. If the vitreous is opened it may partially escape. The foreign body should be located and removed. Metal and stone can be located with the X-ray, but glass cannot. In these severe cases it requires some special training to determine whether there should be an effort made to save the eye or whether it should be at once enucleated.

If the injury is at the corneo-scleral margin, perhaps it would be better to enucleate, as the danger of sympathetic ophthalmia is great.

Copper is especially dangerous, as it is apt to cause suppuration when it comes in contect wiih vascular structures.

Explosions of gun-powder are frequently the cause of serious injury. Under cocaine anesthesia the powder is to be removed with a spud. The powder on the lids is to be picked out and the wounds wet with peroxide of hydrogen, which is something of a solvent.

Injuries caused by chemical agents are usually severe and destructive. Ammonia, lime, caustic, potash, acids, etc., are among the most common. Their action is so quick and escharotic that very often the eye will be lost. If the cornea is burned deeper than the epithelial layer the eye will be forever damaged, while, if not deeper than this, recovery likely will take place.

The destruction of the conjunctiva is followed by adhesions (symblepharon), more or less completely fixing the eye.

Treatment.—First remove at once all offending substance by irrigating the eye profusely with water. In the case of lime some authorities object to the use of water because it will slake the lime, but, owing to the delay in getting something else ready, it is better to use the water.

In the case of alkali, use diluted vinegar, as it is always handy. Or, with lime, you may use a solution of sugar, which forms an insoluble compound with the lime.

If the injury is caused by acid, use a weak solution of baking soda, which is always at hand.

If the cornea is not severely injured, apply ice. It will contract the blood-vessels, limit the inflammation and minimize the exudation. If the cornea is much injured, the ice is contraindicated, and should be replaced by very hot applications intermittingly applied. After the first forty-eight hours, hot applications are nearly always better than cold.

Atropine is a sheet-anchor in injury of the eye, and is usually as much indicated as a splint to a broken bone.

If the conjunctival adhesions are extensive, they may require grafting. If the conjunctiva is too seriously burned the symblepharon may be prevented by passing a probe in the cul-de-sac frequently.

After the inflammatory stage has passed the best stimulant to absorption of opacities of the cornea is dionin; this is a morphine derivative.

It will dilate the capillaries to three or four times their normal size and the lymphatic vessels to ten times their normal size. It is slightly antiseptic. It is used from 1 to 4 per cent. solution. The reaction from it is considerable, the conjunctiva becoming swollen immediately after using it. Remember it in any case where sloughing or the integrity of the cornea is involved.

OPHTHALMOLOGY.

By U. O. JONES, M.D.,
WEST JEFFERSON, O.

This is a subject that possibly all are not interested in, but if I can show that a great many ills can be cured by a proper correction of the eyes, then I will have been paid for the time spent upon this paper.

In the first place, we will take the nerve supply of the eye, and by that show the amount of drainage upon the system at large by defective vision.

The third nerve supplies all of the muscles of the eye except the superior oblique, which is supplied by the fourth nerve, and the external rectus, which is supplied by the sixth.

Dr. E. J. Swift has been investigating the vision of the students at the State Normal School, at Stevens' Point, Wis., and the following is his summary:

1. Only 22.22 per cent of the 216 examined had normal vision.

2. Of those with normal vision, only one · failed to disclose some manifest error of refraction or muscle insufficiency.

3. Thirty-five of the 48 showed manifest compound hyperopic astigmatism in one or both eyes, while of the remainder 4 had simple hyperopic astigmatism and 4 others hyperopia. In most of the cases more or less muscle insufficiency was evident.

4. In 30 per cent. of those examined, the vision of one or both eyes, the most defective when there was a difference, was below 20/30, while between 19 and 20 per cent., nearly as many as had normal vision, were unable to read the 20/40 line a distance of twenty feet.

My method of testing the eye is, first, to place the patient fifteen or twenty feet from the test-cards, and placing an opaque disc in front of one eye, have them begin at top of the card and read as far down as they can with the other eye; then try the other eye the same way. Then place in the frame on one side the Maddox prism, and on the other the chromatic test covered by the opaque disc; then place a lighted lamp twenty feet distant, or the distance I am using for testing; then have them look at the light and move the Maddox prism until one light is directly over the other; then remove the opaque disc and a third blaze will be seen either to one side or the other; then, by placing a prism in front of the chromatic test, if the base of prism is toward the nose we have esophoria; if the base of the prism is out, it is exophoria. Esophoria and exophoria are muscular deviations.

Exophoria means below normal, or a weakness of the internal rectus muscle, and consequently a weakened condition of the third nerve supply, and often a cramp.

Esophoria is the opposite, or above normal, and also a cramp or spasm. There are two kinds of spasm—a tonic and clonic, the first a permanent cramp. Usually, esophoria pains, and there are other symptoms of hyperopia. In this condition, we find headache, stomach trouble, painful menses, wetting the bed, etc. I have relieved just such cases by properly correcting the eyes, if the patient follows instructions.

Clonic spasm is an intermittent cramp, and is often mistaken for astigmatism.

Asthenopia (tired or fading vision), without glasses or with them, comes under the third nerve supply.

In hyperopia the strain is 100 per cent. more than the accommodation required, because of the automatic relation between the convergence and accommodation, and as convergence is not wanted by the hyperope, he practically neutralizes it by sending to the external rectus through the sixth nerve enough power to offset the convergence, thus adding another 50 per cent. to the strain, making the total strain in hyperopia just double the amount of accommodation. Thus the hyperope ot 1 D. in each eye would have a total of 4 D. If the hyperopic condition is more in one eye than the other, we find which is his fixing eye, then, as he will accommodate the same in both eyes, we figure the nerve-strain as if the error was the same in both eyes.

There is no strain in myopia (nearsight) in excess of the normal.

It is really below normal, but the lack of harmony between accommodation and convergence sometimes creates trouble among myopes, who do a great deal of close work, and a correction which makes vision nearly normal for distance, if worn when reading, will restore that harmony and relieve the discomfort.

The accommodation is one of the most remarkable and interesting points about the eye. Nature first made the eye emmetropic, so it was adapted to see distant objects clearly without any effort; but upon coming closer, say to the usual reading distance, which is about thirteen inches, or one-third of a meter, the rays being divergent when they reach the eye, required more power to focus them at the retina.

We take as our standard of measurement of lenses one which will focus parallel rays at one meter. Then one which will focus at thirteen inches must necessarily be three times as strong as our unit. Therefore, the amount of effort required of the accommodation at the thirteen-inch point would be equal to an increase of power of the crystalline lens just three units in each eye. In reading at this point the two must converge in order to not see double. This requires another three units of strain, half being supplied by each eye. All of this force is supplied by the third cranial nerve.

Taking these facts as a basis of calculation, we find the total strain upon the nerve supply of a a normal individual to be one million units per day. Then, when we find defective eyes of the class requiring convex lenses, the application of this same system of calculation show an abnormal strain of 23 per cent. for each unit of error in the two eyes. The natural effects of this strain are as sure to develop weakness in other parts as we are sure the nerves are connected with each other. The most common complaints are headache, indigestion, mental irritation, female troubles, habitual constipation, liver trouble, kidney trouble, irregularity of the heart, and general debility. The remedy is to correct the eye trouble; prescribe rest and the trouble disappears.

I have one or two cases in particular that I wish to call to your attention. The first one, a lady, aged thirty-three years, came to me and said: "I have been the rounds of the oculists and none of them have been able to fit me with glasses, and if you want to try it no pay until satisfied, you may try it." I said, "All right, that is the way I do business." I used the fifteen foot space and found she could not see the test-card at that distance; then at that sitting, by putting on —3.00, each eye, her vision was $^{15}/_{50}$. I told her to wear them one month and come again. At the second sitting I put on what proved to be her final correction, which was — 3.00 ax. 1.80+1.00 ax. 90

(mixed astigmatism), each eye vision $15/20$, and she has had no trouble since.

The second case that I wish to refer to is one that had been the rounds also, and when she came to me was wearing — 25 ax. 90, and was very nervous, with stomach trouble, constipation headache, etc. When making the examination I had to stop and let her vomit, so great was the relaxation; nor could I give her her full correction at this time, because it would be so uncomfortable that she could not wear them at all; so I put on + .25 and told her she would probably vomit more or less for a week, but after that she could stand a great deal stronger lens and suffer no discomfort. If I had not had the confidence and help of her husband I would have failed, for she would not have worn even that weak a lens. However, in two weeks she came in again, and this time stood the examination fine, and at this sitting I put on + .25+.75 ax. 90, with the result that her troubles disappeared and she is to-day happy in the enjoyment of good health.

Dr. McCormack used to use this expression: "What I can't cure with glasses and salt water Dr. Pratt will cut off and throw away." While I think this assertion is a little too strong, yet I believe—and not only believe, but know—that a great many ills can be cured more easily by first correcting the eye-strain, then using the indicated remedy, whatever that may be.

Now just a few words as to the local treatment of eye troubles. I have had quite a number of cases of catarrhal conjunctivitis, or "pinkeye," and the only remedy I use locally in the office is adrenalin chloride, full strength, two or three drops at a time, and have patient keep eye closed. This remedy clears the conjunctiva quickly by its powerful contracting influence upon the blood-vessels. If the patients are in town have them come in twice a day, but if in the country I sometimes give them a small vial and have them use it themselves, and I see them two or three times a week. I also give the patient to use at home an ounce solution composed of boric acid, pure, two grains; zinc sulpho-carbolate, a quarter grain, and normal salt solution. This acts very nicely, although I invariably put glasses on the patient to complete the cure.

SECTION IX.

ELECTRO-THERAPEUTICS.

B. W. MERCER, M.D., PRESIDING.

GALVANISM.

BY J. R. SPENCER, M.D.,
CINCINNATI, O.

This form of electricity was named in honor of Galvani, an Italian, who first discovered it in 1780. Some writers speak of it as voltaic electricity, in honor of Professor Volta, who discovered a new method of generating it, namely, by means of the voltaic pile. Galvanism is produced by chemical action, or the dissolution of metals by chemism. It is termed galvanic or current electricity, to distinguish it from static electricity, which is insulated or stationary. It should be stated at this point that all modern research verifies the conclusion that the different forms of electricity that are known as magnetism, Franklinic and galvanic electricity, dynamic electricity, electro-magnetism or magneto-electricity, are but different expressions for one force, and that it is simply a motion or a vibration of the universal ether.

Analogy and experience prove, in a large measure, that all chemical action is attended by the evolution of electricity, and that electric phenomena are incessant; that electric force is being generated everywhere; that it is manifesting itself throughout the entire universe, and that, owing to the want of a sufficiently delicate apparatus, its presence cannot be detected and its quantity measured.

For the use of the medical practitioner a convenient device for the generation of electricity has been constructed. It is known as a battery. In this apparatus may be found certain metals and solutions which act chemically upon each other, prodcing the electricity. Batteries are composed of one or more cells; each cell is composed of a cup containing two metals, one of which is nearly always zinc, the other metal may be one of several different kinds; usually copper, carbon or platinum is used (See Fig. A). The solution that is most frequently used to produce the chemical action is sulphuric acid and water; a solution of sulphate of copper, bichromate of potassium, and many other liquids or combinations, are used by the different makers of batteries as agents to excite the chemical action. The manufacturers of the different batteries always send with each new instrument a formula of the solution to be used in it.

The chemical reaction necessary to generate electricity in the cells of batteries will vary somewhat according to the elements and solutions used. It is not necessary in this article to study these different reactions, but a general idea can be obtained by studying the steps that take place when zinc and copper are used as the elements, and a solution of sulphuric acid and water is the exciting liquid. When these metals are placed in the acid, the zinc, having a strong affinity for oxygen, will dissolve the molecules of water (H_2O), the oxygen will will unite with the zinc to form oxide of zinc, the hydrogen will escape through the solution to the copper plate, pass along that plate and escape to the atmosphere; then the sulphuric acid will unite with the oxide of zinc, forming sulphate of zinc. At the time, and by the

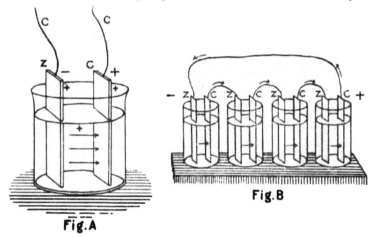

Fig.B

Fig.A

act by which the sulphate of zinc is formed, electricity is generated at the zinc plate; it then passes through the acid solution to the copper plate; when this plate is connected with the zinc plate by a wire, the electricity passes along the copper plate over the wire to the zinc plate, completing a circuit, which is necessary for the activity and usefulness of an electric current. When the two plates are in contact or connected by wires, the circuit is said to be closed; when separated the circuit is said to be broken, or open.

As the electricity in a cell is generated wholly by the action of the acid upon the zinc, its quantity will be proportional to the extent of zinc surface exposed to the acid. Considerable more electricity than can be generated by one cell will be needed in the treatment of disease, so galvanic batteries are constructed with a number of cells; if zinc and copper be the elements used, the copper plate of the first cell will be connected with the zinc plate of the second cell, and the copper plate of the second will be connected with the zinc plate of the third, and so on until the last cell is reached; the copper plate of the last cell will be connected with the zinc plate of the first cell, completing what is known as a compound galvanic circuit, the object being to obtain more zinc surface for the action of the acid. This can be better understood by observing Fig. B.

When electricity is being generated in the cell of a battery, two opposite conditions of that agent manifest themselves, known as positive and negative electricity, marked with a plus ($+$) and ($-$) sign. The electricity leaves the cell over a wire connected with the copper plate, is known as $+$ electricity, and passes on to the zinc plate where it is known as $-$ electricity. There is less potentiality or tension at the zinc plate than at the copper plate, therefore the electricity flows from the copper plate to the zinc. Possibly a better understanding of positive and negative electricity might be gained by thinking of that condition of the current at the copper plate as having a potentiality above a certain state of equilibrium, while at the zinc state the potentiality is below that state.

If the wire connecting these plates be cut, the current will cease to flow, but the electricity will exist at the cut ends of the wire in a static state. The amount of this static electricity will depend upon the strength of the original current before the interruption is made.

The interrupted galvanic current is produced by the successive opening and closing of a circuit during a continuous electrization. These interruptions may be produced in various ways, such as by raising an electrode from the skin and replacing it again, or by any kind of an interrupting apparatus.

When the exciting fluid is an acid the elements in the battery must be removed from it when not in use, or the zinc will soon be destroyed. Most batteries are constructed in such a way as to make this an easy task. If the fluid or exciting agent be an alkali, the elements may remain in it all the time without injury.

After batteries have been in use for a considerable length of time the current will get weak; they are said to have "run down." This condition is known as the polarization of the battery, and is a source of much trouble to the physician in his electro-therapeutic work. There are two causes for this condition :

1. The hydrogen gas that is liberated at the zinc plate by the decomposition of the molecules of water passes through the liquid to the copper plate and along it to the air; in time the copper plate will become covered with a film of this hydrogen gas; in this condition the copper plate is a very poor conductor of the electricity which passes over it in an effort to complete a circuit. On this account the current will be greatly weakened.

2. The hydrogen gas that accumulates on the copper plate has a strong affinity for oxygen, so it passes back to the zinc plate to unite

with the oxygen found there, thus setting up counter-currents or currents of polarization; these interfere with the flow of the electricity as it passes from the zinc to the copper.

The polarization of batteries can be overcome in several was :

1. Lift out the copper plate and brush its surface.

2. Agitate the exciting liquid in any manner; this will prevent the bubbles of hydrogen from adhering to the copper plate.

3. Use a copper plate having elevated points upon its surface, to which the gas bubbles will adhere, and from which they are easily dislodged.

4. Use a set of unpolarized electrodes.

When sulphuric acid is used as the exciting agent in the cells of a battery, it is diluted with water; as soon as the sulphate of zinc is formed it is dissolved in this water. The stronger this zinc solution gets the weaker the current of electricity will become, and will cease to flow entirely when the solution becomes saturated. The battery will do no more work until it is charged with a new battery fluid.

Acid batteries, or batteries containing any liquid in considerable quantity, are not easily carried from one place to another, which is necessary in treating patients in their homes. They are always in need of more or less care, as they will need recharging and repairing from the damage done by leakage, which is not uncommon and very annoying.

These facts have created a demand for dry-cell batteries, and as they are free from the above-described annoyances, and have been perfected in their construction to a point of cheapness and usefulness, they have become quite popular with the general practitioner.

The dry cell is constructed with zinc and carbon, to which is added chloride of ammonia and native peroxide of manganese, all of which is closed in a cover, or they may be made with zinc and chloride of silver.

These cells, with which the battery can be recharged, are manufactured by different firms, and can be bought rather cheaply. The length of time these cells will last will depend upon the amount of work they are asked to perform. The practitioner who has only an ordinary amount of work for a battery will be able to use a dry-cell battery of reliable construction for two or more years.

The chloride of ammonia battery is cheaper than the chloride of silver battery, and is said to be as reliable and lasting. The ammonia batteries have some disadvantages; in common with most batteries, they polarize rapidly when in use, and when the water in the cell becomes saturated with ammonia it escapes in a free state and becomes a slight source of annoyance.

Thermo-Electricity.—This is a continuous current of electricity that is generated by heat in connection with two parts of the same metal or by two different kinds of metal. When two different parts of the same metal are heated, electricity is generated; an example of this is seen when a wire is twisted and heat is applied at the point where the twisted and non-twisted portions come together; electricity will be produced; it can be detected by means of a galvanometer, an instrument which will show the presence of electricity. If one end of a bar of bismuth be soldered to an end of a bar of antimony, and heat be applied at the point of union, electricity will be generated. If the other extremities of these metals be connected by a wire, a circuit will be formed; a galvanometer, placed in this circuit, will show that, when the heat is applied, a current of electricity will flow from the bismuth to the antimony. Should the point of union of these metals be chilled by the application of ice, a current of electricity will also be produced, but it will flow in the opposite direction—that is, from the antimony to the bismuth. These two metals soldered together form what is known as a thermo-electric pair. By their use thermo-electric batteries have been constructed; the heat is furnished by a gas burner or an alcohol lamp.

The experiment of constructing this kind of a battery for therapeutic use has proven to be a failure, as it is expensive, bulky and untrustworthy.

Eye, Ear, Nose and Throat.

CONDUCTED BY KENT O. FOLTZ, M.D.

AMBLYOPIA.

Amblyopia is a term used to indicate a defective vision without sufficient organic or ophthalmoscopic changes to account for the impairment. There are a number of causes for this condition, and it is often difficult to determine the primary cause. Amblyopia may be congenital, reflex, traumatic, uremic, glycosuric, malarial, from loss of blood, toxic or from drug action, from tobacco or alcohol, or the two combined, ptomaine poisoning, or hysterical.

Congenital.—As a rule, no lesion can be detected by the use of the ophthalmoscope, but occasionally an abnormal disk is found. Hyperopia and astigmatism are usually present; and scotomas, especially for colors, may be present. Correction of the refractive errors will often improve the visual acuity, but will seldom give anywhere near the full visual function.

Reflex.—In these cases the cause is usually obscure. Irritation of some of the branches of the fifth nerve, sometimes from defective teeth, may be a factor. Intestinal parasites, nasal or naso-pharyngeal lesions are occasional causes.

Traumatic.—Injuries of the occipital region, the forehead, or of the spinal cord, may cause amblyopia. Fractures involving the optic canal, hemorrhage in the cranial cavity, disturbance or disorganization of the cerebral cortex, with secondary changes in the optic nerve, may be factors in causing amblyopia. An ophthalmoscopic examination may give negative results. The amblyopia may be temporary, but when there is effusion or extravasation into the intervaginal space of the optic nerve the condition is usually permanent. After railroad or street-car accidents an excessive degree of amblyopia is frequently found, and usually is permanent until a jury has rendered a favorable verdict.

Uremic.—This form of amblyopia is not infrequent during pregnancy or in scarlet fever. In the latter case albuminuria is present during desquamation. Both eyes are affected, and sometimes complete blindness results. Cerebral symptoms, convulsions, coma, stupor, vomiting and hemiplegia may occur in severe cases. Pupillary reaction may or may not be absent. In pregnancy amblyopia is usually a late manifestation, occurring near the time of parturition. Ophthalmoscopic changes are often lacking, but sometimes a wooly appearance of the optic disk is noticed.

Glycosuric.—Besides diabetic cataract or retinal hemorrhages, amblyopia may occur without any special fundus changes. The visual field may be normal, or it may be peripherally contracted. Color scotoma is always present. In all cases of color scotoma an analysis of the urine for sugar should be made.

Malarial.—Often no fundus change can be found, but a temporary diminution of vision or even total blindness, sometimes lasting for weeks, may occur. The malarial poison seems to have an influence upon both the optic nerve and retina. The fact that quinine may cause transient amblyopia must also be remembered.

Amblyopia from Loss of Blood.—This condition is more frequently seen following spontaneous hemorrhage than traumatic. Retinal hemorrhages, optic neuritis or atrophy of the optic nerve, resulting in permanent blindness, may result from this type of amblyopia.

Drug Amblyopia.—Many drugs may cause amblyopia. Some of the most active in causing the condition are male fern, iodoform, cannabis indica, alcohol, ergot, tobacco, salicylic acid, santonine, stramonium, lead salts, chloral, carbolic acid, quinine, practically all the coal-tar derivatives, and many other drugs when given in toxic doses.

Tobacco and Alcohol.—Either may cause amblyopia, but as a rule the two agents are associated. Usually found after the age of forty.

Ptomaine.—The poisonous alkaloids in tainted meat, cheese, and sometimes ice cream, not infrequently produce amblyopia.

Hysterical.—Either sex may be affected, but it is most frequently seen in young women.

Simulated Amblyopia.—The most annoying form is the simulated— that is, for the physician and friends of the patient—and often it will tax the ingenuity of the physician to the limit to detect the patient, and prove a normal condition is present.

PHYSICAL WELFARE OF COLLEGIATE STUDENTS.

In our July editorial we called attention to the routine examination of the eyes, ears, nose and throat of school children; to-day we desire to emphasize the fact that many a college and university student is laboring at a disadvantage and is even obliged to abandon his career because of ignorance that his eyes, etc., are defective and that proper attention would secure the unhampered use of his faculties.

The New York State Homeopathic Medical Society, at its semi-annual meeting in Brooklyn, September 24, unanimously adopted the following:

WHEREAS, Eye strain (even with normal vision), nasal obstruction, post-nasal adenoids, etc., seriously handicap a student in his efforts to secure an education;

Resolved, This society respectfully urges upon the administration of every college and school the importance of impressing the above fact upon the whole student body at the beginning of each school year.

Our particular object in writing to-day is to urge each of our readers to exert his active influence in securing this addition to the usual opening exercises of institutions of learning.

No one would for a moment expect the college or school to furnish eye glasses, treatment or expert examinations; but in such institutions as may have a physical director it could be arranged for this official to make such simple tests as will show whether the eye, ear, nose and throat be abnormal.

Adult students are supposed to be intelligent enough to consult competent medical advice once they are apprised that they are (or may prove to be) in need of it.

Although vision is apparently and really normal, there may be an eye strain sapping the nervous energy and manifesting itself only at the point of least resistance; hence eyes should be examined by an oculist—not by an optician or "refractionist" or by a general practitioner—if their use be accompanied or followed by any of the reflex symptoms of eye strain.

Aprosexia is often dependent upon insufficient aëration of the blood;

after an adenectomy or a turbinectomy the student will no longer find it difficult to keep his attention fixed upon the lecture or his book.

We do not mean to say that operations should be recommended or even mentioned in this connection, nor are we saying that they will prove necessary—especially if the case be not a neglected one; medicine and local treatment will often prove sufficient.—*Homeopathic Eye, Ear and Throat Journal.*

Seton Hospital Reports.
By L. E. RUSSELL, M.D., SURGEON.

CASE 118.—Miss B., age thirty years, sister of one of our Catholic priests, from the central part of the State, received an injury at the head of the fibula some three or four years ago, which at times gave some little pain and swelling, but no redness of the tissue until within the last three months, when there developed a tumor, bulging from the outer upper part of the leg, corresponding to the location of the head of the fibula. This growth gave some pain and quite a perceptible bulging of the tissues, extending downward about six inches from the head of the fibula. This lesion had been mistaken by two or three physicians for a ''cold abscess,'' and the patient advised to submit to an opening for drainage. The brother insisted that there was something more serious, and advised the patient to come to the Seton Hospital clinic for examination and surgical interference.

Remembering the experience that we have had in osteo-sarcoma, we very promptly made the diagnosis of malignancy, and instead of sacrificing the leg above the knee by amputation, which possibly might be good surgery, I shall investigate as soon as the patient comes under the influence of an anesthetic by an exploring incision to see if it will not be possible to exsect the upper half of the fibula and remove the osteo-sarcoma, as it remains enclosed in its pseudo-capsule. This capsule or tissue covering of the sarcoma is quite characteristic of this pathological condition.

We make an incision extending over an inch above the head of the fibula to within six inches of the external malleolus. We find on separating the fascia of the external muscle the bulging of the tumor, and the characteristic pseudo-capsule. There is a softened condition which gives warning of the destruction of the head of the fibula. The dissection is extended to the middle of the bone, where the fibula seems to be healthy, and, with heavy bone forceps, we sever the bone and dissect it upward, using care not to destroy the covering, that seems to hold the malignant mass in its pyriform condition? We sever the attachment of the head of the fibula and the tibia, and with the chisel remove the entire mass from its bed.

I have a theory that alcohol, when properly applied in the bed of the sarcoma, will destroy the pseudo-cell, or apparent granular connective tissue. We shall now treat the wound as a partly open wound, packing the cavity with fluffy sterilized gauze, and close the lower part of the incision. I believe that if we have any remedy that is a specific in sarcoma, it is alcohol properly applied against and pressed well into the connective tissue, where it may remain for twenty-four or thirty-six hours, and be replaced by additional sterilized gauze thoroughly moistened in alcohol, until the muscular tissue seems fairly hardened, then we feel that we can safely close the wound with good assurance of an ultimate recovery.

It is the author's opinion that if alcohol be properly used, by hypodermic injection into the malignant tissues, in proper season, it will eventually prove to be the safest and best remedial agent that we can obtain in the destruction of malignant lesions; this with the greatest safety to the patient.

We now open the tumor-like growth, which is about the size of a large pear, and on splitting centrally, we find complete destruction of the upper four inches of the fibula, and all *en masse* in the sarcomatous growth. The lower four inches of the fibula seems to be normal. May we not hope that by this method of dealing with this case we shall be able to give the patient a useful limb, and a new lease on her life?

P. S.—On redressing the above wound, at the end of nine days, there is an entire absence of pus, or any apparent malignancy. We therefore close the incision in its entire length, except about an inch from the central part, from which the tumor was removed, and everything apparently in a healthy condition.

I shall be glad to give a further report of this case in six months or a year hence.

Periscope.

Eclectic Statistics.

The number of Eclectic physicians practicing at any one time in the United States has been greatly exaggerated in several instances. Truth should prevail, and our lowest estimate will show better the strength of our school. It is our desire that the truth, as nearly as it can be ascertained, be recorded herein. To claim 10,000 to 14,000, as has been done, is to fly wide of the mark. At no time has the number ever exceeded about 9,000. At the prasent writing, and at a period when fewer are graduating from all medical colleges of all schools, owing to prosperity in trade and commerce, and changes and uncertainty concerning State requirements, there are something less than 8,000 Eclectic graduates in actual practice. This may look like retrogression, but please remember that this is a clarified list—a list purged of all doubtful and nondescript physicians who have masqueraded as adherents of our cause. It represents the *bona fide* Eclectics, and the estimate is made as low as possible lest we, too, exaggerate our numerical strength.

The appended table revised from a paper read before the National at Los Angeles by Dr. John K. Scudder, shows at a glance how these are distrbuted and comes as near the actual figures as can be readily obtained. It will be observed that in some localities the Eclectic forces are strong. The State societies are unusually well filled, somethiug over 2,300 out of a possible 7,500 being members. It is to be regretted that no such showing can be made by the National body, which now figures only about 520. This should be remedied, and, if possible, every Eclectic practitioner should be induced to join the National. Ohio heads the States with the largest number of Eclectic practitioners, and has an excellent and flourishing State society. Oklahoma, however, has the honor to have the largest State membership in proportion to the number of Eclectics in the commonwealth. This table is timely and useful, and indicates where much work may be accomplished by our National officers :

STATE	Eclectics	In State Society	In National	STATE	Eclectics	In State Society	National	STATE	Eclectics	In State Society	In National
Alabama..	59	....	....	Louisiana	25	....	2	Ohio.........	793	278	67
Arizona....	6	......	1	Maine......	36	26	4	Oklahoma	58	66	8
Arkansas..	196	75	14	Maryland	12	..	..	Oregon..	55	24	8
California	445	80	22	Mas'chu's	107	47	14	Pennsyl'a	246	80	19
Colorado..	58	12	3	Michigan.	308	44	12	Rhode Isl.	12	....	......
Conn'cut.	83	40	8	Minn'sota	80	30	8	So. Car....	6	....	......
Delaware.	6	....	....	Mi'si'sippi	28	.	.	So. Dak.	39	25	2
Dist. Col.	8	....	....	Missouri ..	449	135	29	Tenn'ssee	153	30	12
Florida...	53	14	1	Montana .	8	..	..	Texas .. .	225	85	16
Georgia..	306	150	29	Nebraska.	196	125	12	Utah	15	....	2
Idaho	20			Nevada...	5	....	......	Vermont	35	15	......
Illinois.	813	200	56	N. Jersey.	52	12	8	Virginia.	16	....	......
Ind. Ter.	81	......	1	N. Hamp.	26	26	1	Washi'ton	56	24	4
Indiana .	621	156	58	N. Mex....	12	12	..	W. Virg'.	89	43	7
Iowa........	265	100	21	N. York..	594	200	37	Wiscons'n	143	75	11
Kansas.	306	85	20	No. Car....	12	.	....	Wyoming	8	..	1
Kentucky	131	81	16	No. Dak .	8			Total.	7464	2345	508

Indian Territory and Oklahoma should be combined ; total in the new State, 139. Members in Texas State Society should read 150. The above list is fairly acccurate.—*Eclectic Medical Gleaner.*

"The Three Ages of Women."

The development of disease is so common among civilized women immediately before or after maturity, that it has become convenient for us to speak of *the three ages of woman*, namely, *puberty*, *maternity*, and *the menopause*.

Puberty.—Coincident with the attainment of that age known as puberty, menstruation, or the periodic flow of blood from the female genitals, begins. It is at this period that the evil consequences of the beautifying practices of civilized women first become conspicuous; and it is at this time that medical treatment can do a great deal toward establishing a normal functioning of the reproductive system, thus lessening the individual's liability to future suffering or invalidism.

While neither physical nor psychical distress is naturally associated with menstruation, both are, for reasons already indicated, common in present-day women. "Some pain or discomfort," says Davenport, "is, with civilized women, so universal an accompaniment of this process that its occurrence may fairly be considered normal. It certainly is a fact that the cases among us where no pain is experienced are so rare that they are curiosities."

Although it is not within the power of the physician to render every young subject entirely exempt from the discomforts which now attend menstruation, it is quite possible to decrease these discomforts by the administration of those drugs which augment the functioning capacity of the organs concerned in this process. Moreover, it is possible to promote the development of the reproductive organs to such an extent that they can successfully resist the invasion of disease. To do this, however, the reproductive system should be given attention at the time of the initial menstruation, for it is at this time that disturbances of the monthly visitation fequently have their beginning, and the reproductive system assumes a condition favoring the development of intractable disease.

Indeed, nearly, if not quite, all of the diseases of the reproductive system have for their exciting cause some one of the several anomalies of menstruation, and in many instances these anomalies begin with the establishment of the monthly flow.

Inasmuch as a great deal of the suffering incident to the pubescent period is due to the incomplete development and lowered vitality of the reproductive organs, it is obviously proper for the physician to promote the development of these organs and to augment their functioning capacity and vigor. This can be done by the administration of Hayden's Viburnum Compound.

In addition to promoting the development and augmenting the functioning capacity of the female reproductive organs, Hayden's

Viburnum Compound exerts a beneficial influence upon the nervous system of subjects approaching maturity. In fact, the distinct anti-spasmodic and tonic action of the preparation causes it to be of conspicuous value in the treatment of menstrual disturbances among young subjects.

Furthermore, the administration of Hayden's Viburnum Compound is of added importance in the case of young subjects, for by its administration the menstrual flow can be made regular in occurrence and normal in volume, and the establishment of diseases of the reproductive system can be precluded. In fine, if Hayden's Viburnum Compound is administered at the time of the initial catamenia, the future welfare of the subject is, in large part, insured.

Maternity.—The same conditions which are responsible for the improper functioning of the female reproductive organs, account, in large part, for the difficulty attached to child-bearing among civilized women.

It is seldom that we meet with women who do not approach maternity with extreme fear, and it is equally seldom that they do not experience great suffering during the lying-in period.

While the pain incident to child-birth is frequently due solely to pelvic contraction or other malformations, lack of vitality in the uterus is a common cause of agony. Indeed, the pain of child-birth can be remarkably diminished by imparting to the uterus the proper degree of contractile power previous to the termination of the pregnancy. Moreover, the injuries which commonly occur at the time of delivery are rare in those of vigorous reproductive systems, and this fact renders it doubly important that those approaching motherhood should undergo preparatory treatment.

The administration of Hayden's Viburnum Compound is especially advocated in such instances, because of its tonic effect upon the walls of the uterus. It greatly increases the contractile power of this organ, and unquestionably diminishes the pain attendant upon child-bearing. It is proper, therefore, to use this preparation before and during all confinements.

The Menopause.—The various nervous and mental disturbances which are more or less incidental to the ultimate cessation of the monthly flow, deserve far more attention than they usually receive. It is highly important that these disturbances be corrected with the utmost promptness, for, if unattended to, they may prove a lasting source of suffering.

As a rule, the monthly flow gradually diminishes as the menopause is approached, and, at length, the flow entirely disappears. Again, the flow may be absent for several weeks, when it returns and is profuse. These fluctuations may be sufficient to cause marked systemic disturbances, and they certainly tend to render the uterus incapable of resisting morbid tendencies.

A proper termination of the menstrual function is easily effected by the administration of Hayden's Viburnum Compound, and the normal atrophy of the reproductive organs is seemingly encouraged by the preparation.

On account of the anti-spasmodic properties of the preparation, it is especially serviceable when psychical disturbances are noticeable.

The most gratifying results are achieved when Hayden's Viburnum Compound is administered as soon as indications of a cessation of the menstrual function are recognized. The use of the preparation should be continued until the menopause is well established.—*Southern California Practitioner.*

Bronchitis in Children.

The treatment of this condition is outlined thus by John U. Fauster (*Medical Council*, April, 132–135). The hygienic part consists in keeping the temperature of the room uniform, between 68° and 72°, during the twenty-four hours; sunlight is considered desirable. The child should be kept in bed, so it can be moved about from time to time; if the room is draughty a screen should be kept around the bed. Unnecessary noise and visitors should be excluded. An extra long flannel night-gown should be worn, so that the patient may wriggle about. The food should be given frequently in small amounts; it should be of the blandest character. Water should be given frequently by the mouth, but Fauster does not approve of sponging, as it contracts the superficial capillaries and still more engorges the already impeded circulation. He advises a mustard plaster to the chest; this is to be kept applied until full dilatation of superficial capillaries is produced; the chest should be covered with a cotton jacket; this procedure must be repeated every twenty-four hours.

What We Are Coming To.

"Is the room disinfected?"

"Yes, mother; and I have sterilized the curtains, deodorized the furniture, septicized all the fixtures, vaporized the air, washed my lips in an antiseptic solution, and—"

"Have you septicized the mistletoe?"

"Thoroughly, mother; everything is done. Arthur is waiting now in the hydrogen room."

"Then you may go in and let him kiss you, dear."—*Lippincott's Magazine.*

THE ECLECTIC MEDICAL JOURNAL

A Monthly Journal of Eclectic Medicine and Surgery.

TWO DOLLARS PER ANNUM.

Official Journal Ohio State Eclectic Medical Association

JOHN K. SCUDDER, M.D., MANAGING EDITOR.

EDITORS.

W. E. BLOYER.	H. W. FELTER.	W. N. MUNDY.	R. L. THOMAS.
W. B. CHURCH.	K. O. FOLTZ.	L. E. RUSSELL.	L. WATKINS.
JOHN FEARN.	J. U. LLOYD.	A. F. STEPHENS.	H. T. WEBSTER.

Published by THE SCUDDER BROTHERS COMPANY, 1009 Plum Street, Cincinnati, to whom all communications and remittances should be sent.

Articles on any medical subject are solicited, which will usually be published the month following their receipt. One hundred reprints of articles of four or more pages, or one dozen copies of the Journal, will be forwarded free if the request is made when the article is submitted. The editor disclaims any responsibility for the views of contributors.

Discontinuances and Renewals.—The publishers must be notified by mail and all arrearages paid when you want your Journal stopped. If you want it stopped at the expiration of any fixed period, kindly notify us in advance.

THE SEASON OF GOOD CHEER.*

The season of good cheer—that is what Christmas has been since unnumbered ages before it was called Christmas; and it ought to be doubly so to-day. Can we make it so?

Yes, if we go at it in the right way. It's a question of three things: good-will, energy and pluck, with a strong seasoning of brains throughout the lot.

Intention first. You won't have good cheer yourself unless you're trying to bring good cheer to others. If you've diked yourself in from the flowing tides of human sympathy, your Christmas is bound to be a mockery. The fellow who is too consciously selfish to care how others feel, or too unconsciously selfish to think how they are likely to feel, is always sailing alien seas when the season of good cheer comes round. It's just as well. He isn't built for that sort of freight. He can carry money, and usually does; but the most moderate cargo of human sympathy and human enjoyment would send him to the bottom. If this means you, good-by.

Then energy. If you want good cheer, get out and hustle for it. Don't sit in your office and send kind thoughts by telepathy. Send the unkind ones that way; and trust Uncle Sam's mails with the others. Don't expect your friends to be mind-readers—there are times when you would't like it if they were. If you're thinking of them, let them know it. If you've any good wishes, express them. And do it

* Lippincott's Magazine, December.

now. When good intentions are bottled up too long, they're liable to turn sour; so use yours while they're fresh—and don't worry for fear the stock will get too low.

Then pluck; last but by no means least, pluck. It takes pluck to make good cheer in any quantities; the sort of pluck that can take punishment without wincing; that can moult illusions without losing its appetite, and assimilate a new truth without prophesying the end of the world. You need it in all your business, and especially do you need it here. And you've got a right to it. The world is a good ways from being a garden of the gods, perhaps; but it's a long ways farther from being a house of detention for lost souls. Old Lady Luck may box your ears pretty sharp now and then; but she's got an apronful 'of big red apples for you if you'll only pester her long enough. Try it and see. Keep up your courage; and keep up the courage of others who may need a little boost in that direction. Pass a good thing along.

Good will, energy, and pluck; with brains mixed all through. These are what make good cheer—and this is the season of good cheer. Some day that season will last all the year around—and then we'll call it Brotherhood. ———

RESOLUTIONS AND RESOLUTIONS.

"Lezer's Resolutions.—Resolved: (1) That I won't borrow no trouble nor lend none, nor give none, nor keep none, nor expect none."—*Ex.*

For the beginning of the year this first resolution is one that every one could profit by. In fact, it would be a good idea to have it printed in bold-faced type and hung in the office, place of business or home in a position that would always bring it prominently before the entire force, from the head of the workers to even the transient visitor. It would emphasize the fact that the majority of so-called troubles, while not always "blessings in disguise," are largely evanescent or psychoneurotic, if the term can be used in this connection.

Each and every individual "hugs the delusion" that his personal troubles are of a little more weight or importance than any one else is blessed with, and the more the supposed burden, the happier the person is in his misery. They will inflict their tale of supposed wrongs or woe upon every one they can hold long enough to relate what has been, or they are afraid will be, done to them, and the time will come when none will stop to listen, as the majority of people have enough to do to mind their own affairs, and also are looking for the cheerful optimist rather than the far from cheerful pessimist. There is a trite saying that "all the world loves a lover," and there is a great deal of truth in it. The reason is clear enough ; it is not because the lover is a fool, but because he is a cheerful, roseate optimist. Suppose his dreams are simply "air castles;" while they last he is neither looking for, borrowing, lending nor keeping trouble.

How many are there in the world who feel they are getting their just deserts? Well, how many are there who, if their just deserts were meted out to them according to the opinion of the other fellow, would not be serving time working for the State or sleeping the long sleep? Echo answers, who!

Now for the sake of your own peace of mind and the comfort of those around you, look at the silver lining, not the dark cloud; at the sunshine, not the dark shadows, unless it is for the purpose of comparing your condition with what it might be under—not assumed, but true—adverse circumstances. The world usually judges the value of an individual pretty correctly, and if one possesses merit and a cheerful disposition the result generally is success. Of course, success is a relative term, but, broadly speaking, it means the highest attainment in the vocation of an individual of which he is capable.

Resolutions.—That each and every one of us will do our best, no matter what the line of work.

That we will not look at the dark or pessimistic side of our condition, but will remember how much worse off we might be in every respect.

That we will remember the resolution of Lezer, and relegate trouble to those who delight and are happy in being the down-trodden of this mundane sphere, for surely pessimism is its own reward.

That when any one says unkind things of us, it is a certainty we are of enough value in our respective walks of life to make some enemies, and of necessity some friends.

That the opinion of the majority counts for nothing, but the opinion of the one who is competent to judge correctly is of value to us.

FOLTZ.

THE THERAPEUTICS OF CINNAMON.

Though classed as a remedy of the lesser magnitude, we venture the assertion that if cinnamon were more generally employed it would become a general favorite among the standard, everyday medicines. The carminative properties of cinnamon, both in bark and fluid preparations, have long been duly recognized. Though capable of aggravating an irritable stomach, it may become a stomachic of first importance where employed in atony of the digestive tract. Strongly antiseptic and somewhat stimulating, it also possesses in some degree astringent powers, owing to the tannin contained in the crude drug. Cinnamon is a frequent ingredient of mixtures to restrain intestinal discharges, and the powder or its equivalent in infusion has long figured in the treatment of diarrhea and acute dysentery, though we do not believe it can equal in the latter condition other agents which we now use specifically. It has the advantage of preventing griping when given with purgatives, and it enters into the composition of spice poultice, a useful adjuvant in the treatment of some forms of gastrointestinal disorders.

Every Eclectic who has paid any attention to specific medication knows more or less concerning the value of cinnamon in hemorrhages. The type of hemorrhage most benefited is the post-partum variety, though here it has its limitations. If the uterus be empty and the hemorrhage be due to flaccidity of that organ due to lack of contraction, then it becomes an important agent. Then it strongly aids the action of ergot and should be alternated with it. If retained secundines are the provoking cause of the bleeding, little can be expected of this or any other agent until the offenders have been removed. The cinnamon should be frequently given, preferably a tincture of the oil, though an infusion is useful, but it cannot be prepared quickly enough or be made of the desired strength. Our preference is specific cinnamon, a preparation of the oil in alcohol, in nicely balanced proportions. Oil of erigeron acts very well with specific cinnamon. Other hemorrhages of a passive type are benefited by cinnamon. Thus we have found it a very important agent in hemoptysis of limited severity. In such cases we have added it to Lloyd's ergot and furnished it to the patient to keep on hand as an emergency remedy. By having the remedy promptly at hand the patient becomes less agitated or frightened, and this contributes largely to the success of the treatment. Hemorrhages from the stomach, bowels and renal organs are often promptly checked by the timely administration of specific cinnamon.

In the administration of medicines dispensed in water it is often important that they be made palatable by the addition of some agent. We know of no substance that is so universally liked by children particularly as cinnamon. It is pleasant, warming, aromatic, and, not of least importance, antiseptic. We invariably add it to the indicated medicine in bowel disorders, in common colds, and particularly in la grippe (in which it is credited with specific power even by those who have little faith in medicines), and in typhoid fever. Thus it is that we empty our cinnamon bottle as often as any in the medicine case, and find it to add materially to success in the medication and comfort of the patient.   FELTER.

CAPSICUM.

With us capsicum is a favorite remedy. Its use is by no means new; but it is neglected. As evidence of its virtue we may mention that, to a great degree, it was at one time, if it is not at the present, the key-stone in the arch that supported the practical therapeutics of the physio-medicalists and of the early botanic practitioners.

In the practice of medicine of to-day there is most urgent demand for stimulants. The over-indulgence in food and in drink, the exhaustion due to trouble and care consequent to high-speed living, the seeming necessity of over-work to meet strife and competition in every line of business—the *fast* age brings upon our patrons a depletion that *must* be met by stimulants of some sort. No one realizes this more than the physician. He knows, too, that he, in this instance at least, cannot *remove* the cause, and that unless he supplies the remedy his patient will do so for himself.

We will not argue that the idea of stimulation is to be praised, as there is a possibility, perhaps a probability, unless care be exercised, of whipping poor, tired, abused, exhausted natural functions to death by stimulation. 'Tis here the good judgment of the good physician will prove a blessing to himself and to his patron. But for a short period, at least, in many cases, the stimulant is as absolutely necessary as is the opiate in extreme pain.

In choosing an anodyne we always select the one that we think is least harmful. We should do the same in casting about for a stimulant. In our judgment, capsicum is the most pregnant with good, and at the same time the least harmful when properly used.

We might say much of capsicum as to its local use as a stimulant to the scalp in alopecia and other troubles, to the chest in the compound powder of lobelia and capsicum in the bronchial troubles just now so prevalent, as an efficient gargle in many cases of throat trouble where there is relaxation. The demand is for a local stimulant. With this in view it is frequently an excellent remedy in the later stages of diphtheria, in scarlet fever, any case of relaxed uvula. It is suggested as an efficient application, when properly used, in tonsillitis, relaxation, edema, etc. We all know of its value in the form of a stimulating liniment or embrocation when the skin is unbroken, in chilblains, bruises, rheumatism, and aches and pains generally.

It is especially of its internal use that we wish to speak, and here its field of usefulness is almost boundless, as the demand for a pure and safe stimulant may become prominent in the treatment of almost any disease.

When the digestion fails, appetite becomes poor, there is atonicity and relaxation, capsicum may be added to nux vomica, muriatic acid or other medicaments, or it can be suggested to the complaining one that he use capsicum as a condiment for awhile. It can be used alone in powder or in the form of a sauce or sharp catsup. In throat affections generally where this same atonicity prevails, capsicum should be considered. It frequently quickly allays hoarseness.

In subacute or chronic alcoholism it has no superior as a remedy, no equal in efficiency. Within the past few years we have had some very pleasant experiences from the use of capsicum in the treatment of dipsomania. In these cases we use the infusion *ad lib*. When the desire for drink presses, a cup of pepper tea satisfies. It occasions a feeling of warmth in the stomach, stimulates circulatory and muscular systems, increases the secretions; the craving for whisky is overcome. The patient can eat and sleep—two very necessary things in the cure of these cases. Enough pepper tea will prevent delirium—in fact, it will meet all unpleasant symptoms. In the treatment of delirium tremens we prefer capsicum to all of the hydrate of chloral, etc., imaginable.

In a majority of the cases large doses of nux vomica are an excellent adjuvant. It overcomes restlessness and induces sleep better than any of the so-called hypnotics. If the infusion cannot be given in sufficient quantity, the tincture may be added to animal broths, etc. We believe it will do as well in the treatment of the opium habit, though we cannot speak from so great an experience in this trouble. In acute alcoholism it should be given cautiously, especially if there be *irritation*. In fact, *irritation* is a contra-indication for capsicum in any disease.

It is said that capsicum tends to check abuminuria. It is excreted by the kidneys. Too much of it may cause strangury. In moderate amounts we believe it promotes the functional activity of the kidney, increasing the amount of water. It should do this because of the impetus given the blood current by its stimulation. It is a powerful heart stimulant, increasing the strength and frequency of the pulse. It should never be given when there is acute renal complications of any kind. In chronic parenchymatous nephritis, chronic pyelitis, chronic cystitis with relaxation, give capsicum.

To him who is wearied and worn from sexual indulgence, in prostatorrhea, in spermatorrhea, in functional impotence with atonic guideboards, capsicum may prove a boon. Try it.

In asthenic fevers capsicum is, by far, better than sedatives. We vouch for this. In the anorexia and impaired digestion of the convalescent, give capsicum.

Our older practitioners frequently added capsicum to quinine in the treatment of obstinate malarial manifestations, and usually with much satisfaction. Capsicum, with tincture of myrrh and alcohol, constituted the old compound tincture of myrrh, or the classic No. 6 of the old-timers, and they made name and fame through its judicious use. It was *the* remedy for colics and cramps, diarrheas, etc., etc. There was nothing better in the stage of collapse in cholera, cholera morbus, etc. There is no remedy to us that acts so well its part in the treatment of chronic liver troubles and the complications like constipation, hemorrhoids, etc., as does capsicum. It is a boon companion to nux, chionanthus and remedies of this class. It should not usually be given in acute cases.

We write this not because of anything *new*, but because capsicum is old, tried and valuable, and, from contact with physicians, we do not believe that it is used as frequently as it should be used. We hope to stimulate a study of it, so that it may be given instead of the many more harmful remedies in general use.   BLOYER.

DRY MEALS IN FUNCTIONAL DYSPEPSIA.

If you are preparing tincture of camphor you will not add water to the alcohol, unless you expect a cloudy, flocculent mixture, instead of a clear, perfect solution of the gum camphor. If you expect a perfect solution of proteids in the stomach in digestion, and a favorable action of the duodenal secretions as the pabulum passes onward, on the same lines you rationally will avoid diluting the gastric juice, that the full strength of the digestive solvents may be exerted.

The functions of the digestive juices cannot be expected to be well carried out if they be hampered by dilution. This is a well-known physiological maxim, yet how little is it observed when we come to apply our knowledge to practical use. We study this remedy and then that in indigestion, try first one and then another—unless we are given to shot-gun practice—and probably never stop to inquire what the habits of our patient are as to fluids taken at mealtime.

Unfortunately for the digestion of the populace, it is a fact that ninety-nine out of a hundred people, if not nine hundred and ninety-nine out of a thousand, drink copiously while eating their meals. That this is a stupid and pernicious habit, especially for intelligent—or supposably intelligent—people to indulge in, there is no question. It is a form of slow suicide, for the practice certainly lops off years from the lives of those so indulging. Functional dyspepsia is the probable ultimate result, and dyspepsia, even though functional, must soon or late exert a mischievous influence upon the entire organism. Imperfectly prepared pabulum entails extra burden upon the chylopoietic viscera and kidneys; and in late years, if cancer of the stomach does not finally intervene, organic disease of some of these organs appears as a consequence of the dietetic abuse.

When free taking of fluids at meals is indulged in, the solid ingesta float about for hours in a large volume of inert fluid until fermentation succeeds, the subject meantime often suffering all degrees of discomfort, from which he is not relieved until time for repetition of the process arrives. Thus the nervous dyspeptic becomes a chronic sufferer.

Since the day of Salisbury and his hot-water nonsense, the common people have been greater fools than ever about drinking at mealtime, and the doctors are not much behind. Many who imagine themselves ideal temperance advocates are really very intemperate in this respect, for temperance is not confined to abstinence from alcoholic liquors. When will the profession begin to apply the simplest teachings of physiology to practical use?

Preaching, however, produces little effect in any such case. The proof of the pudding is in the eating. If you have a case of nervous dyspepsia on hand, try the effect of dry meals. Interdict the use of fluids for an hour before and two hours after meals. The most objectionable food will be better if taken dry than the best selected diet if it be allowed to float in a stomachful of inert fluid. It is better, however, to employ some gumption about what a dyspeptic eats.

Also, consider the complications of the case you are treating before you expect startling results. If the patient is suffering indigestion from reflex or organic disease, no diet is likely to do him permanent good until that complication is removed. Reduce your case to one of functional dyspepsia pure and simple, and you can soon cure him without medicine, on dry meals. However, dry meals are eminently proper in any form of indigestion; they ought to benefit any case, though they may not cure it. Let the patient drink sparingly two hours after eating if he then craves drink, but not unless. Fluids hardly ever do good except to relieve thirst, and thirst is often an abnormal craving, due to habit. A mixed diet contains almost water enough for the patient's needs, especially if he is not taking active exercise. Dry bread even contains more or less water. However, drink restriction here is not necessary, except so far as dilution of the gastric juice is concerned.

We struggled along for many years in a blind endeavor to treat dyspepsia successfully. Occasionally benefit could be obtained with some drug, but usually results were unsatisfactory. We have finally found how easy it is by simple measures, when the patient can be induced to follow advice. One day will not accomplish it, but a week or two will, though sometimes a little proper medication may assist sensible precautions as to the taking of slops during meals.

It is best, however, to remember that proper physical effect is often important. Instruct your patient to restrict himself to dry meals and turn him loose, and you will not see him again for a long time, if ever. He is probably prejudiced in favor of medicine, for he has been vitiated by bad example and erroneous popular impressions, and he will probably consult some other practitioner within twenty-four hours, and you will be left with the stigma of failure resting upon you, and with your contention as to drink restriction during meals unproven. He must have some medicine in order that popular fallacy be satisfied, though that ought to be something which will not interfere with nature's efforts. A little colored water will be as good as anything, provided the coloring matter is not prejudicial.

Impress him with the idea that he must have more when that is gone, for you will thus be able to keep him with you, and thus encourage him to persevere in the proper course of cure—the taking of dry meals. Of course, the stomach ought to have perfect rest between meals. Haphazard lunching is one of the worst of practices for sick or well.   WEBSTER.

THE STUDY OF REMEDIES.

It has been asserted by some that cactus has no remedial action whatever upon the heart. This assertion is based upon a series of experiments carried on in a laboratory. The experiments, as we understand it, were made upon frogs and rabbits and guinea-pigs, the experimenter using cactin. The experiments and conclusions are based upon false premises.

It should be understood, first of all, that many remedies have a dual action. There is a wide difference between the physiological or poisonous action of a drug and its remedial action. A physiological action is a poisonous action. Again, no therapeutist would insist that a remedy must possess a poisonous action in order to have a remedial action. No one would think of giving aconite, strychnine, morphine, hyoscyamus or hyoscine, digitalis, ipecac, podophyllin, veratrum, belladonna, and a host of remedies we might mention, with a view of obtaining their physiological when desiring their remedial action.

Again, when experimenting with an alkaloid cr the active principle of a plant, we do not always obtain the same action that we would if the entire plant was used. Possibly the most familiar example of this would be the action of digitalin, and an infusion of digitalis. We are all familiar with the fact that when the diuretic action of digitalis is desired it is best obtained by using an infusion. The degree of dilution of a remedy will also influence its action.

Our attention was recently called to this latter fact in an accidental manner. We had prescribed buchu to be taken in hot water, directing the patient to take it in about a glass of hot water. The complaint was made that the remedy was not having the effect desired. Inquiry elicited the fact that, not desiring to take so large a dose, the amount of water had been reduced about one-half. When taken in the amount of water desired the action wished for was obtained.

Every therapeutist absolutely knows that black haw has a remedial action, yet it can be taken in almost any sized dose, its poisonous action, if it has one, being extremely remote. Yet no one familiar with it will deny but that it has a prompt and very effective remedial action. So it is with cactus. We do not deny the value of the laboratory in investigating drugs, but in this case the experimenter began with a wrong premise, hence his conclusions are wrong. So, in fact, are many of our laboratory drug studies, as well as diagnoses. In the first mentioned, poisonous actions only are studied; in the second many conclusions are reached which are not borne out by clinical investigations.

. You may say this is empiricism pure and simple. Granted it is, empiricism has taught us many valuable truths in therapeutics, and without a knowedge of therapeutics success as a practitioner is impossible. Many mistakes have been and will be made by relying upon a laboratory diagnosis solely; so, too, will many errors be made in therapeutic drug studies when confined to the laboratory and to poisonous actions.

Cactus has a remedial action, and every clinician who has ever given it a test will bear testimony to that fact. It is not a heart sedative as digitalis or aconite, but when we have tachycardia, dependent upon a nervous irritation or erethism—in other words, when it is purely functional—cactus will relieve and relieve promptly.

MUNDY.

BE THOU CLEAN.

In the mad rush now prevailing in the name of science, both enthusiastic youth and prejudiced age are especially apt to forget that the term science is not restricted to test-tubes and artificial laboratories. The scientific work of men whose deeds stand as foundation-stones on which is built a modern superstructure is apt to be forgotten. The young man who reads some of the modern works is apt to think that all outside that book is a fallacy, all behind it vacuity, and that the book in hand began the very scheme of scientific thought. Or, he may believe that the new idea, even if it be a new way of presenting that which is old, has brushed out all the past. He forgets the injunction that has challenged the ages—"Prove all things and hold

fast that which is good.'' This is but one phase of wrong thought
due to one-sided thought or inexperience, but it is enough to serve as
our text, and it is also enough to paralyze the efforts of many good
men.

Whoever believes the word cleanliness is of modern introduction
labors under a delusion. It matters not whether dirt be called by one
name or another, it has long been known as dirt. Nor has it been
scientifically *localized* in modern thought only, for in a general sense
localized forms of dirt have been defined since before the art of printing. Nor has it been left to the modern microscopist to announce
the fact that living dirt under his new name—bacteria or microbes—
produces disease expressions.

In our boyhood's days the term animalculæ covered the whole
multitude of living entities in which the microscope now differentiates
so many forms of living dirt, for as dirt we class matter out of place,
be it vitalized or dead.

Said our observing friend, Dr. W. C. Cooper, to us many, many,
years ago: ''Cholera is caused by living microscopic impurities in
water,'' and he did this by reasoning on observed fact. He argued
from his experience in the disease that this must be so. ''The cholera
germ is generally carried by the water,'' he contended, and he cited
localities where the disease prevailed and others where it was absent,
and noted the difference in the waters used by the respective persons.
Then, at last, he wrote in the *Gleaner* for 1893 an article that sums up
the matter as effectively as possible, if one takes fact for what fact is
worth in science:

''The cardinal fact to be remembered is that forty-nine out of every
fifty cases of cholera are directly traceable to the water drank. In
the one case out of the fifty the toxic principle has gotten into the
system through food, which has been contaminated by unclean hands.
The trouble is to control the habits of the people. Those who are
fortunate enough to live on plateaus where only gravel water is drank,
will escape cholera. Those who have good, perfectly tight cisterns
and who drink *no other* water, unless it be gravel or driven well
water, will also escape the disease. Those who drink ordinary well
water or hydrant water (and the mass of the people do that) are in
perpetual danger, unless this water is *thoroughly boiled* before being
drank. This is troublesome. In the hurry and bustle of life many
will neglect it, and the very poor, who cannot afford ice, will risk a
drink of cool, fresh water rather than drink the warm, lifeless boiled
water. Again, people must travel, must necessarily, for business or
other commanding reasons, visit cities where they cannot control
their dietaries. They are liable to get a drink of contaminated water
at the restaurant, or hotel, or the bar. We know *how* to prevent
cholera, if we knew *how* to get a chance to do it.''

Let us not disparage the work of the man of to-day with the microscope, for he draws yet finer lines when he pictures the microbe and the bacteria; but let us not hesitate to do credit to the man who, from other reasons, *knows* and who tells the story in words unmistakable.

But we may go yet further back in the line of living dirt's definition. Take your "Peter Smith's Dispensatory," 1813. Here the argument is made that the *plague* is due to *invisible insects* wafted by the air:

"In the course of our conversation I asked him what he conceived the *plague* to be, which has been so much talked of in the world. He readily told me 'that it was his opinion the plague is occasioned by an invisible insect. This insect, floating in the air, is taken in with the breath into the lungs, and there it either poisons or propagates its kind, so as to produce that dreadful disease.'"

But some may argue that those who thus spoke *theorized*, because they did not use terms and methods that now prevail. With this thought in my mind, we close the book, lay down our pen and ponder. If such evidence as this be *theory*, what do some others we might name ask us to think of some modern effusions we might mention?

LLOYD.

BOOKS ON THE INSTALLMENT PLAN.

Having had numerous inquiries for the purchase of several of our books on the monthly installment plan, we have decided to send any Eclectic book prepaid as per price list, with approved reference, as follows: On an order of $20.00 or more, $5.00 down and $3.00 per month. On orders less than $20.00, $3.00 down and $2.00 per month. Books to remain our property until fully paid for.

Our latest books are as follows:

Materia Medica and Therapeutics. By F. Ellingwood. Cloth, $5.00.
Medical Gynecology. By A. F. Stephens. Cloth, $3.00.
Diseases of the Digestive Organs. By Owen A. Palmer. Cloth, $3.00.
Treatment of Disease. By F. Ellingwood. Cloth, $6.00.
Nose, Throat and Ear. By Kent O. Foltz. Cloth, $3.50.
Eclectic Practice of Medicine. By R. L. Thomas. Cloth, $6.00; sheep, $7.00.
Reference Book to Specific Medication. By J. S. Niederkorn. Leather, $1.25.
Materia Medica and Clinical Therapeutics. By F. J. Petersen. Cloth, $3.00.

Complete eight-page price-list on request. We will also furnish *any* medical book on receipt of price list. Complete 144-page price-list of *every* medical book sent on request.

THE SCUDDER BROTHERS COMPANY.

Correspondence.

NEWARK, N. J., December 4, 1907.

PROF. JOHN K. SCUDDER, M.D.

My Dear Doctor:—It was with much pleasure that I noted in the ECLECTIC MEDICAL JOURNAL that you were arranging for the building of a new college edifice. I have long desired the multiplying of our schools of instruction, both to strengthen our forces and to develop greater utility for our procedures. But superficial as the advantage may seem, the possessing of suitable and attractive places for the purpose is destined to be of essential importance. Too often has there been a willingness to set up a college and engage in lecturing under conditions analogous to those of a private "select school." I would not despise humble efforts, nor would I establish a class of physicians away from sympathy and the fellowship of the "plain people." Instead, I honor effort, however modest and humble, to develop and improve our knowledge of the art of human healing. But we must be in an attitude to go with the times. The paramount purpose of the American Medical Association is to attain absolute control over every department of medical activity and eject all rivals from the field. This must be wisely met if we would avoid being snuffed out of existence. These, therefore, to sustain themselves, must not be neglectful of externals. There is great—I had almost said vital—need of attractive college buildings.

Eclectic medicine, to have a future, must deserve it. There should be its characteristic procedures and remedies, adherence to principle, fidelity and probity in dealings, and with it all the culture and amenity of well-bred men. Its physicians should be at home with the lowly, and, at the same time, equal to the superiors. I am not so confident and sanguine in these hopes and conditions as I would like to be, for I am old-fashioned still; but I am pleased with every movement that is in the right direction. I regard this proposed action of yours in that light. If the other college enterprises can but follow they will be able take a long step forward. As legislation steadily compresses and restricts opportunity, it will be found necessary for continuing to exist.

As the holidays are nearing us, permit me to anticipate them by wishing you the compliments of the season.

Yours truly,

ALEXANDER WILDER.

The Eclectic Medical Journal

ESTABLISHED 1836.

VOL. LXVIII.　　CINCINNATI, MARCH, 1908.　　No. 3.

Original Communications.

CACTUS GRANDIFLORUS.*

BY WILLIAM P. BEST, M.D.,

INDIANAPOLIS, IND.

"The fresh (green) stems and flowers of the Cactus grandiflorus. Linne (Cereus grandiflorus, Miller and De Candolle).

"*Botanical Source.*—Cactus grandiflorus is a creeping, rooting, fleshy shrub, having cylindrical or prismatic stems, with about five or six not very prominent angles, branching and armed with clusters of small spines arranged in radiated forms.

"The flowers are terminal and lateral, from the clusters of the spines, very large, eight to twelve inches in diameter, expanding at night, enduring for a few hours and exhaling a vanilla-like odor. The petals are white and shorter than the sepals; the sepals are linear-lanceolate, brown without and yellow within. The fruit or berry is ovate, covered with scaly tubercles, fleshy, and of orange or fine reddish color. The seeds are very small and very acid.

"The large flowered cactus was introduced to the medical profession by Dr. Scheele, of Germany; but little attention, however, was given to it until Rubini, a Homeopathic physician of Naples, brought it into special notice as a remedy for heart disease.

"*Action, Medicinal Uses and Dosage.*—Cactus impresses the sympathetic nervous system, and it is especially active in its power over the cardiac plexus. In sufficiently large doses it acts as an intense irritant to the cardiac ganglia, producing thereby irritability, hyperesthesia, arythmia, spasm and neuralgia of the heart, and even carditis and pericarditis.

"According to E. M. Hale, M.D., it acts on the circular muscular fibres of the heart, whereas digitalis acts on all the muscular fibres of the heart. Like the latter, as a secondary effect of over-stimulation, it may induce heart failure. The tincture, in large doses, produces gastric irritation, and also affects the brain, causing confusion of the mind, hallucinations and slight delirium. In excessive doses, a quickened pulse, constrictive headache, constrictive sensation in the chest, cardiac pain with palpitation, vertigo, with dimness of sight, over-

---

* Read at the January meeting of the Marion County Eclectic Medical Society.

sensitiveness to noises, and a disposition to be sad or imagine evil, are among its many nervous manifestations. Melancholia often follows such action. It is generally conceded, however, that the mental, cerebral, gastric and other effects are secondary to and dependent largely upon the primary effects of the drug upon the heart.

"In medicinal doses, night blooming cereus diminishes the frequency of the pulse and increases the renal secretions, and is therefore sedative and diuretic. The special field for cactus is the diseases of the heart, in which it exerts a very decided action, palliating or removing the symptoms, and frequently giving prompt relief. This influence upon the heart is manifested when the disorder is functional ; organic conditions are only benefited in a measure.

"There is no doubt but that the continued use of the drug tends to increase cardiac nutrition and waste, and in this way may benefit cases with structural lesions. The influence of cactus is exerted wholly upon the sympathetic nervous system, through the superior cervical ganglion, expending its force in regulating the action of the heart and controlling cerebral circulation, thus giving increased nutrition to the brain."—(Felter, in " King's American Dispensatory.")

. Scudder says :

"The influence of cactus seems to be wholly expended upon the sympathetic nervous system, and especially upon and through the cardiac plexus. It does not seem to increase or depress innervation (neither stimulant nor sedative), but rather to influence the regular performance of function. I am satisfied, however, that its continued use improves the nutrition of the heart, thus permanently strengthening the organ. It has a second influence which is of much importance to the therapeutist. It exerts a direct influence upon the circulation and nutrition of the brain, and may be employed with advantage in some diseases of this organ.

"Cactus is a specific in heart disease, in that it gives strength and regularity fo the innervation of the organ. Its influence is permanent in that it influences the waste and nutrition of the heart, increasing its strength."

W. C. Abbott says:

"Instable action of the vasomotors, lack of physiological balance, a weak irregular heart, whether the indication be a pulse that is too fast or too slow, too weak or too strong, if the cause is vasomotor instability, as in tobacco heart, the heart of the drunkard, some cases of menopause, over-work, etc., no remedy will do what cactin will do ; no remedy will so quickly restore the equilibrium as this.

"The mistake the unthinking make is to look for toxic effect following (cactus) cactin such as follows the exhibition of decided doses of digitalin (digitalis) and strychnine, and they are therefore disappointed even when enormous doses of cactin (cactus) are used. The man with his frogs, cats, rats and dogs says this toxic effect isn't there—and it isn't. I appreciate Dr. Hatcher's scientific work very much ; there is little doubt of its essential exactness. In fact, his findings on frogs, cats and dogs, even on 'mongrel bitches,' that cactus has no toxic action on the heart, like strychnine and digitalis, is exactly our contention—*exactly*.''

The *Gleaner* for September, 1907, page 339, has the following from Dr. Felter:

"*Raynaud's Disease.*—Cactus has acquired a reputation among Eclectics as a remedy for circulatory disorders that is little known beyond the confines of our school of practice. Notwithstanding that Rubini, and others have from time to time called attention to its action on the heart and blood-vessels, but little serious attention has been paid to the agent except among our own practitioners.

"Rubini early asserted a notable effect upon the vasomotor nerves, and yet but little heed has been taken of this fact in therapy. A recent experience with it in a disease in which the vasomotor nerves are chiefly at fault, if the pathology is at all understood, convinces us that it might have a much wider range of usefulness than is ordinarily ascribed to it.

"It has produced, in our hands, a remarkable restraining, if not actually curative, result in a case of Raynaud's disease, which had lasted from early womanhood to a considerable period beyond the menopause. The case has been seen and treated by many physicians, and was progressively growing worse when we prescribed six-drop doses of specific cactus once a day. The good effect began shortly after the beginning of the use of the medicine. After taking it for a few months it was dropped and the disturbance gradually returned. The good effect had been so marked while taking the cactus that it was resumed, and again with gradual amelioration, until now, considerably more than a year since the patient began the use of the medicine, she considers herself practically cured. However, as a precaution, lest the spasms return, she continues the daily dose. This is, so far as we are aware, the first case of the kind treated with cactus. Electricity gives partial and temporary relief, but does not begin to compare with the effect of cactus in this case."

Lyman Watkins, in speaking of "Certainties in Medicine," says:

"Cactus is another certainty. Cactus is a heart remedy, but not a drug that will cure organic heart disease. Here the statement may be made that many good medicines are brought into disrepute by over-praise, and in the case of cactus some of its over-enthusiastic friends have lauded it beyond reason, and many who have tried it have been disappointed. Like all specifics, cactus is adapted to certain conditions, and it is only when we have the indications that we will obtain results. The field for cactus is that of nervous affections implicating the heart, such as reflex palpitation and excitable heart, a heart prone to run away with but little provocation, tobacco heart, cardiac palpitation of the menopause, irregular heart, and a heart the pulsation of which is abnormally slow. It requires but little thought to discover that nervous influence proceeding from the sympathetic and cardio-inhibitory centres is the field controlled by cactus."— (*Gleaner*, November, 1907, page 449.)

The following from Ellingwood's Materia Medica plainly and succinctly sets forth the result of the observations and experience of those who have studied cactus :

"Specific cactus is prepared from the green stems (and the flowers) of the true species. Although the medicinal effect may be observed from two minims, larger doses may be given, no toxic effect having been observed.

"Cactus exercises a direct influence over the sympathetic nervous system, regulating its action, restoring normal action, whatever the perversion. It acts directly on the cardiac plexus, regulating functional activity of the heart."

Professor W. E. Bloyer, M.D., Cincinnati, O., in Drug Treatise No. 11, issued by Lloyd Brothers, says :

"As has been written before, the administration of cactus has not at all times been followed by the most satisfactory results. This may have been due not to an oversight of the prescriber, as we are told by those who know that it is a very difficult matter to get the true species of the plant from which to make the drug, and that it very frequently occurs that some other species of the great cactus family is foisted upon the unwary, or cheap buying manufacturer. We are also told that once the proper plant be secured that it must be at once, and properly, worked, because of the fact that it contains an abundance of water and quickly deteriorates. We only mention these things to induce the reader to base his study of the drug upon a reliable preparation. . . . In the trial of a drug, next to the *good* drug is the *good* case—that is, a properly selected one—one in which, as we usually state it, the drug 'is indicated.' It is through these 'indications' of the Eclectics and Homeopaths that more and more positiveness in drug action is coming into medicine every day. It is our purpose, at this time, to point out the therapeutic or specific indications for cactus, to place the drug before our readers in such a way that they may have before them the ideas of those who successfully and satisfactorily use the drug. . . .

"Nearly all agree that cactus acts decidedly upon the cardiac plexus of the sympathetic, and that therefore its effects are as far-reaching as are not only the minute distributions of this nerve, but even so far as to the lumen of every capillary of the body. Two things are absolutely essential to the well-being of every mortal ; they are *good blood* and its *good* distribution or circulation. . . . So, then, we will say that cactus under certain conditions is a remedy ; it stimulates the vasomotor centres, the sympathetic ganglia of the spinal cord, and of the heart muscle. Usually it does not disturb the stomach, etc., yet when given in sufficient doses it does produce physiologic or toxic effects. They are irritant in character, even to the production of diarrhea, spasm of the heart, neuralgia, carditis and pericarditis. This is true only of over-doses. Its long-continued use in medicinal doses has no baneful effect. It has no so-called cumulative action, like digitalis and some other drugs.

"Cactus is indicated in impaired heart action, whether functional or structural. Of course, we will not *cure* the latter troubles. But when the pulse is feeble, irregular, quick, irritable, nervous, and the patient complains of oppression of the chest, a grip as of iron upon the heart, and there is fear, apprehension, mental depression, palpitation, worry, hysteria or hypochondria, cactus is the remedy.'' (Copied from *The Gleaner*.)

J. Milton Sanders, M.D., LL.D., Professor of Chemistry in the Eclectic Medical College of New York, states his own case under the date of April 12, 1875.

'' . . . . It was in the early days of November, 1874, that those symptoms made their appearance—at least in an aggravated form—without a note of premonition. Soon after I had taken a short promenade, the weather being cold and disagreeable, I was suddenly taken with a severe pain in the region of the heart and extending across the sternum. Each paroxysm was accompanied with great mental depression, which appeared to be a concomitant of the disease. The dyspnea shortly after became so intense that my case resembled one of congestion of the lungs. Under various kinds of treatment life was barely kept in me, so great was my suffering, mentally and physically, coupled with the fact that nothing more could be done for me. . . . Could not take the least exercise without bringing on paroxysms of intense cardiac pains, accompanied with mental anxiety and dyspnea.''

Dr. Kunze, a colleague of Dr. Sanders, prescribed '' Cactus ounces ss. Sig.: Take ten minims in water three times a day until relieved.''

'' In twenty-four hours afterward I felt less nervous, and in a few days was enabled to take more exercise with less dyspnea following. Cardiac pain not so severe. Pulse reduced to 84, with a better rhythm (it had been 96 and very feeble). Could walk to and from the college with less fatigue, and lecture with less inconvenience. I could also lie down and sleep on the left side again, a thing I had been unable to do for two years past. Improving so very encouragingly I got somewhat careless again in taking the medicine regularly, and therefore when I perceived myself getting worse imagined that the remedy had lost its effect on me, and finally ceased taking it altogether. The fact was I had lost faith in any medicine until Professor Newton assured me that I ought to continue it. This was about the middle of January, 1875. Pain returning with renewed strength, I then suspected that the cactus had done me some good. I then commenced to take this remedy again with more confidence. I took it regularly three times a day in doses of twenty minims. I now felt a slow but assured sense of relief, and after taking the same for three months I ceased to take it any more, as I had got relief from the pain. The throbbing of the heart had entirely subsided; its rhythmic beating was reinstated and synchronously with the steady pulsations of the heart came back the more joyous pulsations of health.''—Transactions of the N. Y. State Eclectic Medical Society, 1876.

To this array of testimony, by men of unimpeachable integrity and ability, it seems useless to add.   Yet we have thousands of educated, active and successful practitioners using the remedy with noticeable effect, and most comforting and satisfactory results.

It will be observed that at no time or place have any one of the above-quoted writers and observers claimed that cactus in any sense of the word "paralleled digitalis" nor strophanthus.   The testimony establishes, as firmly as positive statements can, the therapeutic worth and position of cactus.

LEATHER OR CLOTH BINDING FOR THE MEDICAL LIBRARY, ETC?

BY HERBERT T. WEBSTER, M.D.,
OAKLAND, CAL.

Barzilla Wingate "callates" we all have crazy streaks in us some-wheres, though the crazy streaks don't always break out in the same place.   Probably many of us are cranks, with some particular individual weakness which we love to parade, for our own satisfaction at least, even if it bores our fellows.   After all, this may be a good thing, for it is often the crank who sets people to thinking, and leads some well-balanced thinker to get a better think coming.   This, then, may be considered an excuse for volunteering a little advice upon the topic here considered.

In my time as a student, the great ambition was to get a medical library together as soon as possible.   Now-a-days, possibly, a kit of surgical tools takes precedence, as the young doctor, in these days of surgical craze, is anxious to begin his practice by cutting some one up, thus establishing his reputation as a gentleman of "nerve."   Even then, however, a surgical library is an important desideratum ; and, after deciding what author he wants, the next important question is, what style of binding will he buy?

Some graduates are so endowed with worldly goods that the matter of binding is not of much consequence in a pecuniary sense, and of course such will be apt to choose what is commonly considered as the best.   Uniform leather bindings for all the books of the library will then probably be purchased ; and the practice of adding nothing but such style will be carried out afterward, in order that the library may present an attractive and imposing appearance.   There are others, however, who have reached the limit of their finances at time of graduation, and are not able to purchase half-a-dozen medical works even in cloth, in addition to the text-books they have needed in their course of study.   To such, a handsome and attractive library is out of the question for a time.

I once knew a young man who earned his way through medical college playing a fiddle evenings, in a dive; and, naturally, when graduation day arrived, he had little left except his clothes and the reputation of being one of the best students in his class. He was a '' tony '' fellow, all in all, and managed to keep up appearances for a year or so, and built up a paying practice in a small way; but his diminutive library was made up of cloth bindings principally, because he deemed himself too poor to indulge in what he greatly admired—nice, white-leather bindings. Finally, he appropriated the affections of a charming young lady who had inherited wealth, and after marriage all cloth bindings were soon discarded from his office library, and leather bindings, of uniform size and style, substituted. This shows how taste sometimes runs concerning the matter of medical libraries.

When I was doing a country practice years ago, a young doctor once referred somewhat disparagingly to my library when comparing it with his own, because my books were principally in cloth binding, and presented a somewhat soiled appearance. I improved the occasion by reminding him that it was no great mark of superiority because his books did not appear as though they had been handled; that a library is supposed to be kept for use, and if the volumes in it are too neat in appearance there is very great probability that the owner is not very much given to investigation; and his patients, the philosophical ones, might indulge in some such surmise.

It is true that we learn many practical ideas outside of books, but after all a well-selected library ought to be a great help to every industrious student and physician. It does not matter what the topic under consideration may be, works of reference are almost certain to throw some light on the subject likely to be of value.

If our books are for use, then why expend extra money in furnishing high-priced binding when a cheaper dress answers just as well, if not better? The expense incurred for leather covers, in a fair-sized library, means several more volumes in cloth, and thus a more complete library; for the progressive physician is never done buying books while he lives.

A cloth-bound volume, with good care, will remain in fair condition for thirty years. I now have in my possession a favorite author on therapeutics which I consult almost every day, and have for the past twenty-five years, though I admit that I have recently promised it a new cover. However, I possess several volumes in cloth, frequently referred to, more than thirty years old, which are still in good condition, and I venture that their appearance is superior to that of white-leather covers which have seen as much wear.

No physician will ever be too old to learn, and no physician, who has not become on old fogy, will stop buying books while he is following the practice of medicine. We cannot neglect new publications altogether unless we expect to fall behind the times and occasionally meet those younger than ourselves, perhaps, who are liable to spring something new upon us. It must be a little humiliating for a physician of thirty or forty years' experience to meet a young sprig in consultation who prates learnedly about something which is entirely foreign to his own knowledge; and this is liable to occur to one who has neglected his research into modern medicine for eight or ten years. While in practice, it behooves us all to endeavor to "keep in the swim," and know what is going on about us, even if half of it is nonsensical, new-fangled stuff. If it is considered orthodox and in fashion we ought to know about it, though we consider it more or less trashy, when compared with the solid ideas of former times. The trouble is, that what might have been considered orthodox a dozen years ago may now be regarded as a vagary of antiquity. We live in an age of iconoclasm—an idol-killing age.

What the old practitioner needs to buy every few years these days is a new medical dictionary. So many new terms are being added to the medical vocabulary that one might as well burn the old ones, were it not for the reason that some of the old terms are liable to be dropped from the new ones, thus rendering old ones worth preserving on this account.

I will not attempt to describe an ideal medical library from the standpoint of Eclectic practice. Let it be said though that tastes, special demand, and opportunities vary, A physician's location and the kind of cases he is called upon to treat ought to determine the trend of practice upon which he will need to especially prepare himself. One matter is certain, he should possess a full complement of Eclectic text-books before hunting outside his own field for medical works. This is a provision which some Eclectic graduates neglect. They begin to buy old school works with which to stock their libraries as soon as spare money comes in, to the neglect of their own works of reference, relying on what they have learned in college to keep them in touch with their own school, and thus drift away from the best in medicine into a sort of intellectual fog, from which they are liable to never emerge.

I have known bright Eclectic students, who have graduated with honors, to become very mediocre practitioners by thus dabbling in something they knew nothing about. Text-books from other schools are not objectionable to old practitioners who have become grounded in the essentials of their own practice, but new beginnerrs, who have not yet formed their habits, are better off if they taboo allopathic works for awhile.

My advice to the young practitioner of our school is, keep clear of the heterodoxy until you have learned the resources of your own medical literature. This cannot be done in a day, nor in a year. Know your own resources well before you go rummaging about in foreign fields. When you have practiced close to your college teachings for ten years, with the aid of your own text-books, you will be better fitted to supply anything you may deem lacking from outside sources.

The recent Eclectic graduate who imagines that it would be a good thing for him to attend some other school and graduate before beginning practice makes the mistake of his life. He has had no opportunity to become grounded in any kind of faith, and becomes hopelessly tangled up in all sorts of theories and methods, and he has had no practical experience to enable him to decide as to which are the best. He is, therefore, muddled by a sort of polyglot education, from which he is hardly ever able to extricate himself, and never becomes a successful practitioner. If he desires to become a success · and a credit, let him beware of such a maze of contradictions until he is capable of forming his own opinions from practical experience in his own school.

It is my belief that the bulk of those who leave the Eclectic ranks and go over to the old school are those who have undergone such experiences and have been tangled up in the beginning by old school text-books or by old-school college instruction. They never knew what an up-to-date Eclectic practice consists of, and do not know what they are condemning.

MACROTYS IN LATTER WEEKS OF GESTATION.

BY W. L. LEISTER, M.D.,
OAKLAND CITY, IND.

It is believed by some that if macrotys be used as a *partus preparator* in the last weeks of the carrying period that the woman would be liable to post-partum hemorrhage.

Many years' habitual usage of the agent in cases nearing the end of pregnancy, and with almost universally favorable terminations, has established the conviction that no such untoward result ever follows the use of the agent. Many popular fallacies work their way into the medical mind and the above is one of them.

While in attendance at the Texas Eclectic Medical Association in 1900, one of the visiting professors gave utterance to the belief that black cohosh caused a severe post-hemorrhage in a case wherein the agent had been used preparatorily, having been prescribed by himself.

Occasional echoes have been heard—reflections probably from that publicly-expressed erroneous conclusion.

Macrotys exerts favorable influence upon the reproductive organs of the female and upon the generative organs of the male as well. It is more potent to prevent habitual miscarriage than either partridge-berry or black haw, and both these agents are of good repute.

Macrotys allays irritability of the distended uterus, not by obtund-ing nerves but by assuaging muscular tension. It is tonic and there-fore innervating to the gravid uterus and to its adnexa.

The writer prescribes macrotys in five to six drop doses as often as every three or four hours, beginning this preparatory course as early as four weeks prior to expected climax. Some cases will neglect to apply for the course until a couple of weeks before *accouchement*, or the confinement may precede expectations by several weeks, when the medicine will have been used less length of time by so much. A point observed by the writer is that the macrotys insures enlarged results with those multipara who had suffered inordinately in previous labors, and wherein the muscular structures of the abdomen and those of the uterus as well, were lax and semi-toneless, and wherein the fetus hangs low, causing much urinary and lower bowel distress. In such case enjoin rest in recumbent posture. At same time enjoin the daily use of the agent under discussion.

Barring material urgent complicatioms, such as heavy urine, edematous feet and legs and possibly the body, heart and breathing organs disturbance and macrotys is all-sufficient. In a case wherein the above spoken mal-features present, the writer would again, as he has many times in the past, add equal amount of saw palmetto, but in some picked cases would make the helping-maid rhus aromatica. So confident of favorable outcome in cases submitting to the above course that the writer ceased years ago to concern himself about probable post-hemorrhage, puerperal eclampsia or other untoward, old-time bugaboos the books told about, and that happen still in the practice of the slouch and medical nihilist.

All physicians have favorite labels, and there are a goodly number of true-to-name-and-label products, but the essayist has been partial to the specific medicines. He has used for many years specific macrotys, specific saw palmetto and specific rhus aromatica. No, Doctor, ma-crotys will not cause or even *permit* post-partum hemorrhage.

INSOMNIA.

BY W. H. HALBBERT, M.D.,
NASHVILLE, TENN.

Inasmuch as one of our members has discussed the philosophy of sleep, I have concluded, to avoid a routine that we have drifted into, that I would write a paper on insomnia. The other paper was so ably written that I have felt a delicacy in this, because I could, in no sense, equal it. Do not get the idea now that I regard insomnia as a disease; it is only a symptom of some other lesion or a functional wrong.

I will not in this paper discuss the insomnia which attends acute diseases, such as typhoid, malarial or other fevers, but confine myself strictly to conditions which disturb the function of sleep. I would like to refer, in brief, without trespassing, to the cause of sleep. Why do we sleep? Why don't we go on and on wide awake, and let the ganglionic nervous system take care of nutrition and construction? Now all the activities of the body cannot be going on with full force at the same time. We use in our mental work only a small portion of what is called mental action at one time. Our mind is constantly shifting from one mental effort to another. We are sure that all the activities of the body do not go on with an equal degree and with full force all the time. Playfair and Hammond say that sleep is due to a diminished supply of oxygen to the brain. Pryer says that the oxygen is used up in a different manner than when awake, and says that a material which he calls "weariness material" is accumulated in quantities corresponding to the intensity of its activities, etc., and which lays hold of the oxygen during sleep. This is very plain, and I know you understand it as well as I do.

The only wonder is that some bacteriologist hasn't found a specific germ which early in the evening eats up a part of the oxygen, just leaving enough to preserve the body through the night. There is a great deal of difference between stupor and sleep. You can paralyze and stupefy the brain with medicine, such as chloral hydrate, hyoscyamine, and the various preparations of opium; but this is not sleep. You cannot make any medicine which, when given, paralyzes the nerve centre, produces normal sleep. Again, Foster says sleep is the diastole of the brain. To some extent this is true, but not wholly. The brain may not sleep, but a degree of refreshment may be obtained by giving the muscles a complete rest. As against this we can also at least assume that the brain cells during repose are re-building, doing their complex work, as the salivary and other glands when in a state of rest are building their mother ferments, old material of the brain waste-matter is being carted away, carried to the trash-heap, like old brick, mortar and rotten wood, disposed of by being burnt and the poisonous gas enclosed in safety sacks to be cast off from the system by the lungs, kidneys, skin or bowels. While we have another line of carts entering the structure with new material, placing as the workman does his brick, bolts, mortar, etc., in the shape of lime, iron, phosphates, etc., and all the organic constituents just where each is needed.

This beautiful study of the equilibrium of the human body can be equalled nowhere in nature. The supply in the healthy body is just equal to the demand. No friction, no check, no disturbance, everything in perfect harmony. Every movement governed by a fixed law. Where there is loss there is equal gain. This is loss, nutrition and construction. Both fluids and solid tissue, enjoying a · ceaseless activity, ever changing, yet always the same. Call it retrograde metamorphosis, or any other name you will, remembering these changes take place in muscle, nerve, gland, cartilage, brain, spinal cord and nerves by the work of the ganglionic nervous system. This highly organized system controls the work of nutrition and construction. This does its work when the rest of the body is, as it were, exhausted or partially so, reparation by the lost elements by active assimilation of new material prepared by digestion.

We are conscious of the active work of the cerebro-spinal system, and feel when this system becomes exhausted then we become wholly unconscious of the active work of the sympathetic nervous system. When this activity is predominant, we fall asleep. It is then we sleep, Just at this stage of work when the assimilative system begins its vigorous work, exerting its predominating power over the cerebro-spinal, we find that there is an irritable condition of the abdominal viscera, which causes increased flow of blood to the part; this irritation is caused by a fixed law—*Ubi iritatio ibi fluxus*—where there is irritation the blood flows—the law that governs in this case.

This increased action of the sympathetic lessens the power of all the other activities of the body. For the want of these exciting elements, we soon become unconscious. The elements necessary for the day's work having been consumed, the nutritive and constrictive elements are needed for repair and nutrition. The carts and laborers are sent to the abdominal organs for new material, consequently there is less blood in other parts of the body. All other parts of the body are comparatively inactive, and this includes the brain, muscles, and the excretory organs. This work of assimilation cannot be well done until the other activities are lessened. Should the cerebro-spinal system continue its active work, the sympathetic could do but little in nutrition and constructive power, consequently there would be at an early day a worn-out body, worn out for the want of nourishment. When one predominates the other must be quiet. It is true there is a lessened circulation in the brain with a decreased supply of oxygen, yet there may be too little of this and consequently sleeplessness. The body may sleep for a short time from sheer exhaustion when there is too small a quantity of oxygen for the brain, but in a few hours the cerebro-spinal system must assert itself for an increased supply of oxygen, and the equilibrium being destroyed, the sympathetic not being able to supply the demand, there is loss of nutrition and constructive material, loss of sleep, for the body in this case only sleeps from exhaustion, not being able to sleep while the brain is active.

An increased activity of the brain causes an increased flow of blood to that organ, then diminishing the flow to the abdominal viscera. In this we not only lose sleep, but our power of assimilation also suffers. We should learn to control our brain-work and give it a rest, using will-power as the circulation is lessened and the brain gets its rest in a state of partial unconsciousness—sleep.

I believe that there must be, if anything, an increase of the quantity of oxygen during sleep, as there is during the predominating activity of the sympathetic a greater necessity for a larger quantity of oxygen, to aid in the assimilating process. This ebb and flow, this periodicity, cannot be explained, but we know that when one works the other system is at rest. We see the necessity for this periodical rest for each system, but cannot understand the how. The new-born child sleeps almost continuously for six weeks, because of the predominance of the sympathetic system. Over-eating, worry, anger, hatred, etc., may banish sleep, may overpower the force of the sympathetic for a time, but when it does it is at the cost of the whole organism, and must finally yield to the recuperating power of necessity.

Anything that depresses the nerve centres, such as loss of blood, over-eating, exhaustion, tired or worn-out by over-exertion, hot drinks, a drink of brandy or whisky, will produce sleep. The condition which follows excessive cold or heat is not sleep, but stupor. In this condition the brain is in more or less a state of congestion which renders it unfit for mental action. On the contrary, anything which excites the nerve centres produces wakefulness. There can be such a storm of excitement of the nerve centres as to absolutely prohibit sleep day or night, the patient finally dying from exhaustion, or becoming insane. Excessive mental strain which we find among business men and students, persons laboring under great trials, sorrow, anxiety, over-work the brain until this mental labor inhibits or lessens the assimilating power, until the system is worn out, as it were. This necessarily breaks down the entire working forces of the body, until at last the mental activities are an insane wreck.

There are a number of acute diseases which prevent sleep, none of which will be referred to in this article. There are many lesions of the nerve centres which cause insomnia, and but few medicines which can be used without detriment to the patient. You have a patient, who, when she retires, say at 9:30 or 10 P.M., drops off into a sound sleep because of the exhausted and tired feeling, sleeps sound one, two, or at the most, three hours, wakes wide awake suddenly and remains sleepless until about 5 A.M., when apparently almost worn out, has another hour of sound sleep. During the waking hours there is no worry, keeping perfectly quiet, no restlessness whatever. This is kept up for two, three or four weeks, when the patient sleeps perfectly sound for two or three nights, for eight or nine hours, when the insomnia returns again for several weeks. We have this cause for this —the patient is not getting enough oxygen to the brain. In this case the patient has the power of deep concentration on a subject, but has not the power to stop the mental work at night, but keeps it up until he is completely exhausted, when a few hours' sleep follows. This patient is not nervous and there is no passive congestion. This condition may last for five, ten, fifteen years without wearing the patient out. This is because there is no worry and there is rest for the muscular system. We will give this patient an oxygen-carrier, one that will only do normal work. Give five grains of kali sulph. 3x at 4 and 8 P.M., and we will have him permanently cured in less than a week. Now if he is nervous and restless, flouncing from one side to the other, possibly shedding a few tears now and then—men cry as well as women—for fear something terrible is going to happen, kali sulp. 3x will not relieve this patient until we have given kali phos. 3x for several days, three grains every three hours, and then we will get good results from the kali sulph.

Again, we have the same amount of sleep in the same way, except there is another nervous lesion. The patient in this case worries and is irritable, easily offended. I treat these patients with specific staphysagria for a week or more and then give the oxygen-carrier, or both can be alternated. I am sure that no good results are obtained without this specific medicine. Those are about the only medicines for this condition, and they will never fail you.

Let us not forget that in any of these functional troubles causing insomnia, that tea, coffee and heavy suppers must be prohibited, and that no opiates are to be taken. What we want to do is to produce natural sleep, and we must be careful not to have the patient disturbed.

Again, we have a patient who gets sleep just as the ones just mentioned, but who wakes suddenly and takes some time to find himself —can not locate himself, appears frightened. Give this patient specific rhus tox. This will give relief at once, and with proper care will make a permanent cure. This remedy should not be confounded with matricaria, all of which indications are somewhat similar, except in matricaria the patient will have these symptoms during sleep as well as when awake, and in addition one other symptom—the head is almost continually covered with perspiration.

In the indication for belladonna there is perspiration of the head and a dull, stupid, sleepless state, and no nervous excitation. For belladonna we have a state of passive congestion to remove. In not a few of the patients who pore over work they have an expression of wild delirum and talk it as well as look wild, give specific hyoscyamus. I would use a small dose every few hours, one or two 'drops.

Again, we have a patient who is laboring under a high nervous tension, whose muscles are twitching; give ammonia bromide in small doses, say five grains at a dose, every four hours. I would not, for lesions which are only functional, give an opiate at any time. In other words, I would not undertake to force sleep on the patient at all unless there was danger of insanity or death.

There is another type of insomnia in which the cerebro-spinal system is at such a high tension—cyclonic, if you please—that there is neither sleep nor rest day' nor night. I do not mean the hysterical patient; neither do I refer to that caused by some reflex action. Somehow the storm centre is in the brain. There is no anger, grief, or fear, or business loss, but there is no sleep. I have seen these patients almost insane—indeed, showing evidences of insanity. I would give this patient, besides a carefully restricted diet, a teaspoonful of powdered capsicum, a good article mixed with eight ounces of hot water. This is to be taken at one dose at night. This is one of the best of sleep-producers for this specific wrong, and will, every time it is given, produce a quiet normal sleep. One dose of this, for only a few days, each night at bedtime, makes a permanent cure. This condition is caused by too much blood to the brain, and the medicine, by its local irritation, causes an increased flow of the blood to the abdominal viscera, thereby relieving the brain. This theory caused me to use this medicine for this, and it has never failed me.

PAIN is often present for months after a fracture of the leg, especially in elderly people. This is mainly due to the formation of the callus and needs no operative interference. Of course, a subacute osteomyelitis must be kept in mind.—*American Journal of Surgery.*

PROGRESS IN MEDICINE DURING 1907.*

By O. A. PALMER, M.D.,
CLEVELAND, O.

After somewhat careful survey of the field of medicine for 1907, I find that there have been no remarkable discoveries, but a perfecting of many principles that render the practice of medicine of more value to diseased sufferers. It is hardly proper, in a paper of this kind, to mention the smaller details, but to take up the main questions that have been discussed and improved upon during this time.

The discussion of the treatment and causes of tuberculosis has received as much attention as any other branch of the subject, and the most striking fact that has been demonstrated is that the want of oxygen is one of the greatest causes of consumption, therefore of the most value in its cure. For this reason they are advocating sleeping out of doors and in tents. This mode of treatment is of some value, but statistics show that it has not rendered the service that it should, especially to the advanced sufferers.

After a careful investigation I have fully determined that suboxygenation is the main cause of consumption or tuberculosis. Without a doubt every individual should have his lung capacity examined, and if not up to the standard the means of developing the lungs should be resorted to at once.

When we think that one person out of every three dies with pneumonia or tuberculosis, and in some instances very suddenly, we should be on the alert to determine the exciting cause, as well as a successful treatment. As it has been determined that the majority of people are not getting the amount of oxygen that belongs to them, it is of the greatest importance to educate them to properly handle the quality and quantity of air necessary to run the natural processes of the human body. The greatest question is the subject of prevention. It is beyond a doubt that consumption can be prevented, so that our greatest good to the people would be educational.

Dr. Wright's opsonic index methods have received considerable attention during this year, and no doubt in time will be of great service. These methods are not yet practical, and will have to be simplified to a great extent to come within easy working bounds. Much has been said and much could be said upon the real value of these methods, but I call attention to them only as a part of the year's progress.

Much has been written during the year upon the subject of causes

*Read before the Northeastern Ohio Eclectic Medical Association, December 12, 1907.

of diseases, as well as upon the subject of diagnosis. That the thinking part of the profession is returning to the natural processes of the human body to seek for the main causes of disease can be readily seen.

We have no fault to find with chemical analysis and the microscope as aids, but they do not tell us how the body changes in order to produce the results that they bring so accurately to our minds. The human body is governed by natural laws, and whenever they are broken abnormal changes must come.

Physiological chemistry, as well as the pathological changes, have been so carefully studied that they render valuable knowledge in determining diseased conditions of the body. That the subject of diagnosis has been placed upon a firmer foundation during the year there is no question, and we are at a point in the history of medicine where we can safely say that diagnosis is not a science of guesswork, but founded upon exact information.

The subjects of bacteriology and pathology have received their share of attention and have given us some new information, but nothing of importance beyond what was known.

What interests us the most is advancement in the successful treatment of disease. Much has been said by a certain portion of the profession in regard to the use of remedies, holding that they were of no practical value, but the more advanced thinkers and careful investigators along the line of materia medica have fully demonstrated that the use of remedies is of special value when properly prescribed, and materially assist nature in overcoming diseased conditions.

The use of physiological methods for the treatment of disease, as well as the use of electricity, has engaged the attention of a great portion of the profession, and no doubt they are of value when properly used. The discussion upon these subjects during the year, as well as their advancements, have been somewhat interesting and instructive. The length of my paper prevents me from entering into a minute discussion of these subjects, but they do not take the place of properly prescribed remedies, but are only assistants, and should be used only by those who thoroughly understand the methods of their use.

I am happy to say that the Eclectic profession stands upon exact and therefore a firm foundation, because their remedies of cure are selected according to the language of the diseased processes, which never fail to give the proper indications when properly observed by the physician.

In many respects harmony in the profession has been on the increase during this year, and if all of the good qualities of the three main branches of the profession could be combined into one greater medical profession, I think all would be willing to admit that we would be in a better condition to convince the people that the practice of medicine was not a failure, but a success.

It is a fact that the laity are considering the profession unable to handle many of their ills, and 'are seeking all sorts of advertised remdies and surgical appliances for relief. The profession is suffering because of our past errors, and in order to make good each one must exert himself to demonstrate that our accurate methods are able to give them satisfaction if the directions are followed.

Materia medica has received its share of careful study during the year, and has furnished its share of success to the general practice of medicine. I cannot finish this paper with any more appropriate sentence than to state that the efforts of the year have placed the materia medica in a better condition, so that our means of relief are much improved.

SEVEN NEW REMEDIES.*

By A. L. SWARTZWELDER, M.D.,
CLEVELAND, O.

At this meeting I desire to call to your attention the leading uses for several of the newer remedies. I believe it behooves us, as a school, to lay hold of the good in all branches of the materia medica, remembering we are but a part of the sum total of the healing art under the banner Eclecticism. Other men are busy learning to better their condition in the realm of medical knowledge, therefore we should better ourselves lest we take second place as healers of the ills of the people.

For the moment let us consider *Aspirin*, one of the grandest remedies we now possess for the relief and cure of acute or chronic rheumatism, with or without cardiac complications. It is administered for the same conditions you would use a salicylate, without their untoward, bad manifestations; and also quicker cure.

A few hours after administering the first dose your patient will perspire freely, feel easier and be in every way improved, and after several doses will notice the disappearance of the agonizing pain.

Aspirin is also indicated in rheumatic eye affections, with the addition of local application of tresotar around the painful eye. In cases of chorea you can expect grand results from aspirin if faithfully followed for a length of time. Aspirin not only relieves this class of cases, but assists in curing cardiac complications due to rheu-

------

* Read before the Northeastern Ohio Eclectic Medical Association, December 12, 1907.

matism, which removes all fear regarding its action on the heart. The average dose is 10 to 15 grs. every three to six hours, as needed to give relief.

Alypin.—Another remedy deserving of attention is alypin, as a substitute for cocaine, not causing the habit or the disagreeable features attending the latter in operations. It is indicated wherever cocaine is desired, such as eye, nose and throat work. Strength of solution about the same as cocaine.

In the use of this drug the anesthesia will be just as great and in addition the avoidance of the toxic symptoms of cocaine and post-operative hemorrhages as well as blanched tissues for the operation. In dental practice it is the remedy to relieve pain par excellence. A trial will convince of its merit.

Agurin.—This is a compound salt containing 60 per cent. of theobromine; it has been used as a diuretic for several years. The cases in which agurin is especially indicated are those of dropsy due to heart disease. If albuminuria is also a complication a marked decrease of albumin will be apparent, as well as a better action of the heart.

Sajodin.—In iodine we have a good remedy for syphilis, yet it has its disadvantage in upsetting the stomach in large doses; therefore we can use in its place the tasteless sajodin, which readily passes through the stomach without nausea or loss of appetite, and its action is just as great. It is indicated in all cases where potassium iodide is required, such as secondary and tertiary syphilis, asthma, arteriosclerosis, chronic bronchitis, gastric and glandular enlargements. Dose is 5 to 15 grs. three or four times a day, in powder, capsule or tablet form.

Protargol.—The next remedy we desire to investigate is better known, being used extensively. I refer to Protargol. It is indicated wherever nitrate of silver can be used, yet without its irritating effects added to all its beneficial qualities. In gonorrhea of the urethra, female genitals, or eyes, it is the remedy that will certainly hasten a cure, as it destroys the germ without irritating the tissues. In cases of ulcers it stimulates granulations and the healing process. The strength of solution needed varies with the locality of the disease, but is similar to nitrate of silver.

Many cases of slow-healing wounds can be hastened by powdered protargol. Cases of cutaneous disease of microbic origin can be cured when allelse fails by ointment of protargol. An investigation and use of this valuable remedy will convince you of its merits.

Veronal.—In the practice of medicine no remedy stands more in need than one which will quiet and give sleep to the nervous, hysterical, sleepless patient, and in veronal we find an admirable remedy.

The rest it gives is refreshing and natural in every way, with none of the untoward effects of morphia. In cases of great pain and sleeplessness veronal can be combined with small doses of morphia, overcoming the bad effects of the latter remedy. Veronal is thought well of in neurasthenia, vomiting of pregnancy by enema, sleeplessness of la grippe, mental over-exertion, whooping-cough, epilepsy, chorea, etc., where a quieter and hypnotic is needed. Dose is 5 to 7½ grs., which acts inside of half an hour if taken in warm milk, and is prolonged four to six hours, or longer, in some cases.

Alphozone.—The last, but not least, of the remedies I desire to consider with you is alphozone, one of the greatest, non-irritating germicides we so far possess. It can be used in every case where peroxide of hydrogen is indicated, but with more certainty of success. It being in 1 gr. tablet form gives it greater convenience in handling and carrying with you in your case.

Alphozone is called for in all septic wounds, ulcers, slow-healing surfaces, chancres and gonorrhea, open boils, carbuncles, bed sores, cancer sores, etc. In typhoid fever, cholera, diarrhea, and dysentery, it is a splendid adjunct to destroy the germs causing the disease by allowing the patient to drink freely of the solution of alphozone. After curettements if septic odors exist, by using alphozone on cotton swabs much further trouble will be avoided. In conjunctivitis, nose and throat work it is valuable as a germicide. The ordinary strength of 2 grs. to 4 oz. is sufficient in ordinary dressings of wounds. As a spray 1-2000, as a dusting powder 1 to 20 parts of alphozone to 100 parts of diluent ointment, 50 to 500 parts of petroleum for skin diseases, eye work 1-3000. A further study of this valuable remedy will prove its great merits.

HEART DISEASES AND THEIR CAUSES.*

BY E. F. DAVIS, M. D.,
CLEVELAND, O.

The subject is so large and great that I hardly know where to begin or where to end. But I will say in the beginning that rheumatism is the cause of 60 per cent. of all heart diseases we have in this climate, and rheumatism is endemic all along the lakes from Buffalo to Duluth, and a fearful disease it is. Hundreds of people are dying from this disease yearly, with quite a number of people with their arms and hands all drawn out of shape, and they, perhaps, would be better off if they were dead than to live in this horrible condition.

* Read before the Northeastern Ohio Eclectic Medical Association, December 12, 1907

Now the question seems proper to me to ask, how to prevent this disease, and prevent heart complications, which are so frequent and fatal. We have a certain atmospheric condition in February and March that exposures of a few months, especially during the nights, will develop malaria or rheumatism. Now, in my opinion, this disease can be prevented in the following manner :

First, have your patients wear very heavy flannel underclothing, heavy woolen socks, and heavy shoes or boots, so as not to get chilled in any way. Keep the body perfectly warm, and the circulation will go on correctly and properly. Keep the stomach and bowels well regulated, and use a hot soda bath every four to six days, and take a little quinine, perhaps, every three to six weeks during these months, which will neutralize any malaria which may be accumulating in the system, and you will be very apt to go through the bad spring months without having rheumatism.

If you have chills, and followed by pains in your feet, swelling in your hands, etc., also pains in your back, with an increase of the pulse and temperature, you have rheumatism on hand. Now the great question is the quickest method of a cure, if you have got the disease. I recommend the following :

Put your patient to bed and give him the following medicine :

Fluid extract of colchicum seed	3 drachms.
Fluid extract of bryonia	½ drachm.
Fluid extract of veratrum viride	12 drops.
Salicylate of sodium	3 drachms.
Fluid extract of phytolacca decandra	40 drops.
Distilled water	6 ounces.

Mix thoroughly, and give a teaspoonful every two hours, until it loosens the bowels, then give in smaller doses as occasion may require.

Also use the following external application if the extremities are much swollen :

Alcohol	6 ounces.
Oil sassafras	2 drachms.
Oil of wintergreen	2 drachms.

Mix and rub the painful parts every four to six hours, and surround the limbs with flannel.

If not materially better in three days, give the patient twenty-four grains of quinine in divided doses in addition to the other remedies, and you will be surprised to see the rapid improvement. If you wish to change your remedy after five or six days, give cimicifuga and gelsemium, which is almost a specific for this disease.

The quicker you cure your patient the less likely you are to have heart complicatioi   This disease usually affects the fibrinous and muscular tissues of the system. There seems to be an increased amount of fibrin in the blood, and in order to prevent the adhesions of morbid growths and accumulations of almost every description from inflammation on the outside and within the heart, it seems to me that if there is anything in Professor Watson's theory that mercury bridles the lymph, it would be necessary in small doses, though I have seen many cases die from these heart complications where mercury had been given to produce slight ptyalism during the treatment. I think if given at all it should be given very early.

A young man of twenty years had three different attacks of inflammatory rheumatism within six years. I cured him, or relieved his symptoms very soon, but after a long time he had chronic rheumatism with serious heart complications, suffered from shortness of breath, palpitation, pain in the region of the heart, etc. Well, my treatment failed to do any material good, and he went to a dignified professor in this city, and several other doctors, but he finally died. His mother requested me to open his chest that she might see the heart, as all of the doctors said he had a very bad heart. Well, Dr. Granger and myself went to make an autopsy, but inasmuch as she sat right down beside the corpse and watched every move that was made, we concluded not to cut any more than we possibly could conveniently get along with. Dr. Granger opened up the thorax, I then called the attention of the mother to the size of the heart, about three times its normal size. The pericardium was attached to the upper part of the heart, and the lower part contained a dirty fluid. The doctor then cut down through the right auricle and tricuspid valve into the right ventricle, and there we discovered an embolism or a fibrinous growth two-eighths of an inch thick and three-eighths of an inch wide. I had him pull it out until we could carefully examine it, and it was about four and one-half inches long, extending from the surface of the right ventricle to the pulmonary arteries. This was undoubtedly started from a fibrinous deposit on the ventricle. The growth was symmetrical, straight in the middle and thickness, and had all of the appearance of a piece of fresh raw beef. The tripsicud valves were also hardened from the deposit.

I will report another case of a girl, eleven years of age. She had heart disease. She was pale, anemic, with a very feeble heart. I treated her for about three months. The treatment was ineffectual. Then they went to a certain professor in the city and he brought her before the class of students, and delivered an eloquent address on aneurism of the aorta, which was the disease she was laboring under. Well, they continued their treatment for about six weeks, and she died. I was invited to the post-mortem, and upon the removal of the heart they found a calcareous deposit within the lower part of the heart about as large as the end of my finger. The heart appeared perfectly normal and healthy otherwise, the liver was healthy, and nothing else to be found like disease. The aorta was all right. Gentlemen, I merely mention this case to show you how easy it is to be mistaken in the diagnosis of the diseases of the heart.

JAMES KILBOURNE.

By HARVEY WICKES FELTER, M.D.,
CINCINNATI.

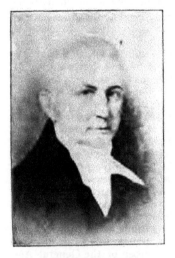

JAMES KILBOURNE.

James Kilbourne, pioneer, was born in New Britain, Conn., October 19, 1770; died April 9, 1850. In early life he suffered the hardships of farm life and apprenticeship. Afterward, through the kindly offices of the son of his employer, who became Bishop Griswold, he acquired a knowledge of classics and mathematics. During the fourth year of his apprenticeship he was given entire charge of the business—that of a clothier. November 18, 1789, he married Lucy Fitch, daughter of John Fitch, of Philadelphia, the inventor and builder of the first steamboat in the world. In 1800 he took orders in the Episcopal Church and formed a project of emigrating to Ohio. In 1801-2 he explored the new country, and arranged for the purchase of land enough for forty families. In the spring of 1802 he commenced his journey, the first three hundred miles by stage to Shippensburg, Pa.; then, carrying a heavy pack, walked over the Alleghanies to Pittsburg, one hundred and fifty miles. From there he continued to travel on foot about one thousand miles. Selecting a location he returned to Connecticut, and formed the "Scioto Company," and closed the contract for sixteen thousand acres of the land selected. In the spring of 1803 he started with a portion of his company for the new home in the "Far West," now Worthington, Ohio. On May 5, 1803, the first tree was felled. The balance of the party arriving, land was cleared and seed sown. Cabins were built, a blacksmith shop, school and church edifice erected, and the town laid out. He again returned to his former home, and brought his own and other families. St. John's Episcopal Church, the first in Ohio, was organized; and Kilbourne served as rector, and organized several other parishes. He became general manager of the colony, and published, in 1811, the first newspaper in Franklin County, the *Western Intelligencer*. In 1804 he retired from the ministry. Upon the organization of the State government he was appointed a civil magistrate and an officer in the militia. In 1805 he explored the south shore of Lake Erie, and selected the site for the city of Sandusky. In 1806 he was appointed a trustee of the Ohio College at Athens; in 1808 one of the commissioners to locate a site for the Miami University. He successively became major, lieutenant-colonel, and colonel of a frontier regiment. He became president of Worthington College, and in 1812 was sent to Congress, and again in 1814. Here he gave the interests of the great West his especial care, and "was the first to propose donation of land to actual settlers in the Northwest Territory, and drew up a bill to that purpose." On the breaking out of war with Great Britain, he was persuaded by friends and urged by the President and his Cabinet to embark in the manufacture of woolen clothing for the army. In the face of previous failure of others under similar circumstances, he invested all his ready cash; and when the war closed, there being no protection on woolens, the company lost heavily. However, he kept in the business until 1820, when the factories at Worthington and Steubenville were closed. At fifty years of age, with a large family, most of them young, he found himself deprived of all his accumulations made throughout a long and busy life. He took up his surveying instruments, and, with his customary energy, pursued the work of a civil engineer for more than twenty years. He surveyed more of Ohio than any three men in the State. This secured him a competence. He was appointed by the governor to select the lands granted by Congress for the Ohio Canal. In 1838-9 he was a member of the General Assembly. On July 4, 1839, he presided at the great convention held at the laying of the corner-stone of the State capital. He declined further public offices, except that of assessor for Franklin County, which he held until 1845. During the six years ending with 1848, he delivered more than one hundred addresses on State and national policy. He was always the friend and champion of Reformed Medicine, and was president of the Board of Trustees of the "Reformed Medical College of Ohio," and was active in securing the charter for its successor, the Eclectic Medical Institute of Cincinnati. Colonel Kilbourne's first wife died soon after going to Ohio. In 1808 he married Cynthia Goodale, the first female white child to set foot on Ohio soil. His son, Dr. James Kilbourne, Jr., was a teacher in the "Reformed Medical School of Cincinnati." Colonel Kilbourne "lived to see the forest where he cut the first tree grow into a flourishing city." We are indebted to his grandson, James Kilbourne, of Columbus, the recent (1901) Democratic gubernatorial candidate, for items and portrait of Colonel Kilbourne.

Texas Eclectic Medical Association.

PROCEEDINGS OF THE TWENTY-FOURTH ANNUAL MEETING.

L. S. DOWNS, M.D., EDITOR.

The Texas Eclectic Medical Association met October 23, 1907, at the Commercial Club Rooms, Dallas, Texas, in the twenty-fourth annual session. There were between seventy-five and one hundred from different parts of the State.

The meeting was called to order at 10 o'clock by President J. A. Lanius, of Bonham. A welcome address was delivered by City Attorney James J. Collins, acting for Mayor Hay, and the response was made by Dr. H. H. Blankmeyer, of Honey Grove, which was well received, and was printed in full in the Dallas *Daily News*. Annual reports of the treasurer and secretary were submitted.

TREASURER'S REPORT.

"In submitting to you this, my tenth successive annual report, I want to, first, assure you that I have exerted every effort to keep intact our full membership by urging every member to pay his or her dues. As you all know, two years in arrears for dues, surrenders or lapses the membership of a member, and when it is realized that a lapsed member adds nothing to our numerical strength, it becomes all the more important that each member understand, and safeguard the interests of our chosen school of medicine in the future by keeping his or her membership in force.

"This question of numerical, as well as relative strength, with our school in the future, in this great State, is a matter we should begin now to give the closest attention. Authoritative data must be collected and compiled for ready reference. Ready preparation is the imperative demand of the hour when it is realized that we occupy a position I deem most critical—are engaged in *the* battle that will decide our future existence, and our success in this contest depends upon the loyalty of our membership.

"I am pleased to report that three delinquent members were reinstated during the year.

"For your information I submit the following statement of the Association's finances :

RECEIPTS.

At the close of the last meeting, October 9 and
  10, 1906, there was on hand . . . . $ 51.00
Collected during the year up to October 19, 1907 . 348.24

Total in treasury $399.24

DISBURSEMENTS.

Since last meeting up to October 10, 1907 . . $287.22

Present balance $112.02

"Of the amount expended, $235.45 was used by your Legislative Committee, an itemized account of which is shown in my books which the Auditing Committee will inspect, and report to you. During the contest that was waged during the last Legislature, it is gratifying to me that our membership was not called upon to contribute to a fund to pay the expenses of its Legislative Committee, having ample funds on hand to meet every legitimate need, and at one time four committeemen were sent to Austin, and as many as two at a time, several times.

Respectfully submitted,

MARQUIS E. DANIEL, Treasurer."

The report showed the Association to be in a healthy financial condition, while the Secretary's report declared there is a membership of nearly 150. Regular committees were named on Press, Credentials, Auditing, Necrological, Resolutions and Arrangements. A special committee to judge papers and award prizes offered by publishers of various medical books was named as follows: Prof. J. K. Scudder, Drs. C. E. Frazier and E. H. Cowan.

The program under the sections designated was taken up (that of Materia Medica and Therapeutics being postponed because of the absence of the chairman); Section of Practice of Medicine, Chairman C. H. McQuistian, Valley View; Section on Obstetrics, Chairman R. W. Fowler, Pottsville; Section on Gynecology, Chairman C. E. Frazier, Weatherford. One of the distinguished visitors at the meet. ing was Prof. J. K. Scudder, M.D., of Cincinnati, Ohio.

October 24, 9 A. M., business was resumed. Resolution by Dr. M. E. Daniel, that the Association authorize its Treasurer to admit all its delinquent members now and during the coming year on the payment of $5. Carried.

Resolution by Dr. M. E. Daniel, that Dr. S. M. Carlton, of Thornton, Texas—an ex-president, and who has attained the ripe age of seventy-seven years—be exempt from further payment of dues. Carried.

SUPPLEMENTAL TREASURER'S REPORT.

Collections, dues and initiations during session . $183.00
Expenditures' approved 70.05

Net gain in receipts $112.95
Total now in treasury . .   —$224.97

Section work was then resumed as follows: Materia Medica and Therapeutics, Chairman M. A. Cooper, Leakey; Diseases of the

Nervous System, Chairman S. D. Donaho, Sherman; Eye, Ear, Nose and Throat, Chairman J. M. Watkins, Luling; Surgery, Chairman W. E. Bridge, Gober; Diseases of the Skin, Chairman Charles Dowdell, Ft. Worth; Business Side of Practice, Chairman George A. Taylor, Bettie; Miscellaneous, Chairman A. Helbing, Bonham.

The officers elected are as follows:

G. W. Johnson, San Antonio, President; C. D. Hudson, Waco, First Vice-President; C. E. Frazier, Weatherford, Second Vice-President; M. E. Daniel, Honey Grove, Treasurer; L. S. Downs, Galveston, Secretary; W. R. Fowler, Pottsville, Corresponding Secretary; J. M. Watkins, Luling, and C. E. Frazier, Weatherford, representatives to meeting of National Association.

Upon motion of Dr. Blankmeyer the Texas Association approved the plan to affiliate with the National Association, making State members also members of the National with a per capita basis of $2 per year.

Resolutions were adopted thanking the Commercial Club, the *News*, and the various speakers for courtesies extended, and the report of the Credentials Committee, recommending the names of fifteen new members, was adopted. The Auditing Committee reported all books and accounts in good condition. Prof. John K. Scudder, of Cincinnati, Ohio, was elected an honorary member. He made a very strong address, lauding the conditions of the Association in Texas.

Dr. M. E. Daniel, President of the Texas Examining Board, was present and explained how to verify under the new law. Secretary Downs was voted his expenses to the meeting. The president delivered his annual address, and the newly-elected President, Dr. Johnson, took charge of the meeting, naming the following committees for the coming year:

Press—P. A. Spain, Paris; H. H. Blankmeyer, Honey Grove; Jason Tyson, Santa Anna.

Credentials—D. W. Holmes, Bellevue; W. R. Fowler, Pottsville; J. P. Rice, Fredericksburg.

Auditing—Charles Dowdell, Fort Worth; S. F. Donaho, Sherman; J. N. White, Queen City.

Necrology—C. H. McQuistian, Valley View; H. W. Gates, Waco, B. B. Beakley, Hylton.

Resolutions—M. E. Daniel, Honey Grove; Gus Helbing, Fort Worth; J. A. Lanius, Bonham.

Arrangements—J. H. Mitchell, Dallas; L S. Downs, Galveston; O. T. Mitchell, Renner.

Legislative—C. E. Frazier. Weatherford; J. M. Watkins, Luling; C. D. Hudson, Waco.

Prizes were awarded as follows: For the best paper before the

Association, Dr. H. H. Blankmeyer, of Honey Grove; for the best organized section, Dr. McQuistian, of Valley View; second best section, Dr. Charles Dowdell, of Fort Worth; best paper on eye, ear, nose and throat, Dr. J. M. Watkins, Luling; on practice of medicine, R. E. Sawyer, Bokchito, I. T.; on gynecology, G. W. Moore, Gent; surgery, Dr. E. H. Cowan, Crowell; on obstetrics, Dr. W. R. Fowler, Pottsville; materia medica, C. M. Williams, Rosebud; on skin and anatomy, Dr. Jason Tyson, Santa Anna; business side of life, Dr. S. D. Donaho, Sherman; miscellaneous, P. A. Spain, Paris.

The secretary was instructed to offer the papers to the ECLECTIC MEDICAL JOURNAL for publication.

After a very interesting and prosperous session, the Association adjourned to meet in Dallas, October, 1908.

G. W. JOHNSON, M.D., President.

L. S. DOWNS, M.D., Secretary.

PRESIDENT'S ADDRESS.

By JOHN A. LANIUS, M.D.,
BONHAM, TEXAS.

Having been honored with the presidency of this association at your last meeting, I realized at once the great responsibility that I had accepted. My mind at once reflected to the lamented Scudder, Goss, Howe and others, who have passed into the great beyond. I was made to say: Wonder if they are not watching me to see how well I will carry out their plans and how well I will preach the great doctrine they had founded years before many of us were born.

Friends, I am proud to say that not only during this year, but for the past ten years, your servant has ever expounded the greatest medical doctrine known to man—Eclecticism. Yes, it sounds so sweet to me, it does away with calomel and cinchona tea.

To be president of an association that such men as the above, and Lloyd, Durham, Webster and others have fought so long for—yea, I repeat, is an honor that cannot be excelled though you were President of this great republic.

As to how well I have filled this great honor and trust that you have entrusted to me I leave you to judge. During the year I have written for the association some seven hundred letters, gotten up four hundred circular letters, three hundred programs, two hundred postals. It has seldom been that I wrote a letter without mentioning this meeting. To the officers and others who have co-operated with me, I now wish to express my thanks, for had it had not been for your co-operation this meeting would have been a complete failure, I feel we can safely say that at least four thousand letters have been written by the Eclectics of the State wherein there was mention made of this meeting. The results of such an effort we shall see before we close.

On entering my new duties I heard the thunder roar, I saw the great illuminating flashes of lightning, which extended from Red River to the gulf and from Arkansas to Mexico. I realized at once that one of the greatest cyclones that had been for years was on us, with no cellars for escape. Johnson, of San Antonio, gave the signal; Daniel and myself responded. The qusstion presented itself, where are all of our men? A further investigation revealed that they were all asleep. The terrific thunder continued, and finally Blankmyer, Frazier and Watkins awoke and arrived on the scene in time to assist in bridging over momentarily the greatest fight ·Eclecticism has ever had in this State, but to our sorrow, the Governor, in his fury, saw fit to burn the bridge we had helped to build. I was made to ask how long we had slept. An angel of the "Regs." answered by saying that since you won the victory in 1901. I at once realized that we had slept while the enemy had worked, and a miserable state of affairs we had slept into. The only remedy that I can offer, friends, is for every true believer in Eclecticism to wake up at once and show your colors. I hear one say that I do not believe in such; it will injure you financially; I have got to look out for No. 1. To such I appeal, brother, be what you are; if you are a believer in Eclecticism and her principles, for Heaven's sake do not sacrifice principle for dollars and cents. Eclecticism is not dead in Texas—yea, never. When all history has passed into oblivion and time shall be no more, Eclecticism shall shine as the only true way of combating the different ills of mankind. A brighter day is before her and ·she shall soon take her place as the the leader of practical medicine. The medical world is turning to the action of drugs, and our materia medica is full of rich remedies that have been thoroughly tried and proven to be curative when rightfully applied. An Allopath was telling me not long since that we had them skinned a country block when it came to materia medica and therapeutics. We, as Eclectics, are both timid and envious. Why should I envy my brother? Push him higher up the ladder if he is worthy. But if he is after self-honor alone when the honor could be made to glorify Eclecticism, such a one should be sent to the "Regs." at once for he is an honor to them working under the wings of Eclecticism. Brother, be what you are and let the world know it.

Our cause should be advertised more in the next two years than it has in the last ten. Why do I say this? To illustrate, you accumulate one thousand dollars and from some misfortune you lose it. You will find that it is a greater burden to accumulate the second thousand than it was the first. We worked, fought and almost bled to secure our own board of examiners. The misfortune came by our sleeping on our rights, and we lost. By comparison you can see that we must be up and doing. We should never lose an opportunity to let the world know what we are. If you run a card in the local paper say what you are; also in your stationery, cards and such, and for heaven's sake when you allow your name to be put in a medical directory do not allow it to be followed by a blank or simply an "R.," but put "Ecl." after it. I feel I can safely say you cannot take Polk's Medical Directory, 1906 edition, and find one-third of the Eclectics, not only in Texas, but the United States. Brother Eclectic, why is this? Are you ashamed to own your father? Or is this simply neglect?

Knowing that there are no others our superior, I suggest that you remove all timidity and have self-confidence, and whenever an opporaunity presents itself apply for places of trust. Why should we not? Are not we each of us taxpayers, and should we not reap some of the honors as well as the "Regs."? I hear one say that I applied for so-and-so at one time and failed getting it. It is useless to ask for such with the "Regs." in the majority. To such I would ask if he did not have half a dozen "Regs." for company who had suffered defeat also, and further I would state, should you suffer defeat I believe Eclecticism in your community has been glorified by your having applied, and you would not know whether you had lost or gained if you had not applied. We are entitled to and should have a chair in the State institution at Galveston. I recommend that we ask for a chair on materia medica and therapeutics. Methinks I hear one say that would benefit one of our men there. It is so; it would not only benefit one Eclectic in Galveston, but it would benefit our cause and every Eclectic in this State. As to who would secure an appointment to this place if we were successful, you know not but that you would be the lucky man. Away with such "bosh!" Let's pull together for the place and get it, and trust to the good Lord that it will be filled with a good man. We should select our men for public offices and let them know that we are working in their behalf. I would further suggest that we make an effort to establish a medical college and hospital in this State. Yearly young men are going to Allopath schools for convenience. There means a limit. I feel an Eclectic college could be put on a paying basis in this State at once. I further suggest until we have a college of our own that we urge every young man or woman with good literary qualifications, who contemplates attending a medical college to investigate Eclecticism and to attend one of her institutions. Further, I feel each member of the State Association should be a member of the national organization, and to accomplish this I feel that we should ask the National to accept those who are members of a State organization on the payment of a two-dollar fee. To make myself more plain, I feel our constitution and by-laws should be so changed that when one joins a State organization it makes him a member of the national body. I reeommend that the Texas delegation at Kansas City, next June, make an effort to have such passed.

Again thanking all who have co-operated with me, and assuring the one who will follow me my co-operation and all the assistance that I can give him as a true Eclectic, I will refrain from further addressing you.

May this meeting be one of the greatest ever held by this association, and may each member find his stay here exceedingly pleasant and profitable.

DENGUE—BREAKBONE FEVER—DANDY FEVER— THREE-DAY FEVER—ETC.

By J. M. WATKINS, M.D., LULING, TEXAS

The fancy and various names for this disease go, in a measure, to describe the character of the disease. The intense pain characterizes the name "breakbone," while the peculiar gait, stiffness of joints, etc., of the patient give it the name "dandy."

Definition.—This is an acute specific infectious disease, occurs epidemically, confined chiefly to the tropical and subtropical climates, and is characterized by two separate and distinct paroxysms of fever, with usually two days of intermission, there being in most cases an eruption of the body or a roseola rash.

History.—The first accurate description of this disease was given by Brylon, which occurred in Java in 1779, in which he termed it articular fever. In 1780 the first known of it in America was in Philadelphia, and was described by Benjamin Rush. In the early part of the nineteenth century it appeared as an epidemic in various parts of the world—Spain, Brazil, India and West Indies. In the latter part of the nineteenth century it appeared in Turkey, Greece and the United States, and has been seen as far north as Philadelphia, New York and Boston. The more recent epidemic was in 1885, when Texas was visited by an epidemic in various places, and in 1897 Texas was again visited by another epidemic along the coast, as well as Louisiana, and at the present time it is prevailing in many places in Texas.

This disease is no respecter of persons; neither age, sex, race nor position has any influence in warding off the disease, the exception being, if any, the negro or Mexican, they not being by any means immune from the disease. The disease seems to be milder with these two races than the white, and my observation has been that blondes suffer more than brunettes. Why this should be the case I don't know. My observation has led me to this conclusion.

Etiology.—The nature of this infection is not yet known. Dr. Graham has conducted experiments to ascertain the cause of the infection, and as a result of his experiments he believes that the disease is propagated by the mosquito (the Culix Fastigans) carrying the parasite from the sick to the well. Dr. McLaughlin, in his experiments, isolated a micrococcus which he believes to be responsible for the infection.

Symptoms.—There is an incubative period from two to four days, with no premonitory or prodrome symptoms whatever. The disease is ushered in by a chill; this may or may not be marked, with rise in temperature, with at first extreme frontal headache, then extending to base of brain, temperature running 103°–104°, and even 105°, pulse very rapid. There is an intense aching of back and legs, with darting pain through elbows and knees. There is nausea and frequently vomiting; the vomiting is very intense; usually neither food nor water can be retained. In the cases in which the pain in the hypogastric region is very marked the nausea and vomiting is much worse.

There is a general muscular soreness and stiffness of the joints; the lymphatics are painful and swollen, and especially the glands of the neck, and sometimes even the tonsils are involved.

The first or primary fever lasts from three to five days. About the third day the rash makes its appearance, though not in all cases, which lasts until the intermission; the intermission is usually about two days, when the second fever returns with equally as violent a chain of symptoms as in the primary stage, which will last usually about two days, and is attended with the same rash as the primary stage. In cases in which the rash does not appear in the primary stage of the fever, it is almost certain to appear in the secondary fever, though the duration of this fever is from seven to ten days. Convalescence is very slow, their physical condition being very much impaired.

The total disgust for food is very marked in this disease. With the high temperature there is very little desire for water; in fact, water is about as repulsive to their stomachs as food—except lemonade. With some the bleeding of the nose is a very marked symptom, chiefly among children. Diarrhea is quite frequent, especially during the secondary fever.

The tongue is usually coated with a dirty, nasty white coating.

Diagnosis.—In an epidemic as we have just passed through there is but little difficulty in making a diagnosis. The suddenness of the attack, the aching of bones, soreness of muscles and stiffness of the joints, with the peculiar excruciating frontal headache extending to the base of the brain, and the soreness of the eyeballs, make a diagnosis very easy.

Prognosis.—The prognosis is usually good; very few die with this disease.

Treatment.—Having just passed through an epidemic of this disease, in which fully 98 per cent. of the population of our town has been affected, I have endeavored to find some remedy or remedies that would relieve the sufferer, shorten the attack and modify the conditions generally. And in giving my treatment I will confine it chiefly to the drugs with which I am most successful. The first step in the treatment is a warm bath (100°), the body being rubbed thoroughly (while in bath) with sodii bicarb., followed with a thorough rubbing with a Turkish bath-towel; then give four or five grains of acetanilid comp. or antikamnia. This in a majority of cases will reduce the temperature to 100° or 99°, relieving the excruciating headache, puts the patient to perspiring, and they feel reasonably comfortable. Then the patient gets the following to cleanse out the bowels and to flush out the kidneys:

Potass. nitrate	2 drachms.
Salts Rochelle	2 ounces.
Aqua	q.s.
Sol. sodii. phosph. q.s . . , . .	6 ounces.

M. S. Tablespoonful in half-glass of hot water every two hours until the desired results have been produced. Then a powder which contains:

Codeine sulph. . ·	3 grains.
Antikamnia	2 scruples.

M. Ft. charts No. 10. Sig: One powder every two or three hours, as needed to reduce pain and keep the temperature reduced.

These powders will keep the skin in a good active condition and will be sufficient to control the temperature. If these powders do not relieve the excruciating headache (but they nearly always do), then I give a few ten-grain doses of sodium salicylate every three hours. At the expiration of the primary fever quinine is given in this manner: Start at one o'clock at night and give four or five grains of quinine bisulphate every two hours until nine o'clock A.M.. Repeat the same dose the next night in like manner. With this treatment I have been very successful, and after having tried many other remedies. This treatment is given for adults and not for children. The children would get: Aconite, ipecac, gelsemium, jaborandi, elix. pep. (or simp.) aqua, q.s. M. Sig.: Teaspoonful every two hours for fever.

This prescription is varied, of course, to suit the individual case. Some would get cimicifuga, bryonia ; but bryonia is not tolerated by the stomach in dengue; neither is gelsemium. Phytolacca acts very nicely in some cases. The nausea and vomiting in these cases are not easily controlled, being very persistent at times. I find that the codeine usually relieves the stomach disorders given with hot water. Allow no ice nor ice drinks during the nausea and vomiting stage, but hot water freely.

I have given quinine in the primary stage, but only to aggravate the condition. Have never seen any good results derived from its use until the period of intermission. Gelsemium seems to be specifically indicated, but it seems to aggravate the stomach disorder which so frequently accompanies this disease. The baths in this fever are very essential, and all my patients get two baths per day, one about noon and the second about six P.M.

MEASLES.

BY R. E. SAWYER, M.D.,
BOKCHITO, OKLA.

In speaking to you on the disease, measles, I hope you will not expect me to take up, separately, all of the twenty-nine divisions into which this disease has been separated ; for, in so doing, I fear much valuable time would be lost and little gained by such a minute treatment of the subject. Therefore, in treating this subject we will only speak of it in the common acceptation as measles, discarding all synonyms and minute parts where unnecessary divisions have been made.

Measles is an acute, contagious and infectious disease, attacking most frequently the young, but no age is exempt. It is characterized by a coryza, conjunctivitis, sore throat, difficult deglutition more or less hoarseness and general catarrhal symptoms, with a characteristic papular eruption.

The history of this disease is both interesting and instructive. Until about the year A. D. 900, this, with other eruptive diseases, were all classified under one great head. About this time Rhazes, an Arabic physician of recognized authority, gave quite an extended description of smallpox and measles in the same paper. During the next few hundred years much was talked of eruptive fevers and their classification, but not until the close of the seventeenth century, or about the year 1670, had any advancement been made, except in a general way, and measles, with scarlatina, were yet considered one and the same thing.

As to the etiology of this disease, we know nothing more than we know the dwelling-place of the stars. As far back as we have any history we read of these eruptive fevers, but usually spoken of without any distinction, one from the other.

The habitat of measles is found in almost every land. It made its first appearance in America soon after the arrival of the first colonists and liked the climate so well that it has been with us ever since that period. It found its way to the great Northwest in 1829, and to the Pacific Coast about the breaking out of the Texas Revolution.

In classifying this disease two divisions will be made—the one of a catarrhal, and the other of an eruptive stage. The early symptoms of the catarrhal stage are those of a cold, with a dry, irritating cough; the mucous membranes of the nose, throat and bronchial tubes are early affected. More or less photophobia is present, with eyelids swollen and red, later taking on a gummy exudate, almost sticking the lids. Snuffing and sneezing, with a thin watery discharge from the nose, is always present. In from twenty-four to forty-eight hours this discharge becomes muco-purulent, and cold air sniffed through the nostrils causes a painful burning sensation. Loss of appetite, tongue coated with thin whitish fur, nausea, vomiting and general gastric disturbances, followed with a diarrhea, which shows clearly the extension of the catarrhal symptoms. Sibilant and sonorous rales are usually present, the patient complaining of severe headache, shivers with chilly sensations playing up and down the spine. The fever ranges from 101° to 105°, being higher in the afternoon and continuing high until the fourth day, when the eruptive stage begins.

This stage begins with Koplik's spots, which may be seen on the hard palate twenty-four, and sometimes forty-eight hours before the eruption appears on the face, which is first seen on the neck, temples and at the edge of the hair, extending to the face, forehead, body, and last to the lower extremities. In eight or nine days the rash is all gone, leaving a bluish mottled appearance all over the body,

Treatment.—The treatment of measles, as a rule, is very simple, many cases passing through successfully without any treatment except a few hot teas and baths. As the disease makes its appearance the patient should be kept in the house and well protected from the damp air and cold winds. If the fever is high and the patient is nervous, have him put to bed and given spec. jaborandi, asclepias and gelsemium, of each, one drachm; aq. dist. q. s. ounces four; teaspoonful every hour until the fever begins to cool. If the arotids care full and throbbing, then add spec. veratrum, drops 15 to 20, to the above mixture and continue as above directed. If the patient continues nervous, tossing from one side of the bed to the other, every little noise increasing the irritation, and with fever high, then order hot sponge baths to be given, with the water at a temperature of 100°, while internally give spec. aconite drops 15, nepeta drachms two, aqua dist. q. s. to make four ounces. A teaspoonful is given every hour until free perspiration is produced. If the patient is very young, frail and anemic, cocoa-butter applied with a vigorous massaging of the entire body will be found beneficial ; this, of course, should follow the hot sponge-bath.

For the bronchial complications you will find the silk jacket, carefully oiled and dusted with compound emetic powder, to give splendid results. Where the bowels are distended, with nausea and vomitng present, the old peach-leaf poultice applied to the epigastrium and extending over the entire abdomen will give good results.

This paper, though not intended to be a complete treatise of the disease, briefly outlines an uncomplicated case, giving one line or mode of treatment.

STIMULANTS AND THEIR INDICATIONS.

By D. L. HESS, M.D.,
MERETA, TEX.

A medicine which possesses the property of being capable of producing a quickly diffused and transient increase of vital energy and strength of action in the heart and arterial system, and of exciting and increasing the organic action of any or all of the different parts of the animal system, is termed a stimulant.

Stimulants act by calling out the nerve force which is apparently latent, but not increase that force any; in fact, the remote effect is to cause exhaustion, especially if their use is persisted in, and pushed to the point of over-stimulation.

Some stimulants are diffusible, and their action is transient, such as ammonia, ether, amyl nitrite and alcohol; while others are more lasting in their effects, as strychnine, capsicum and opium in small doses.

Stimulants may be divided into two principal classes, to-wit, cerebro-spinal and vascular, which may be further subdivided into hepatic, cardiac pulmonary, nervous, renal, uterine, lymphatic, etc.

Cerebro-spinal stimulants are those that, when given in medicinal doses, exalt the functions of the brain and cord, invigorate the action of the heart, and promote nutrition, secretion, and excretion. These remedies are useful in atonic dyspepsia, atony of the bowels and bladder, cardiac weakness, emphysema, neuralgia, paralysis, phthisis, and in the latter stages of long-continued fevers and in wasting diseases.

Among the principal members of the group are nux vomica, strychnine and belladona.

Vascular stimulants are those that strengthen the action of the heart and blood-vessels; they are, therefore, advantageously employed in weakened conditions of the central organ of circulation, in transudation due to blood stasis, in hemorrhages, in dropsies which are caused by an atonic condition of the blood-vessels. Among the principal members of this group are alcohol, preparations of ammonia, digitalis, ergot, nitroglycerine and apocynum cannabinum.

Stimulants call out the vital forces, and, as it were, whip them into more vigorous action, and in many cases of collapse will assist to carry the patient safely over the critical period.

If large doses of stimulants are given, the stimulating effect will be followed by a condition of relaxation, and, if the stimulant is pushed too far, to a state of exhaustion.

Stimulants will act secondarily as diaphoretics, diuretics, expectorants and cathartics, through their secondary relaxing effects.

The action of a stimulant is on the nerve structures, and this accounts for the brief duration of the effects in the case of certain drugs that are classed as stimulants.

In the latter stages of pneumonia you will find stimulants of especial benefit, and almost indispensable, especially in the severe cases; many times the patient would succumb to the disease if not for the timely employment of stimulants, and here you will usually find that strychnine or alcohol are the best adapted to the occasion.

In bronchial affections you will find an appropriate place for an alcoholic stimulant; by its stimulating influence on the mucous membrane of the bronchial tubes it causes the expectoration to be thinner and to cough up; at the same time, by its stimulating effects on the nervous system, it increases the expulsive power of the lungs.

In the latter stages of all continued fevers you will find that the administration of a stimulant will be of great advantage to your patient; it will call out the latent nerve force, and by so doing will tide your patient over a critical period in which he might have succumbed to the disease if the stimulant had not been administered. You will find this the case more so in typhoid fevers and typhoid conditions than in any other condition that you might meet up with.

During the administration of an anesthetic the use of a stimulant is a great aid towards preventing collapse, and if you will administer a hypodermic of strychnine before you commence the anesthetic your patient will bear the anesthetic much better and will come out from under the anesthetic in a much better condition than he would have done without the administration of the stimulant; and in the case of threatened heart failure during the administration of an anesthetic a little amyl nitrite to the nostrils for the immediate effect, and a hypodermic of strychnine for the more lasting effect, is a very valuable procedure, and will frequently be the means of preventing an untimely death.

In all toxic diseases, such as diphtheria, the use of alcohol should be begun as soon as depressing symptoms make their appearance, and continued in doses regulated by the degree of prostration.

In acute gastro-intestinal diseases the depletion is often so great, and there is so little absorption of food, that patients must in certain cases be sustained by alcohol or strychnine for several days, until the system is in a condition to assimilate the nourishment that is taken, when the natural forces of the body will be able to take care of the patient.

Indications.—If you have a weak pulse, which is rapid; weak heart action, labored breathing, more or less prostration, with a moist skin, system in a general state of relaxation, or patient is weak and exhausted, a stimulant is indicated, and should be given regardless of what you might see fit to name the disease. When the patient is in a condition of collapse a stimulant is always indicated, and should be faithfully administered; when the patient has been chilled and the internal organs are in a state of congestion, the administration of a stimulant will give your patient relief.

However, on the other hand, be exceedingly careful not to over-stimulate the patient, for the reaction resulting from the over-stimulation would leave the patient in a worse condition than he was before using the stimulant.

With a strong and bounding full pulse, high temperature, flushed face, dry skin, scanty secretions, and patient restless, a stimulant is contra-indicated, and should never be given when these conditions are present.

COUP-DE-SOLEIL.

By S. D. DONAHO, M.D.,
SHERMAN, TEXAS.

Synonym.—Sun-stroke, heat-stroke or asphyxia.

Definition.—Thomas says a stroke of the sun. Generally, any affection produced by a scorching sun.

The term sun-stroke is applied to a condition of nervous prostration caused by excessive heat.

We have the same from exposure to heat, hence the term heat-stroke.

Sun-stroke is so common in the United States during the summer months we would expect to find it described in all works on practice, but, strange to say, we see but little written on the subject save by the newspaper men. There is a great deal said in the papers from the North and East during the heat of summer. But the medical journals don't have much to say, if anything. I don't see them all, and those I read don't say much on the subject.

Of the eight, volumes of the "Annual of Eclectic Medicine and Surgery," only one volume says anything on the subject, and that only a short paragraph.

The literature of the disease is confined almost exclusively to the daily papers, which report the attacks of the disease and the deaths from it as they would the killing of a man in some way.

Etiology.—The predisposing causes of the disease are such as enfeeble the frame and oppress the nervous system ; thus we find it to occur most frequently after attacks of sickness.

When one is not at himself the use of whisky and beer, etc., exposure to excessive heat, such as the rays of the sun, the temperature being from 95° to 105° in the shade. Furnaces and laundry-boilers are the direct causes.

Pathology.—Owing to the excessive heat of the body, putrefactive changes occur very early. If a post-mortem is held it should be done at once, as the high range of temperature will cause destruction of the tissues. The left heart is found to be contracted and the right engorged. The venous trunks filled with dark semi-fluid blood. There is also venous engorgement of the brain.

Professor Scudder said : "It is my opinion that the action of heat on the brain is productive of cerebral syncope, or partial paralysis of the nervous system, and that this, by enfeebling the action of the heart and lungs, caused the engorgement of the latter and difficult respiration."

Symptoms.—The first are a feeling of weight or tension in the head, with considerable heat at the surface, and dizziness. If severe, the patient will soon lose control of his limbs and falls to the ground unconscious.

In the more severe cases the patient suddenly falls unconscious while walking along the street, or attending to his business, and though there may be brief returns of consciousness, it is not complete for several hours, or the patient may die in a short time after the attack. If he don't he is a long time getting well. Sometimes he will complain for years, when he gets a little too warm. There is in some involuntary discharges of urine and feces ; in others, nausea and vomiting.

Diagnosis.—There is but little trouble in making a diagnosis. The exposure to heat or the rays of the sun will help us in making a correct diagnosis. One might make a mistake in the case of apoplexy, but if he will notice the difference in the two cases he need not make a mistake.

Prognosis.—The prognosis is favorable in mild cases. But in severe cases, where the pulse is from 130 to 150, with a temperature of 110° to 115°, there is not much chance of recovery unless seen early and the case yields to treatment at once.

Treatment.—Preventative should be used, especially with those who use beer and strong drinks—such as wet cloths, sponges or green leaves worn in the hat. If dizziness is felt and perspiration scanty or absent, he had better go to the shade. If the attack is mild we may need only stimulants. Belladonna, nux vomica, cactus, carbonate of ammonia, nitrate of glycerine and such remedies as are indicated. Aconite, rhus tox, gelsemium, ipecac and an infusion of the peach leaf or the young twigs of anything indicated. Low muttering delirium I would use kali phos., five grains of the 2x trituration in four ounces of water. Dose, a teaspoonful every two hours in alternation with other indicated remedies.

Professor Tascher, of Chicago, says: ''The most efficient means in the treatment of a case of sun-stroke is to put the patient in a cold bath, and if necessary add ice to the water to abstract the bodily heat more rapidly. I have frequently seen cases that were unconscious, with muscular twitching all over the body, weak, thready pulse and a temperature ranging from 108° to 111°. Necessarily the treatment must be begun before the excessively high temperature has injured the nervous system to such an extent that disorganization has set in.''

Professor Thomas, of Cincinnati, says: ''In severe cases and where the temperature is very high, strip the patient of all clothing and sponge him with hot water ; at the same time have two or more assistants fan him vigorously. Any one who has not pursued this course will be surprised how rapidly the temperature will be reduced. The sponging with hot water determines the heat to the surface and the fan secures evaporation.''

Chronic Cases—Silica, dose two to three grains of the third trituration, three or four times a day. It prolongs the intermissions between the attacks, and in incurable cases it may lessen the frequency of the attacks by half or more. Scutellaria, in the specific medicine, dose from one to twenty drops.

(*To be continued.*)

Seton Hospital Reports.

By L. E. Russell, M.D., Surgeon.

Case 119.—Man, twenty-five years of age, referred to the Seton Hospital clinic on account of a deformity of the left knee-joint—a partial luxation of the condyles of the femur outwardly.

The general appearance of the patient would hardly suggest a tubercular condition, yet when we come to examine the left leg there are several tubercular ulcers extending from the foot up to the knee; evidence of necrosis along full length of the femur, with the greatest lesion centering at the knee-joint.

This patient has been prepared for any operation upon the leg or knee that we may decide upon while he is under the influence of the anesthetic. I think, inasmuch as the limb has been of absolutely no service for two or three years, and the evidence of active tubercular destruction within the knee-joint, that there is but one problem in the question of surgical interference—that is to at once remove the leg by amputation sufficiently above the knee-joint to allow the manu- facture of an artificial leg to have room to make a useful artificial joint. Our method of amputation in this case will be the "double flap," making the anterior equal in length with the posterior, because the skin tissue is diseased at this point, and we must modify the length of the posterior flap.

The limb can be amputated readily and safely without the use of a tourniquet, or rubber constrictor, if it is held high above the body for a few moments to make it anemic. The anterior flap is cut through the skin and fascia of the heavy muscles, turned backward to about the point which we select for the severance of the bone.

The bone, after the soft parts of the anterior surface are removed, is carefully severed with the saw, and as it comes apart the distal end is pulled forward for the purpose of freeing and taking it out of the field from which we make the posterior flap. Just at this time we form the posterior flap, using the bistoury, cutting from the upper line or angle of the anterior incision downward, backward and across the posterior part of the limb, reflecting the posterior skin flap equal in height to the anterior. We extend the incision well down into the muscles, but not deep enough to sever any important blood-vessels, which are approached by a transverse incision corresponding to the line of the severed bone.

Our hemostats are ready; we cut down onto the blood-vessels, they are immediately grasped by the hemostat, and at the conclusion of the amputation the femoral artery is grasped by hemostats, separated from its surrounding tissue, and carefully ligated with Tait's silk, the end of the ligature cut within a half-inch of the knot, leaving the ligature to be encysted or absorbed, instead of the older method of having the ligature protrude through the end of the flap, and weeks afterwards withdrawn.

Quite often I re-saw, or shorten the femur, say an inch shorter than its first severance, but before doing so push back the periosteum, so at the completion of the amputation the periosteum can be pulled forward and sutured over the end of the bone. I deem this of considerable importance, especially in these cases of a tubercular condition, as it is desirable to limit the time of trauma of the osseous tissue to the shortest possible period. I also suture through the fascia of the severed muscle with catgut, pushing the cut end of the muscles upward, using the continuous suture, approximate and fix the muscles so that they may be immobolized as much as possible, at the same time obliterating space or cavity.

The heavy skin, fat and fascia ends of the flaps are immobilized and their edges coaptated by the over-and-over-suture of silkworm-gut, which acts as a splint, holding the outer tunic in close apposition, pushing outward the inner, holding all in line until union takes place, which is, as a rule, by first intention, without pus, complete within ten days.

The ligatures that we applied are only to the active bleeders, possibly one or two points beside the femoral artery.

Our patients thus far have made a very speedy recovery, without the use of any antiseptic, except the gauze bandages and dressings moistened in alcohol.

I want to say to you that I witnessed an amputation by Professor Von Bergmann in the Berlin clinic. He and his assistants had over two dozen hemostats pinching the bleeding points, which were afterwards replaced by ligatures, while in this case two ligatures are all that seems to be required, with the method which we have adopted in suturing the severed ends of the muscles. I commend this method, because it fixes the traumatic tissue in an immobilized manner. The patient in two or three days will be able to raise the limb without the aid of assistance.

Soft soap very energetically applied to the tissues with a scrub-brush, carefully shaving with a sharp razor, and a cleansing of the skin with alcohol, constitute the regular preparation of these cases for amputation. Inasmuch as they all make good recoveries, without pus. I see no necessity for dabbling with antiseptics and a multiplicity of details, as practiced in some of our hospitals. What I want to do is to simplify all the details of an operation, cutting out entirely the non-essentials.

Eye, Ear, Nose and Throat.

CONDUCTED BY KENT O. FOLTZ, M.D.

PENETRATING WOUNDS OF THE EYEBALL.

Two general classifications can be made of penetrating wounds of the globe, viz., surgical and accidental. The former are usually the result of premeditated measures for the relief of some morbid condition, and will not be treated of in this article.

Accidental penetrations are the kind that cause worry and annoyance to the physician, because the object doing the damage is either dirty, carrying infection, or so blunt or dull as to produce considerable bruising of the tissue surrounding the point of entrance. Another unfavorable feature in the accidental punctures is that the elective point of entrance is not always where the skilled operator would select for the traumatism. The iris, or lens, may be injured, or what is still worse, the selected point may be in the ciliary region—the danger zone—of the eyeball.

Any penetration of the cornea or of the ciliary region by a comparatively blunt object, unless the velocity is sufficiently great, will produce so much bruising of the surrounding tissue that ulceration is pretty certain, even if the object is surgically clean. On account of this tendency a guarded prognosis is always advisable, for the destruction of tissue through ulceration is often excessive, and the removal of the globe becomes necessary. It is true that in many instances the eyeball may be saved, but vision is lost and the atrophy following the inflammatory and ulcerative process is considerable, the result being an unesthetic appearance. This might not be of any especial importance, but there is always the danger of sympathetic inflammation of the fellow eye resulting in blindness.

Another point to be taken into consideration in cases where the eye is positively destroyed so far as useful vision is concerned, is the time necessary for complete recovery from its injury. If the patient is a laborer, and every day lost from work means privation to himself and family, what is gained by keeping him from work for weeks in the attempt to keep a shrunken, sightless globe in its socket? After an honest endeavor to save the eye, and it is found to be hopeless, why not remove it? In a week or two the patient can resume work, and is also saved much pain.

I do not advocate the immediate removal of an injured eye, as it is always best to try to save it if possible, but when it is found impossible to preserve vision, and delay in removal not only endangers the fellow eye but also means weeks of suffering, I cannot see humanity, charity nor good sense in waiting until the danger signal is raised in the other eye.

THE PREVAILING SORE THROAT.

Just at present we are having a grip, follicular tonsillitis, follicular pharyngitis or sore throat, according to the diagnosis of the consultant. No matter what it is called, it certainly is causing plenty of employment for the doctors and annoyance to the patients.

Usually there is a more or less severe chill as a premonitory symptom. The fever following is not always proportionate to the severity of the chill, and, although there is usually considerable aching of the back and legs, as well as headache, some of the cases complain more of a general lassitude. In the first class the headache is nearly always throbbing in character, but in the second type it is usually either a dull pain so described as a heavy feeling.

Inspection of the oro-pharynx and pharynx reveals a reddened zone along the soft palate, and some exudate covering the crypts of the tonsils, or over enlarged pharyngeal glands. The tissues show congestion, either active or passive, and in nearly all cases present a glazed appearance.

The patient complains of a feeling of soreness, stiffness or rawness in the pharyngeal region, and usually of a dry, hacking cough. In some instances the cough is more or less continuous, but frequently '' comes on in spells.''

Treatment.—The season remedy or remedies, so far, have been bryonia and cimicifuga. This has been the basis of treatment in the majority of cases so far. For the cough, either ipecac or lobelia, in small doses, gives the most relief. Not infrequently minute doses of morphine, in combination with one or both of these drugs, will be a valuable aid. By minute doses, I mean from gr. 1-128 to 1-1000. This may read like a ''pipe dream,'' but give it a trial, and you will find it is a reality.

Headache and Eye-Strain.

Parker (*St. Louis Medical Review*, August 1907) is firm in his belief that one-fourth of all the educated people in America suffer from various kinds of disturbances more or less due to eye-strain, and that in most cases these defects are remediable by proper treatment, and that the early discovery of these defects is the prime factor in the maintenance of health. He is convinced that the profession at large has not been awakened to the possibilities of the functional disturbances that have been brought about through ocular defects.

The author quotes from the records of the medical inspection staff of the New York City Health Department, which show that from March 27, 1905, to September 29, 1906, of the 99,240 children examined in the schools of the Borough of Manhattan, 65,741, or about 65 per cent., needed some form of medical treatment. Of these 99,240 children, 30,958, or about 30 per cent., required correction of defects of sight. In most of these cases the trouble could be ascribed to some form of eye-strain, which caused more or less headache, and concludes : In the city in which he resides they have compulsory vaccination, which has very materially lessened the percentage of smallpox ; organized crusades against tuberculosis ; established resident quarantines against measles, diphtheria, scarlet fever, whooping-cough, etc.; have passed laws by which text-books are supplied free to the pupils, but the eyes, that are so essential to make this great country of ours keep her position in the foremost ranks of progress, have been and are now being grossly neglected. If such is the condition in the schools of other large cities, what must, the author asks, be the situation in onr own schools, and if such is a fact, is it not criminal that we sit quietly by and make no attempt to correct such conditions by having laws passed which will enable the child to have proper protection ?— *Journal of Ophthalmology and Oto-Laryngology*.

Periscope.

Alkaloids Versus Galenical Preparations.

No one will attempt to deny the value and efficacy of alkaloids in a great many conditions, but to hold that active principles separated from their natural plant combinations are always preferable to Galenical preparations, does not harmonize with pharmacological facts. Let us bear in mind that the active principles of plants usually exist in combination with some plant constituent, and that in the manufacture of Galenical preparations simple solution and separation are the only processes employed, while to obtain active principles chemical decomposition of existing combinations is necessary and must precede the formation of alkaloidal salts.

Some of the so-called active principles on the market are not definite chemical substances, but varying mixtures of a number of bodies, in reality purified solid extracts. If an aqueous solution of the alkaloids of aconitum be heated they are broken up into one or more acids and simpler bases. These decomposition products occur in varying proportions in most, if not in all, commercial "aconitines," and their action is variable. The official tincture of aconite, if properly made, is more stable and reliable than any "aconitine" on the market, as solution in alcohol hinders decomposition.

Commercial "emetine" is really made up of three distinct alkaloids, cephaline, emetine and psychotrine; the first two are almost identical in action, while the last one is almost inert. The separation of these alkaloids is so difficult that it is unlikely they will be made use of in the near future; besides, they are not used for action after absorption, but merely for local effect on the alimentary canal, and Galenical preparations of ipecac root are much less liable to produce purging or other toxic symptoms, while they are but little slower in emetic action.

The active principles of digitalis and ergot are mostly glucosides, and consequently very unstable and difficult to isolate in a pure form. "Digitalins" and "ergotins" on the market are all mixtures, in varying proportions of the native glucosides and their decomposition products. Many of them are practically inert after a short time, as glucosides do not form salts, and after separation decompose more rapidly than when in their natural plant relations.

The alkaloids found in drugs used as simple bitters are inferior to the fluid Galenical preparations made from these drugs, because their action depends on their ability to excite the sense of taste, and solutions containing all the soluble plant constituents do this more effectively than the pure alkaloids. Quinine and strychnine merely as bitters are inferior to the fluid preparations of cinchona and nux vomica. Aloin is less certain in action than aloes, and pure crystalline aloin is practically inert in the bowel.

The alkaloids of opium exist in the gum in combination with meconic, lactic and sulphuric acids. Their action on the bowel is chiefly local through their depression of the ganglionic cells of the plexus of Auerbach and Meissner. The opium itself, or its Galenical preparations, is more slowly and therefore more continuously absorbed and gives more local effect than any of the opium alkaloids. If relief of pain chiefly is the result desired, the alkaloids are preferable, but for local bowel action in lessening peristalsis and secretion, the Galenical preparations excel.—*Practical Druggist*, January, 1908.

— --

Real Versus Fictitious Medical Education.

The opening address of Dr. Willis G. Tucker, before the Albany Medical College, printed in the *Albany Medical Annals*, and reproduced in *Science*, issue of November 8, 1907, is one of the most sensible papers on medical education that we have read for some time. Its whole trend is common sense and real education on the one hand, as against a fictitious and inflated mass of educational require-ments and equipment on the other. It argues strongly for the small medical school and its democracy as opposed to the large school and its trust-like methods of aristocracy. The speaker questioned the sanity of the critic who said at a conference of State medical exam-ining boards, recently held in Chicago, that of the one hundred and fifty medical schools in this country, only six were what they ought to be, and pertinently asks if we are to assume that the school with which the critic is associated is one of the six that are "what they ought to be," and if his opinion is the one to be taken on the sub-ject. We would like to reproduce the entire article, so replete is it with good horse sense, but we will content ourselves with the follow-ing quotations, since it evidences some of the just opposition that is arising in reference to the absolutism of the American Medical Asso-ciation.

"Whatever others may think, I shall not hesitate to raise my voice in opposition to such utterances as the following." Says the *Journal of the American Medical Association*, in its issue of September 14, 1907, in the leading editorial.

"Stronger safeguards should be placed about admission to medical practice in many States. The examining boards should be given supervision of all medical colleges within their respective States, with authority to pass on the entrance requirements of prospective medical students, and to issue or have issued to medical students entrance cer-tificates. They should have the right to inspect the medical college and to close such as are not properly equipped or are not doing satis-factory work. . . . Without this right the boards are not in position to protect the public from incompetent physicians."

And this is the utterance of a journal which is supposed to repre-sent the profession of the United States, but which, under its present management, is, in the opinion of some, representative of commercial-ism in medicine in a pre-eminent degree. It floods the mails with cir-culars urging graduates of the schools against whom it brings this general charge of incompetency to ally themselves with the associa-tion and to subscribe to the *Journal*, and it solicits the advertisements of the colleges with unwearying persistence. In the issue in which this editorial appears, I find the advertisements of no less than ten medical schools, which, according to its own statistical tables, pub-lished in its issue of May 25, 1907, ranked in the lowest class, as judged by the percentage of failures before State examining boards during the year 1906. Now, I do not hesitate to say that, in my opinion, there is not an examining board in any State in the Union which could safely be invested with such authority as the *Journal* recommends. . . . In many of our States men of only average ability are drawing salaries and exercising a little brief authority under the laws in places often secured through political influence. What shall be thought of a proposal to place the medical schools of this country under their absolute control? . . . Physicians should be banded together that they may promote the interests of the profession in proper ways, but any action that looks like closing the doors or putting up the bars for the purpose of lessening the number of medical men and restricting competition, ought not to be tolerated. Dr. Tucker goes on and scores the idealists as follows: ''They pursue their investigations with a foot-rule and hour-glass, place implicit faith in statistics, and would reduce all to a system. They would determine the competency of a student to enter upon the study of medicine by the special courses he has taken and the hours devoted to each, and whether his work is to be counted or not, is to be decided by a measurement of the floor space of the recitation rooms and laboratories in which he has been instructed and the cash value of the apparatus employed. They would measure his subsequent progress by mathematical computations in which the factors are forty or fifty divisions of the medical curriculum, each subdivided into lectures, recitations, clinics, demonstrations and laboratory work, and the value of each determined by a laborious conversion of these into hours, which must be so apportioned as to preserve a certain ratio, and the sum total of which must not fall below a prescribed minimum. And whether this instruction which he has received has been good or bad is to be determined by a consideration of the population of the place in which the medical school is situated, the value of the buildings and apparatus, the ratio of students to floor areas, the number of cases treated in affiliated hospitals and dispensaries, and other such data.''

The doctor also shows that under State control, in many States, and he probably was thinking of New York when he said it, ''The laws are so framed as to apply to physicians of established schools of practice, while irregulars of many kinds and 'healers' are exempted from their provisions, but however effectual they may be as restrictive measures, laws are much less effective in elevating the people in any direction than many enthusiasts would have us believe. . . . I think that our medical schools themselves may be trusted in a greater measure to bring about needed reforms and advance medical interests than some noisy reformers who clamor for more and more stringent laws, seem to suppose. It seems to me to be time that the medical profession asserted its dignity once more and resented the imputation that so large a number of its members are so incompetent or unworthy that the public needs further protection by special legislation.''

These sentiments have been frequently expressed in the past in the editorial columns of the *Medical Century*, and have been its contention ever since it was started.—Editorial, *Medical Century*.

To Stimulate Germ-Destruction.

The defenders of the body against the germs of disease, or at least certain of them, are the white blood-corpucles, or "leucocytes," which engulf intruding bacilli and destroy them. It used to be believed that every leucocyte had a natural appetite for intruders, and would attack them on sight, but the experiments of Prof. A. E. Wright, of London, seem now to have proved that without the action of some peculiar substances in the blood serum they could not perform that function. These substances—for there may be several, one corresponding to each class of diseases—Professor Wright has named opsonins, from the Greek word *opsono*, "I prepare the banquet," since their action appears to be upon the microbe rather than upon the devouring corpuscles, and may be likened to that of some sauce or condiment. The amount of any particular opsonin in the blood may be obtained by a method devised by Prof. Wright, and is denoted by what he calls the "opsonic index." This index may be increased by inoculation with minute quantities of the same bacteria that causes the disease. The "opsonic index" is determined by ascertaining the number of bacteria engulfed or devoured by the leucocytes as compared with the number devoured by those of a normal healthy man, since it has been found that the activity of the opsonins is practically the same in all healthy persons. Thus, to say that a person has an opsonic index of 0.6 toward a particular disease means that where the normal man's blood could dispose of 100 microbes, that of the subject could devour only 60. All this we learn from an article on "The New Microbe Inoculation," contributed by Prof. R. K. Duncan to *Harper's Monthly Magazine* (New York, July). Professor Duncan goes on to tell how, in the case of a person suffering from these diseases, deficiency in a particular opsonin may be remedied. He says:

"This was the great problem for Professor Wright, and he has apparently solved it by the renascence of a discredited method, which, illuminated by his genius, now bids fair to become one of the most valuable assets in medicine. In a word, he inoculates the patient with an appropriate dose of the dead micro-organisms which, when alive, are responsible for the infective process; for example, dead staphylococcus microbes to combat boils and acne, dead pneumococcus microbes to combat localized pneumococcus infection, dead tuberculosis microbes to combat localized tuberculosis.

"The reason for this treatment and for the phenomena that are afterward observed seems to depend on two facts: First, in this—that the opsonin in the blood will unite with the dead innocuous microbes as well as with the living vicious ones; next, the disappearance of the opsonin, through union with the dead microbes, stimulates the body cells not only to the production of more—an excess of—opsonin. . . . It may be asked why is it, then, since the microbe is 'hoist with its own petard,' that it ever gets a foothold in the body? The answer is that in normal people such microbes do not get this foothold, but that in certain other people there is lacking a quality of opsonin-producing power; then, too, when the microbes do win entrance they have a way of ensconcing themselves within a fortalice of protective material, or of erecting barricades of destroyed tissue, so that corpuscles and opsonin together find difficulty or impossibility in handling them.

"In practice, the man is inoculated subcutaneously with a standardized emulsion of dead microbes; thus, we read of Wright inoculating a patient with 2,000,000,000 dead staphylococci, or of one of his students inoculating another patient with 2,000,000 dead pneumococci, and it may seem that it would be quite an undertaking to count so many. The matter, however, is not so difficult as it looks. We have said that normal blood contains about 5,000,000 red blood-corpuscles to the cubic millimeter; why not, then, mix equal quantities of blood and microbes, and, under the microscope, count the proportionate number of each? In every cubic centimeter, then, of his microbic emulsion the investigator knows the microbic content."

Although not all germ diseases, apparently, are subject to cure by the action of opsonin, certain affections seem to yield to them easily; and in all cases the determination of the opsonic index bids fair to be a wonderful aid to diagnosis, as indicating resisting power of the organism. Thus, although in systemic tuberculosis opsonic treatment appears to fail on account of the fact that the patient is continually inoculating himself with the products of his own disease, the opsonic index will often show whether or not a suspected case is really tuberculosis or not. Says Professor Duncan :

"Remembering, then, that this man Wright and his work are together a product of the ultimate science and training of our day, if a man has a daughter over whom the doctors shake their heads, 'There are no microbes, but we do not know, it is not unlikely, we are inclined to think that it is incipient tuberculosis,' surely it would be wise, it would be helpful, to have this opsonic index taken. But to get it intelligently taken is the serious difficulty. Wright's laboratories in London are crowded with students from every quarter of the civilized world—from Russia and Sweden to Hindustan and Japan—but it takes time to provide men adequately trained. Some of the great hospitals in this country have already taken steps to inform themselves by bringing over from London one of Wright's assistants to demonstrate his method, and they are, doubtless, by this time more or less prepared. Not adequately prepared, for therein lies one great practical difficulty; the determination of an opsonin index takes more than an hour, and to spare this time, short though it seems, is of serious difficulty to an overworked hospital. Still, the General Hospital of the City of Toronto has deemed it advisable, even at this early stage of the discovery, to establish within its gates a department of opsonic inoculation, and has appointed as director of this department Dr. G. W. Ross, one of Professor Wright's most brilliant students. One of the great houses concerned with the manufacture of pharmaceutical preparations has already sent over to England, to study under Professor Wright, a member of its own staff; for with the establishment of this method of treatment there will fall upon these manufacturers the duty of providing for physicians the dead microbic inoculating material.''

On every side it is seen that the attitude of the educated and intelligent part of the medical profession toward this opsonic philosophy is one of waiting, of suspended judgment, and of extreme respect.—*Literary Digest*. July 13, 1907, p. 49.   M.

A Body of Leaders.

What is needed in this country to-day is concerted action, unity among men belonging to the same vocation or calling. When a united medical profession will present suggestions for the welfare and health of communities in this country as a body, such suggestions will go far towards fulfilling the social mission of medicine as a higher pofession.

Concerted action is needed. Every Eclectic physician should feel the need of affiliating with the local society; and of taking part in the deliberations of the larger, national organization. One of the ways in which the physician fulfills his obligations towards his fellow-men, aside from preventing illness and curing the sick, is by the good the community derives from the concerted action of medical men as a profession, banded together for work that requires the combined strength of all. Each unit counts. Do not withhold your support and encouragement from the local and national Eclectic organizations. Attend the meetings, take part in their deliberations, listen to the opinions of others; it will brighten and clear your mental vision on many subjects. Be lavish with your opinions and views; they will do good, even when you may be inclined to think they are not worth while. Somebody will be benefited.

The Eclectic body of physicians has done as much good in this country during the past seventy-five years as any similar body of professional men, and every Eclectic physician has reasons to feel proud of the achievements of his school. Progress has set a high pace for itself, and it is proper that the Eclectic physicians take care not to lag behind. During the next few years many questions of vital importance for the preservation of health and life will have to be settled. The Eclectic physicians must be found grouped together in a harmonious body, ready to take up any question of preventive medicine, health legislation, medical education, etc., which properly belongs to its sphere and contribute towards its satisfactory solution.

The means for that end have already been inaugurated. At the last meeting of the National Eclectic Medical Association a committee on organization and legislation was appointed, and we believe this to be one of the most important moves which the national organization has made in recent years. The men on the committee, as a body of leaders, are the peers of any who have ever led a great movement. Every State in the Union is represented on the committee. We must help this representative body of men, for their work is ours. We should hold ourselves in readiness to rally to their support whenever they issue a call. Above all, do not neglect to write to the representative from your State, or to the secretary, if you have any suggestion to make that will prove helpful in their work.

The Committee on Organization and Legislation of the National Eclectic Medical Association is constituted as follows:

Chairman—W. J. Pollock, 748 W. Chicago Ave., Chicago.
Secretary—J. K. Scudder, 1009 Plum St., Cincinnati.
Arkansas—G. A. Hinton, Hot Springs.
California—J. P. Dougall, Douglas Bldg., Los Angeles.
Chicago E. M. S.—W. J. Pollock, 748 W. Chicago Ave., Chicago.
Cincinnati E. M. S.—C. G. Smith, 224 Dorchester Ave., Cincinnati.
Connecticut—S. B. Munn, Waterbury.
Colorado—B. F. Richards, Masonic Temple, Denver.
Florida—S. F. Smith, Leesburg.
Georgia—John H. Goss, Decatur.
Illinois—John Dill Robertson, 481 W. Monroe St., Chicago.
Indiana—C. G. Winter, 14 W. Ohio St., Indianapolis.
Indian Territory—See Oklahoma.
Iowa—P. L. Price, Milo.
Kansas—C. I. Welch, Clifton.
Kentucky—J. C. Mitchell, 1004 Fifth St., Louisville.
Maine—Henry Reny, Biddeford.
Massachusetts—John Perrins, 107 Botolph St., Boston.
Maryland—George W. Fisher, 1510 Linden Ave., Baltimore.
Michigan—C. S. Sackett, Charlotte.
Minnesota—S. E. Sanderson, Minneota.
Missouri—E. A. Mendell, St. Joseph.
Nebraska—E. J. Latta, Kenesaw.
New Hampshire—Lillian J. Bullock, Manchester.
New York—D. P. Borden, 384 Ellison St., Paterson.
New York—E. H. King, Saratoga Springs.
Ohio—J. K. Scudder, 1009 Plum St., Cincinnati.
Oklahoma—B. K. Wood, Anadarko.
Oregon—H. L. Henderson, Astoria.
Pennsylvania—C. J. Hemminger, Rockwood.
South Dakota—W. E. Daniels, Madison.
Tennessee—George M. Hite, Nashville.
Texas—H. H. Blankmeyer, Honey Grove.
Vermont—P. L. Templeton, Montpelier.
Washington—G. W. Overmeyer, South Bend.
West Virginia—C. W. Seeley, Wileyville.
Wisconsin—C. E. Quigg, Tomah.

—Editorial, *Chicago Medical Times.*

THE ECLECTIC MEDICAL JOURNAL

A Monthly Journal of Eclectic Medicine and Surgery.

TWO DOLLARS PER ANNUM.

Official Journal Ohio State Eclectic Medical Association

JOHN K. SCUDDER, M.D., MANAGING EDITOR.

EDITORS.

W. E. BLOYER.	H. W. FELTER.	W. N. MUNDY.	R. L. THOMAS.
W. B. CHURCH.	K. O. FOLTZ.	L. E. RUSSELL.	L. WATKINS.
JOHN FEARN.	J. U. LLOYD.	A. F. STEPHENS.	H. T. WEBSTER.

Published by THE SCUDDER BROTHERS COMPANY, 1009 Plum Street, Cincinnati, to whom all communications and remittances should be sent.

Articles on any medical subject are solicited, which will usually be published the month following their receipt. One hundred reprints of articles of four or more pages, or one dozen copies of the Journal, will be forwarded free if the request is made when the article is submitted. The editor disclaims any responsibility for the views of contributors.

Discontinuances and Renewals.—The publishers must be notified by mail and all arrearages paid when you want your Journal stopped. If you want it stopped at the expiration of any fixed period, kindly notify us in advance.

RESINOIDS OR "CONCENTRATIONS."

There is an old saying, and an apt one, too, that "history repeats itself." It is interesting to note in following up our editorial in the February JOURNAL on polypharmacy, that there is a consistent attempt being made in some sections of Allopathic literature to laud the virtues of certain plant products newly introduced to them under the name of "concentrations," as though the term were something new. It is new to the Allopath, but old history to Eclecticism.

Our friends of the Allopathic school, in their efforts to appropriate much of the research work done in the past fifty years by Eclectics and Homeopaths, have been unable in the majority of cases to separate an alkaloid from a plant. This is nothing new to Eclectics, who demonstrated years ago the fallacy of that scheme.

The next effort is naturally to talk of a so-called "active principle" of a plant under the name of a "concentration." This is again history over and over. Many of our readers yet with us went through the "concentration" craze, which from 1850 to 1870 nearly wrecked our school of medicine.

For the sake of history and the younger generation, we reproduce two striking editorials from this JOURNAL, which express about what our Allopathic brethren will discover before they have wandered much in the old Eclectic track.

"In 1855, much of Eclectic medicine was an unmitigated humbug. It was the day of the *so-called concentrated medicines*, and anything having a termination in " *in* " was lauded to the skies. It was claimed that these resinoids were the active principles of the plants, and as they would replace the old drugging with crude remedies and teas, they must prove a great boon. But they did not give success, and finally, after trying them for awhile, the practitioner would go back to the crude articles and old syrups and teas with success, or he would settle down to podophyllin catharsis and quinine."—From editorial by JOHN M. SCUDDER, M.D.; in ECLECTIC MEDICAL JOURNAL, March, 1870.

"The so-called concentrated remedies are especially condemned. Thousands of dollars have been taken from our hard-working physicians for these powders, having no more medical properties than so much powdered charcoal or sawdust. One of our prominent manufacturers, who has sold them for fifteen years, confesses that there are not more than a dozen in his list which are valuable, and it might even be reduced below this. Another stated that the more honest the manufacturer, the poorer the medicine ; that the rogue who dried and bottled the extract really sold the best medicine."—JOHN M. SCUDDER, from article in ECLECTIC MEDICAL JOURNAL, August, 1870.

These are enough for our purpose, but we could give others stronger if necessary. We presume our Allopathic brethren will, however, prefer to travel over the old worn-out Eclectic road and find out for themselves. They wish to make old Eclectic history into new Allopathic.

The reputation of both the Eclectic and Homeopathic schools during the past thirty years has been staked on the general reliability of pharmaceutical preparations of definite strength, the detail of manufacture and menstruum being appropriate to each plant remedy.

This is necessary, because few of our plant remedies yield *alkaloids*, while so-called *concentrations* do not represent the full medicinal value of a plant, the delicate structure not being susceptible of desiccation.

Our readers are familiar with the many editorials in this journal from time to time on "the spirit of the plant." In nine cases out of ten this is lost in making a so-called resinoid or a "concentration."

We shall follow this series next month on another fad, "the fallacy of physiological drug study."   SCUDDER.

THE THERAPEUTICS OF ASCLEPIAS.

Asclepias is not so well known to the younger physicians as it is to those whose practice reaches back into and beyond the days of specific medication. It is a drug of the lesser powers, but may be relied upon to act kindly and efficaciously when indicated. The therapeutic field of asclepias is not wide, being restricted most largely to diseases of children, and particularly to those of the respiratory organs. Always safe and usually effective, it should have a more general use than is accorded it.

Asclepias was an important remedy in the practice of the botanic physician and the early Eclectic, for they saw in it the qualities of a direct diaphoretic, and of which there are but few. But they employed it in large doses and in decoction. Specific medication has demonstrated that it acts best in the small doses, and specific asclepias is the preparation now chiefly employed. The perspiration induced by it more nearly resembles normal insensible perspiration than that brought about by any other medicinal agent, corallorhiza perhaps excepted. Asclepias favors more largely the elimination of solid matters with a minimum of liquid secretion, and is often indicated, though copious transudation is already taking place. It may be used when fever is high, but is more effective when the temperature is but moderately exalted. It works well with the special sedatives—aconite when the pulse is rapid and small, and veratrum when the pulse is full and bounding. The chief indication for asclepias is a slightly moist skin, or an inclination to moisture, with a strong and vibratile but moderately rapid pulse. Then it becomes a valuable adjunct in the treatment of various respiratory troubles. Its domestic name—pleurisy root— attests its reputation in painful inflammation of the pleura. Here it may well follow the use of bryonia, the latter drug being more useful in the early stage of the disease. During this winter we have found it the most generally useful agent in controlling the bronchial irritation and the attacks of acute bronchitis in little children. It assists the special sedatives to reduce the fever and lessen pain by establishing true secretion from the skin. Expectoration is favored by it, and nervous excitation is lessened. In pneumonia and broncho-pneumonia it should have a wide use as an auxiliary agent, and we have known it to be the only medicine required in mild cases of measles, as well as other exanthemata. In the severer cases we invariably find indications for its selection. In respiratory disorders it should be exhibited in the acute stage, and where large areas of the lung seem involved. It seems specifically adapted to those areas supplied by the bronchial arteries. In the convalescent stage, when dyspnea and suppression of secretion and expectoration are threatened, it proves a remedy of first importance. With or without specific lobelia, it forms a good remedy for coughs when dry and there is a sense of constriction. Asclepias might be more advantageously employed for the relief of recent colds than many of the more powerful and often harmful agents that find extensive use in such conditions. Being one of our best agents to modify catarrhal discharges and bring them as nearly to normal as can be accomplished, asclepias should be more widely employed in catarrhs of all character when brought on by recent colds. As a remedy for the '' snuffles '' or acute nasal catarrh in infants it divides honors with matricaria and euphrasia. We invariably find one of these three indicated in that complaint. Asclepias is a drug of much value in the gastro-intestinal disorders of children with mucoid or catarrhal discharges, a weak stomach, some tendency to flatulent colic and nervous impairment.

The indications for asclepias may be summed up briefly as follows : Pulse strong, vibratile and moderately rapid ; pain acute, and dependent most largely upon movement ; skin moist, or in some cases hot and dry ; urine scanty ; face flushed ; marked vascular excitement with increased arterial tension ; serous inflammation, and acute catarrhal disorders of the respiratory or gastro-intestinal tracts due to recent colds. While pre-eminently a child's remedy, it is equally serviceable in the respiratory disorders of older patients. In most instances it will be used to re-enforce the action of the special sedatives, and the dose ranges from a few drops to a drachm of specific asclepias well diluted and given every one or two hours. If prompt sweating is to be encouraged it may be advantageously administered in hot water.

FELTER.

WHO USES THE ECLECTIC REMEDIES?

One of the principles of the early Eclectics was the selection of remedies to best serve their purpose, regardless of their source. In this way the fathers drew from Homeopathy, Allopathy, and wherever else came a remedy of value. In turn they endeavored to give back to the world from their own field, for they did not care to be considered as either parasites or sponges.

One of the misfortunes of the Allopathic physician of that date arose from the fear that a remedy introduced by an Eclectic should find place in his practice. Consequently, the very best remedies developed were for a long time out of his reach. This fact, if one speaks conservatively where harshness might be indulged, accounts for much human suffering that could have been avoided, and many unnecessary deaths. Although a few Eclectic alkaloids such as berberine and sanguinarine, a few resins such as those of podophyllum and cimicifuga, a few compounds such as compound sarsaparilla syrup and compound syrup of rhubarb and potash, had drifted into the outside, the introduction of specific medication found the dominant school resisting anything Eclectic in either name or setting. In some respects this is not surprising, for, as a rule, a dominant party resists every outside innovation, be it good or be it better than the plank in their own platform.

But, as time passed, the success of Eclectic physicians, the fairness of Eclectic writers, the elegance of Eclectic pharmacals, began to appeal to the rank and file of the dominant school. The study of Eclectic methods, principles and medicaments that began spasmodically with a few of the more friendly members of the Allopathic profession, spread to the many. The unfortunate pessimism of certain aged leaders of the dominant school, who have become discouraged over the action of their new remedies and lost faith in their old ones, finally approached professional despondency.

Medical agnostics, such discouraged leaders as these naturally become, and, rationally, infidelity as concerns medication, next followed. Dependent, not on the practice of medicine but on medical politics for a living, it mattered little whether the more conspicuous of these men believed in the curative value of drugs or even understood how to use them. To the physician—so-called—practicing in a laboratory with test-tubes and chemical apparatus, sickness is a thing afar off.

Not so with the rank and file to whom the sick look for relief, and who are employed to cure disease, not to decry medication. They could not face an appealing mother and say, "there is nothing in my profession but the art of diagnosis; I can tell what ails your child, but there is no cure for disease." The practicing physician must know what to do and how to do it or pass the child over to one who does know. Beside such as these the man who calls himself a physician and preaches medical nihilism is a conscienceless fallacy. To such as these came at last the thought—our teachers who told us that all outside our school was irregular, now tell us that all inside it is worthless. Our old materia medica has been abandoned once because it was vicious, and yet again because it was illogical; our lingering remedial agents are made of haphazard remnants thrown together like crazy-quilt patchwork.

One hundred thousand conscientious physicians of the dominant school are now questioning their leaders' methods of the past; they are also studying the living present, and are confronted with the future. They are freely questioning the assertions made by men who first claimed to teach them how to practice the only orthodox medicine, and next, without replacing it with anything tangible, abandoned the very remedies they asserted were to be used in regular practice. These physicians are now of necessity studying what lies in the outside; their honor, their conscience, their practice, their professional success demand it.

No longer does the word Homeopathist or Eclectic in souud or print give them a shudder, nor do they accept that remedies effective in the hands of more than ten thousand cultivated, intelligent, successful, systematic practitioners that the people trust are to be ostracised because some men do not know how to successfully use them.   It is perceived by these thoughtful physicians that seventy-five years have been systematically devoted to the development of the Eclectic practice of medicine and to Eclectic medicaments.   No cry of nihilism is heard by Eclectics, be they of the rank and file, or be they leaders.   As an evolution the process of drug study has progressed both as concerns remedies and in practice.   Confidence in their drugs and success in their application are evidenced in the result of Eclectic medication.   The physicians are gentlemanly, courteous, and they as freely give of their treasures as they have thankfully received of others.   One by one, an Eclectic specific medicine, or valuable compound thus becomes known to a member of the Allopathic school; it helps the recipient and credits Eclecticism. The medical nihilist ceases to be an authority under such influences as these.   We speak advisedly when we say that Eclectic physicians would be more than gratified could they know the esteem in which their medicines are held by a host of fair physicians of the dominant school who depend on them in their practice, and who are fair enough to credit Eclecticism for their excellence, and who are fast learning that a system of medication that has progressively evolved for seventy-five years is not to be denied them in their necessity because the leaders of their school know little or nothing about either the practice or the remedies.   LLOYD.

ORIGINALITY.

Judge: "You said the defendant turned and whistled to the dog. What followed?"

Intelligent Witness—"The dog."—*Ex.*

While the above quotation may seem, and is, foolish, there is "more truth than poetry in the item." Too many persons do, think, act or follow the customs, thought and precepts of others, particularly if they are considered "authority." What is authority? Who is authority? Well, one may say truthfully that the word of any person who has had experience in a certain line of work is an authority. This is true in a measure, but only as it applies to the individual case. Every emergency, every condition in business or professional lines calls for a specific handling of the situation, and authority or precedent is valuable only in so far as it aids in avoiding errors or in protecting against gross incompetency.

Nature has never turned out two objects mathematically the same. There is always a variation, slight in many instances it is true, but always present. No two persons have the same brain formation, consequently do not see, think or act alike. Now, why should any one individual locate and claim as his especial pinnacle a position from which to dictate to others, often his superiors mentally, how they should act in a certain affair which may present? Some rules can, of course, be formulated which will absolve a person from liability, but still we must remember that these rules are elastic, and not like those of the Medes and Persians.

In the practice of medicine especially is it incumbent upon the physician or surgeon to bear this in mind. Here there is a dual personality—the physician, the patient. The two should work synchronously, but often do not, and the result is "rag-time" to both. The physician must use his own "dome of thought" and do that which is best for the patient. He alone can judge of the requirements of the case. What value is the opinion of some one hundreds or thousands of miles away in this specific case? Aside of certain general rules of conduct, his opinion is of no value whatever. Each and every case is in a class by itself, and must be so treated. The environment, physical condition, severity of attack, nature of the lesion, and hereditary disposition must be taken into account if the best results are to follow. Who can do your thinking for you under these circumstances?

Brains and how to use them is the secret of success in any vocation. The ability to think is what constitutes originality, and the more the ability in this line the more successful the individual. Do not think you know it all. Self-complacency has caused more failures in business and professional lines than anything else. Profit by the labors of those who have had more experience than you, but remember you must do your own thinking. Much can be learned from unexpected sources, and it is not a sign of superiority to ignore the truth from the most humble of your patrons. FOLTZ.

SEASONAL REMEDIES.

This is the season of the year when catarrhal affections of the respiratory organs prevail. As a natural consequence, our attention is directed toward those remedies which have a direct influence upon the mucous tissues. As in the study of remedies under any conditions we are guided solely in their selection by the predominant symptoms presented and not by the name of the disease—in other words, no matter what may be the name of the disease or in what organ or tissue it may be located, the same symptoms prevailing—the indicated remedy will either relieve or prove curative. Prof. J. M. Scudder used to talk and write of the epidemic remedy, and we frequently notice that at certain seasons of the year or in certain years certain conditions seem to present themselves or appear dominant, no matter what may be the nosological name of the disease.   Thus we have seen duodenal catarrh prevail to such an extent as to almost assume the proportions of an epidemic.   Again, the catarrhal influences seem to affect the larynx, at other times the nasal cavities, or it may be the bronchial tubes.   Under such conditions it is but natural that during the prevalence of these diseases the remedies should partake of a similar character.   Granting this premise to be correctly taken, we find at the present time our indications in all acute cases presenting themselves at this time pointing strongly to asclepias tub., bryonia, rhus tox, phytolacca, and occasionally macrotys.   It is hardly necessary to point out the special indications pointing to each remedy.   We are all familiar with them.   Our aim is to again call attention to the epidemic or seasonal remedies, a fact so often called to our attention in the past.   MUNDY.

Surgical Note.

In cases of intestinal paresis following an attack of appendicitis, or injury of the abdominal viscera from any cause, followed by a tympanitic condition of the bowels, we have a remedy of much value in eserine salicylate as an adjunct treatment to aid the normal paristaltic action of the bowels.   I would suggest in these cases the hypodermic injection of 1-50 grain of eserine salicylate repeated every three or four hours, according to indications.   We occasionally have intestinal paresis following extensive surgical interference in the pelvic cavity, where the intestines are exposed, or where adhesions have taken place that require prompt aid, and I think eserine the remedy, aided by the high rectal enema of glycerine, turpentine and soapsuds, or warm linseed oil in large injections.   I should like a report from our men on the success attained by the use of this remedy in intestinal paresis.

                                                        L. E. R.

Medical Note.

In acute arthritis from whatever cause—as a rule from specific infection—I believe there is no medication better locally than to use say a pound of Epsom salts carefully spread on aseptic absorbent cotton, extending two inches above and below the joint, and over all a flannel roller bandage, and where necessary a plaster-paris cast to completely immobilize the joint.   In a few hours the tissue around the incased joint will take on an active perspiration, and after the absorption of the salts by some means the pain will subside and the arthritis gradually disappear.   L. E. R.

Errata.

January JOURNAL: Page 10, footnote, New York should read *New Jersey;* on page 12, footnote, Thompson should read *Thomson.*   F.

The Eclectic Medical Journal

ESTABLISHED 1836.

VOL. LXVIII.   CINCINNATI, APRIL, 1908. ·   No. 4.

Original Communications.

ASCLEPIAS TUBEROSA.

BY JOHN WILLIAM FYFE, M.D.,
SAUGATUCK, CONN.

Asclepias was a favorite remedy with many of the early Eclectics, and Dr. Wooster Beach used it in several of his valuable compounds, but it was employed in medicine at a much earlier date. So far as I have been able to ascertain, Dr. Schoef was the first to introduce asclepias tuberosa to the medical profession as a remedial agent. Cutter recommended it in 1785, and later Barton wrote approvingly of it. In 1810 Professor Thatcher referred to it as having been successfully employed in "pleurisy and other fevers."

Although asclepias was a well-known remedy long before the time of Wooster Beach, its present usefulness is the result of its adoption and development by the Eclectic school of medicine. The early writers on asclepias indiscriminately recommended it in all inflammatory diseases, but Eclectic study and investigation soon narrowed its leading use down to diseases of the serous membranes—"when the skin is hot, but inclined to moisture, the face flushed, and the pain sharp."

Many of the early Eclectics extensively employed asclepias for the purpose of "promoting perspiration and expectoration in diseases of the respiratory organs, especially pleurisy, inflammation of the lungs and catarrhal affections," and one Eclectic writer said that "we do not need to inquire the cause of pleurisy, for if there is pleurisy there should be asclepias."

Dr. Grover Coe, in his work on "Organic Medicine," spoke of asclepias as follows:

"No other remedy with which we are acquainted is so universally admissible in the treatment of diseases, either alone or in combination with other indicated drugs. In fact, we can think of no pathological condition that would be aggravated by its employment. It expels wind, relieves pain, relaxes spasm, induces and promotes perspiration, equalizes the circulation, harmonizes the action of the nervous system, and accomplishes its work without excitement—neither increasing the force or frequency of the pulse nor raising the temperature of the body. It is of especial service in the treatment of affections involving the serous membranes, as pleuritis, pneumonitis, etc. No one agent manifesting so little excitement in its operation is capable of successfully meeting so great a number of indications.''

The best results are obtained from asclepias when the temperature is but moderately increased, and the skin is inclined to moisture, although it is many times of value during high fevers. Asclepias is a remedy of marked curative ~power in a wide range of abnormal conditions, but its extreme freedom from injurious effects under all circumstances has led many physicians to think it lacking in therapeutic power. If, however, such practitioners will test it in a severe case of pleuritic pain, administering from fifteen to thirty drops of the specific medicine in hot water, a few doses thus employed will remove from their minds all doubt of its medicinal properties. No other remedy with which I am acquainted, under such circumstances, can equal its relieving effects. In pneumonia, pleurisy, bronchitis and other wrongs of the respiratory organs, asclepias is employed with splendid results. When administered early it often constitutes the only needed medication. As a means of removing the effects of la grippe it is one of our most efficient remedies. If the effects are characterized by nervousness, it quiets the nerves, and if derangement of the stomach is a prominent feature it relieves the stomach irritation, and thus makes for recovery.

In rheumatism asclepias exerts a decidedly corrective influence, and in nervous irritability its effects are markedly soothing in character. In insomnia, when given in hot water at bedtime, restful sleep is often secured through the influence of this medicament. Coughs aud colds also come within the curative range of asclepias, and in all forms of colic it can be prescribed with perfect confidence that its action will be positively beneficial. In all such cases it should be administered in very hot water—so hot that it has to be taken slowly.

While asclepias does not interfere with the action of other remedies, it is usually better to employ it singly, and if other drugs are needed use them in alternation.

The dose of specific asclepias (or a good fluid extract) is from one drop to one drachm, but in many cases it may be employed with advantage as follows :

Asclepias . . . . . . gtt. x–dr. ij.
Water . . . . oz. iv.

Teaspoonful every hour to every three hours,

A BAD BURN AND ITS TREATMENT.

By H. L. HENDERSON, M.D.,

ASTORIA, OREGON.

On January 26, 1907, a young man, aged twenty-six, while employed as a locomotive engineer on a logging railroad, and while running his engine, the engine left the rails and rolled down a seventy-foot embankment, turning over twice, completely wrecking it, and in its tumble carrying the unlucky engineer with it. In the fall several steam-pipes were broken, gauges knocked off, etc., so that the wrecked engine was literally a seething cauldron. From this horrible torture the unfortunate engineer was soon dragged by his less injured companions. He at once walked a distance of half a mile, without assistance, and was at once swathed in cotton smeared with the white of egg. The accident happened at near the noon hour. The place where it happened was nearly twenty-five miles from the nearest doctor. I was immediately sent for, but did not reach the unfortunate sufferer until nearly midnight following the accident. I at once arranged for and removed him to the hospital in this city. When I removed the cotton dressing that had been applied by his comrades, I found the destruction of tissue to be enormous. It was of the Dupuytren fourth degree in severity, and the area involved was so great that I at once gave warning that the case was almost necessarily fatal. The whole back, from the coccyx to the occiput, was burned through the skin and fascia and one leg and one arm seemed to be almost entirely cooked, the skin and fascia afterward sloughing off. I found the young man to be an exceptionally pure-blooded fellow, he never having so much as used tobacco, with no family taint whatever to impede his ability to recuperate.

The suffering of the poor fellow was not as great as one might expect, the burns being so deep that the sensitive nerves were all destroyed. During the whole progress of the case I was only compelled to use anodyne remedies but twice. To make a long story short, I used antiseptic remedies as local applications, and in due course of time all the burned tissue sloughed off, and after about three months from the time of the accident, the burned surface was covered with apparently healthy granulations, and skin grafting was resorted to to help cover the denuded surface. His companions, to the number of nine men, willingly offered themselves as subjects, and at the first séance I placed *two hundred and sixty grafts*, on an average of two to each square inch of surface. I applied gutta-percha tissue as covering, and applied gauze and cotton dressings. After a few days all the grafts that I had applied seemed to entirely disappear, and a crop of

enormous granulations seemed to develop. Great jelly-like masses
covered the denuded surface as thick as the thick part of a man's
hand, from which poured in great quantities a sero-purulent fluid,
which seemed destined to drain away all the life and vitality of the
poor fellow.

One day, while sitting in the dressing-room, watching the trained
nurses carefully cleansing this jelly-like mass, the idea struck me
that that surface needed *pressure* to hold those granulations in check.
I am not specially sensitive to revolting things in surgery, when I
conceive that they are necessary for the benefit of my patient, but
there is one thing on which I have thus far been able to draw the line,
and that is, the use of a curette to scoop away superflous granulations,
as is directed by the authors of standard text-books on surgery. So
I was casting about for some method to control these granulations,
as I had failed to do so with the classical applications. I at once
called for an ordinary Martin rubber bandage, and applied it, almost
enveloping the whole body, in order to reach all the affected area.
After the lapse of twenty-four hours, on the removal of that bandage,
I found that it had done good, so far as the condition of the granulations was concerned; but it being practically air-tight, the smell that
had developed was unbearable, so that I could see that pressure would
accomplish the desired result, but that the Martin bandage was not
the thing to get that pressure with, to the advantage of the patient.
I at once wired to a supply house to send to me at once fifty yards of
a rubber webbing, three inches wide, such as is sometimes employed
as a bandage in varicose veins. In due time the webbing arrived and
was applied, using one-half of the supply each time, so that the part
that was taken off could be immediately washed and dried, ready to
be applied the next day. The improvement of the patient was simply
marvelous, so far as his general condition was concerned, and the
granulations at once lost their exuberant character.

Now the most surprising feature of the treatment developed. All
the grafts that had been applied several weeks before reappeared, and
cicatrization rapidly progressed. Two more sittings of grafting finally
closed the burned area, making in all nearly five hundred grafts applied.
He was burned in January, and was discharged from the hospital,
cured, on October the first. I did not resort to the use of the barbarous
curette during the progress of the case. The point that I wish to
emphasize in the case was the application of the rubber webbing, after
the granulations had formed, and their rapid absorption as a result,
thus permitting the grafts to do their work and stop the exausting
discharge that threatened to drain away the life of my patient. The
grafts prevented the formation of contractile cicatrices that would have

certainly rendered the patient a cripple, deformed by their contraction ; but to the contrary, he is now able to do a mans work, and do it with pleasure. This case taught me that it matters not the extent of a burn, occasionally a patient will get well in spite of the text-book statement that if one-third of the surface is involved death must follow. I am very sure that in this case a far larger fraction of the surface than one-third was involved, and yet the patient is well and strong to-day.

HOW TO COMPLY WITH THE MEDICAL LAW OF TEXAS.

By MARQUIS E. DANIEL, M.D.,

HONEY GROVE, TEXAS,

President State Board of Medical Examiners.

There being many physicians residing in various portions of the United States, legalized to practice medicine in Texas under former laws, which entitle them to verify under the new medical law, and in answer to many inquiries coming from without as well as within the State, is my apology for giving publicity to this notice.

The information to follow is based strictly upon the latest rulings of the Attorney General of Texas.

Physicians who at any time were qualified to practice medicine in Texas, regardless of present residence, are entitled to verify under the present law, unless barred by evidence that fraud was practiced in securing their legalization, and the further evidence of " conviction of a crime of the grade of felony or one which involves moral turpitude or procuring or aiding or abetting the procuring of a criminal abortion, or grossly unprofessional or dishonorable conduct of a character likely to deceive or defraud the public, or for habits of intemperance or drug addiction calculated to endanger the lives of patients."

One year is allowed in which to comply with the law, and the time limit is *July 12, 1908, after which date all rights to practice will cease, and can only be re-secured by examination before the new Board*. There are five classes entitled to verification, designated as per methods of legalization under previous laws.

CLASS I.—*Those legalized by years of practice*, who were practicing medicine in Texas prior to January 1, 1885, should send to the Secretary, affidavits of citizens sufficient to establish that fact and will then receive verification licenses.

CLASS II.—*Those legalized by District Board certificates between January 1, 1885, and July 9, 1901*, should send the original certificate or certified copy of same, together with evidence of their registration in some District Clerk's office, to the Secretary, and will then receive verification licenses, providing said medical certificates were *recorded prior to July 9, 1901*, and provided further that in the event the owners of said medical certificates changed their location after date last mentioned, they must show evidence of registration in county of last residence and a District Clerk's certificate of registration must be furnished, providing registration both before and after July 9, 1901, as under said law, to have been legally registered at all times, registration was required in each county to which licentiates might have moved.

CLASS III.—*Those legalized by registration of diploma between January 1, 1885, and July 9. 1901*, should proceed exactly as in Class II. The same rule applies to both alike, throughout, except that it is not necessary to send diploma for inspection, but an affidavit from the dean of the college of graduation testifying to the issuance of the diploma. This secures the Board against bogus diplomas.

In some instances certified copies of diplomas are sent, which is not objectionable, but the dean's affidavit is sufficient.

CLASS IV.—*Those legalized by registered certificates issued on reciprocity, under the Act of 1901 (the three board law) between July 9, 1901, and July 13, 1907*, should send medical certificate or a certified copy of same, to the Secretary, together with District Clerk's certificate of registration and verification licenses will be issued, providing said medical certificates were *recorded prior to July 13, 1907*.

CLASS V.—*Those legalized by registered certificates issued on examination under the Act of 1901 (the three board law)* should proceed exactly as in Class IV, and verification licenses will be issued providing medical certificate was *recorded prior to July 13, 1907*.

Under the Act of 1901 all physicians who had registered upon diplomas from January 1, 1891, to July 9, 1901, were required to verify before one of the three State Examining Boards created by said Act, but inasmuch as the Attorney General has ruled that every physician, regardless of how or when legalized, must verify under the present law, I have included this class with Class III. However, State certificates thus secured are accepted for verification, *provided they were recorded prior to July 13, 1907*. From this explanation physicians can easily determine their status under the new law.

Legalization on one basis is all that is necessary, even though a given individual may possess the necessary credentials to qualify under any one or all the classes mentioned ; only one legal credential is necessary.

The verification fee is fifty cents, and must accompany the application. Send all applications, credentials and fees to the secretary of the Board, Dr. G. B. Foscue, Waco, Texas.

After receiving the verification license it must be recorded by or before July 12, 1908, to be valid. To have same recorded, proceed as follows: Take verification license to District Clerk in *person;* he will record same in the Medical Register, on a page devoted to you, and take your oath as to your age, post-office address, place of birth and school of practice. But if it is impossible or impracticable to do this in person, then it will be necessary for you to go before a notary public or some one authorized to administer oaths (non-residents would better go before a clerk of a court of record) and make out an affidavit something like the following:

State of ———, ——— county.

This day personally appeared before me, the undersigned authority, Dr. ———, who, being duly sworn by me, deposes and says that he is the owner of the accompanying medical certificate, issued by the State Board of Medical Examiners of Texas, dated ———, numbered ———, and that his age is ——— years, post-office address ———, place of birth ———, school of practice ———.

Send this affidavit with verification license, together with the recording fee of one dollar, to District Clerk of county of residence, or if a non-resident, to any District Clerk, and it will be recorded same as if presented in person.

Inasmuch as it is not, as yet, known to but few of the district clerks, it will save time to call said clerk's attention to the ruling of the Attorney General, under dates of December 20, 1907, and January 6, 1908, which authorizes said record to be made when medical certificate is accompanied by the foregoing affidavit.

This same method of registration holds good in recording certificates issued under the present law upon examination and reciprocity. Licenses issued under the present law must be re-registered on every change of residence to a new district or county.

By way of general information, I will state that only such applicants are admitted to the regular examination of the Board as are graduates of four-year colleges, said colleges being in good standing in the *national college organization of the school to which it belongs,* and the fee is fifteen dollars.

Texas reciprocates only upon the basis of actual written examination; that is Texas recognizes only such certificates from the States with whom she reciprocates as were secured upon written examination and the fee is twenty dollars.

The present Board is being maligned for not verifying such certificates as are barred on account of not having been recorded within the limits mentioned.

The Board can exercise no choice in the matter—is merely the instrument through which the law may be complied with—but would be pleased to see a test case go through the courts which would forever settle the matter and make its work less burdensome.

CHRYSANTHEMUM LEUCANTHEMUM.

By HERBERT T. WEBSTER, M.D.,
OAKLAND, CAL.

In the August number of last year's JOURNAL I called attention, in an editorial note, to "White Daisy." At the time this was written I was sojourning at a farm-house in Oswego County, New York, where works of reference on botanical subjects were entirely wanting, and possessed no means of identifying the plant; not being a botanist, I was able to refer to it only under the name it was generally known in the vicinity.

In correspondence with Dr. Fearn, who was then visiting in West Virginia, he suggested that it might be chrysanthemum leucanthemum, as my description of the plant to him did not correspond with that of bellis perennis, the common wild daisy. Upon reaching a destination where works of reference afforded light on the subject I became convinced that this was the correct view; that the plant was a chrysanthemum, and not of the daisy family botanically, though it is commonly known throughout the East as white-weed, ox-eye daisy, white daisy, etc. The flower resembles, somewhat, that of the daisy, but the plant is entirely different. It consists of a single delicate stalk, bearing at its apex a single flower, with yellow centre and white corolla. The stalk is arborescent, and from twelve to fifteen inches in length. It grows among the tall grasses of the meadows, which assist in supporting it; and the flowers are so numerous, in many localities, showing upon the surface, as to impart a whitened appearance to the landscape. The plant is found from Canada to as far South as Virginia at least, and from the Atlantic to the Mississippi. I believe it possesses valuable medicinal properties; in fact, I know that it does, though it has not been very fully investigated as yet.

In my own family I have on hand a case of lymphadenoma, which, in March and April of last year was in an extremely debilitated condition. The patient suffered excruciating pains in the head, neck and other parts, from pressure of swollen glands, was anemic and feeble, with stubborn intermittent fever—temperature between exacerbations ranging from 94° to 97° F. Taking of food, even of the most bland, was followed by extreme gastric distress, and appetite was entirely absent at all times, with loathing of nourishment. Dizziness and fainting frequently occurred upon moving about, though the patient was too nervous to remain long in one position, or even a recumbent position, much of the time. Insomnia was so persistent that little sleep occurred, day or night.

After exhausting all my own resources, as well as those of eminent counsel to no avail, and coming to the conclusion that the end was near at hand, I decided at length to try a change of climate, and took the patient to her old home in New York, arriving there about the middle of May. Here appetite and digestion slightly improved, but debilitating night-sweats soon set in, and the insomnia persisted.

The patient's brother, an observing farmer, had great faith in "white daisy tea" in obstinate sweating, as the result of its beneficial action years before in his own case and the effect he had observed in others under his own observation since, and suggested that it be given a trial. A decoction of the green plant was prepared, and administered in tablespoonful doses every two or three hours during the day and until bedtime. The result was more than was hoped for, for the night-sweating ceased within two days, restful slumber followed at night, and permanent improvement soon became marked. Within a fortnight the patient was eating and appropriating a general diet satisfactorily, improving in flesh and strength, and was soon able to attempt a pleasure trip down the St. Lawrence River and through the New England cities, occupying several weeks, which proved a complete success in everything anticipated.

In September we returned to Oakland, and the patient has since remained in passable condition, though of course the chronic disease is not eliminated. Certainly, we must ascribe some of this improvement to climatic change, but there is no doubt that the medicine deserves much credit for turning the tide in favor of at least temporary recuperation, for it was the only drug taken during absence. Since return a tendency toward relapse in night-sweating and insomnia has once recurred, but a saturated tincture of the green plant of the chrysanthemum, in minute doses, promptly dispelled it.

In conversation with Dr. Fearn, who returned soon afterward, I recently learned that he was having considerable trouble with a case similar in some respects to mine, though not one of lymphadenoma. The patient was a female, somewhat past the climateric, who had been sleepless, debilitated and exhausted by profuse perspiration, continuing day and night, during a period of about four months, and nothing thus far had afforded any lasting benefit. The chrysanthemum was suggested here, and the doctor was supplied with an ounce vial of the saturated tincture for trial. A report of very favorable character soon followed, and prospects now seem to indicate that it will prove the principal remedy needed to restore the patient to health. She is already greatly improved, and the insomnia and night-sweats have disappeared.

As this is, to my knowledge, the first report ever made upon chrysanthemum leucanthemum as a medicine, and as we have as yet given it but little trial, of course it is impossible to at present outline its field of therapeutic action, beyond its value in profuse perspiration of chronic nature. That it is specific in controlling obstinate relaxation of the sudoriparous glands there is no question, for this was well proven in domestic practice long ago, and there is no doubting it; and we may prescribe it here with full confidence.

However, there may remain considerable to be added as time progresses; much may be developed in the future which we cannot at present attempt to predict. It possesses some of the influence ascribed to such old nervines as cypripedium and scutellaria, though it differs materially from both in its influence upon the nervous system. It also resembles pulsatilla somewhat in its influence upon the mental sphere, yet is not a substitute for that remedy. As a medium for relaxation of the sudoriparous glands it ranks with picrotoxin, atropia, agaricin, etc., though its influence is more permanent, apparently, than any of these agents, while it seems to augment vitality something akin to the influence of echinacea, though it is not a dynamic antiseptic in any sense, so far as I have observed.

It will be much in evidence in the meadows of the greater East next June and July, and I would suggest that country-practitioners tincture a small quantity, for future use and experiment. Pack a quart Mason fruit-jar with the green plant, when it is in blossom, and cover with best drug-store alcohol. Allow it to stand two weeks or longer. After fourteen days, it will be ready for use. Add a teaspoonful of this to four onces of water, and order a teaspoonful every hour in stubborn and protracted relaxation of the skin attended by perspiration.

We will not find the remedy indicated very often, but when the proper indication is present it will serve profitably. It might prove useful in the night-sweats of phthisis.

INTERSTITIAL FIBROMA COMPLICATED WITH AN ULCERATIVE COLON.

By C. WOODWARD, M.D.,
CHICAGO, ILL.

Practitioners who make a pretention of ability to treat chronic conditions know that, in order to be successful, three important features must be considered, namely : The removal of cause, a properly adapted treatment, and sufficient time in which to restore the part and general health to a physiologic state—three features that conform very little to operations, but which specifically indicate a long and judicious course of treatment in order to strengthen normal functions. There are few diseased conditions of the system that require the application of these three features more than fibromata of the uterus, for the reason that they are usually complicated with one or more of the following conditions : Subinvolution, endometritis, mal-assimilation, muco-colitis, weakened metabolism and diminished elimination. To treat fibromata of the uterus successfully, all of the complications must be corrected during the treatment, as will be exemplified by the following case :

Mrs. C. M., aged thirty-nine, was delivered of a male child in her thirty-first year by forceps, which resulted in a slight laceration of the cervix and quite an extensive rupture of the perineum. An anesthetic was employed during puerperium, and consciousness was fully restored before the accoucheur stitched the perineum, but, she claims, seriously shocked her nervous system. Her bowels were retained for ten days, and when evacuated with the aid of oleum ricini and enema, she suffered extreme toxemia, and to one part of fecal matter was attached a scab-like piece of mucous three-eighths of inch wide and five inches long. For eight years she was under medical attendance most of the time, either for the bowels or uterine diseases.

Several eminent surgeons had examined and diagnosed her trouble as interstitial fibroma of the uterus and advised an operation, to which she did not consent, however. Early in 1907 a physician lent her a copy of Intra-Uterine Medication, and after reading it she was anxious to be treated according to its instructions, confidently believing that she might recover without submitting to an operation. Leaving her home in Kentucky, she called at my office July 6, 1907, and was examined. The conditions disclosed were as follows : Base of tongue coated a brownish color, pulse 92, temperature 99°, and her complexion dark as that of an Indian, an interstitial fibroma in the left side of the uterus about two and one-half inches in diameter, depth of uterine cavity seven inches, deflected to the right side of the pelvis and discharging a profuse sanguinolent exudation. Further examination proved muco-colitis and an ulcer five or more inches long situated at the superior descending colon; at this location a dull pain was felt most of the time, and was quite severe whenever scybala were passing.

Treatment.—The treatment consisted of advising the quantity and quality of food, the diminished use of butter and sodium chloride, the proscribing of salted meats, fish and all kinds of canned and anti-septically preserved foods.

These remedies were prescribed to 'restrain the degenerative growths, correct the muco-colitis, assist nutrition, and strengthen and heal ulceration of the colon:

> Hamamelis dis. . . . . . . oz. iss
> Specific hydrastis . . . . . . dr. i
> Aqua dis. q. s. . . . . . . oz. iv
> M. Sig.: One teaspoonful every three hours. Eight pro-tonuclein tablets were given daily.

For eight years her bowels had scarcely moved without assistance. It must be apparent to all that the greatest causes of muco-colitis are the stimulating physics and relaxation, resulting in weakened peristalsis and followed by distension from overeating. Patients who manage their bowels as described cause them to acquire hyperemia and hyper-esthesia—conditions which are easily aggravated by iron or any irritant remedies, and especially acid preparations. Here, I will state that I have never found any combination of remedies for controlling the hyperesthesia, restraining excessive mucous and strengthening peristalsis equal to the following slightly alkaline, antiseptic and stimulating laxative:

> Tri-strength infusion of senna . . . oz. ii
> Specific belladonna . . . . . . gtt. vii
> Rye whisky and glycerine, aa, . . . oz. ii
> M. Sig.: One to two teaspoonfuls in a glass of cold water before breakfast every morning during the summer months, and warm water in the winter.

Experience with the modern method of irrigation has proved that we can successfully cure fibromata by temporarily inducing anemia of the uterus, inhibiting one or two menstrual flows, thus controlling the supply of nutrition to the growth. The local treatment consists in cleansing out the uterus every third day for three months with a 50 to 75 per cent. solution of peroxide of hydrogen, alternated with a 1 per cent. solution of lysol, then followed by a solution of iron sulphate, five to eight grains to the ounce, after which a six-ply absorbent gauze, with a string attached, saturated in one part each of specific hydrastis and thuja to six parts of sterilized water, is inserted, by the use of a sound, to the base of the uterine cavity, followed by a large dehydrating pack placed against the cervix, both to remain forty-eight hours. On alternating days following an enema, the ulceration of the colon can be reached through the rectal speculum by long dressing forceps, with oxygenated and other mild antiseptics. A rubber tube is passed through the rectum and these remedies landed into the transverse colon, or above the sore, to be retained as long as possible :

Specific hydrastis	.	.	.	.	.	.	dr.	i
" calendula	.	.	.	.	.	.	dr.	i
Aqua dis. q. s.	.	.	.	.	.	.	oz.	viii

This treatment induced so much anemia of the uterus at the expiration of thirty days that menstruation was partly inhibited ; at sixty days the flow was merely a color ; at the end of three months she failed to menstruate, but the fibroma had diminished from two and one-half inches to about one inch, and the depth of the uterine cavity to four inches. She returned to her home and all treatment ceased, except the protonuclein tablets, and at the expiration of thirty days she menstruated, and has done so regularly ever since ; her evacuations are also natural.

In the modern method of uterine irrigation we have a specific treatment with which, when necessary, we can cause congestion of the uterus that will overcome amenorrhea and by the application of a different class of remedies induce its anemia, thus diminishing the supply of nutrition to various growths.

Eclectic practitioners who are applying this method have written stating that it has increased their reputation for curing female diseases and given them an appreciable advantage over their competitors.

LIBRADOL FOR CRACKED HEELS.

By C. PICKET, M.D.,
DUNNING, NEB.

Whoever drives horses in a muddy country becomes familiar with a condition called "grease heel," which consists of a deep crack just under the pastern joint. This is extremely hard to cure. A similar condition is sometimes found in man, the foot from some cause becoming very rough, the black roughness or dead skin being difficult to remove. After a few days there appears a crack in the skin in what we might call the corner of the heel. Inflammation now follows until the one who suffers describes it as feeling like a severe burn, especially at night. The writer has quite an experience in this line, for he, like most other doctors, lets anything run on until it becomes unbearable. The crack seldom exceeds three-quarters of an inch in length, is not wide but deep, and is as red as fire, the borders partaking of the same red color. This condition will not yield to any application in common use, such as a wet pack or elm-bark or flaxseed poultice. We went the rounds, the pain still increasing until it was suggested that libradol be used as an application. For a short time the pain increased and decreasingly continued for about one hour, then it disappeared, and in a few minutes thereafter we were sleeping as sweetly as a babe. The libradol was left on for four days, being renewed once a day until the parts were white and free from redness and pain. Since that we have treated several patients afflicted in the same way, and in each case with success. To every physician we would say, libradol will cure cracked heel, if properly applied and kept on the parts until it has effected the cure—say three or four days.

MEDICO-LEGAL.

By E. S. McKEE, M.D.,
CINCINNATI.

THE American International Congress on Tuberculosis and the New York Medico-Legal Society will meet in joint annual session at Chicago June 1, 2 and 3, 1908. The local committee of arrangements is Dr. Denslow Lewis and Dr. Thomas Bassett Keys, of Chicago, and Dr. E. S. McKee, of Cincinnati. The latter takes the place of Dr. Nicholas Senn, lately deceased. The permanent officer of both societies is Hon. Clark Bell, LL.D., 39 Broadway, New York.

Practicing Physician as Druggist.

In State vs. Moorman, Michigan, also in New York and Oregon, it has been decided that a practicing physician cannot keep a drugstore or sell or give away drugs which he has not prescribed.

Chinese Selling Opium.

The Appellate Court of the State of Illinois has sustained the State Board of Pharmacy in the case against Yee Wa, Chinese laundryman, prosecuted for selling opium. In handing down its decision the court held that opium is a drug, and not an ordinary article of merchandise, and that a place where drugs and medicines are sold is a drug-store, in the ordinary meaning of the law.

Come High.

It is frequently said, and sometimes repeated, that every man can be bought, provided only that the price is high enough. However true this may be, we always like to see doctors bring high prices. Some really munificent fees were received by alienists for expert testimony in the Thaw trial. Dr. Carlos F. McDonald, $6,300; Dr. Austin Flint, $5,380; Dr. Wm. Maybon, $3,987, and Dr. Robert C. Keruf, $3,102.

Pertaining to Prescriptions.

A very learned court, Bruendi 102, Wis., p. 48, held that the word " prescribe," as applied to the act of a physician, means to " advise, appoint or designate a remedy for a disease." The same view is taken by the Supreme Court of Alabama, which court says that to prescribe means to " direct as a remedy." A prescription, then, appears to be a matter of advice. It may be simply oral, as where a physician advises a patient to go and drink a bottle of Pluto water. The advice may be committed to writing so that it requires the skill of an apothecary to read and compound the advice. It seems erroneous that the prescription is the property of the physician who gives it, as some have claimed. The physician has given his advice either gratuitously or for consideration, and it no longer abides in him. In the case of the Chicago Board of Trade vs. The Christy Company, 198 U. S. 236, the Supreme Court of the United States held that certain quotations collected by the Board of Trade, and communicated to certain telegraph companies under an agreement that they should be distributed only to certain persons approved by the Board, were entitled to protection by injunction from use by certain others. If we apply the principle of this case to a prescription, such prescription might perhaps be delivered to the patient with a similar contract and consideration that it should be held confidently for the use of the patient alone, and even that it should not be repeated. The opinion of a court has this merit, at least, that as a rule counsel are heard on both sides of a question, and then the judge, presumably impartial and honest, renders his decision as best he can.

The Pupil—Poetic, Prosaic.

" It may be that the wise and painstaking student who first essayed to write up a description of the organ of vision may have had a sweetheart whom he consulted constantly on that which interested his host; and on one occasion, when he was looking down into her soulful eyes and reading his fate in their liquid depths, imagined that he saw an image there which resembled an infant, and at at once called it 'pupa,' a baby, 'pupilla,' a little baby, and that has been the name of that little opening in the iris ever since. Had he been possessed of the ready pen of the 'Autocrat of the Breakfast Table,' methinks he would at once have laid at the feet of his darling something like this :

> " I look upon the fair blue skies,
>   And naught but empty air I see ;
> And when I turn me to thine eyes,
>   It seemeth unto me
> Ten thousand angels spread their wings
> Within those little azure rings."

The above is quoted from the entertaining and instructive writings of Dr. A. N. Ellis, of Maysville, Ky., special oculist to the U. S. Pension Department, on "The Pupil in Health and Disease."

A new conception of the pupil is thus suggested, and the very neat and appropriate little verse quoted by Dr. Ellis reminds the writer of a verse by More, which recalls a slang expression, very aptly describing the all-too-prevailing custom of the age and race in spite of Roosevelt's advice and example.   It runs as follows :

"Look in mine eye, my blushing fair,
Thou'lt see, like old, thine image there;
And when I look in thine I see
Two little images of me.
Thus in our looks some propagation lies,
For we are making babies in each other's eyes."

More also said : "The minds of some of our statesmen, like the pupil of the human eye, contract themselves the more, the stronger light is shed upon them."

VESICAL CALCULUS IN A CHILD OF SEVEN YEARS.*

Extraction Through the Natural Ways.

TRANSLATED BY DR. G. G. WINTER,
SHELBYVILLE, IND.

P. Angéle, of Antiles, whose parents were farmers in very good health, was born in 1898.   She has a sister four years old, in excellent health.   Born at term, nourished by breast for twenty-two months, the youthful patient endured easily several successive cases of bronchitis without trouble.   At two years, after one of these repeated attacks of bronchitis, it was noticed that she was crying while urinating ; this pain was more or less calmed by numerous and various treatments which were necessary to touch the cause.

In August, 1904, that is, at six years of age, she was brought to the Hospital General, medical ward, on account of the pain at micturition.   Diagnosis : Vulvo-vaginitis.   Injections with a special catheter were held proper.   The pains, however, remained just as violent.   The girl was always wet at the genital organs with fetid pus.   The injections were, nevertheless, continued up to the day when the mother, in introducing the catheter, asserted that she felt, at the point of the instrument, a body which she thought was a stone.

About January 30, 1905, she returned the child, who was then introduced into the surgical ward.   An examination was made under chloroform anesthesia.   To our great astonishment, in a spasm of cries and pain, during the chloroform excitation, a jet of urine spurted forth

* Reported by Dr. César Roux, of Nice, in Gazette Médicale de Paris.

from the urethra, the orifice of which became suddenly obstructed by a large calculus. Notwithstanding the dilatation was of the size of a 50-centimes piece, through which was presented the urethral sphincter, it could not pass out. We prepared ourselves to seize the foreign body, when suddenly the calculus disappeared ; the patient returned to a complete resolution, the bladder completely emptied itself, the liquid not bringing the calculus forward. It had gained the low vesical bottom again.

We injected two hundred cubic centimeters of boiled water. The child, purposely half-awakened, uttered new cries and made efforts at expulsion under the influence of the pain. The calculus again fell upon the orifice of the urethra. At the same time she expelled some urine. We seized the calculus between the teeth of dressing forceps, and, debridling it hurriedly above and below, finished the operation. We extracted a big calculus, in the form of a bottle, with a neck and

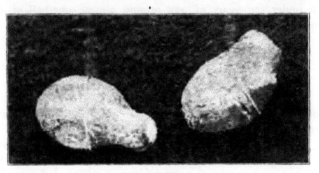

Vesical calculi removed—natural size.

an enlarged part four centimetres in length and two centimetres in breadth in its middle, and in weight 7 gr. 9.

Vesical lavage was done and then we introduced sound for measurement. The following day the sound had evacuated itself. There was still some incontinence of urine and pain at micturition. The bladder was irrigated with permanganate of potassium, 0.25 per cent.

February 2 the incontinence had disappeared, but the pain persisting. On the 7th, at night, pains became aggravated. The child uttered fearful cries, and informed the nurses that she was going to expel another stone ; in fact, in the bed was found, in the midst of small gravel, a second calculus, analogous to the one which had been extracted six days before. It had the same amphorical form and weighed 7 gr. 50. After some days of rest the child left the hospital entirely cured.

The two calculi were of the same weight, form and length and the same volume. They were composed of a swelled-up mass in ovoid form, resembling a pigeon-eye, of which one pole proceeded through a neck. This extremity of the calculus ended in each one with a facet, oblique from above to below with one, from below to above with the other, in such a manner that the two facets adapted themselves exactly, as if they originated from the fractures at this place, having been one primitive calculus which then must have presented the form of dumb-bells.

The chemical examination showed that the calculi were formed from triple phosphate of calcium. At the intersection, three visible concentric zones indicated that the solid substances of the urine had deposited themselves upon the initial calculus in the form of successive layers.

Urinary lithiasis is very frequent in youth ; according to statistics, children under ten years of age present almost one-half of those published.

THOMAS VAUGHAN MORROW, M.D.

By HARVEY WICKES FELTER, M.D ,
CINCINNATI.

Thomas Vaughan Morrow, M.D., the "Father of Eclecticism in the West," and founder of the Eclectic Medical Institute, was born

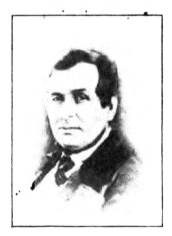

at Fairview, Ky., April 14, 1804, in the same house in which, four years later (June 3, 1808), Jefferson Davis was born. His father, Thomas Morrow, was of Scotch descent. Tradition has it that the origin and name of the family dates back to about the year 1326 A D., when Robert Bruce brought over the French architect, Thomas Moreau, to repair Melrose Abbey. A custom of the family from that day to this is to name the eldest male child Thomas, Dr. Morrow having a son and grandson of that name. A singular coincidence is that Professor Morrow, his father, and Professor Morrow's son were all born on

THOMAS VAUGHAN MORROW, M.D.

the same day of the month (April 14).

The Morrows lived in Edinburgh, Scotland, and from there went to Ireland, and settled near Monkstown, not far from Belfast. About the time of, or a little before, the French and Indian War they emigrated to the New World, settling in Winchester, Va. They took part in the war, and were with Washington at Braddock's defeat. The Morrows removed to Kentucky just after the Revolutionary War. Jeremiah Morrow, once governor of Ohio, was a first cousin of Dr. Morrow. The mother of Dr. Morrow was Elizabeth Vaughan, of English descent, but Roman Catholic in faith. After settling in Kentucky, there being no Catholic Church near, she worshiped at the Methodist Church, though to the day of her death she is said to have continued to count her beads. The Morrow ancestors were Scotch Presbyterians, and Professor Morrow was a devout Methodist.

Dr. Morrow was educated at Transylvania University, at Lexington, Ky. Going to New York, he attended and graduated at a regular medical college, and also from the Reformed Medical College conducted by Dr. Wooster Beach. Subsequently he held the chair of Obstetrics in the latter institution. After graduation he practiced in Hopkinsville, Ky. Two circumstances determined him to leave the South. He and his family had a great repugnance to slavery. A brother of Dr. Morrow's and a son of Henry Clay, who was killed at Buena Vista, were bosom companions. Clay's antagonism to slavery filled them with intense hatred for it; and Dr. Morrow declared he would never marry in a slave State.

Shortly after a disagreeable incident happened. He was boarding in the hotel at Hopkinsville, his office being near by. There was in the place a young man named ¯Pennington, of excellent family connection, who had become dissipated and the subject of several escapades. Young Pennington, with some associates, planned a robbery of the horses in the hotel stable. Dr. Morrow was putting his horse in the barn when he overheard the plot, and warned the proprietor. On a certain night the attempt at robbery was made, and the perpetrators caught and made to suffer punishment for the crime. Pennington afterward found out that Dr. Morrow had informed the proprietor of his intention to rob the stable, and he swore vengeance against his life. Shortly after, as Dr. Morrow was returning from camp-meeting, riding through a lonely dell, Pennington jumped out from the bushes, and attempted to shoot him. His pistol, however, failed to discharge. Morrow jumped from his horse, and took after him. Wherever the doctor went, he carried a cane with a concealed spring-knife in the end. Knowing his anatomy well, Dr. Morrow thrust the dagger through the ham-strings of one of Pennington's legs, crippling him for life. After this episode, Pennington still threatened his life, and Dr. Morrow removed from the State. Subsequently Pennington committed a murder, and threw the body in a sink-hole. The murder was a mystery, yet Pennington fled to Texas. After two or three years' search the detectives heard of a crippled man in the Indian Territory, and, as suspicion pointed to Pennington, they instituted search for him, and found him fiddling for the Indians. His crippled leg and skill with the violin, both of which were well-known, led to his identification. He was brought to Kentucky, tried, and hanged.

Professor Morrow was a large, handsome man, over six feet tall, and weighed about two hundred and fifty pounds. His hair was coarse and black, and his eyes blue. He seemed to have come of a race of physical, as well as mental, giants. A brother was six feet and four inches, and a nephew six and one-half feet tall. The family furnished some good orators; and the doctor, though not an orator, was a vigorous and strong speaker, using excellent language in all of his discourses. There was no more ardent Whig in America than Dr. Morrow. When, in May, 1830, the Reformed Medical Society of the United States, of which Dr. Wooster Beach was president, expressed, in a resolution, the expediency of establishing ''an additional medical school in some town on the Ohio River, or some of its tributaries,'' Thomas Vaughan Morrow stepped forward to emancipate the West from medical bigotry. Through the invitation and efforts of Colonel James Kilbourne, a medical school, known as the ''Reformed Medical College of Ohio,'' was established in 1830 at Worthington, Ohio; and Dr. Morrow, though a young man, was placed in charge. He threw himself into the work with such zeal and spirit that he soon gathered around him a body of competent associates, some of whom have become inseparably linked with the history of the greatest medical reform of modern times.

The new school, under the master-hand of Morrow, who possessed great firmness of purpose and rare executive. ability, prospered remarkably, until the seven-year financial crash, beginning in 1837, compelled its intrepid leader to curtail expenses, discontinue the issuance of the *Western Medical Reformer*, the official organ of the school, and to close the infirmary in connection with the institution. Internal dissensions and the green eye of jealousy came in for a share in wrecking the undertaking. Though sued in the courts, and in the face of the opposition of medical opponents, and a suspicious populace, culminating in a mob attack upon his school, Dr. Morrow remained steadfastly at his post, even after his colleagues had forsaken him. For ten turbulent years he remained at the helm as president of the infant institution, and at the same time carried on a large practice among the best families of the place. Notwithstanding that many felt that the cause of medical reform was crushed, the hopeful spirit and indomitable will of Professor Morrow would not entertain the idea of a lost cause.   In fact, he never regarded the Worthington enterprise as a failure, and time has abundantly proved that, though apparently a hopeless undertaking, the school had been in operation long enough to disseminate far and wide, through its graduates, the new principles and practices of the reformers, and in its death it only awaited a glorious resurrection elsewhere.

Shortly after 1840, Dr. Morrow contemplated the union of all reform medical bodies, and proposed a national committee, with subcommittees, to raise one hundred and fifty thousand dollars for a great medical university, with hospital attached, and a corps of competent professors, devoted to Reformed and Botanic medicine.   In several quarters this was looked upon with great favor.   But the wedge of disunion was entered by Dr. Lanier Bankston, of the Botanico-Medical College, of Forsythe, Georgia, attributing to Dr. Morrow ulterior motives.   The South seemed unwilling to ally itself with the platform proposed by Dr. Morrow—that of promoting the leading interests of the common cause by a willingness to adopt all improvements, whatever their source might be.   Consequently, Dr. Morrow bent his efforts toward the perfection of the reformed system alone.   The school at Worthington having closed, Dr. Morrow was persuaded to remove to Cincinnati, where his restless desire to further the cause led him, in 1842, to plan a second institution, the Reformed Medical School of Cincinnati, which finally became our Alma Mater, the Eclectic Medical Institute.   Here Dr. Morrow bent all his energies to accomplish his task.   After delivering courses of lectures for a little over two years, a charter was obtained, and the first Faculty appointed, with Professor Morrow as Dean and Professor of Theory and Practice, in which capacity he served until, in 1850, his useful and eminent career was cut short by a fatal attack of dysentery.   His remains now rest in the Wesleyan Cemetery, of Cincinnati, marked by a suitable monument.   Dr. Morrow was a manly man of excellent judgment, uncompromising honesty, and an exceptionally successful practitioner. Among his patients were many noted men; for Dr. Morrow's standing was high, Governor John Brough, Father Collins, of St. Xavier's College, and Archbishop Purcell being patrons.

Before becoming Dean of the Faculty, he had delivered about forty courses of lectures; consequently his ripe experience as a teacher served him to good advantage before the rapidly-increaeing classes at the Institute. In his teaching he had embraced the whole range of college departments.   Though it has been said that Dr. Morrow wrote but little, the pages of the *Western Medical Reformer* are replete with sound and well-written articles upon the principles and practice of the new movement and upon the treatment of diseases, and fairly bristle with pointed editorials from his pen.   After his death his writings upon diseases and their treatment were collected and published, together with his own, by Dr. Ichabod Gibson Jones, his former associate in the medical school at Worthington, in two volumes, under the title of "Jones and Morrow's Practice of Medicine."

Dr. Morrow was the first president of the National Eclectic Medical Association.   While at Worthington, he was one of the incorporators of the Worthington Female Seminary.   Before Dr. Morrow's death his chair was divided, Dr. Joseph Rodes Buchanan taking Physiology, Institutes of Medicine, and Medical Jurisprudence ; and after his death Pathology and Theory and Practice of Medicine was taught by Dr. Morrow's life-long friend, Dr. I. G. Jones. Many to whom we have written, whether of our own or opposite faith in medicine, for material for sketches, have made it emphatic that Dr. Morrow was "truly a great man."   Dr. Morrow married Isabel Greer, of Worthington.   His son, Mr. Worcester* Beech Morrow, is now an attorney at law in Cincinnati, and kindly furnished some of the items for this sketch.   Of the character and attainments of Professor Morrow let a Committee of Five, expressing the "Sentiments of the Medical Class," reply : "Dr. Morrow we consider profoundly versed in all that pertains to his department—as one vast digester of the medical doctrines of the age—and as amply competent to make plain, philosophical, and instructive what hitherto, in pathology, has been but confusion, contradiction, and absurdity.   We regard his almost unparalleled experience in the various modes of medication, at the bedside of the sick— his scientific acquisition in the department of practice, and his long and laborious experience as professor, as having so qualified him for the duties of his chair that he is placed above comparison, and is regarded by this class, and will be regarded by subsequent classes and the profession at large, as a man of rarest talent, a teacher of the greatest success, and a pillar in whose sustaining capacity the Eclectic Medical Institute can confide in all the storms she may encounter from jealousy, envy, or malignity, as she rises to an inestimable position in the work of medical reformation."

————•••————

THERE is such a condition as idiopathic swelling of the liver—an acute hepatitis—due to an unknown cause.   The condition gradually subsides without treatment.—*American Journal of Surgery.*

* The original spelling of the name of the Woosters.

ANNUAL REPORT OF THE SETON HOSPITAL.

Medical Staff.

Surgeons and Gynecologists,
L. E. RUSSELL, M.D.   J. S. HAGEN, M.D.

Physicians,
R. L. THOMAS, M.D.   THOMAS BOWLES, M.D.
L. C. WOTTRING, M.D.   E. R. FREEMAN, M.D.   V. L. BELL, M.D.

Oculist and Aurist,
K. O. FOLTZ, M.D.

Electro-Therapeutist,
OTTO JUETTNER, M.D.

Pathologist,
JOHN L. PAYNE, M.D.

Resident Physician,
VICTOR P. WILSON, M.D.

Internes.

1901-1902—G. H. Knapp,
C. G. Patterson,
Susan R. Cooper,
A. O. Barclay.

1902-1903—W. F. Weikal,
C. W. Beaman,
A. J. Kemper,
P. A. Kemper.

1903-1904—G. D. Callihan,
P. E. Decatur,
J. G. Sherman,
C. P. Krohn.

1904-1905—G. E. Dash,
C. M. L. Wolf,
Wm. A. Ellsworth,
C. J. Otto.

1905-1906—M. F. Bettencourt,
A. T. Rank,
C. L. Hudson,
A. J. Johnson.

1906-1907—Nellie Van Horn,
D. E. Rausch,
A. C. Jenner,
J. C. Shafer.

1907-1908—C. C. Hamilton,
E. W. Horswell,
C. C. McCaffery,
G. W. Sauter.

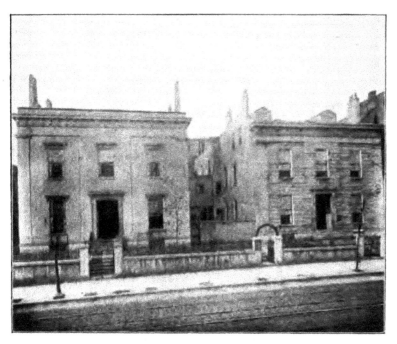

SISTERS AND NURSES HOME. LAURAL MEMORIAL HOSPITAL.

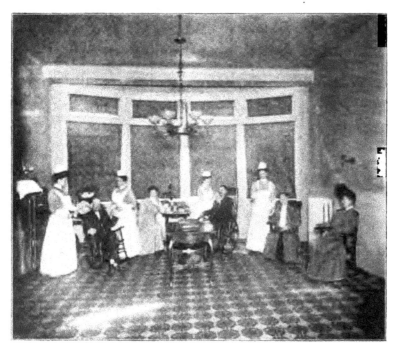

SUN PARLOR—McDONALD BUILDING.

Physicians Treating Patients During the Past Seven Years.

Allen, S. E.
Arndt, D. C.
Bacharach, F.
Bates, M. L.
Behymer, E. T.
Berry, J. T.
Bonifield, C. L.
Bowles, T.
Bloyer, W. E.
Bramble, D. D.
Brown, R.
Caldwell, J. A.
Carr, A. H.
Cassello, J. B.
Church, W. B.
Cook, L. E.
Crowe, W. F.
Denman, D. M.
Domhoff, L.
Dowling, F.
Drury, A. G.
DeCourcy, Carroll,
DeCourcy, Paul
Evans, J. C.
Feid, L. J.
Felter, H. W.
Fitzpatrick, T. V.
Francis, R. W. C.
Freeman, E. R.
Foltz, K. O.
Ford, S.
Forchheimer, W.
Grear, Louis
Grimes, J. F.
Hagen, J. S.
Haines, W. D.
Harding, W. O. C.
Heflebower, R. C.
Hines, H. H.
Hocker, E.
Hoppe, H. H.
Huffman, L. D.
Hunter, F. A.
Hunt, E.
Jenkins, J. O.
Johnson, A.
Julier, C.
Juettner, Otto.
Keefe, E. M.
Kiely, W. E.
Knapp, G. H.
Maloney, J. J.

Marcus, J. E.
May, E. S.
Meade, C. C.
Meyer, C. T.
Miller, Jno.
Miller, R.
Mitchell, G.
Noble, H.
Orr, G. B.
Payne, J. L.
Pearce, C. T.
Quinn, J. D.
Rattermann, F. L.
Ravogli, A.
Reed, Chas. A. L.
Riggs, A.
Rogers, S. T.
Russell, L. E.
Russell, C. W.
Sattler, Eric.
Sattler, Robert.
Savage, W. E.
Schwab, E.
Scudder, J. K.
Shriner, W. W.
Smith, C. G.
Smith, E. O.
Souther, C. T.
Sparks, C. M.
Spencer, J. R.
Stewart, T. M.
Strouse, Lee.
Taylor, R. E.
Thomas, L.
Thomas, R. L.
Timmerman, J. D.
Turner, W. S.
Twitchell, H.
Ulery, D. M.
Van Horn, B.
Walker, E. W.
Watkins, L.
Weaver, W. B.
Werner, W. L.
Wenning, W. H.
Wilson, V. P.
Wintermute, R. C.
Winton, C. F.
Wottring, L. C.
Yates, E.
York, J. F.

Number of Patients Admitted.

1900	.	.	.	.	.	.	139	1904	.	.	.	.	.	.	267
1901	.	.	.	.	.	.	177	1905	.	.	.	.	.	.	214
1902	.	.	.	.	.	.	231	1906	.	.	.	.	.	.	282
1903	.	.	.	.	.	.	243	1907	.	.	.	.	.	.	369

Total 1922

The Seton Hospital was started with a modest beginning in 1900 at Eighth and Cutter Streets, with a capacity of ten beds. In 1901 a three-story addition was added, with the financial aid of the Eclectic Medical Institute. This added sixteen rooms and a well-lighted amphitheatre for surgical operations, seating over 100 students.

The location of the hospital in the west end of the city in a thickly settled neighborhood filled a long-felt want, and professional friends soon filled it to its capacity, necessitating turning away of many cases in the winter of 1906 and 1907.

In the spring of 1907, the Sisters of Charity had an opportunity of purchasing the Presbyterian Hospital property on Sixth Street and Kenyon Avenue, west of Mound Street. This included four buildings and complete equipment.

The Seton Hospital was removed to the new location in June.

The building at 626 West Sixth Street is used as a Sisters' and Nurses' Home. The building at 618 West Sixth Street (The Laura Memorial Hospital) is used for children's and obstetric wards and private rooms for medical cases.

The McDonald building on Kenyon Avenue is devoted exclusively to surgery. It faces on the proposed Bathgate Park, bounded by Kenyon, Cutter, Barr and Mound Streets.

The first floor is devoted to the Seton Dispensary, which is open daily from 8 : 30 to 10 : 30 A. M.

The second floor embraces a male and female ward, with a capacity of twelve patients each. The third and fourth floors embrace an excellent, well-lighted operating room, sun parlor and twenty-eight private rooms.

The building is almost new and is modern in every respect, and was erected at a cost of $75,000.

The new location has given us an opportunity of enlarging our Training School for Nurses.

The Seton Hospital will receive any case excepting contagious diseases, and is open on the same terms to any reputable physician.

For particulars in regard to rates for private rooms or ward service,

Address, SISTER FLORENTINE, *Superior*,

618 West Sixth Street,

Tel. West 2614.   Cincinnati, Ohio.

Texas Eclectic Medical Association.

PROCEEDINGS OF THE TWENTY-FOURTH ANNUAL MEETING.

L. S. DOWNS, M.D., EDITOR.

EMPIRICISM AND DOGMATISM IN MEDICINE.

BY P. A. SPAIN, M.D.,
PARIS, TEXAS.

In medical parlance the terms dogmatism and empiricism are frequently encountered, and hence a little discussion of the relative meaning, and application of the two terms would not be out of place.

The word empiricism gets its root meaning from the Greek, "*peira*," meaning "a trial," and hence in medicine would give us the germ idea of a practice based upon trial or experiment.

The word dogmatism gets its root formation from the Greek, "*dokes*," to think, and hence, as applied to medicine, its germ idea is a practice based upon thoughtful or theoretical suggestions. Expanding upon these two ideas, we may say that the empiric gives treatment because it has been tried and seemed successful; the dogmatist says something else is better because it is based on good principles. Empiricism says experience is my guide; dogmatism says reason is my guide. The fact is, both plans are subject to the broadest latitude of error, and both plans are fraught with much that is good.

It is very hard sometimes to meet the argument of a man when he says : "This is right, I've tried it." All sorts of authority, high and low, in empirical ranks, stand by this proposition. The old woman with her catnip and garlic teas will challenge every college professor in the land on that proposition; she has tried them. The faith healer, the charmer, the rubber, the fellow with 30-X triturations and dilutions all stand by the proposition, "I've tried it," and the common mind allows no question of such authority. The history of violations of this authority is sometimes written in blood.

We sometimes hear it said that experience is the test of theory. In a great measure, this is true, but is no more true than the counter-proposition that theory is the test of experience. Each one is the test of the other; each is the looking-glass through which we view the truths or fallacies of the other. Each plan of research, when followed in its exclusiveness, will lead us into the gravest of errors.

Many of the greatest mistakes in the medical history long bore the sanction of experience until some pungent logician arose and flayed the practice into disuse. So, likewise, many of the theories of would-be scientists have been condemned to the haze of mysticism by the tri-square of experiment.

There is this difference between the practical operation of empiri-cism and dogmatism. 'Empiricism is the sole field of the ignorant man, and every honest physician realizes that his bump of ignorance is considerably larger than his bump of actual knowledge.

Our ignorance usually keeps most of us largely within the empiric field. We all remember the old adage that "Experience is a dear school, but fools learn in no other," and that hits the most of us. So few of us are trained to think. We cannot grasp or comprehend a broad theory. Logical sequences are usually beyond the ken of the average man. Experiment alone can appeal to their beclouded visions. But to the mind of the truly educated physician both the fields of empiricism and dogmatism are alike open, and to such a mind both are alike unsatisfactory until one corroborates the other. The greatest man in medicine is undoubtedly the profound thinker, the profound theorist, who has equal respect for experimental methods.

Mediocrity is usually content to tread the paths of custom and stick well to the traditions of the fathers. Thus it is that the body of humanity is slow to evolutionize itself into better standards. No country is a progressive country in which the customs and traditions of ancestry are held too sacred for violation. China is a fair example of this condition.

Positive and negative electricity meet with the evolution of fire. Empiricism and dogmatism are the positive and negative of poles of medical research, and their union produces the fire of truth. Theo-retically, the pure empiric is the man who does much and stops to think but little ; the pure dogmatic thinks much and does but little. Both extremes alike become the sport of the other, and both are equally ridiculed by broader and more liberal culture.

Men in all ages have been disposed to become extremists on one side or the other. As a result, the man with theories and the man with experimental facts, so-called, have always been in constant war-fare, when the real truth could be found by harmoniousty blending the two.

It would be unjust to claim superiority to either course in pro-moting the world's progress. Dogmatism represents the triumph of mind over matter in the solution of intricate problems, while empiri-cism represents the constructive force that is constantly putting in practice the findings of dogmatical research. The purely dogmatic is full of errors until he is trimmed down by the practical experimenter. The purely empiric does much of his work in old-fashioned and often bungling methods until he is dragged out of them by the man who teaches him the principles underlying his business. Dogmatism solves the problem of a better way ; empiricism is the proof of the solution, and the result is finished science, the hope of the world, at least in its material career.

Columbus was, to his contemporaries, an unwelcome dogmatic, a theorist until he actually proved by his own experiment that the world was a globe and subject to circumnavigation. Socrates, Aristotle, Galileo, Newton and others like worthy were considered in their day as arrant dogmatics full of heresies. The dogmatist has ever been the martyr in history. The man who goes on and does things in an empirical way just because somebody before him did the same is rarely ever disturbed in the even tenor of his way. It is the man who thinks and theorizes and searches for ground principles until he is convinced of a better way who drinks the hemlock or goes to the stake or guillotine for mere opinion's sake. The inconoclast, the man with opinons, the man who is ready to violate the traditions of the fathers, the man who founds a new system of philosophy, or looks into the future and seeing new vistas of beauty and utility attempts to lead his fellows thither—this is the man who is so often hounded to his death by the anathemas of the sticklers for the old régime.

THE DOCTOR AND HIS MEDICINE.

By W. O. B. REMY, M.D.,
WILMER, TEXAS.

I would be gratified, indeed, if I were able to command language to portray to your minds all that this subject means in its fullest sense, but I shall only attempt to say some things and those in a general way. The question that suggests itself to our minds is, What is the doctor? As Emerson said of the gentleman, '' he is a man of truth, lord of his own actions, and expressing that lordship in his behavior, not in any manner servile either upon persons or opinions or possessions beyond his manhood first and then gentleness.'' He is charity in its broadest significations, true benevolence, earnest well-wishing, and active well-doing. It is not merely in service, but in dollars and cents.

I am sure the doctor has laid his highest offerings upon the altar of sweet charity. With open hand and heart he ministers to the afflicted, with sympathy active and alert, day by day and night after night. His ministrations are commanded by the indigent. The true doctor stands for patriotism, devotion to country, in war, in peace, in prosperity and adversity. In all the glorious annals of our country's military history he occupies a conspicuous place. Never does the tocsin of war sound and the trumpet call to the field of sacrifice and suffering that the doctor does not respond. With death upon every side, he stands like a granite mountain, a restoring refuge for the wounded.

The true and loyal doctor does not endorse the oppression of the weak by the strong, and lends no acceptance to the doctrine that might makes right. With the last drop of his unselfish blood he would defend his native land against hostile invasion, or sacrifice himself in the protection of the laws and the preservation of her institutions. But to more properly picture the true, ideal doctor, we will endeavor to show some of the infallible signs that make the highest standard of perfection.

He is courteous, kind, considerate and obliging. He is a friend true and tried, both to the sick and the poor. He prescribes alike to the righteous and the unrighteous; to all classes and conditions of society he is the same. He so studies human nature that even the humblest or vilest among men may enter his presence without fear or trembling. He knows no isms, no schools, no creed. Values the friendship of all reputable physicians. He does not endeavor to build up a practice by abusing a fellow-practitioner. He attends strictly to his own professional work. If he possesses real merit he relies upon that alone to secure to him a full measure of success,

He is strictly loyal to his patients. He reveals nothing that would in any way injure his reputation among men. He works unceasingly and unselfishly for the recovery of his patients. He does not magnify his patient's malady nor manufacture imaginary ills in order to secure patronage. He does not in any way retard his restoration in order to extort from him an unnecessary fee. He does not boast of having performed miraculous cures in order to exploit his own name and fame. He strives not simply to restore in the shortest possible time the body to health and vigor; he aims, moreover, with equal diligence to guarantee to the sufferer peace and tranquility of mind. His patient's welfare is, indeed, to him of supreme importance. He is charitable; no other class of professional men so perfectly exhibit in their lives this cardinal virtue. When friend and kindred fail to comfort and console, and all others have forsaken him, the dying patient can turn to his physician assured that in him he has a friend, steadfast, immovable, always abounding in charity, year in and year out. Often without the slightest hope of pecuniary recompense, the physician as an angel of mercy ministers to those in penury and destitution. Some can say that the county has provided a home and a physician, but is it fair to deprive a man of his choice among physicians simply because he is poor? Is not the humblest creature in the lowliest hut as much entitled to his choice of physicians as the wealthiest citizen in the costliest mansion?

The true doctor is a man whose moral and Christian character is above reproach. His word should be as good as his bond, his character should be as gold tried in the fire, he should cultivate a conscience, void of offense toward God and toward man.

The physcian looks not upon the wine when it is red, for, as a physician, he knows full well it at last biteth like a serpent and stingeth like an adder. He into whose hands are placed the lives of human beings, of all men should possess a steady hand and an unclouded intellect.

These are some of the tangible signs that mark the physician, While much more can be said, I will for the present pass to the second part of the subject.

THE DOCTOR'S MEDICINE.

The question is of considerable importance. It is the doctor's weapon of warfare, whereby he may be able, by the proper application of means and remedies, to rob the grim monster, death, of its victim.

The doctor that understands therapeutics best, as a general thing, is the most successful as a practitioner. He may be a bright scholar, understand theory, and to all outward appearance a fine physician, but if he is lacking in the knowledge of the remedies and means to successfully combat and treat the pathological conditions, he is a failure. To be ever ready is to be resourceful. There lies the chief difference between the Eclectic physician and the Allopath or regular school. Meet them in consultation, and you will find it to be the fact that the majority know but little in regard to remedies besides calomel, quinine, bromide, morphia, iodide, the mineral acids, and a few others. Ask them about passiflora, macrotys, bryonia, echinacea, thuja, etc.— almost any of the specific medicines—and they will tell you they never used them and don't know. The skilful physician is able for the emergencies, and should not be at a loss to know what to do. Life, in many cases, depends upon the quick and immediate action of the proper remedies and means used. No time to wait and discuss theory and bugology. But the doctor should be able to treat the patient at once. As to the kind of medicine used, that is a matter of choice. He has the whole world of remedies to choose from, mineral or vegetable preparations, liquid or powder or tablet form. I am rather partial towards the fluid preparations, from the fact that they are quicker in action and will give better results than either tablets or pills. Tablets are too hard—take too long to dissolve in the stomach—and are not easily assimilated. If used at all they should be previously crushed and then dissolved in water before taken. So when choosing a medicine for continued every-day use, he wants to use that kind of preparation that he can rely upon giving the very best results. He wants to be thoroughly acquainted with the preparation he uses, and he becomes so by constant every-day use. He wants to choose that which is easiest handled, and not too bulky to carry. In my opinion, the preparations to meet the requirements of the up-to-date Eclectic physician are the specific medicines. The more I use them the better I like them.

You will never fail to get the effect wanted if given in proper doses. Whatever the Eclectic physician ought to do, in my opinion, is to dispense his own medicines, especially if he is doing much of a country practice. And even in the city it will pay.

I was at one time acquainted with a doctor who dispensed his own medicine, seldom ever wrote a prescription. While he was not any better doctor than the other physicians, he made more money than any two doctors in town. We are all aware of the fact that among druggists there is a great deal of counter prescribing done, and the only way, in my opinion, to correct that is for the practitioner to dispense his own medicine. He knows then just what he is giving. No substitution, he can expect results wanted. Make a careful diagnosis, painstaking, no hasty work about it; too many doctors are careless in examining their patients. It will pay to carefully go over the case and find out what is the matter. This ostentatious display of methods to impress the patient is not the thing. Be thorough; the doctor that will do that will certainly establish for himself a reputation. I can't tell how many have said to me in regard to Dr. So-and-So: "He never pretended to examine me; never even looked at my tongue. All he did was to give me calomel and quinine, that made me awful sick."

The doctor should not pose as a know-all or a cure-all doctor, but be able for the emergencies. As I have said before, by his courteous, kind and considerate manner, gain the friendship of all classes.

There is a very important matter connected with the practice of medicine, which by many is greatly neglected, and that is collecting their bills. The doctor should be a good collector. The doctor, as a general thing, who is careless in collecting will be in dispensing. We should unite on that one point. Outside of worthy charitable cases, make the people pay or not practice for them. Let them know that just because you are a doctor they have no right to your time and skill without remuneration, and that in a reasonable time, at least during a lifetime, and a short one at that.

Collect your bills, so that you can be able to pay your own bills; you can then be better prepared to give your patrons good service. If you are all the time financially pressed you can't give yourself that much-needed rest and recreation that every hard-working physician is entitled to, in order to be active in the work and not dull and sluggish. Lastly, but not least, let us regard mankind as one vast brotherhood ; especially the physicians should be brothers.

As each of us know the hardships we have to undergo amid the desolating plague, the physician and surgeon goes forth braving all dangers and enduring every hardship.

In his merciful work he makes no distinction between the high-born and the lowly, friend or foe, at whose call for help he feels it his duty to respond ; no danger, no loathsome disease repels him. He is found on the battlefield attending the sick and the dying. Every where he is a Good Samaritan. The tireless searcher of that knowl-edge that will more speedily cure, abate and prevent disease—no hour is set apart for repose. While others are resting from the labors of the day the physician is rising to bring hope and relief to the chambers of the sick. So when life's duty is done and life's race is run, with a clear conscience he may wrap the draperies of his couch about him and lie down to pleasant dreams.

DROWNING.

By H. H. BLANKMEYER, M.D.,
HONEY GROVE, TEXAS.

In the *Chicago Medical Times*, November, 1906, I read Professor H. K. Whitford's article on drowning, which to me was very interest-ing. You know it is, as he there states, a commonly accepted fact :

1. That a drowned person under water five minutes cannot be restored to life.

2. That a drowned person going into the water *alive* has his lungs filled with the fluid.

3. That a person drowned must not be resuscitated by the use of heat.

To all three of these accepted ideas he takes a most emphatic oppo-site stand, and with convincing argument. He argues that a person can be restored to life even if apparently dead *an hour* or more, and all this time under water, so long as decomposition or breaking down of tissue has not taken place, and he quotes cases that he has actually resuscitated, while two other doctors failed, and all three patients were drowned at the same time and in like manner. He argues that a person going into the water alive *never* gets any in his lungs while drowning, because as soon as two or three drops touch the epiglottis it will spasmodically contract and close the entrance of the trachea, which, as you know, is the passage to the lungs.

Therefore, a person taken from the water with water in his lungs was most likely dead or unconscious *before* entering the water, and therefore the generally accepted evidence that the person entered the water dead, if the lungs are found free of water, according fo Dr. Whitford, is false. He argues that to-day men are serving penitentiary sentences upon the circumstantial "water in the lung theory" who may be innocent of murder.

The water you have seen come from the mouth of a drowned person when rolled over a barrel or held with feet elevated was from the stomach, and not the lungs.

Dr. Whitford argues that to resuscitate a drowned person heat should be used and not withheld. In drowning, the body becomes chilled, and naturally the blood thickens and the capillaries become clogged ; therefore, it would be the height of folly to cause artificial respiration and try to make the heart force congealed blood to flow through frozen capillaries. Get the capillaries and blood in condition first and *then* perform artificial respiration. Don't that seem reasonable ? What engineer would ever think of making steam and power if he knew the pipes were filled with mud and ice before he would get such ice or mud in condition that it would move and allow the steam to circulate ?

"Here is the main point of this paper that I wish to bring forward." If Dr. Whitford is correct in his views—and I like them better than any I have ever heard—" *haste is not necessary in restoring a drowned person.*" It will be difficult to make the friends of the drowned person see it as you do, and most likely you will hear criticisms about you for not working with the body as soon as it is taken from the water and losing time waiting for water to be heated ; while to cause artificial respiration before the capillaries are ready would be to only injure a good heart trying to move blood before it is in a flowing condition. You might satisfy the friends by busying yourself with the body and getting ready for the hot bath, or by using friction, but *don't* attempt artificial respiration *until* your case is ready.

The actual method of artificial respiration is not the essential feature. You all know the Paris or Laborde method of drawing out the tongue and jerking it rhythmatically. It is claimed this produces an artificial hiccough, which excites the diaphragm to contract and the heart to resume its function. Hot fomentations to the epigastrium assist.

The Sylvester method is to draw the tongue forward, move the arms from side of body upwards until they nearly meet over the head, and then slowly bring the arms down until the elbows meet over the abdomen; repeat this movement sixteen to eighteen times per minute.

Marshall Hall's method is to place the body flat on abdomen, press on back with hands gently but intermittently, then change the position of the body from face downward to side or farther, then back upon abdomen again, doing this about sixteen times per minute.

The Michigan method is to place the body face downward, with forehead upon the forearm; stand astride the body and grasp it about the shoulders, raise chest as high as possible without removing head from arm, holding it about three seconds; then place body upon the ground again, press lower ribs downward then upward, gradually increasing force, for ten seconds. Suddenly let go and repeat lifting as before.

Dr. H. K. Whitford's common-sense, practical method is to restore the normal temperature of the body first. This, he writes, is best accomplished in a bath-tub with the stopper so arranged that the water will gradually and slowly escape, allowing more hot water to be added from time to time, and thus keeping the water at one temperature. While the patient is in the tub the stimulation can be increased by pouring the hot water from a height of five or six feet on the body, avoiding the face and spine. If a bath-tub is not handy, use blankets soaked in hot water, repeating as often as necessary to get body and circulation back to normal. If you are where hot water or blankets are not to be had, then do the best you can with friction to get normal temperature of the surface and capillaries. When you have caused as much stimulation as you can toward normal circulation, then draw the tongue forward with a tongue-forceps, or by use of your fingers and a cloth; raise the spasmodically closed epiglottis with your finger and give free passage of air through the trachea to the lungs. *Then*, cause artificial respiration by any method best known to you, and if the blood current has been properly prepared it will not take more than five or ten minutes' work at artficial respiration to accomplish happy results.

UTERINE DISPLACEMENTS.

By C. E. FRAZIER, M.D.,
WEATHERFORD, TEXAS.

Carefully studying the literature of some dozen or more journals that come to my hand weekly and monthly for the past year, and from personal experience, I have been endeavoring to gain some new ideas for the Association this year. I have kept this subject in mind hoping that I might be able to give you something in addition to the text-book descriptions, but I fear I have not much to offer.

The general displacements are, as we all know, forward and backward, downward and twisted, designated respectively as anteversion and -flexion, retroversion and -flexion, prolapsus, and torsion, also classified as movable and immovable.

Many medical treatments have been suggested, each, doubtless, possessing an element of merit; but that none have ever been proven specific is apparent by their number and diversity. That good, common-sense uterine tonics do good there can be no doubt; especially is this so when the uterine displacements are the result of muscular weakness or functional inertia.

Among the legion of medical remedies whose advocates advance the strongest claim for it as a specific, and whose use has in my hands been the most disappointing, is sepia 3x or 6x. When I first read about sepia I procured some, but I have had uniform failures in every case where I have used it for uterine displacements. I have found that the good old macrotys, helonias, and kindred uterine tonics are about the best medical treatment. Glycerine and calendula tampons were formerly used extensively for certain displacements, but the benefits derived from their use have been so doubtful that they are now about abandoned by the majority of physicians, although in some special selected cases tampons still have their place.

Taxis manipulated in the knee-chest position for retroversion and -flexion and in the dorsal position for anteflexion and -version, and absolute rest in bed, will sometimes effect a cure. The patient should be instructed that there should be no lifting of anything for weeks or months after a replacement has been effected; and it is always well to keep patient quiet in bed a good while. There are some cases where the round ligaments are so stretched, either from gestation or tumors, that they will not resume their normal conditions without surgical interference, and this state of affairs, unfortunately, occurs in a large number of cases.

The method of surgical procedure seems to be handled differently by, and according to the caprice of, each authority, but I have yet to learn of a better way than that described by a writer in the *Chicago Medical Times* about a year or two ago. The method is an old one, and I am not sure that the writer in this instance claimed originality, but at any rate he emphasized and elaborated what appears to me to be the best operative procedure in vogue at present in this line of cases, namely, opening the abdomen in the median line, bringing up and attaching the uterus to the abdominal parietes. The sutures will be absorbed and adhesions will be formed which will hold the uterus in place.   The supporting ligaments of the uterus are sometimes also shortened in this operation. In the median line very little or no hemorrhage will be encountered, and on the whole the operation can be performed with comparative safety to patient and certainty of desirable results.

(*To be continued.*)

Seton Hospital Reports.

BY L. E. RUSSELL, M.D., SURGEON.

Case 120.—Mrs. M., widow, thirty-five years of age, husband dead five years ; has three children, the youngest seven years of age. This patient confesses to a few accidental excursions.   Recently there has been irregular menstrual conditions, a missed period, a recurring menstrual flow, and then an intermittent bleeding for a few days ; also a very sudden enlargement in the left pelvic quadrant extending to the crest of the left ilium ; soreness and pain quite constant. The patient sought the services of an abortionist, who for a paltry sum attempted to produce abortion by the introduction of instruments, and after three attempts in about as many weeks the patient developed a severe pelvic peritonitis.

It was just at this time that the regular family physician was called in to take charge of the case, and as this was the physician's second ectopic case presented at the clinic this winter, the diagnosis was very readily made out, and the patient placed in bed in the hospital for about a week, attempting to reduce the tympanitic condition manifest in the abdominal cavity, and prepare the patient for the laparotomy. We make a liberal median incision, about six inches in length, and, as we approach the peritoneum, it shows a black, mottled condition—positive evidence of destructive inflammatory conditions.

On making the intrusion within the abdominal cavity there is extensive adhesions of omentum, bound down in the left pelvic quadrant ; much of this omentum is destroyed and in the nature of gangrene. We shall therefore ligate and take away all that has been destroyed.

We now have a mass about the size of a man's double fist ; there is a blood-clot, gestation-sac, placenta, and all the débris that makes a clinical picture in so aggravated a case of ectopic gestation. As the destruction advanced the fundus and posterior part of the womb is found to be denuded of its peritoneal cover and bound by adhesive inflammatory exudates to intestines. The condition in the pelvis is such that we deem it the safer plan to remove the uterus and appendages, giving us free drainage down through the vagina. We therefore place about two feet of plain gaze, spread out to protect all pelvic trauma, with one end projecting through the vagina to act as a constant drainage.

————————

Eye, Ear, Nose and Throat.

CONDUCTED BY KENT O. FOLTZ, M.D.

FOLLICULAR TONSILLITIS.

Synonyms.—Lacunar tonsillitis, cryptic tonsillitis.

In this type of tonsillitis there may be only a few of the crypts affected, or the entire gland may be involved. In the latter condition it is really a parenchymatous tonsillitis.

Etiology.—The anatomical structure of the tonsil is a factor in causing this form of tonsillitis to be quite common. The crypts are deep, and their openings being small, any change in the character of the secretion, or irritation of the surface of the gland will be liable to cause retention of secretion by constricting the openings. This retention will produce irritation of the crypt walls, increasing the amount of secretion, which being retained soon undergoes decomposition, forming a nidus for infection. A subnormal condition of the system may also be a predisposing factor. Sudden climatic changes are important factors.

Symptoms.—Pain is a characteristic and constant symptom. The pain is increased by any motion that causes movement of the pharyngeal muscles. A sharp neuralgic pain, passing from the throat to the ear and sometimes to the cervical region, is frequently complained of. The voice is changed in quality. There may be an irritating cough which is usually reflex in character, the result of inflammatory pressure on the recurrent laryngeal and phrenic nerves. There is an almost constant desire or effort to clear the throat. Usually but one tonsil is affected at a time.

Not infrequently it is almost impossible to swallow either liquids or solids, and sometimes when the effort is made there will be regurgitation of the material. Middle ear disease may result through extension of the inflammation to the vault of the pharynx and Eustachian tubes.

Inspection of the tonsil is often difficult in severe cases, as the patient cannot open the mouth sufficiently to give the examiner a good view of the faucial region. When possible to get a good view, the surface of the tonsil appears deeply reddened and edematous, with whitish or yellowish points, indicating the mouths of the crypts. If there is a profuse inflammatory exudate, there is a sero-fibrinous material covering more or less of the surface, and resembling a membranous inflammation. Febrile symptoms vary, but usually there is an increase of temperature, the skin dry and warm, and more or less nausea.

As the disease progresses, especially as suppuration occurs, there will be chills, the skin will be clammy, face pallid and with an anxious expression, and mental dullness. The tongue is heavily coated, usually a pasty or dirty colored coating, and the breath is characteristically offensive. Thirst is constant, and especially annoying on account of the difficulty in swallowing.

The usual clinical symptoms of an inflammation are found in this type of tonsillitis. Constipation, scanty, high colored urine, with an excess of urea and urates, and sometimes some albumin. In the later stages the glands at the angle of the jaw are usually enlarged.

Diagnosis.—Usually not difficult if the case is seen early and is one of moderate severity, but sometimes, quite frequently, in fact, in the milder attacks the true condition is overlooked. It is especially of this class of cases I wish to speak. The tonsils may not be much enlarged, and the affected crypts are hidden by the anterior pillars of the fauces, so unless a careful examination is made the morbid state is not seen. The tonsils should be brought into view, either by causing the patient to gag, or by drawing the anterior pillars aside with a blunt hook. When this is done there will usually be revealed the affected crypts.

Prognosis.—Favorable if seen early and proper remedial measures are instituted, as then there is seldom suppuration.

Treatment.—Evacuation of the crypts is necessary. This can be done quite thoroughly by wrapping a small pledget of cotton tightly around the end of an ordinary cotton carrier and pushing this into the crypt. With a rotary motion the probe and cotton should be withdrawn, when the crypt will be found free from the accumulated material. After each crypt has been cleansed, the patient is ready for the usual treatment indicated in tonsillar inflammations. Unless these crypts are emptied, the reparative process is slow, and suppuration is more liable to occur than when proper cleansing is done in the beginning of the affection.

The Significance of Subconjunctival Ecchymosis.

Diagnosis and then prognosis are reached by an intelligent interpretation and analysis of the aggregated symptoms before us. Hence to judge aright the importance of a symptom, it is necessary to consider the causes which produce it and the relative importance of results which may follow. It is with this thought in mind that the subject of this paper is offered.

Idiopathic ecchymosis of the conjunctiva is comparatively frequent. A blotchy, uniform hemorrhagic spot in the conjunctiva with sharp uniform limitation of outline. It is distinguished from inflammatory redness by the absence of any network of vessels.

The suddenness of its appearance is alarming to the patient, though generally there is an absence of pain or much irritation.

In his efforts to reassure the alarmed patient, the physician usually makes light of it and dismisses it as an occurrence of little importance. In fact, the text-books on the eye devote but a few lines to it. But I am of the opinion that in many cases it is of serious significance, sufficient to justify at least a brief consideration.

Ecchymosis of the conjunctiva may result from various causes. It may follow great bodily exertion, sneezing, whooping-cough, local injury, and at times fracture of the base of the skull.

A predisposition to a rupture of the conjunctival arteries is found in those with weakened or brittle arteries in general. Hence more frequent among older people, or in those with arteriosclerosis or atheromatous softening; therefore, where there is loss of elasticity with high arterial tension, or a consequent diminution of resistance with added blood pressure.

This tendency to lack of elasticity and weakening is likewise associated with gout, syphilis, lead poison, alcoholic abuse, nephritis, rheumatism, and is also found in typhoid and scarlet fever. This is not local but general.

Why the rupture is more frequent in the conjunctival vessels, is probably because of the delicacy of this structure and the lack of tissue support, and hence of resistance.

It will thus be seen that the conjunctival ecchymosis is as a rule a complication which follows some definite predisposing cause, associated with a lessened arterial resistance, either temporary or permanent. This being general and not local predisposes to similar hemorrhages in any other part of the body; in the brain (apoplexy), inner eye, heart walls, kidneys, etc.

The majority of cases coming under my observation have been in persons over fifty years of age, where the predisposing causes mentioned above are most likely to be found.

In connection with this subject has been, to me, another interesting fact. Last summer I had five cases of conjunctival ecchymosis within the short space of three weeks' time. We are all aware of that strange and unexplained law of coincidence, where several cases of cataract, strabismus or enucleation follow at short intervals. In these last-mentioned cases there could not be any special predisposing cause to explain, for they have nothing in common. But in the conjunctival hemorrhage, in the class of patients it is most frequently found, there is generally a similar underlying cause : brittle arteries and increased arterial tension. So in my five cases mentioned I can readily believe that some atmospheric or telluric influence, which regulated atmospheric pressure at that time, was the real cause of the increased arterial tension, and the hemorrhage was a natural result of the combination of conditions present.

This view may perhaps be more readily accepted when we recall the well-known effects of variations in atmospheric tension in balloon ascensions when high altitudes with rarified air are reached, where hemorrhages from the nose, ears and even eyes are recorded. The inner pressure is greater than the outer ; the equilibrium is disturbed and hence the hemorrhage is outward. In the compressed air of the caisson, in bridge building, the hemorrhage is inward, as in the spinal cord or brain tissue. But in neither of these cases is the defect universally uniform; some are more easily affected than others, depending upon the arterial condition and capacity of resistance of each individual.

The reasons for the presentation of this paper and the conclusions which follow will now be evident. They are :

1. Conjunctival ecchymosis is a result of increased arterial tension with a weakened resistance, which is probably general as well as local.

2. Such cases are of serious import and prognostic significance. When they occur the situation should be carefully investigated, the conditions thoroughly explained to the patient so afflicted and, if examination shows increased arterial tension with indications of arteriosclerosis or athermatous degeneration, the patient should be carefully instructed and warned to avoid anything which could aggravate or intensify such predisposition, and thus be enabled to avoid as far as possible the occurrence of a more serious cerebral hemorrhage which might easily terminate fatally ; for truly, as a celebrated surgeon has said, "A man is as old as his arteries."—JAMES A. CAMPBELL, M.D., in *Homœopathic Eye, Ear and Throat Journal*.

Dr. H. Marion Sims, the father of gynecology, said : "For severe dysmenorrhea I have found Hayden's Viburnum Compound of great service." See notes by Marion Sims, Volume No. 2, of Grailly Hewitt, on Diseases of Women. Few drugs employed in the treatment of diseases of women have gained the commendation of so excellent an authority, and like expressions since the time of Sims have been uttered by many of the best men in the medical profession. Hayden's Viburnum Compound has stood the test of time for twenty-six years, and is the recognized standard viburnum product by which imitators would measure.

Periscope.

Staphisagria and Mistletoe.

Specific staphisagria is prepared from the seeds of delphinium staphisagria, commonly known as stavesacre. The medicinal action, if the agent be carefully administered, is as reliable as any of the specific preparations.

In a general sense, staphisagria acts upon the prostate gland. It is not curative in the entire range of the diseases of this organ, but for certain conditions it is very reliable.

In prostatorrhea its influence is not so marked as in chronic cases of spermatorrhea. In chronic gleet I have been enabled to do more in the complete cure of the cases with this remedy than with any other single remedy, having succeeded nicely even in very protracted cases. It is not ordinarily advised in the acute stages of inflammation of the prostate, but in cases of subacute or chronic enlargement with chronic irritation it is useful, especially if combined with saw-palmetto. I have certainly found these two remedies to work very nicely together.

In urinary irritation, common to old men with prostatic enlargement, with frequent desire to urinate, it overcomes the desire and the subsequent tenesmus, producing a sensation of restored tone. This result will occur if there is any inflammation of the bladder, provided it is combined with thuja or with chimaphila.

There is a class of these stubborn conditions that will yield to a combination of these three remedies, with perhaps the addition of gelsemium or cimicifuga if the nerves are involved, and will induce results most highly satisfactory.

I should like to have reports of the use of this remedy in the treatment of irritability of the vesiculæ seminales and of the prostate ducts, not uncommon between the ages of forty-five and fifty with men who have been excessive and dissipated in their habits..

The remedy has been recommended in prolapsus of the bladder-walls where an operation was impossible and where there was a long train of distressing symptoms.

In the treatment of certain forms of impotency I give this remedy with saw-palmetto and avena. It increases sexual power when imperfect and arrests excessive prostatic discharges.

It is a remedy for nervous excitement and nervous irritability which depends upon sexual irritation or upon any disease of the genito-urinary organs. It should be given for certain forms of mental depression which occur in conjunction with hysteria or hypochondriasis, especially if accompanied with violent outbursts of passion.

Mistletoe.—I have been inclined to believe that this remedy has been disappointing with many users, because of the fact that the fluid preparations were not made from the green plant. Furthermore, it must be given in sufficient doses, and in many cases it is best to 1epeat these doses frequently until a mild physiological action of the remedy appears.

If we were to compare its influence with that of many other well-known remedies, we should find some point of resemblance quite marked between it and ergot. It produces contraction of the involuntary muscular fibre the same as ergot, but it does this without causing irritation, in medicinal doses.

It also acts upon the circulation of the brain, overcoming engorgement and excessive fullness of the circulation. It should be administered with positiveness when there is an undue flow of blood to the brain, with intermittent headaches and a tendency to a flushed condition of the face which appears and disappears frequently. If this condition be present with hysteria, or where there is a tendency to epilepsy, with other nervous manifestations, it will be found especially efficacious.

I am inclined to think that a very happy combination in these cases can be made between this remedy and gelsemium. Not only in these cases but in painful conditions, such as those conditions which produce a sensation of tearing or rending pain, or where there are rheumatic or neuralgic pains. Some writers have claimed that in these cases it is an ideal pain subduer, especially where the pain is not extreme.

There are conditions accompanied with the above symptoms when amenorrhea or dysmenorrhea are present, in which from its influence upon the uterine muscular fibre, conjoined with its influence upon the central nervous system, and especially upon the capillary circulation of the central nervous system, it should be selected as an ideal remedy.

Dr. Brodnax, in his time widely known as a medical writer, told me that he had given this remedy in the form of an infusion for a number of years, as an oxytocic. He began when the pains were feeble and administered it in frequent doses, expecting that it would increase the pain, promote dilation and normal expulsive effort. His opinion confirms that of others, that the remedy produces a normal, intermittent uterine action, while ergot produces spasmodic contractions, which have but little resemblance to the regular, normal pains. It seems to exercise its full force upon the larger muscles of the uterus, causing the fundus to contract while the cervix remains soft and dilated.

No observations of any untoward results have been made. It does not seem to produce those painful contractions which bring on disaster, as ergot may do.

Quite a number of other valuable observations have been made concerning the action of this remedy. One writer has recently used it in the treatment of chorea, especially those cases which were of long standing and very persistent—not amenable to usual treatment. He gave five drops of the fluid extract of mistletoe every two hours, with satisfactory results. Other physicians have used the remedy as an antispasmodic in the convulsions of childhood, with good results.

Dr. Tascher, at one time Dean of Bennett Medical College, was convinced that this agent had considerable merit in the treatment of diseases of the heart. He gave twenty drops four or five times a day where there was hypertrophy with valvular insufficiency, accompanied with dropsy of the extremities, slow, weak pulse, difficulty in breathing and an inability to rest in a reclining position. In one or two cases he was astonished at the result. The pulse became full, strong and regular, there was relief from the difficult breathing, the patient was enabled to lie down and there was a greatly increased flow of urine and serous discharges from the bowels with increased action of the skin, which resulted in very decided relief of the dropsical symptoms.

I have not observed any claim of this kind made by any other writer, but Dr. Tascher was a very close observer and a successful physician. I have confidence in his statements and believe that the remedy should be tried so that we may determine whether it is of benefit in this class of cases or not.

This remedy may be given with excellent advantage combined with strychnine, during the latter stages of typhoid or other asthenic fevers where the heart's action is weak, rapid and irregular, and where there is a tendency to collapse.—FINLEY ELLINGWOOD, M.D., in *American Journal of Clinical Medicine.*

Professional Strife.

It so happens that all medical men are not gentlemen either by birth or training. This is indeed unfortunate, for it is accountable for much of the unseemly bickerings between individuals of our profession. Such disputes, in due course of time, produced a "Code of Ethics" by which each member of the profession is supposed to govern himself. Quite naturally it is an amplification of the "Golden Rule," and as such it should be an efficient and safe guide. But it is a fact mnch to be regretted that some members do not adhere to its teachings, except when "the other fellow" is concerned. This is particularly noticeable in their associations with the patients of other physicians. Competition being keen, some men are always in need of patients and are constantly grasping for those rightly belonging to another. Such action produces discord, and frequently engenders strife. Sometimes a " free-for-all fight " ensues, in which the partisans of each take sides, and there is a genuine neighborhood row. As a result, the entire medical profession is brought, in a measure, into disrepute. Such conduct is unseemly, and should be strongly condemned. Let us be gentlemen!

Furthermore, many a dispute between a client and his medical adviser is begun and continued by a lack of dignity and discretion on the part of the latter. It is quite true that there are some men who regularly "dead beat " the medical profession ; but the experienced practitioner can readily separate the goats from the sheep, and it is far better to drop them at once than to carry them along to the inevitable controversy with its bitterness, and frequently unsatisfactory ending. Many times the physician wins ; but even then his moral standard of humanity in general is appreciably lowered, though he may be unconscious of such result. It is better to believe in the justice of our fellow men.—*Los Angeles Journal of Eclectic Medicine.*

Therapeutic Optimism.

The careful reader of medical journal literature must admit that the trend of medical thought is swaying toward the usefulness of drug therapy.

The theory of the uselessness of drugs in combating disease is being more and more controverted in many quarters. In its place there is the tendency to study more closely those agents which, in days gone by, were given with such implicit confidence.

The reign of drug therapy is once more on the ascending plane of medical thought and action. In order that it should attain and hold its rightful position we must cast aside all of the old dogmas that prevented advance in times past. We must realize that we are not to combat a name ; that under each name, or diagnosis, if you choose to call it, are gathered together many conflicting conditions ; that almost invariably the various patients' classified under one generic term may every one need something different from the rest to enable them to successfully contend with their departure from the normal or health, and regain what they have lost.

The term *diagnosis* should have two entirely different meanings for the accomplished drug therapist. The first is that, by connecting all the various symptoms into one harmonious whole, he is enabled to give a name, according to prescribed medical nomenclature, to the disease for the benefit of patients and friends. The second is that, by dissecting the various conditions which go to make up its entirety, he can intelligently treat them by the appropriate remedies. These two meanings should be clear-cut and entirely separated; not allowed in the slightest degree to invade the realm which belongs to each distinctively.

Much of the therapeutic nihilism is due to the fact that drugs have been said to be useful in certain diseases, without any distinctive reason why any particular one should be used in preference to the others. Such teaching could only result in an indiscriminate use of the drugs recommended with a very small chance of a successful outcome.

Therapeutic optimism must be brought about by a different line of tactics. Drugs must be carefully studied, and their action in the various parts of the human economy more closely defined. The idea of prescribing at a name must be abandoned. We must desist from declaring that such and such drugs will cure such and such diseases, but must rather inculcate the thought that each patient is in a class by himself and must be so considered and treated.—Editorial in *Journal of Therapeutics and Dietetics.*

Protecting the People in California.

The California State Board of Medical Examiners does not regard practice of medicine, materia medica or therapeutics, branches worthy to be examined in. Anything that pertains to the art of medicine, its application in disease is non-essential. Here are ten questions taken from the last examination held in that State December 3, 4 and 5, 1907:

1. Name the layers of the retina.

2. Describe a septic tank and explain the principles involved.

3. Describe the phenomena of indirect cell division or karyokinesis.,

4. Define colostrom, emmetropia, diapedesis, hemolysin, lochia, osmosis, alexins, atavism, zymogen.

5. Give ten different varieties of pyogenic organisms and their microscopical characters.

6. State the morphology of the specific organism of plague.

7. Give formula for chloroform.

8. Give formula for boric acid.

9. Name CH_3OH.

10. Name $C_2H_5O.H$.

We could give ten more questions of equal practicability from this examination. This is protecting the people of the Golden State with a "vengeance that is mine," saith the California Board. How many physicians of any school of ten, five, or even two years' experience in actual practice could answer these questions? There is no practicability whatever in them, and to say that an examining board of any State is a protection to the people by requiring candidates to answer them and to omit the essential, practical questions of the application of materia medica for the cure of the sick is worse than farcical, it is sheer imbecility. We would wager a 100 to 1 shot that not a single member of the California State Board of Medical Examiners even with six months' preparation could answer 50 per cent. of the questions propounded in this last examination. It is not in them. As for us, we would prefer to be a theologian and know many things that are not so than to be able to answer this tommyrot."—*Medical Century*.

Kill Therapeutics?

Dr. Reed made the proposition to the A. M. A. that the various State examining boards exclude therapeutics from their tests of candidates. Dr. Reed is a bit behind the procession, for this exclusion is at present made by some of these boards. The reason advanced is that it will do away with the objections of homeopathists and eclectics to a single board, by placing their candidates on an absolute equality with the others, since the only difference in the teaching of the three schools is in this one department.

To this we may object that it will not do away with the distrust these gentlemen manifest toward any board controlled by the regulars. They feel that under no circumstances would they receive an impartial examination from their enemies. Moreover, this would not apply to the other and possibly more numerous practicians of osteopathy, Christian science and innumerable others, who have in law and equity as much claim for consideration as the two sects named, and whose differences with us are by no means confined to therapeutics.

There are other and more fundamental objections. Every teacher in medical schools knows well that the student cannot be induced to give attention to any branch except those on which he must stand examination. No matter how essential it may be to his success in practice, he studies solely with a view to passing those dreaded exams. They are an obsession to him. He thinks of them by day and dreams of them by night. He logically reasons that he must first acquire the legal right to practice, and the how to practice is a topic for future consideration. The more difficult the trial the more he must exclude all that does not directly aid him in meeting its requirements and concentrate his powers upon them.

Our third objection is based on the foregoing : The exclusion of therapeutics nullifies the original object of the creation of these boards, and their only excuse for conttnued existence—the protection of the people against unqualified practicians. It makes little difference how proficient a doctor may be in the fundamental branches of a medical education if he is ignorant of the best methods of treating the sick. He may be all kinds of a good anatomist, chemist, pathologist, bacteriologist and several other ists, and yet be utterly at a loss and useless as a practicing physician—and yet it is precisely that and nothing else in which the community has an interest in him and his qualifications. Instead of excluding therapeutics from these examinations we would suggest that all else except this branch and diagnosis be excluded. The rest could be taken for granted—the medical colleges surely look out for them—what interests the public, in whose name and for whose protection these boards were called into existence, is the ability of the doctor to recognize and treat diseases.

In our boyhood we had pointed out to us in Philadelphia a row of rather ordinary houses, which went by the name of Morris' Folly. It was said of them that the builder had seven stories of cellars, and by the time the structure reached the surface of the ground his means were exhausted and he could only place these mean buildings over the magnificent cellars. *Verbum sapienti sat.*—Editorial in *American Journal of Clinical Medicine*.

Music as a Remedial Agent.

While the therapeutic effects of music in a general way have long been recognized and accepted by the profession, its specific action had not been studied until recently, when several French and German scientists conceived the idea of adapting it to various abnormal conditions of the nervous system.

The investigator has found that music, according to its character, will modify the blood pressure, pulse rate and respiration, according to the condition and susceptibility of the patient. This theory is borne out in a way by the report of cases in the army in which hemorrhage was relieved when soldiers were carried to within hearing distance of music. All careful observers are familiar with the stimulating, as well as soothing effects of music upon many, or indeed, most individuals ; in fact, this agent is being quite generally utilized in asylums and institutions for the treatment of nervous diseases. The employment of certain chords and harmonies for certain abnormal conditions is only another progressive step in psychic medication.—*New England Medical Monthly*.

THE ECLECTIC MEDICAL JOURNAL

A Monthly Journal of Eclectic Medicine and Surgery.

TWO DOLLARS PER ANNUM.

Official Journal Ohio State Eclectic Medical Association

JOHN K. SCUDDER, M.D., MANAGING EDITOR.

EDITORS.

W. E. BLOYER.	H. W. FELTER.	W. N. MUNDY.	R. L. THOMAS.
W. B. CHURCH.	K. O. FOLTZ.	L. E. RUSSELL.	L. WATKINS.
JOHN FEARN.	J. U. LLOYD.	A. F. STEPHENS.	H. T. WEBSTER.

Published by THE SCUDDER BROTHERS COMPANY, 1009 Plum Street, Cincinnati, to whom all communications and remittances should be sent.

Articles on any medical subject are solicited, which will usually be published the month following their receipt. One hundred reprints of articles of four or more pages, or one dozen copies of the Journal, will be forwarded free if the request is made when the article is submitted. The editor disclaims any responsibility for the views of contributors.

Discontinuances and Renewals.—The publishers must be notified by mail and all arrearages paid when you want your Journal stopped. If you want it stopped at the expiration of any fixed period, kindly notify us in advance.

NEW POSTAL RULING AFFECTING SECOND-CLASS MATTER.

We have received a copy of the recent amendment of the United States Postal Regulations regarding the privileges of publishers of second-class matter, affecting especially the sending of sample copies and determining the length of time a subscriber can be carried as such after his paid-up subscription has expired.

We quote the following relating to subscribers:

Paragraph 3, Sec. 436, Postal Laws and Regulations: "A reasonable time will be allowed publishers to secure renewals of subscriptions, but unless subscriptions are expressly renewed after the term for which they are paid within the following periods,* they shall not be counted in the legitimate list of subscribers, and copies mailed on account thereof shall not be accepted for mailing at the second-class postage rate of 1 cent a pound, but may be mailed at the transient second-class postage rate of 1 cent for each four ounces or fraction thereof,. prepaid by stamps affixed."

(* The period allowed for securing renewals of subscriptions differs, according to frequency of publication. The time allowed weekly publications is one year; semi-monthlies, three months; MONTHLIES, FOUR MONTHS, etc. The amendment goes into effect April 1.)

From the above it will be observed that this new ruling goes into effect April 1, 1908, and the Government will allow us four months, April, May, June and July, in which to collect delinquent subscriptions to the ECLECTIC MEDICAL JOURNAL. We would be compelled to affix a two-cent stamp on each *delinquent* copy after July 31.

Many of our subscribers have already paid their subscriptions for 1908, and we are satisfied that many more will help us comply with the new regulations during the next four months. We are giving the notice publicity now in order that no one may be offended later on. *A formal order for renewal for the current year is necessary.*

This amendment to the postal regulations at last solves the perplexing question whether subscribers should receive a publication a year or two or more after they have paid a subscription, or whether names should be dropped immediately on expiration of subscription. No solution to this question that pleased all has ever been reached by any publisher.

If a subscription was discontinued at expiration the publisher was, in many cases, berated and lost the patronage of the subscriber forever afterwards; if subscriptions were continued indefinitely, hoping that some day the subscriber would pay up, he was in many cases sorely disappointed, and was, in addition, sharply criticised for sending the periodical after the term for which it was paid. Hence, we welcome this new ruling. It places the responsibility where it belongs, and as Uncle Sam's shoulders are broad, he will hereafter take all the blame.

SCUDDER.

WHAT OF OUR FUTURE?

Those who have not kept in touch with medical education for the past twenty-five years cannot realize what great strides medicine has made towards becoming a science in fact as well as in name.

A quarter of a century ago any one who desired to study medicine, no matter what his preliminary education, could enter a medical college, and if at the end of two years he could pass his examination he became one of the units of a "learned profession." It mattered not whether he could speak grammatically or spell correctly, he belonged to, and represented, a scientific profession.

Then he studied seven branches for five months and returned the following year for another five months, the second year being a repetition of the first. To-day, every student must have a diploma from a first-grade high school, or its equivalent, before he can begin the study of medicine, and the two-year course of five months each has been lengthened to a four-year course of eight months each. The seven branches of the former times have been doubled and trebled, and the faculty of seven increased many times.

Well-equipped laboratories for chemical, histological, bacteriological and pathological research are necessary to every institution that does the work of a first-class medical college. With the increase of these various departments the expenses of a medical college have correspondingly increased, though the tuition to the student has not increased in corresponding ratio.

The future of Eclecticism rests with the Eclectics of this country. We must have more students in Eclectic colleges if we are to supply the calls that are constantly made for Eclectic practitioners. I am sure if the 7,500 Eclectic physicians could realize that the very life and prosperity of our school depended upon an army of recruits each year, our colleges would soon be filled.

We *must* have more students to-day than we had twenty-five years ago if we wish Eclecticism to maintain its high standard and continue the good work that has already been accomplished. That Eclecticism is as popular to-day as it ever was is shown by the constant call for Eclectic physicians from every part of the country, and our colleges are unable to supply the demand. How are the colleges to get these prospective students?

A little thought will convince any physician that they must come from our practitioners. Professional ethics forbids the college from advertising, and even if this were allowable the young men that are to make up our classes would never see them, so it remains for the individual doctor to recruit our institutions. Now what are some of the methods that can be used by the physician in securing students. I will mention three, and no doubt any wide-awake practitioner will think of others.

First, he can secure a list of the high school graduates from his locality, and mail it to some one of the Eclectic colleges.

Second, he might insert, with propriety, in his local paper, a notice like the following:

"THOSE INTERESTED IN THE STUDY OF MEDICINE.

"I would like to communicate, personally or by letter, with any young man or woman of high-school qualification who contemplates the study of medicine. I have something to say which I believe will be to the advantage of any such person."

This means will enable our men to get in touch with prospective students who can be directed to some one of our institutions.

Third, he can talk Eclecticism, using discretion, of course, to one or more bright young men, and thus stimulate a desire to study medicine.

This is certainly not asking too much of the individual physician, for I take it for granted that every one who practices our system is surely interested in the perpetuation of our school, and it can only be perpetuated and further disseminated by a large number of yearly recruits.

Now do not imagine for a moment that the colleges are flying the distress signal, and that we fear a dissolution in the years to come. Not a bit of it; but we believe that Eclecticism still has a mission to perform. While not perfect, and while there are still great problems yet to be solved in curing the sick, we still contend that Eclecticism is the most rational system of medicine practiced to-day, and that the principles upon which the system is founded are as true as the eternal, and there is no reason why Eclecticism should not march the highways of life, even to the ends of the earth, if her children will only awaken to the possibilities that are open to them as well as the responsibility that is upon them and do a little work for the cause.

Remember, Eclecticism can only be taught in Eclectic colleges, and every student that you let get away to other schools is lost to Eclecticism.

A *little* work, and just a little time on the part of our practitioners will mean much for a forward movement of our cause. *Will you do it ?*

THOMAS.

BACTERIOLOGY STILL LACKING.

For many years bacteriologists have been studiously delving in their special field to demonstrate the *fons et origo* of disease. No doubt their labors have resulted in some things that are valuable and practical, both as regards preventive and restorative medicine, but much seems to be still lacking ; many matters which ought, it seems, to have long ago been cleared up, still remain in obscurity, if not in complete mystery.

Strange to tell, those among our most common infectious diseases seem to be the ones where the greatest difficulty lies in pointing out the specific germ upon which the infection depends. We now possess fairly clean-cut ideas in regard to typhoid fever, diphtheria, yellow fever, tuberculosis, bubonic plague and some other infections, but the more common diseases, such as measles, scarlet fever, rotheln, chickenpox and whooping-cough, with all their frequency of occurrence and opportunity for study, have remained, after many years, still a mystery. Something seems behind them which the microscopist fails to detect.

Apparently, improvement must be made in apparatus, technique, or in method of investigation, before these matters are satisfactorily settled. The object is a worthy one, and it is to be hoped that newer developments will ultimately result in a clearing up of these problems.

The bacteriologist is seldom a successful physician or progressive thera-peutist, yet he is engaged in a worthy vocation, one which tends to the enlightenment of the entire profession, and it is to be hoped that some time we will be fully informed as to the *materies morbi* of each and every infectious disease now known,

One fact is encouraging, and that is the enthusiasm and optimism of the bacteriologist is unquenchable. He is absorbed and engrossed in his specialty, and. never gives up the fascinating line of investiga-tion. He is an untiring faddist, and promises to yet unfold a tale.

It is a pity that the subject is so technical that we cannot all take a hand, but if we were to do it practical medicine would eventually go to the dogs. The profession cannot afford too many bacteriologists, because it needs a few practical minds to apply. what little .the science has taught us to useful purposes, besides considerable more that has been learned without their aid.

It still appears as though the most scientific physicians, as the term is usually understood, are the least successful ones, when it comes to the treatment of the sick. It seems difficult for science to get at the bottom of the secrets of life. When it comes to delving in the vital processes of the human economy, all so-called science has thus far proven rather crude. It still seems as though the successful physician is born, not entirely made. Scientific research is amusing to many and unfolds some interesting details, but so far as curative measures go it is still a '' little raw.''

It cannot be gainsaid, however, that bacteriology has resulted in much that is beneficent. Through it we have learned to follow typhoid fever to its secret fastnesses, and have learned to combat its epidemics by proper preventive precautions. We have learned where to look for its origin, and know how to shut off the source of its defilement in many instances. Bacteriology has led the way to serum inoculations in the treatment of diphtheria, and these promise something more reliable, perhaps, in some instances, than other measures at command. Though this measure is attended by failures, and probably is abused in many instances, it is apparently a step in the right direction. Maybe we have advaced in the preventive treatment of tuberculosis through bac-teriological research ; time will tell. We know a little more about the origin of malaria than we once did, though not as much as we would like. Our knowledge of yellow fever has doubtless been improved. We knew, before the days of bacteriology, that rats were in some way connected with the spread of bubonic plague ; we know no more now than before of any successful treatment. Will bacteriology teach us any better way of meeting it successfully ?

And when we have learned more about the specific germs of our more common infections, will our treatment of their ravages be improved? Let us hope so. We already possess knowledge of their management—we, us and company—which we may view with considerable complacency. Will some upstart in the bacteriological line point out, some time, a better way? Let us hope, in all sincerity, that our best resources will yet be improved upon. We are open to conviction, and will welcome a better way, if it can be shown to us. Nevertheless, we can afford to wait patiently, for we know of some good things already, which we have evolved by patient observation and experimentation, not due to the revelations of the microscope or the developments of the serum manipulator.

In short, we have accomplished enough in our own way to encourage further industry in our own field. The time may come when we will not be needed so much as in the past, but we feel that we are still useful in our own particular sphere. When the bacteriologist and his brother worker, the serum experimenter, has shown us a better way to treat all diseases we will be out of the race, and it will be time for us to quit our particular line of business. It will be time to merge. Will that time ever arrive?   WEBSTER.

AUTO-INTOXICATION.

This term is overworked. It is so convenient to fill a hiatus in pathology and diagnosis the temptation is strong to resort to it frequently.

New conceptions as to pathology and etiology naturally require corresponding readjustment of our practice. Recent advancement, resulting from adoption and exploitation of the germ theory of disease, has accordingly been followed by corresponding changes in medical practice. "Equalizing the circulation" is a phrase that served long and well in suppressing to curious laymen prone to propound embarrassing questions.

By common consent to meet such changes we have now a substitute phrase better reflecting the newer light. Instead of equalizing the circulation, if it ever was really done, we have very largely turned attention to "sterilizing the intestinal canal." Nothing is more characteristic of many enterprising physicians than their readiness to accept new remedies and procedures in advance of complete demonstration of their efficacy. Without waiting for proof that such sterilization is necessary or possible, these are making the attempt with great zeal and unanimity. We are all agreed that our bodily well-being is menaced by foes within as well as without ; that life is a warfare, with continued existence depending on the exercise of eternal vigilance. Nevertheless, it has passed into an axiom that ''Self-preservation is the first law of nature.'' Either endowed by the Creator originally with design, or evolved by the necessities of environment, as you prefer, all living creatures are possessed of some means of defense against their enemies. The presumption is, therefore, that nature has not left us defenseless against our microscopic antagonists. It is fair to conclude, also, that her work is in no need of such extreme supervision as sometimes advised. Auto-intoxication is associated in our minds especially with the débris and filth passing along the intestinal canal, which is regarded and often referred to as a sewer. With this conception of its function, flushing it has naturally become a routine procedure. Profession and laity are so generally committed to this view that the propriety of unloading the bowels is taken for granted, so it is hard to persuade any one that there can be any valid objection to clearing out the *prima via*. Occasions for this are far the most frequent of any that arise in medicine. Invariably is this made part of the preparation of the patient for a laparotomy ; and nine times in ten a cathartic is the first drug exhibited in any case of illness. Exception must be made on behalf of our homeopathic confrères. Many surgeons of this school habitually operate without previously disturbing the bowels in any way. They also medicate all cases of severe illness with careful avoidance of physic. The results they secure amply justify the omission. In journals and society proceedings the allopaths regularly deplore the statistics of pneumonia and typhoid fever, leading many to abandon drug therapy altogether. Among the few who contend still for something of merit in drugs, a majority offset the good of all other measures by senseless and always injurious attempts to unload the bowels. It took a long, long time to establish the fact that powerful drastic cathartics increased the mortality of all grave cases of disease. A compromise on milder remedies in smaller doses is a very evident improvement. Further betterment is checked for a time by this unwarranted assumption of auto-intoxication. Putrefaction is not so common in the intestinal canal as many suppose ; consequently, we are not taking great chances if we interfere less with its contents and nature's method of disposing of them. CHURCH.

CURIOSITY.

It was during the dessert course. He had been sitting next to her for the last hour and a half, and was deeply conscious of the beautiful contour of her arms and shoulders.

"Do you know," she said suddenly, "I've been in misery for a week. Sometimes I could almost scream with the pain."

"Why, what is the matter?" he exclaimed sympathetically.

" I was vaccinated a while ago, and it has taken dreadfully."
His eyes fell and his gaze was curious. But he saw no scar.
" Why, where were you vaccinated ? " he asked, impetuously.
She raised her eyebrows and smiled sweetly. "In New York,"
she replied.—*Cornell College Widow.*

There is curiosity and curiosity. Some types are annoying, impertinent or impudent. Others are friendly, sympathetic, or for the purpose of actual knowledge. Another or last type is simply polite interest.

We are all familiar with each of the types and their subdivisions, but few of us have much use for either the first or last type, and usually but little for the second classification if the questions are regarding personal affairs, which cannot have any bearing on the subject, but are prompted only for probing into secrets that should be kept inviolable.

Curiosity is a component of every individual, but there is reason in all things. Curiosity to add valuable knowlegde to your own stock is all right, provided you injure no one in so doing ; but curiosity to know another's private affairs simply so you can gossip about them or use the information for selfish ends is contemptible. The polite curiosity is usually harmless, as the answers to questions are usually not heard, but, nevertheless, these same questions are an annoyance to the one interrogated.

Physicians of a necessity are compelled to question their patients more or less in their professional capacity as physicians, but they should not transgress their authority in so doing and ask questions irrelevant to the subject. Also all personal matters volunteered by the patient, as well as those gained by direct questioning, should be kept secret. Such secrets are usually not obtained through idle curiosity, but because one or both of the parties interested in the examination believe it will be of value in understanding the patient's condition.

The doctor should restrain his curiosity to the professional side only, and never allow the other types to obtrude, for almost always there will come a time when trouble will result from the idle form. It may not be serious, but it is very liable to be annoying. FOLTZ.

GASTRIC DIGESTION.

The gastric juice is especially active in the digestion of proteid substances and reduces them to soluble peptones. The enzymes are pepsin and hydrochloric acid. The per cent. of pepsin in gastric juice varies according to the character of the food, and is small when the diet is chiefly carbohydrate. About four hundred and eighty grains of pepsin are secreted by the stomach in twenty-four hours, an average of two drachms for each meal,

The gastric juice contains from 0.2 to 0.3 per cent. hydrochloric acid. The gastric glands secrete pepsinogen or pro-pepsin, which is later converted into pepsin by the action of hydrochloric acid. The chief cells of the gastric glands secrete pepsinogen, and the parietal cells hydrochloric acid. Pepsin results from a combination of these two elements. Pawlow, by his experiments, has shown that hunger will produce a flow of gastric juice, or that indigestible substances when introduced into the stomach will stimulate secretion. This he calls "appetite juice." This fluid is of strong digestive power, and may be provoked in the stomach of a dog, after which it can be removed through a fistulous opening, prepared beforehand, and has proven an effective remedy in cases of asepsis. Juice from the stomach of a dog for internal administration may, at first, seem revolting, but, after all, it is no more disgusting than pepsin from the stomach of a hog.

Normally from fifteen to twenty pints of gastric juice are secreted in twenty-four hours, about five or six pints for an ordinary meal. It is secreted gradually and is reabsorbed or passed through to the duodenum so that there is never a very large quantity of this fluid in the stomach at one time, except in cases of pyloric obstruction or gastric dilatation, when the contents of the stomach may reach large proportions. As much as three gallons of fluid have been removed from the stomach by lavage in cases of this nature. The secretion of gastric juice is influenced but not altogether controlled by the central nervous system, and the sight of food or its keen anticipation will, in the fasting stomach, cause an increased flow of digestive fluids. It is well known that mental emotions such as fear, anger, anxiety or grief will diminish or arrest the normal secretion, and that mental worry alone is a frequent cause of gastric indigestion. The stomach digests proteid substances only; fats are dissolved, the areolar tissue and albuminous cell walls digested, thus freeing the oleaginous matter, but no further action upon fat occurs in the stomach.

With the exception of adipose tissue, flesh is principally digested in the stomach. Milk undergoes coagulation by a special ferment, rennin or prexin; the coagulum is then digested by pepsin. Eggs are digested in the stomach with the exception of the fats, which pass on for further digestion below. Vegetables when well cooked are disintegrated and their proteid constituents digested. Contrary to the popular opinion, vegetable protieds are not as readily acted on by the gastric juice as animal proteids. Raw vegetables, about which so much has been said as an article of food for consumptives. may possibly be of some benefit, but unless very finely·subdivided before eating are practically indigestible. Raw vegetables and fruits frequently pass through the alimentary tract unaffected by its juices. All proteids are not completely digested in the stomach, but are there prepared for digestion in the small intestines.

Absorption from the stomach is not as extensive as formerly supposed. Gastric digestion requires from two to four hours for its completion, but absorption by the stomach walls begins soon after ingestion, and the two processes, digestion and absorption, are going on simultaneously. As soon as the food is rendered soluble, portions of it begin to pass the pylorus, and the stomach should be empty in four hours. Pathological conditions may delay digestion, and the character of the food has an influence upon the rapidity of this process.

WATKINS.

THE CHICAGO OCTOPUS.

The *Journal of the American Medical Association* has a department on pharmacology which devotes its energy in a large measure in exposing the presumably fake preparations on the market, the methods used by the manufacturers in exploiting them, and in passing upon the merits of the new and untried remedies offered to us. The *Journal* undertakes the task of acting as sponsor for the medical profession, and it presumes to be pure and untainted in all things, no suspicion of anything unprofessional or unethical in it.

The object of the department of pharmacology is certainly commendable, for we are all aware that our offices are flooded with literature commending this and that preparation and containing the·endorsements of physicians of presumed ethical standing. In a recent issue we note a long harangue upon the methods of Lehn and Fink in advertising their products, especially " Purgen," whatever that may be. Under " Correspondence," we note a tirade against *The American Journal of Medical Sciences* for advertising Antikamnia, Seng, Cactina and other products.

It looks somewhat like a case of " the pot calling the kettle black," for in the same journal we find advertised "Sajodin, a substitute for Potassium Iodide;" " Novaspirin, used in rheumatic and gouty conditions, influenza and neuralgia when all other forms of salicylic acid medication are badly tolerated by the stomach." . . . " Soreness of the throat, cold in the head, obstruction in the nose are promptly relieved by Coryfin—prolonged menthol action improved. It is applied to the painful area in headaches of all kinds, etc. Samples and literature supplied by —— Company."

We are not objecting to the advertisements of either journal. Had they a better system of therapeutics the criticisms would be unnecessary, yet they seem to us paradoxical, when taken in conjunction with the advertisements quoted from the pages of the critic. Does it make any difference where the article is made or by whom patented?

I am not an extensive user of patented or proprietary medicines, and fail to see any difference between those patented in Germany or made there and those of American manufacture. It looks like a case of Germanophobia, or the blind following of presumed authority. We see no difference in the methods of advertising of the manufacturers, either. A closer study of pure materia medica and therapeutics would relieve many physicians of the necessity of relying on the manufacturing pharmacists for ''specific remedies for specific diseases.'' MUNDY.

A Pleasant Laxative.

The physician is called upon to prescribe for constipation oftener perhaps than any other trouble. We will not discuss the cause here of this trouble. But I will call your attention to a remedy I have been prescribing and using for a good many years—and with success. I first learned of it in this way. One of my patients, long a sufferer, returned from her vacation and her first greeting was, ''I have got rid of my bowel trouble.'' She told me she had been advised to eat three or four English walnuts after each meal; they relieved her. I began to use them myself, and to prescribe them for my patients; they did the work. I can say they are a very pleasant and a very successful remedy. I believe the laxative principle lies in the skin that covers the meat—this principle, according to my observation, acts upou the liver. I may say I have seen parrots in captivity carefully peeling off this skin before they swallowed the meat. Before getting your patients into the habit of taking strong cathartics prescribe about six walnuts after supper, always using with them a little table salt.

FEARN.

Special Lectures.

The junior and senior students at the College have been having considerable interesting work this winter in the way of special lectures. During January and February special lectures were given on Mental Diseases every Monday afternoon by the Staff of the Longview Asylum.

Professor W. E. Postle, Superintendent of Shepard's Sanitarium at Columbus, Ohio, gave a very instructive course of twelve lectures on Nervous and Mental Diseases.

Professor Dickson followed with his usual course of twelve lectures

on Medical Jurisprudence, and Professor J. P. Harbert, of Bellefontaine, Ohio, gave a special series "On the Use of the Ophthalmoscope
in Diagnosis."

Professor Heidingsfeld, a member of the City Hospital Staff, has
been taking our senior class in small sections and giving them bedside
instruction in the wards every Thursday morning on Skin and Venereal
Diseases. Dr. Hiedingsfeld has also given several lectures in the
evenings at the City Hospital to the seniors of the various colleges.
His lectures were illustrated with colored stereopticon views, and
proved very interesting as well as instructive.

Commencement Exercises.

The sixty-third annual Commencement Exercises of the Eclectic
Medical Institute will be held at the Scottish Rite Cathedral, Wednesday evening, April 29, at 8 P.M. All of our former graduates and
their friends are cordially invited.

On Wednesday morning Professor Russell will hold a surgical
clinic at the new Seton Hospital from 10 to 12, and in the afternoon
at 2:30 the annual meeting of the Alumnal Association will be held
in the College Lecture Hall.

IN MEMORIAM.

WHEREAS, In recognition of the loss we have suffered by the death of our
class-mate, Daniel F. Oswald, and of the still greater loss felt by those who
were nearest and dearest to him, therefore be it

Resolved, That it is but a just tribute to the memory of the departed to say
in regretting his removal from our midst we mourn for one who was in every
way worthy of our respect and regard; and

Resolved, That the class of 1908 of the Eclectic Medical Institute has lost
one of its most proficient members and Eclecticism a zealous advocate, and one
who by reason of his admirable personality was eminently qualified to pursue
his calling; and

Resolved, That we sincerely condole with the bereaved family on the dispensation with which it has pleased Divine Providence to afflict them, and commend
them for consolation to Him who orders all things for the best, and whose chas-
tisements are meant in mercy; and

Resolved, That this testimonial of our respect, sympathy and sorrow be forwarded to the bereaved family of our departed class-mate, and that a copy be
sent to the ECLECTIC MEDICAL JOURNAL for publication.

D. EDWARD MORGAN,
CHARLES C. McCAFFREY,
H. F. POHLMEYER,
J. W. BOWERS,
Committee.

The Eclectic Medical Journal

ESTABLISHED 1836.

Vol. LXVIII.　　　CINCINNATI, MAY, 1908.　　　No. 5.

Original Communications.

ACONITE—ACONITUM NAPELLUS.

John Fearn, M.D., Oakland, Cal.

Aconite has been used as a medicine for many years, and yet for a long time it never took that place in therapeutics to which its great merits entitled it. For this mistake I believe there are at least two reasons:

First, men have been more interested in its physiological and poisonous properties than in its therapeutic power.

Second, the very great difference and strength of the drug and its preparations.

There are several reasons for this difference in quality and strength. First, there has been carelessness in gathering the root; not only poor qualities have been collected, but roots of entirely different nature have been gathered and sold for aconite. Second, it has been gathered without reference to the natural habitat of the plant. We all know that plants will seem to thrive in soils which are not likely to develop their peculiar qualities, and this is especially true with regard to narcotics. There may be big plants, and yet in the alkaloid-bearing plants there may be very little of the alkaloidal strength. The same applies to other medicinal constituents. Hence the pharmacist considers it absolutely necessary to assay the different batches of root that he may discover their alkaloidal strength, which is one factor in drug energy.

In reference to this matter Dr. Shoemaker, quoting from Murrell, says the English aconite is many times stronger than the German, and that the French is very variable. Then, again, years ago there was not that care in pharmaceutical work that we find to-day. In a drug-store owned by the present writer he gave special attention to the preparation of tincture of aconite. First there was an effort to get the best root the market afforded; second, percolation was not deemed sufficient. It was macerated for a long time in the proper menstruum, when it was carefully percolated. One old druggist working in that store said he had never seen such strong aconite, and that it was not safe for a stranger to use it, it being so much stronger than the U. S. P. aconite. Our people know how their success is conserved by the specific medicine which is their established standard.

For many years our Homeopathic friends had practically almost a monopoly of the use of this drug. And Bartholow tells us that owing to this great use of this remedy by the Homeopaths, a prejudice has been created against it. What a comment on human weakness that prejudices should have kept this grand remedy in the background for years! But our old school friends are fast outgrowing such childish methods.

I think it safe to say that no one man ever did more to popularize the use of this drug than the late John M. Scudder. His students are scattered over the world, and they know when and how to use aconite.

Physiological and Poisonous Action of Aconite.—Aconite is a terrible and deadly poison. It acts on the vaso-motor nervous system. It is a heart paralyzant. It seems to act first on the terminal filaments of the sensory nerves, and afterwards on the nerve trunks; it destroys reflex activity and voluntary power. If sufficient be taken —and it does not take much—there will be increased tingling in the lips, mouth and throat, diminished pulse and respiration, frothing at the mouth; the voice, sight and hearing are lost, muttering delirium ensues, and death ends the scene.

If a large dose has been taken science knows no certain remedy or antidote. The most powerful stimulants may be given. If the poison is thought to be lodged in the stomach the stomach-pump may be used.

Specific Symptomatology.—Have we any guiding symptoms for the use of this drug? Most certainly we have. Aconite is the remedy for *asthenia.* The pulse is small, frequent, often easily compressed; there is difficulty in the capillary circulation; there is lack of tonicity in both heart and blood-vessels; there is increased temperature, and in the early stages there is coldness and chilliness. In acute cases this chilliness alone is indication sufficient for the use of the aconite. Some of my medical friends push this remedy in the case of the full, hard, bounding pulse. I know we have better remedies for this condition.

What Preparation Shall We Use?—In my hands the safest,

quickest and best acting remedy we have ever used is the specific medicine aconite. Many use aconitine, and I believe them when they tell me they get good results with it. I have tried the alkaloid; but I come back to my first love. Specific aconite is a perfect remedy. If you will be careful about the dose you have nothing to fear, even with the most weakly babe. The safe dose and the effectual will be from two to ·not more than five drops to four ounces of water, a teaspoonful of the dilution at a dose.

As an adjuvant in treating cases of fever where I want to get quick action of the skin and a kindly action on the stomach, I add to the preparation dr. i to .drs. ii of spir. niter dulc. In many cases, especially in chronic cases, I prefer to use the 1x dilution of the specific medicine aconite and I would strongly advise this course. A little more can occasionally be added to the glass, and yet this is not always needed. Many close observers say that they get even better and more kindly results from the dilution.

I cannot leave this part of the subject without adding a warning against using this remedy too freely. Some advocate using ten drops of specific medicine aconite to four ounces of water. This I am sure is a mistake, especially in the case of children, who suffer from such heroic dosage, but cannot describe their misery.

Therapeutic Action.—Aconite is a stimulant to the sympathetic system of nerves. As Scudder tells us, it increases the power of the heart to move the blood; at the same time it places the blood-vessels in a better condition for its passage, and yet we place this remedy among special sedatives. Will it sedate? Give this remedy where you have a rapid, small pulse and see how soon it will bring down the number of pulse beats, and at the same time increase the strength of the individual beat.

In conference with a very intelligent physician of the dominant school some years ago, the call for aconite was to me very clear. But when I mentioned the remedy the physician complained. "Aconite is a sedative," he said; "you may try it, but I will take no responsibility." The remedy was given, the patient improved, and the doctor was impressed. Thus we see this remedy has a very wide range of usefulness.

In the early stages of fever frequently this is the only remedy indicated. We do not know the disease. Why should we wait? Give the remedy. At your next visit you may find it has done its work so well that nothing else is needed.

Take the feverish, fretful babe. The highly sensitive nervous system has been impressed, you don't know how. Dentition may be in process; it may have taken cold. The skin is dry, the mouth hot, the pulse small and rapid. Here the full strength specific medicine is too strong even to dilute. Add ten drops of Ix dil. of specific medicine aconite to three ounces of water, give teaspoonful doses every twenty or thirty minutes. The skin softens, the fever goes down, the little one sleeps. How nice! Yes, and how true.

In simple croup with the aconite indications, using it with the cold pack to the throat, I regard aconite as one of the certainties in medicine, and I know of nothing that will compare with it.

In tonsilitis you may give the remedy internally. However, the quickest way to get relief is to use it with the steam atomizer. There will be sufficient of the remedy absorbed used in this way, so that it need not be given by mouth.

In excessive action of any of the excretory organs aconite is a grand remedy; such excess may be of the bowels, the skin or the kidneys, in diarrhea, dysentery, polyuria, or excessive sweating, acting in these cases by toning up capillary circulation and mucous surfaces, and the dose is so small there is no trouble to get the patient to take it. I remember well my first case of summer complaint for which I prescribed aconite. I added a few drops to a vial of water. It was tasteless; it looked so weak that I came very near throwing it away and giving an old compound. I gave the medicine. The result was satisfactory.

In any case of bowel trouble, given the aconite symptoms plus stools largely of mucus, I would rather trust aconite plus small doses of ipecac than anything I know of. I can freely bear out Ellingwood when he says aconite given early retards exudation, suppuration, induration and hypertrophy, and thus it becomes a grand remedy in pnuemonia where the constitution is feeble. If there is but little expectoration and that is mucus, add ipecac.

In suppression of menstruation from cold, this remedy, with the addition of macrotys, aided by warmth, usually leaves nothing to be desired. Aconite is one of our best remedies in rheumatism. In many cases it will cure alone, and why not? According to Webster, through its action secretion is encouraged, skin and mucous membranes become moist, the action of the kidneys is increased, and thus it is the opponent of those conditions which cause rheumatism.

Aconite as a Heart Remedy.—I wish to call attention to the use of aconite in heart troubles. I have for a good while in my own mind and practice looked upon aconite as a heart tonic. Owing to opposition by many physicians I have said nothing about it in my writings and teachings. But as I continued its use on these lines I am more and more impressed with its value. Hughes in his manual of pharmacodynamics well says: "Aconite in its action is quite different from that of the so-called arterial sedatives, which in large doses knock down fever by prostrating the heart's energy. This remedy brings down rapid action of the heart by giving help in the muscular motor sphere, so that the rapid feeble pulse gives way to the slower and normal pulse beats, so that its action on the heart resembles that of cactus." With this I fully agree. And I want to say no one need fear weakening the heart by this remedy if they are only careful about dosage. Do not overdose. I have given aconite many times in typhoid fever, but given alone I have had no good results as a rule in this disease with aconite, except it be as a heart tonic.

Aconite has long been used as a pain obtunder in liniments because of its specific influence on the peripheral nerves. For this purpose it can be combined with chloroform; say five or six drops of specific medicine aconite to the same amount of chloroform, mix and apply to the seat of pain. In this way relief often follows quickly in cases of pain in the stomach, bowels, local neuralgia, lumbago or sciatica.

We can trace the action of aconite when we give it, not mechanically, but intelligently. Give it for relief of acute chills and coldness in the early stages of disease. The arterioles under the influence of the vascular nerves have contracted, cutting off peripheral blood supply. Hence the coldness. Aconite acting through the sympathetic nerves flushes these cutaneous arterioles, the patient becomes warm, the chills are gone, perspiration becomes free.

It is doubtless a fact that giving the simple remedy we can get a better knowledge of the individual characteristic action of the remedy. On the other hand, with our present limited knowledge of many remedies, we can at times certainly make useful combinations. For instance, in pneumonia, according to indications, aconite may be combined with ipecac, bryonia or lobelia; in rheumatism with rhus, bryonia or macrotys, or, when there is much pain and not sufficient bowel action, with colchicum.

In cardiac trouble, where there is not only the characteristic weakness, but irritation shown by the varying and uncertain pulse, aconite can be combined with cactus.

Eclectics have always taken a pardonable pride in the success which attended their efforts against blood-letting. We must never forget that in that fight we had noble helpers in our Homeopathic friends. These men never tired in publishing to the world that in aconite they possessed a remedy which had all the energy without the inconvenience of bleeding. So that in an early day aconite with them took the place of the lancet.

In conclusion, if you ask me what remedy I place first in my list of essentials in the fight with disease, with the single exception of water, I say specific medicine aconite.

A RE-STUDY OF SCILLA MARITIMA.

Brose S. Horne, Gas City, Ind.

This plant grows near the seashore in sandy and sunny places, being indigenous to the basin of the Mediterranean from Syria westward to the coast of the Atlantic. This drug has been frequently subjected to chemical investigations, but the true active principles are still unknown. Vogel's and Tiloy's "scillitin" was exploded. Sanderer and Marais (1857) obtained certain compounds that they supposed were alkaloids, but Tiloy proved the non-existence of such a body in squill. The presence of certain crystals in squills was discovered long ago. Schroff, in 1864, showed that these substances were "very fine and sharp-pointed needles of oxalate of calcium."

One of our very late authorities gives the constituents of squills to be, scillitin (?) skalein, calcium oxalate, sinestine, scillipicium, scillitoxin and scillin. One authority, who is charmed by the new love, Alkaloidal Medication, gives scillitoxin (glucoside) as an emeto-cathartic; says it slows the pulse and raises arterial pressure; diuretic in cardiac dropsy; stimulant expectorant when secretion is free but not expelled (dropsy with dry, harsh skin, parched tongue, feverish lips, contracted features).

I never could understand from the use of this so-called constituent how the above indications could be produced from clinical evidence. We have undisputed evidence to show that scillitin in four-grain doses destroyed a dog of medium size in twenty-four hours. Some claim the virtues of squill can be extracted by water, alcohol and vinegar. It has been analyzed by different ones with varying results. There is a bitter principle, but not obtained pure—scillitin. Merck claims to obtain three compounds of this class, scillipicium, scillitoxin and scillin (see U. S. D., 1907).

Clinical evidence shows that not one of these products represents the full drug. A poisonous dose of squills produces violent vomiting, colic, purging, and a few report blood in the urine. It will produce rapid breathing, a cold skin, coma and convulsions. The older experimenters claimed that they found inflammation and erosion of the stomach and hemorrhagic transudation about the heart and lungs, and in the kidneys and brain. Later experiments show that the drug does not produce any lesion of the stomach, nor any inflammation of the kidneys and bladder, but the lungs and pleura were congested.

In other words, the poisonous effect of the drug produced a congestion of the lungs and pleura.

The so-called medicinal (?) doses of squills, as used by the old school, exert a diuretic action, relax the bowels and cause a reduction of the pulse beat, but increase the tension of the pulse. The continued use of these large doses impairs the appetite and digestion. Some claim the drug will excite the pulse, and urge this as an objection to its use in all inflammatory troubles. Others claim this is not the case. The truth of the matter is that squills, like many other drugs (a point that many seem unable to comprehend in the "old school," Robert Bartholow excused), has a different action in a small dose than it has in a large dose—the so-called medicinal dose of orthodox medicine.

This drug has an elective affinity for the mucous membrane of the lungs. In proper doses it excites (shocks), thus promoting the secretory process. In old-school medicinal doses it produces great shock to the nervous system, producing nausea and diminishing the action of the pulse. Dr. Coxe's old time hive syrup shocked many a young one into the grave, and no doubt some of my old-school ancestors helped in an innocent way to do it. Dr. Horne, of Edinburg, Ssotland, believed in the diuretic power of squills, but he maintained that the only way to get the full diuretic effect was to vomit with it—puke it out, I suppose. My grandfather believed the same, and remained true to his medical ancestor. I find Dr. Beck (1861), of New York, indorses the treatment.

It was the abuse of squills that has caused it to be sadly neglected in our day. The diuretic puke-cure with squills was far more dangerous than Thomson's universal puke-cure with lobelia. One class escaped punishment when they did kill (innocently, of course), while the other class was persecuted by orthodox medicine and accused of killing when they did not do so.

Squills is an old drug. It was used by the Greeks and by their followers in Rome, Arabia and Europe. In combination with honey and vinegar it was anciently employed in dropsical affections. At one time it was praised as a great remedy for spongy and ulcerated gums, ulcerated throat, etc. One ancient writer said it was a good remedy for debility of the digestive organs in small doses, but he fails to give the exact dose. I do not intend to repeat, "parrot-like," the authorities of the past and of the present as to the use of this drug, because facts show that a poisonous dose has been advocated as a medicinal dose for so long that very few can speak from true observation, reason and experience as to the use of this drug in its truly medicinal dose.

Scudder, whose writings have saved me from following the teachings of a pseudo-science, and gave me a new hope and a new life in medicine a thousand and one times in my humble life, was the cause of my investigating scilla maritima. In "Specific Medication," page 236, as if he felt dissatisfied with the record of the past, he says: "In minute doses it relieves irritation of the mucous tissues and stimulates secretion. *Though it has been so extensively employed, it needs to be re-studied.*" That is exactly the point, "it needs to be re-studied." I do not wish to appear as advocating a dynamic action of this drug. Such a theory of drugs is beyond my humble comprehension. As Hale (Edwin M.), who was one of our greatest Eclectics, although he sailed under Homeopathic colors, said: "Hahnemann and some of his radical disciples teach that the action of drugs is dynamic, meaning of an imponderable, immaterial force. This theory must be discarded. The idea of a dynamic force is abandoned by all scientists. There is no dynamic force except that exerted by the human soul. Medicines, even in the minutest quantity, act on the animal organism by means of their ultimate molecules coming in contact with the various tissues of the body."

If one wants any theory of how drugs act, I am inclined to believe that Dr. Cooper, the medical sage of Cleves, comes nearer advocating the most reasonable theory in his " shock theory." With a large dose we may get too much "shock." Let us "shock" the sluggish organism by slight taps frequently repeated until it revives the function.

The provings of squills show that it has an elective affinity for the lungs, that under certain pathological conditions it "makes for cure."

Scilla in old-school therapeutics is classed as expectorant and diuretic. We find that in its mildest operation (small doses) it excites the muciparous glands of the trachea and bronchi, and also the urinary secretion slightly. In a large enough dose this drug will produce inflammatory symptoms resembling bronchitis and pleuropneumonia.

The presence of inflammatory action is held by the old school to contraindicate its use. In this particular drug the simile is correct. In small doses, say one drop of the first dilution, it gives good results. This is not Hahnemannian conclusion, for we find before his time that it was much used in pnuemonia and pleurisy. Hughes, in speaking of this drug, says: "I know of no other medicine that has the same characteristic range of action as that of scilla." I have myself used the first dilution for coughs. I cannot understand why it is that the new schools of medicine have not used scilla more than they have, unless it is from prejudice of the poisonous use of it by the old school. Scudder gives an indication for its use: "Cough with secretion of a yellowish muco-pus, mucus rattling in the chest, scanty urine, feeble circulation."

One Homeopath gives as indications: "A whooping-like cough, sounding loose, with sneezing and watering of the eyes and nose. Catarrhal affections with loose-sounding cough; more expectoration in the morning; wheezing breathing." Clinical evidence demonstrates that an active inflammatory process does not contra-indicate scilla in a small dose. This drug should play an important part in the treatment of acute bronchitis. Hale always used scilla in this disease, and the one guiding symptom was "profuse watery urine which scalds." In the treatment of broncho-pneumonia, after aconite or veratrum has been given, scilla comes in very well, when there is a great rattling in the chest and the patient is unable to raise the sputum.

In fact, it is more prominently indicated than bryonia. Bryonia does better in pleuro-pneumonia. In a case where there is weak pulse, hot, dry skin, dry spasmodic cough, which appears to pain greatly, great dyspnea and struggling for breath, due to an obstruction of the bronchioles, also the sputum is frothy, glairy, red and difficult to detach, give squills, I say, one drop or more of lx dilution every hour or two. One authority found that one to three drops of this ticture in glycerin was superior to all other medicines in the later stage of this disease, "when the right side of the heart becomes distended and the heart's force declines, threatening failure." When heart failure threatens in these cases, larger doses, say three or four drops of the 1x dilution, should be given, and in this way we sustain the heart by the secondary effect of squills.

This dose will positively remove "the small, quick, irregular pulse, the cold livid face and extremities," and suffocative attacks from large accumulations of mucus in the bronchi. It was their action that the old school was endeavoring to get, but their excessive doses frequently overreached the mark and bad results ensued from poisonous action. In ordinary cases of broncho-pneumonia, after the proper sedative has been used, give minute doses of squills. Later on in the disease, if heart failure threatens, give it in larger doses until you get the secondary effect.

Squills can be used to good advantage in pleurisy. Its action resembles that of bryonia, having many sypmtoms in common. Whenever the pleuritic effusion is accompanied with capillary bronchitis, caused from exposure to cold, or the result of eruptive fever, this drug will do good.

It will reward any practitioner to re-study squills in a small dose and test it at the bedside. It is with much sorrow that I find even the new school writers overlook the worth of this drug. Ellingwood overlooks its important indications, as do Locke, Thomas and others. Of course, all of the old school men are unable to understand it as a curative agent in reasonable (small) doses. Scudder desired a restudy, and Hale (a shining light in true Eclecticism) discovered its true worth and made a brilliant plea for its use in a proper manner. This drug should be used in a very small dose at first (say in 1x dilution). A study should be made of its secondary effect in drop doses. A pronounced (old school) dose is never desired. I have used squills for eight years in a small dose, and it has demonstrated its worth to me at the bedside. The first dilution is not "delusions" of Homeopathy. The dose of the fluid extract of squills for an adult is from one to five minims, according to orthodox medicine. He who must use large doses should leave squills alone. *"Give the smallest possible dose until you get the desired effect."*

ARTHRITIS DEFORMANS.

W. B. CHURCH, M.D., CINCINNATI.

Professor Webster's comment on the arthritis deformans paper of October, in the December JOURNAL, is in his usual lucid and trenchant style. He is no mean authority, and always shows an intimate knowledge of his subject that makes any communication from him welcome. Much that he writes very strongly enforces the reason for writing the original article, which was a hope to rescue some of these cases from the limbo of hopelessness to which they have been consigned, and many more from frittering away time and money on antirheumatics. The cases he cites are directly in point, and most will agree with his suggestion that trophic disturbance is an important etiological factor. His remedies, too, are well chosen; but, with all deference to his judgment and keen penetration, which I have long held in high regard, I venture to take issue with him when he advises young practitioners not to follow my "example in forcibly breaking up joints stiffened from arthritis deformans." I shall continue to teach some of them that it is the proper thing to do. At all events, I cannot agree that a given procedure is justifiable in an old practitioner and unadvisable for a younger one. I would have each one act on Davy Crockett's motto: "Be sure you are right, then go ahead."

The pathology, correctly given by the learned professor, does not support his contention. It is quite true that the disease is especially characterized by degeneration of the articular cartilages, which disintegrate at points of contact and proliferate at the joint margin, often eventually developing bony outgrowths which serve to lock the joints. But the conclusion that "forcibly breaking up such structure leaves little probability of return of normal elements, and it is hardly probable that joint function can ever be restored," is hardly justified. It will be admitted by all that such restoration cannot be brought about without such preliminary breaking up. As in all similar cases, more "trouble" is likely to ensue from non-use. Even in neurotic cases, the hysterical knee, false ankylosis, and muscular wasting often follows long-continued disuse; while massage, with passive motion and electricity, bring about normal conditions. It has often happened that a subacute, or chronic case of ankylosis, with more or less swelling, pain and sensitiveness, has been cured by a fall or accidental injury which forcibly flexed the joint. In joints, as elsewhere, functional activity favors trophic processes. When a joint is locked, its function is suspended, only to be resumed by unlocking it. This removes obstructions to the circulation, the first step toward improved nutrition.

The influence of massage afterward is well known to promote the circulation, with all that this implies. Nature is endowed with wonderful resources when conditions are made favorable, and Professor Webster cannot set a limit to the degree of restoration which is now possible.

Fortunately, evidence is available on this point that will be more conclusive to most physicians than any based on theory. One of the cases cited in the October JOURNAL is still under treatment. Reference to page 521 of the JOURNAL will show the condition when first brought to my notice, and the improvement shown at the time of writing the article. Attention is particularly called to the condition of the phalangeal joints of both middle fingers, and to the statement as to evidence of renewal of cartilage, as shown by disappearance of pain, tenderness and grating noise on motion. The improvement has been more rapid since. The bony outgrowths are nearly absorbed, and the fingers have straightened out and become almost normally flexible, affording conclusive evidence of "return of normal elements," and restoration of joint function. That which has been done in a small joint can be done in a large. The ankylosis that results from arthritis deformans is rarely, if ever, bony; but a fibrous ankylosis can restrain motion completely; and it is this form that we are considering, due to organization of inflammatory exudate, inside or ouside, or both, of the capsule. It often results from fibrous adhesions and cicatricial contraction outside the capsule, nearly always in inconvenient and disabling positions. Much benefit will always result from breaking up such adhesions, if followed up with proper treatment to maintain flexibility. Therefore, physicians everywhere, young or old, are urged to give their cases the benefit of the measure, which, if heroic, is also successful.

LOCAL HYPEREMIA.*

U. N. Mellette, M.D., Holdenville, Okla.

Just now much interest is being manifested in the new doctrine of artificial local hyperemia as taught and practiced by Prof. Bier in the treatment of indolent ulcers, chronic joint ailments and other intractable conditions heretofore indifferently met.

As yet I've had no case suitable for the verification of this new doctrine; but because it makes clear some matters which I long ago stumbled upon, and met, in a bungling way, the elucidation meets my hearty approval and confidence.

And it recalls with pleasure the same feeling of approval and confidence I experienced on reading the first edition of Haig's "Uric Acid as a Causation of Disease," which explained so vividly conclusions I had already arrived at relative to sick headache (being myself a victim), and because of such conclusion had already discarded meats, coffee and pie, and adopted precautions as to renal functions and the restraint upon a vigorous appetite.

But, at the risk of some measure of circumlocution, I desire to point the cause of, and course of reasoning which led me, in the long ago, to the simple conclusion which now makes one marvel that an adverse belief should ever have had entertainment.

A few days before the close of my second session (now fifty years ago) our Professor of Surgery had concluded his regular course of lectures in advance of other members of the faculty, but continued to put in his daily hour on supplementary subjects. And one of these subjects was leg ulcers, and pointing a finger he said: "I want you young gentlemen to understand from the very outset that neither man nor angel knows how to make a salve or lotion that will heal a sodden, water-logged ulcer on a swollen leg. First, the swelling must be removed, and the normal circulation restored to the part before amendment can be hoped for, and that condition can best be secured by *bandaging* and *position*."

Next, the fact must be recalled that Indiana, which was to be my field of labor, was a heavily timbered State, and of consequence furnished an ample crop of sore shins. And all wanted to be cured,

---

* Read before the Hughes County Medical Society.

of course, but some rebelled at the restraint imposed, while others balked at the requirement of cleanliness, deeming that an effeminate superfluity not to be submitted to.

In visiting one of my early cases I chanced to meet the oracle of the neighborhod, and as we rode down the lane together he volunteered the following pronouncement:

"Doc., ef I am destertute of larnin' I'm older than you, an' tell yer now that you'll never cure them legs onless you skarryfy and cup 'em, 'kase that blood is p'izen, an' you must get it out."

But I knew the victim would kick like a steer at that proposition, and besides it would deter others, and so adversely affect the contribution. Besides, after all, there was not much the matter with the blood aside from too much carbon and too little oxygen, and isn't there some other way?

Come to think—when my feet are warm they fill my boots, but when very cold they shuffle about like loose seeds in a gourd, and why not supplement Prof. Howe's "bandage and position" with a frequent *hot bath*, lasting until the feet and legs become as red as beets, and so *dilate* the sodden and obstructed capillaries and allow the bad blood to pass out and good blood to pass in?

The next day I fabricated an excuse for calling again, and put the inspiration to the test. Then, in order to deplete the sodden tissues, a piece of cotton batting was saturated with glycerine and applied, and rendered better service than the present-day antiphlogistine. Then with bandage carefully applied and limb well elevated improvement was perceptible in twenty-four hours. And this continued steadily except when interrupted by some indiscretion.

Other cases came, and with them, of course, many set-backs, and some failures—not due to the plan or principle, however, but usually to poverty or ignorance, and sometimes chargeable to the common cussedness of mean human nature, as when a fellow celebrates his thankfulness by a drunken lay out.

Well, it is easy to realize what the Bier plan will do without waiting for the demonstration; for there must be temporary venous engorgement, and, of consequence, temporary dilatation. Then, on removing the obstructing bandage, the heart force, supplemented by gravity and massage, will empty the vessels while still in a state of dilatation, and again permit nutrition to resume its function.

Even my plan was a notable success in its way, though it never occurred to me as bringing about a state of local hyperemia and so feeding the part; but simply as a means of securing capillary dilatation, and so removing obstruction to, and offering facility for, the restoration of normal circulation.

And the cumbersome way in which the result was brought about deterred imitators and left the field to myself.

But now, with the new light, the field is widened and the way made clear and easy for all.

I venture no special outline of Prof. Bier's work, since the mere mention of local hyperemia makes clear what the bandage will do for the parts adapted to its application, while dry heat or hot bath may have to serve elsewhere.

But let us go a little further and see what more the bandage-ligature may do for us. Say you've just had an obstetric case; the work is over, the babe is at the breast, and the exhausted mother has fallen into a peaceful slumber, and you have quietly gathered up your belongings, but in order to be assured that all is well you touch the pulse softly before replacing your gloves, and discover— post-partum hemorrhage!

Your hypodermic syringe is quickly in hand, but you've forgotten adrenalin. However, here is ergotole, and there is opium and gallic acid, and next the womb is kneaded to arouse it to a sense of duty.

Finally, the danger is passed, but those miserable cramps in the legs and feet continue, and finally the old woman proposes cording the thighs, and with ill-concealed contempt permission is given, and some of the cramps abate, then cease. You knew the opium would do it—yes, but it was an ugly coincidence.

Next, a man goes to mill. The road is long, the water low, the grinding slow, and it is nightfall when he returns, famished because of no dinner. But the good wife provided for that contingency by setting aside an ample dish of pot-pie with dumplings, string beans, new potatoes, cucumbers and gooseberry pie.   .   .

About midnight he awakes, feeling that everything inside was afloat, and sicker than a dying calf. The doctor is sent for, and the process of emptying begins, in two directions, and becomes most thorough. The doctor was absent and all medicaments in the house had been swallowed and ejected.

Finally the storm abated, but the cramps became terrific. However, the ubiquitous ·old -woman and string were there, and *did the work*. But how?

Uric acid is a waste product, always present in the blood and tissues; and, like drift wood in a swollen stream, glides smoothly on. But when the water is shallow and the current week the debris is apt to jag bank or bottom.

And so, when the blood-vessels are depleted, whether by hemorrhage or draining off the blood serum, the microscopic crystals of uric acid impinge upon the capillary walls, and the muscles set up an injunction, and the victim sets up a howl. But loosely cord the limb, and by so doing dilate the blood-vessels—then sit on the fence and see the injunction dissolve.

PROGRESSIVE PARALYSIS OF THE INSANE.

LYMAN WATKINS, M.D., CINCINNATI.

General paralysis is characterized by its gradual and insidious approach and by its resemblance, in the beginning, to many other nervous disorders. Insomnia, headache, mental depression and irritability, conjoined with loss of appetite and digestive troubles, are among the first manifestations of general progressive paralysis, and frequently lead to errors of diagnosis in the beginning. The mental symptoms which may suggest the approach of paresis are many and varied, and consist of slight memory lapses, temporary confusion of ideas and words, small and inconsequential actions which attract attention only because different from the usual behavior of the patient. He appears to ignore the important affairs of life and to. magnify trifles. Later, as the disease progresses, he is confused in business and makes mistakes in monetary affairs, his memory of faces fails. he becomes lost and commits acts against the proprieties and decencies of life. In the beginning the patient realizes that his mind is failing and strives against it, but later pays no attention to his symptoms and grows negligent, sullen and depraved. After the disease is fully developed—and its development may consume a period of months or years— the symptoms become exaggerated and the progress more rapid. Progressive enfeeblement of mind and body is plainly evident, but actual paralysis is rare, though special paralyses of groups of muscles about the. face and throat may appear and disappear. The Argyll-Robertson pupil is pathognomonic, while the pin-hole pupil and a lack of harmony in the regularity and size of each pupil is common. Apoplectiform convulsions are of frequent occurrence in the course of general paralysis, a spasm of this nature sometimes being the initial symptom of the disease. Those cases marked by frequent paretic spasms are attended with more rapid mental failure and a greater number of paralytic phenomena. Delusions, hallucinations and absurd conceptions are coincident with advancing physical debility. One peculiarity of this disease is the occurrence of periods of remission, when the patient regains his normal mental condition for a time and may resume his usual occupation. These periods of remission may continue for several months or a year, but in time the malady reappears and resumes its inevitable progress.

Pathologists have heretofore asserted that progressive paralysis of the insane was always of syphilitic origin. But recently some exceptions have been noted. Fournier has termed the disease para-syphilitic. He claims that it is due to degenerative processes the result of an impaired vitality of the neurons which causes premature decay and atrophy, the whole trend of the symptom-picture being one of gradual degeneration of body and mind concomitant and equal. One writer states that general paralysis is due to *syphilization* and *civilization*, because it is more frequently found in large cities and more frequently affects men. Green says that this disease has been ascribed to alcoholism, but claims that in countries where intemperance is rife yet syphilis absent general paralysis is unknown. Kraft-Ebing has shown that eight general paralytics who exhibited no external signs of syphilis possessed an immunity to this disease, for they could not be inoculated with the virus. Morbid anatomy reveals cerebral atrophy with thickening of the meninges; the weight of the brain is diminished one-third in some extreme cases. There is usually hemorrhage into and distension of the ventricles. Microscopically there is destruction of the neurons and an increase in neuroglia cells. The destructive processes are more marked in the frontal and central gray matter and in the island of Reil. At the base of the brain and in the medulla degenerative processes implicate the nuclei of nerve origin, and the third nerve is usually affected early in the disease, thus accounting for some of the characteristic ocular symptoms. The destructive processes are of great extent and general.

Treatment offers very little hope in this disease. Neurons once destroyed are never regenerated.

———•———

CHAMOMILLA.—Useful in spasmodic conditions attending teething in infants. Child is irritable, fretty, peevish. The remedy must be given in small doses. Chamomilla may be combined with aconite in these cases. Dose: one-half teaspoonful of the 3x dilution in one-half glass of water, a teaspoonful of the mixture to be given hourly. Chamomilla is also useful in infantile colic or diarrhea, where there is great irritability and restlessness; diarrhea with green, watery stools, with colic, thirst, bitter taste or bitter eructations. It is also useful in hysterical conditions.—*Journal of Therapeutics and Dietetics.*

ICHABOD GIBSON JONES, M.D.

By HARVEY WICKES FELTER, M.D., CINCINNATI.

Ichabod Gibson Jones, M.D., was born in the town of Unity, Waldo County, Maine, June 18, 1807, and died of consumption at Columbus, O., March 14, 1857, aged nearly fifty years. Of his pre-

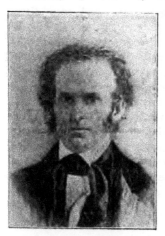

ICHABOD GIBSON JONES, M.D.

liminary education nothing is known, except that his qualifications in later years would indicate that he had received a liberal education. After a preparatory course of medical study, he had conferred upon him, at the Medical Department of the University of New York, the degree of Doctor of Medicine, in 1830, and in the same year was appointed a professor in the Reformed Medical College of New York. Filling this position with great honor to himself, he was invited to a professorship in the newly established Reformed Medical College at Worthington, O., where he gave great satisfaction as a teacher, and began the practice of medicine. Here he married the daughter of Colonel James Kilbourne in 1833. His territory of practice having now extended to Columbus, he took up his residence, in 1834, in that city, which became the field of his active labors until his death. While there, he served for awhile as physician to the Ohio Penitentiary. This in itself was a distinguished honor in those days and one rarely held by an irregular physician.

In 1850, upon the death of his close friend, Professor Morrow, at the earnest solicitation of the faculty and friends of the Institute, he was induced to accept the chair of Theory and Practice of Medicine in the Eclectic Medical Institute. He was also selected by his colleagues to prepare for publication the manuscript of the late Professor Morrow. This he did, adding to it another volume of his own, issuing the two-volume "Jones and Morrow's American Eclectic Practice of Medicine," which was long a favorite work with Eclectic physicians. The work of his chair proving too arduous for his rapidly declining health, and wishing to take better care of his interests in Columbus, in 1853 he resigned his active connection with the Institute, being made Emeritus Professor of Theory and Practice of Medicine, which distinction he retained until the disruption of the faculty, in 1856. He then espoused the cause of the Eclectic College of Medicine, he being one of the editors of the *College Journal*. At the time of his death he was vice-president of the Ohio Eclectic Medical Association. Said Professor Scudder, who was a great admirer of Professor Jones: "He was a typical pioneer, large, active, strong, the type of a noble man and a gentleman, and one that made his mark in every pursuit."

Dr. Jones was an exceedingly energetic man, and even disregarded his physical condition in his zeal to give his attention to his practice and worthy public movements. He took great interest in medical students, was regarded as an exceptionally fine and thorough teacher, and sternly opposed to acts and influences immoral in their tendency. As a physician he took a first rank, being regarded the foremost Eclectic physician of his day, was kind and exemplary, and a friend, abiding and sympathetic. A zealous and true friend of medical reform, a man of deep and profound research, and a consistent Christian, his early death cast a gloom upon those who knew him. He was one of those whose strong character exercised a great influence over those with whom he came in contact—one who was regarded as great in the hearts of his associates—a true type of "nature's noblemen."

Strictly Germ Proof.

The Antiseptic Baby and the Prophylactic Pup
Were playing in the garden when the Bunny gamboled up;
They looked upon the Creature with a loathing undisguised—
It wasn't Disinfected and it wasn't Sterilized.

They said it was a Microbe and a Hotbed of Disease,
They steamed it in a vapor of a thousand odd degrees;
They froze it in a freezer that was cold as Banished Hope,
And washed it in permanganate with carbolated soap.

In sulphuretted hydrogen they steeped its wiggly ears;
They trimmed its frisky whiskers with a pair of hard-boiled shears;
They donned their rubber mittens and they took it by the hand
And 'lected it a member of the Fumigated Band.

There's not a Micrococcus in the garden where they play;
They swim in pure iodoform a dozen times a day;
And each imbibes his rations from a Hygienic Cup—
The Bunny and the Baby and the Prophylactic Pup.
   —Arthur Guiterman, in Stuffed Club, Denver, Colo.

Texas Eclectic Medical Association.

PROCEEDINGS OF THE TWENTY-FOURTH ANNUAL MEETING.

L. S. DOWNS, M.D., EDITOR.

BREECH PRESENTATION.

H. H. HELBING, M. D., ST. LOUIS, MO.

The subject assigned me was "Deciduoma Malignum," but as I encountered a stubborn case in obstetrics recently, I thought it would be of more benefit to this Association than would a. paper on the other subject.

It is not my purpose to take up the etiology, diagnosis and prognosis of this condition, but to merely enumerate my experience in this one case, and in that way help some of you over some difficulties in your practice.

In the first place, this patient was thirty-four years of age, and was a primipara. Her mother had difficulty in her two labors, both instrumental deliveries, although the babies weighed but little more than two pounds. The patient herself had fallen in early life, and had injured her spine, although examination revealed no deformity of the pelvis—only that it was small. I was first called Monday morning, October 14, and discovered that the patient was having false pains. Examination revealed that not only was there no dilatation, but that the cervix was standing out prominently, indicating that parturition would not take place for several days. Gave chlorodyne tablets to relieve pain. Was called again that night about 9 P. M., by the nurse, who had just arrived. Found conditions the same as in the morning.

Was called again Wednesday, October 16, 7 A. M., and found pains regular, about five minutes apart, but no dilatation taking place. Examination revealed an abnormal presentation, but too high to determine positively the position. After two hours I decided to give H. M. C. per orem. No. 1 was given, after which patient slept three hours. At bedtime another was given, and patient slept until 2 A. M. This was Thursday, October 17. Pains from this on to 7 A. M. were severe enough to keep patient awake. At this time I found that the os had not dilated, although the presenting part had pressed a little lower—in fact, had engaged in the superior strait—so that I was now enabled to determine the presentation

I had during the progress of the case been giving sp. gelsemium and caulophyllum, and I now began the use of quinine in addition to the above.

I returned at intervals during the day, and in the afternoon, finding that the os was not dilating, and there being little advancement in the presenting part, I decided to call Dr. A. F. Stephens. After consultation, we decided to put her under H.M.C. and endeavor to get more relaxation before attempting forcible delivery. I gave her, at 6:30 P.M., a hypodemic of No. 1 H.M.C. In fifteen minutes her pains had subsided and she was snoring loudly. I decided to stay with her until 10 or 11 o'clock. At 10 P.M. I made an examination and was surprised to find the os dilated to about two inches in diameter, although she had been sleeping soundly during the dilatation. I thought it wise to remain for two reasons: First, to be at hand should spontaneous delivery occur; and second, to observe the effects of H.M.C. At 11 o'clock she began to rouse a little when each pain came on. At 12 she began to complain during each pain, but dropped off to sleep immediately after it had passed. At 12:30 I gave another hypodermic, inasmuch as she could not sleep any more. This controlled her until 5:30 A. M., at which time another No. 1 was given. An examination revealed the presenting part in the inferior strait and the os slipping back over the hips of the child. At 7 A.M., concluding that spontaneous delivery was out of the question, and that the parts were sufficiently relaxed to effect delivery without much injury to the soft parts, I sent for Dr. Stephens, who, upon arrival, coincided with my opinion, and we immediately went to work. Patient was still sleeping soundly, but could easily be aroused. She would protest against any efforts on our part, so we gave her chloroform and effected delivery after great exertion on the part of both of us. It required a half hour's work and the use of about two drachms of chloroform.

The legs or feet of the child seemed to be wedged above the brim of the pelvis, and were brought down with great difficulty, after which delivery was comparatively easy. We were agreeably surprised at the progress of the labor, although profoundly under H.M.C. The patient expressed herself as not feeling anything after going under the first hypodermic. The patient seems to pass into a state of hypnosis, and has hallucinations, so that it is wise to warn the friends of this fact, so that they will not be frightened. I am now using H.M.C. as an anesthetic in surgery, and while it does not profoundly anesthetize the patient, still it lessens very much the quantity of ether or chloroform necessary, and I have found by the use of ether that the patient will not suffer with vomiting following the operation.

CARE OF MOTHER BEFORE LABOR.

M. B. MOREY, M. D., GONZALES, TEXAS.

If it were possible, we would wish to have care of this mother about three generations in the past, or rather forces and circumstances that have made her what she is to-day; but as this is impossible, we are most wonderfully thankful that to-day in America all things are tending along lines of development most desirable for her that is to be the mother of American men—the most perfect specimens of manhood that tread the globe to-day, any way you may so consider them.

Then if we are to care for this mother after labor, we at least want her through the whole period of gestation, and we publicly announce that we cannot take cases that we cannot have six weeks or two months before confinement.

Sometimes it is our lot to be called hurriedly, and when we enter protest be told, "Well, you are here and you cannot help yourself;" but these are exceptions and not the rule.

We will say now, if this paper is to be confined to the few days after labor, we have nothing to say, for the whole nine months' care is to prepare for these last few hours. All the work is done, and we now simply expect results. If our patient has been obedient and followed instructions, even as near as she understood them, we need have no fear.

We are Eclectics, and that explains our use of medicines in these cases—just what is indicated. We are working to accomplish certain results—that is, to have an easy, uncomplicated labor. A few medicines we use in a general way. Aletris cordial seems to meet the most indications in the early monthis of pregnancy, and is the best for an all-round prescription. We always use specific mitchella the last two months, three-drop doses in water three times a day. Other medicines we use as needed. Cascara and rhubarb we prefer as a laxative, although we often permit our patient to choose the laxative when needed, so they do not use calomel, and we only allow the minimum dose of podophyllin. Quinine we use when there are malarial complications, but only in the small dose, and we wish to say here that more accidents occur from malaria than from the use of quinine. If we think there is a weak, lax condition of the uterus, we give strychnine, the small dose three times a day for several weeks before confinement.

We insist on a daily bath, neither cold nor hot, but pleasantly warm, and a walk of a half to one hour every pleasant day the last

three months. No beer or intoxicants are allowed. If they persist
in this we refuse to take the case.

In food we insist that they use fruit, vegetables and cereals. The
white meats such as fish, bird or chicken, we allow at all times; usually these cannot be had every day. Beef or heavy meats we only
permit once or twice a week, and then sparingly. We forbid fasting
as we do feasting, because of the effect on the child, as it produces
a morbid appetite.

This to us is like building a beautiful structure. We now have
to go in and occupy it, and yet the care of this woman for a few days
more may mean the weal or woe of this patient for the rest of her
life.

After labor we cleanse thoroughly and put her to bed on her back
for the first few hours, then the most restful positions for the patient. We watch the contractions and see that all organs are in place.
If it can be afforded, use only absorbent cotten and sterilized gauze
in these cases. We use bandages. We also bind up the breasts and
keep the milk out except when in use.

A warm sponge bath each day, if there is muscular soreness, and
a rub with alcohol and hammamelis after, should be given. We recommend the use of the commode for the first call of nature, and
always give a laxative on the second or third day. We always leave
a cake of Lloyd's Asepsin soap with these patients, not for the babe,
but for he use of the mother on herself.

Now is the time to correct any abnormal conditions of the uterus
and have the patient get up well. If there has been any prolapsus
we keep her in a reclining position for most of the first month, and
allow no lifting or hard work for three months. In food, we allow
no meat or eggs for the first week, but almost anything else they
wish, and often give them a dose of quinine each morning as a prophylactic, and if we fear any septic conditions use specific echinacea.

Always teach your patient that motherhood is the grandest office
woman can fill, and that every thought, word or act of hers may make
or mar the future of her unborn child.

To Break up a Cold.—Take of bayberry (bark of the root)
oz. iv; ginger (powdered), oz. iv; capsicum, oz. ss.; cloves (powdered), dr. vj; mix; add a teaspoonful to a cupful of hot, sweetened
water; a little milk makes it more palatable. This dose may be repeated every hour or two. Try a cupful of the above after taking a
long drive some cold winter's day. Useful in the chill of pneumonia.
—*Journal of Therapeutics and Dietetics.*

SPECIFIC PAROTITIS, CYNANCHE PAROTIDEA, ANGINA MAXILLARIS, OR MUMPS.

C. H. McCustion, M.D., Valley View, Texas.

I don't expect to present anything new on this subject, only a résumé of facts with which you are no doubt familiar.

Mumps is a disease of very ancient lineage. We find a very clear description of it in the writings of Hippocrates. It is peculiar to all seasons, all countries and all people, though it prevails most frequently during childhood and adolescence. It is as prevalent in Algeria as in France, and much so in Europe as in America.

Its power of expansion is not to be compared to measles or whooping-cough. Its contagion is more restricted, often confined to a single school, asylum or garrison, though in exceptional instances it may include entire provinces or communities.

The greatest epidemics appear in spring and autumn, which seasons appear to be most favorable to the spread of the contagion.

Of its bacteriology much is known, but little exact knowledge. The trend of modern thought is in favor of some family of the diplococci.

So far as actually known, its propagation depends solely on contagion. The contagious element is present even before any swelling of the gland occurs, and extends far into convalescence. Contact is, in the main, esential for its expansion. The contagium is not very volatile.

Mumps is an epidemic disease, though it may be endemic to certain localities. Idiopathic cases are rare. We have a remarkable idiopathic parotitis following injury to the abdominal or pelvic viscera, the cause of which is unknown. We may have an inflammation of the parotid gland occurring as a complication to typhoid fever, pneumonia and other infectious diseases, all of which should not be confused with the specific form now under discussion.

One attack, if double, usually confers lifetime immuuity, though relapses are on record.

The incubation of mumps is quite variable, extending from a minimum of six days to a maximum of twenty-six. During the period of incubation no sypmtoms of any consequence appear. The invasion is more or less abrupt, and is characterized by pain and swelling just below the ear, with elevation of lobe on one side midway between the mastoid process and ramus of jaw. The swelling rapidly extends forward and backward, soon giving the patient a decidedly asymmetrical appearance. The elevation of temperature is usually slight, though in severe cases it may reach 104 degrees. There is stiffness of the jaws and painful deglutition. The salivary secretion is diminished and usually of an acid reaction. In children the attack is ofttimes ushered in with a severe attack of earache.

About the second or third day after attack the other gland becomes involved and passes through the same process, though the other gland may remain unaffected, as in single mumps, but such a course does not confer immunity.

From four to eight days after attack all symptoms gradually abate and the patient is none the worse from the experience. While such is usually the case, it is by no means always so. The other salivary glands may become involved.

So frequently are the seminal glands involved that we are inclined to consider it a special localization of the disease rather than a complication. It is rare prior to puberty. It is for the most part unilateral. This metastasis is an object of serious import, as it may be followed by sterility or impotence. It usually appears with the decline of the maxillary swelling. Orchitis may be followed by considerable atrophy and the individual remain virile.

Among other complications may be mentioned mastitis and inflammation of the vulvar glands. Ovaritis is a rare complication, as is also urethritis, carditis, rheumatism and meningitis. Orchitis may terminate in suppuration, as do the salivary glands at times; but this termination is due to the invasoin of some pyogenc organism, as the germ of mumps is not of a pyogenic nature.

Various disorders of the circulation, skin, kidneys and nervous system may arise as complications. Those of the nervous system are at times very grave, e. g., convulsions, paralysis, etc., The ears and eyes are not exempt.

While the prognosis of mumps is favorable in the main, yet the principles of prophylaxis should be adhered to strictly.

The treatment of uncomplicated cases of a mild form is mainly hygienic. All cases, however mild, should be confined to the bed during the course of the disease and placed on a restricted diet to lessen the risk of a possible metastasis. The remedies usually indicated are phytolacca, aconite, macrotys and acetate of potassium. I always preface my treatment with a mild but thorough purge. In this, as in all other diseases,*specific medication* should be our watchword and *specific diagnosis* our guiding star.

All hail to the day when the glories of Eclecticism will envelope the globe and paralyze all opposition with its dazzling splendor, and the bones of old Aesculapius roll over in Greece and acknowledge the tribute to his fame—*the unfurled banner of Eclecticism.*

CHLOROFORM IN. OBSTETRICS.

W. H. GORE, M.D., ELIASVILLE, TEXAS.

The first use of chloroform in obstetric cases, so far as I have been able to learn, was in Queen Victoria's time. She heard of it being used among the peasantry cases and decided to have it given her at her next confinement, which was done, we are told, with entire satisfaction.

The use and mode of using chloroform in difficult labors seems well etablished among all observers.

My own experience has been that ordinary cases do not need chloroform at all, and are better off without it, only in difficult cases, and then the smallest amount that will serve the present purpose, just enough to take off the sharp edge of pain, and when the patient is nervous and apprehensive, and then only during the pains.

I have a little cotton or soft cloth in a cup or glass, and pour on that about a teaspoonful, rub a little vaseline about the mouth and nose to prevent irritation, and have her inhale as she feels the pains coming on. Give only during a pain. Push the anesthetic toward the end of the second stage, withdrawing the chloroform as soon as the head is born. It should be used according to circumstances in complicated cases.

Boisliniere says: "In eclampsia it has given surprising results in the hands of some observers. It does not, however, cure eclampsia, which is caused by certain poisons in the blood; it only prevents the irritation by the poisons on the cerebro-spinal axis, the integrity of which it preserves, thus checking the explosions of the convulsions and their dangerous results, such as cerebral or pulmonary edema and apoplectiform effusions."

Chloroform is accepted or rejected with much reserve by most French observers, but strongly advocated by most German and English scholars.

Most American physicians and obstetricians use it to-day, and it has proved of such signal service in eclampsia that it is now very frequently used, either alone or jointly with morphia, veratrum and other antispasmodics, greatly reducing the mortality.

The same authority says, give chloroform at the onset of every convulsion. Suspend if the patient becomes livid. Watch the respiration. If it becomes irregular it is the most important sign of danger.

Charpentier says that it should not be adopted to the exclusion of other remedies nor absolutely rejected, and that if it fail in a great many cases there are others where it renders valuable service.

Dupaul, who is a strong opponent of its indiscriminate use, states that its full anesthetic dose in eclampsia has several times proved fatal by intensifying the state of coma and cyanosis.

Lusk says, except in cases where labor is nearly at an end, the giving of chloroform should be restricted to the period of pain and restlessness, which is often the preliminary sign of a fresh seizure.

My experience is that ordinary cases of labor do not need it, only as stated above, those that are nervous and restless and have severe cutting pains, and in complications; then it should be used according to circumstances.

The only evil effects that I have been able to observe are that there is more tendency to post-partum hemorrhage and cyanosis of the child.

Eye, Ear, Nose and Throat.

CONDUCTED BY KENT O. FOLTZ, M.D.

ACUTE CATARRHAL CONJUNCTIVITIS.

The spring and autumn are especially productive of catarrhal conditions of the mucous membranes, and the mucous membrane of the eye is affected almost as often as that of the upper respiratory tract. The sudden variations in temperature are largely the cause for this condition.

An acute catarrhal conjunctivitis may be primary or secondary. If the former, it usually runs a short course even without treatment; but if secondary, especially if the result of extension from a rhinitis, the morbid state may become subacute or chronic unless attention is given the nasal cavities. For this reason an examination of the nose should be made in all cases with a catarrhal inflammation. It is also best to examine each case carefully to exclude the presence of a foreign body embedded in the bulbar conjunctiva, cornea, or the conjunctival surface of the lids. Not infrequently foreign bodies will be found which are the cause of the inflammatory action, and any treatmeat would prove ineffectual as long as the exciting cause remained.

The name "pink-eye" is often used to designate this affection of the eye, but may as well be applied to any other ocular condition characterized by increased redness of the mucous membrane. "Pinkeye" means nothing, describes nothing but redness of the mucous membrane, and is about as definite as saying " a person has skin disease." Unfortunately, too many writers are careless in their selection of terms, hence this designation.

If not infected, the course of an acute catarrhal conjunctivitis does not vary from the simple acute catarrhal inflammations of other mucous membranes, the various stages being well marked.

Diagnosis.—Having eliminated foreign bodies as a cause of the inflammation, and if no rhinitis is present, the diagnosis and prognosis are easy. If rhinitis is present, it will modify the prognosis only as regards time of cure, as this complication may retard recovery or even be an active factor in causing the condition to become chronic, especially if the nasal affection is one in which there is considerable thickening of the inferior turbinal bone. In conjunctivitis the congested blood-vessels are freely movable, which may be determined by pressing the lower lid against the eyeball and moving it upward and downward. The secretion after the initial stage is thin watery mucus. If the attack is severe, there may be hemorrhagic areas showing in the mucous membrane of the lids.

The secretion does not become purulent unless infection occurs, although in some cases it comes very close to purulency, but the mucous characer predominates in all the cases.

Treatment.—In uncomplicated cases the use of the boric acid wash and also the following:—Lloyd's hydrastis, dr. ss.; solution boric acid, dr. jv; Sig. two drops in the eye every three hours—will be all that will be required. When the nasal cavities are affected they must be taken care of. Such internal medication as is required should be used.

The Removal of Tonsils from the Standpoint of Preventive Medicine.

This seems to be pre-eminently the day of preventive medicine; its height is not yet reached, the pendulum still swings on. The faith of each and every community in the efficacy of preventive medicine must be advanced by education; the progressive physician is the greatest factor in this educational campaign.

The conditions resulting from and accompanying enlarged tonsils require a consideration at our hands. I will not enter into a detailed description of the anatomical relations of the tonsils. An enlarged tonsil is a diseased tonsil. By pressure it interferes with the circulation to the middle and internal ear. By pressure on the Eustachian tube its functions of equalizing the air pressure in the middle ear and draining the middle ear of mucus are interfered with. Tinnitus often results, and also, in case of middle ear diseases with either mucous or muco-purulent discharge, the mastoid is much more likely to become involved, or progressive deafness may result without mastoid trouble.

That enlarged tonsils predispose to tonsillitis, diphtheria and other throat diseases in various forms, is recognized by all. In some forms of tonsillitis the substance in the crypts forms an excellent culture for the various kinds of bacteria, and in children who have frequent attacks of gastric and intestinal trouble, the cause can often be found to be located in the tonsils, and an individual attack explained by the swallowing of a quantity of these bacteria that have been breeding in the tonsil. The extreme vascularity of the tonsils and the ease with which they become infected make them the avenue of entrance whereby the infecting element of many systemic diseases enters the blood. The fact that rheumatism is so prone to accompany or follow tonsillitis has led some to believe that the rheumatic poison reaches the blood through the tonsils, and is therefore a tonsillar disease.

Tuberculosis can be introduced into the system through the tonsils. Robertson found 8 per cent. of tonsils removed to be tubercular. The tubercle bacillus is thought to enter through the crypts which empty into the supratonsillar fossa and then involve the tonsil. The general infection is through the blood current and the bacilli thus find their way to the apex of the lung.

Tonsillitis has a tendency to recur at least once a year, and with each attack the tonsil becomes larger. Peritonsillar abscess or quinsy is another form that is almost sure to recur if the diseased tonsils are not removed.

Diseased tonsils are usually accompanied by adenoids as well. It is among growing children that the bad results of enlarged tonsils and adenoids are particularly apparent. The face has a vacant look, the mouth is open and the little one appears inattentive and hard of hearing. The backwardness of such children is not due to natural dullness but to a diseased condition of the throat and nose. Children with obstructed throats and noses sleep with open mouths and snore loudly. Their restlessness and night terrors are but evidences that they do not sleep well. Every one whose nose has been obstructed by a cold in the head, knows the effects of a night of broken rest, The head aches, the throat is dry and there is a feeling of general misery. This shows in a measure how the little one feels night after night till the trouble is removed.

The most troublesome form of diseased tonsil is not necessarily the enlarged tonsil. Oftentimes the flat submerged tonsil may be diseased and contain a ramification of diseased crypts deep down in the neck. A large tonsil with open crypts gives less trouble than a small one the spaces of which may be filled with decomposing foul smelling débris which keeps the throat inflamed. Many an annoying cough and many an irritable throat and offensive breath are due to diseased tonsils.

Greber, of Jena, who made an extensive study of the tonsils in health and disease, has come to the conclusion that in civilized life the tonsils are not only useless but dangerous. He advises that all children have their tonsils removed whether they are troublesome or not. He considers such a course as beneficial as vaccination for smallpox. It is certainly a fact that such a course would greatly lessen the mortality among infants, and many children would enjoy much better health.

It may seem an extravagant claim, but there are those who contend that more deaths result from diseases directly traceable to diseased tonsils than from appendicitis.

The public in general and the public school authorities in particular should understand and appreciate these facts and, recognizing the harm that may come from enlarged and diseased tonsils, insist on their removal.

The unreasonable prejudice (and all prejudice is likely to be unreasonable) of many people against having the tonsils removed from their children's throats, is lesesning, but is still in many cases found to be very decided. They seem to feel that the tonsil has some vital function to perform which they do not understand, and that its removal, even when badly diseased, will in some mysterious way interfere with the well-being of the child. The sooner this ungrounded belief is uprooted, and the removal of diseased tonsils becomes universal, the better for the race, and just so soon will a certain proportion of school children, now dull and listless in their work, become more attentve to their studies and accordingly accomplish better work and also improve greatly in facial expression. And this will not be all. The liability to deafness, middle ear disease, mastoid involvment, gastric and intestinal disorders will be greatly lessened; and who can estimate the decreased mortality that will thus be accomplished?— H. A. HARRISON, in *Homeopahtic Eye, Ear and Throat Journal.*

SCUTILLARIA.—This is a valuable remedy for nervous patients, more especially for those female patients who are passing through the climacteric. Use a preparation made from the fresh plant. Scutillaria is a bitter tonic, creates appetite, builds up the patient and at the same time quiets the nerve centers. Try it instead of some fashionable dope. Dose of fluid extract or ticnture, fifteen to thirty drops. —*Journal of Therapeutics and Dietetics.*

Periscope.

Cancer and Its Successful Treatment.

One of the first physicians to make a business of treating cancer was Dr. Fell, of London, who treated it locally with chloride of zinc and bloodroot. His formula is known to physicians the world over. Dr. Marsden, of London, treated the disease locally by arsenic mixed with mucilage of acacia. These men treated cancer as a local disease; their methods were crude, yet they cured some cases, and their treatment offered some hope to the victim of cancer, while a surgical operation offered none at all.

Later on Dr. Thomas W. Cooke, surgeon of the Cancer Hospital, London, England, who from his long years of experience, became convinced that a surgical operation was not a cure for cancer, published a book on cancer, and was the first, I think, to advocate the treatment by constitutional means, and in this book gave the results of his treatment. He was at least trying to cure cancer, and did cure many cases. It remained for a distinguished physician of London, by the name of Dr. J. Compton Burnett, to teach the profession how cancer of the breast could be intelligently and successfully treated. In 1888 he published a book, "Tumors of the Breast," with a record and treatment of cases cured. He has pasesd to his final reward, but he has proved by a mass of reliable evidence that cancer of the breast can be cured by internal remedies.

What Dr. Burnett was trying to do in London, the writer of this article began to do in the United States in 1869. I treated a case of cancer of the breat by internal means alone, and cured my patient. The remedy I used was phytolacca decandra. I treated cancer as a blood or constitutional disease, and have never seen any reason to change my views from my own experience. I am of the opinion that 95 per cent. of cases of cancer can be cured by medicine if the treatment has been commenced before any surgical operation has taken place or the X-ray treatment used.

I have kept a careful record of my cases, and I find that of all cases of cancer, both external and internal, I have treated, 80 per cent. of them have been cured permanently. The reader must bear in mind that most of them had been cut out or burnt out with a caustic; thus it is that they were well-developed and oftentimes in the last stages before I saw them at all. It is not one time in a hundred that I get a case to treat until after another treatment has been tried. The reader must bear this fact in mind in considering my percentage of cures. It has been claimed by some "would-be" critics that I have deceived myself all these years, and that what I thought was cancer must have been something else. In reply to this, allow me to say that cases have come under my treatment that had been examined by professors in the medical colleges of Philadelphia and New York, by prominent surgeons and by others using the microscope, and diagnosed as cancer before they came under my care. If I was deceived, then some of the leaders in the profession have been fooled also.

For many years the leading specialists in the treatment of cancer have treated cancer as a local disease, and treated it with some form of caustics or escharotics. Some have used plaster made of arsenic, but it is very painful, and only a small surface can be treated, for fear of absorption of the arsenic and getting the poisonous effects of the remedy. Caustic potash had its day, and has been put aside as too painful. Chromic acid, chloride of zinc, chloride of chromium and carbolic acid have been used in various forms. Solid extracts of poke root, red clover and sheep sorrel have been used, but these vegetable extracts did not go deep enough; they only acted on the surface. Any application that contains carbolic acid strong enough to do any good will almost invariably leave a scar after the wound heals up. I have always tried to avoid leaving a scar after I had used any local treatment: I have seen patients so marked that they carried the scar through life. All the above remedies and others that I might mention, except arsenic, have been thoroughly tested by me, and I know what they will do and just how much may be expected of them. It has always been my purpose when I use anything of this kind to cause my patient as little pain as possible.

The chloride of chromium is the least painful of any, but care must be used in selecting the cases, for in many cases it will not go deep enough. Chloride of zinc will go deeper into the body of the growth than any other caustic except carbolic acid. When I speak of the latter I mean a 25 per cent. solution. I do not place so much dependence on the use of caustics in the treatment of cancer as I did ten and twenty years ago. I am learning to depend more and more upon internal remedies and mild local remedies.

The treatment of cancer locally by caustics is a crude method and a relic of the dead past. In ten years from now any doctor who claims to cure cancer by local means with caustics will be a back number. The doctor of the future will depend upon internal remedies almost entirely.

While some physicians have claimed to treat cancer as a blood disease, they have rang the changes of all the alteratives, trying to find a remedy that would act upon cancer, but they lost sight of the important fact that cancer was not an ordinary blood disease, but a specific disease peculiar to itself. Some of our doctors and pharmacists, acting on the theory of its being an ordinary blood disease, like scrofula and erysipelas, compounded half a dozen alteratives of different kinds, hoping some one of those remedies would hit the mark. All the different varieties of sarsaparilla have no effect upon cancer at all. Corydalis, yellow dock and tag alder are very good remedies for some things, but have little effect upon cancer. Very much was expected from red clover, but cancer patients have taken gallons of it, and it had no effect upon the cancer. Of all the vegetable remedies, the phytolacca stands in the front rank, for I have learned by many years of experience that it does have a positive remedial effect upon some forms of cancer. Taking them in the order of remedial value, hydrastis comes next, then thuja and baptisia tinctora, and, lastly, arsenic has been used internally, but it is best adapted to cancer of the lips in the form of iodide of arsenic. Conium maculatum sometimes relieves the pain of cancer, but does not seem to check the growth of the disease. As echinacea is such a fine remedy in depraved conditions, one might expect very much from it in the treatment of cancer. I will say that I used a hundred pint bottles of the remedy in different cases of cancer, yet while it relieved the pain in the last stages of the disease, it did not retard the growth of the cancer at all. 'I am satisfied that lime in some form does have a remedial effect on cancer, as I have proved to my own satisfaction. The carbonate or the fluoride of lime are the forms I use it in the most. The chloride of potassium is another remedy that acts upon cancer, especially the soft tumors of the breast. The bellidis perennis (the English daisy) is indicated in breast cancer caused by injury. The thuja in cancer following vaccination. In cases where a patient has been saturated by all kinds of alteratives until the blood becomes thin, a good preparation of iron will always improve the general health of the cancer patient.

In this article I can only briefly outline a general plan of treating cancer. To go into details of the various forms of cancer would fill a good-sized book. I have at different times reported cases of cancer treated and cured to the medical journals. In some cases my attention has been called to the fact that one of my formulas has been used by a doctor to cure all forms of cancer. This is pure quackery, as he might as well take an "eye-wash" and try to treat all diseases of the eye with it.—E. G. JONES, in *Albright's Office Practitioner.*

The Business Side of a Doctor's Life.

Every now and then, says the *Southern Clinic,* we wake up from our treadmill service and find that we are very close to the man with the muckrake, when we compare our financial intake with that of the average business man or skilled laborer! Our carpenter gets four or five dollars a day when he is jobbing about our premises, and puts in a very short day at that, and spends very little brain force while earning his money. The pretty part of it is that he gets his pay cash and has no anxiety to keep him awake.

The operator who sets this page on his linotype machine can easily make six or eight dollars a day with his own hands, though, unlike many artisans, he has a head full of brains, which he uses to our advantage, as our readers can attest from the freedom from errors usually seen in the *Clinic.* But when night comes he can rest without danger of being rung up at any hour to do an odd job of composition.

Our plumber who picked up his trade while hanging around an old-time tin shop will not think of doing any kind of a piddling repair job on any property of ours unless he picks up five or ten dollars for a few hours' work in which a negro laborer at about $1.50 a day does all the work practically. Now, we are not growling about the charges that these people make, but we are alluding to the fact that they get good prices and collect their money cash. In other words, they do not work for charity, sentiment nor love, and leave their bill to stand, or be cut down, or never collected. They collect ample pay for their services, get the money and enjoy it in this life, instead of waiting to be rewarded in a better world. Now, as humiliating as it is to say so, the average physician does not collect from his incessant and trying work as much as five dollars a day, though he may book five thousand a year. The truth is, the doctor is a poor business man. He is so taken up usually in assuaging the pains, both physical and mental, of his unappreciative patients, that he forgets to demand and collect what is justly due him when he renders the service. It is a bad habit that too many of us drop into of being indifferent about promtly collecting our bills. It encourages our patients to neglect payments and makes them feel that we do not value our services very highly, and they will place a low estimate on our value accordingly. The only men making any money in the profession are those who put aside all sentiment and make the practice of medicine a business for what there is in it. The old time once-a-year rendering of bills, or the hope that gratitiude will stimulate the payment for our services, if relied upon now, will make a pauper of any physician who is dependent upon his practice.

If you have been in the old rut, brother, get out of it to-day, or get out of the profession and make room for somebody with gall enough and sense enough to make as much money as a job carpenter or an average machinist.—*Oklahoma Medical News Journal.*

Consumption and Schools.

The confinement of large numbers of children in schools unquestionably make the schoolroom a source of danger from contagious or infectious diseases. A susceptible child exposed to consumption is exceedingly liable to contract the disease.

No teacher known to be afflicted with consumption should teach in a school.

No pupil known to be afflicted with consumption should attend a school.

No employee known to be afflicted with consumption should be allowed to work in the school.

The schoolroom should be well ventilated. The best uses should be made of he poorest facilities of ventilation.

The schoolroom should be flushed with fresh air during intermissions by opening windows and doors.

Children should not be permitted to use any pencil or other article belonging to another which is liable to be put in the mouth.

Children should not be permitted to use slates.

Children should not be permitted to spit on the floor.—*Med. Review of Reviews.*

DIGITALIS.—Relaxation, weakness, dilatation of the heart muscle. Should never be given until compensation has failed. If given during the stage of compensation, will hasten the death of the patient. Digitalis is a powerful remedy, and should never be given by a physician who is not competent to make a thorough physical examination of the patient. Digitalis is a slow acting drug, requiring two or three days to exert its full physiological or mechanical action, and should therefore cannot be depended upon in an emergency. The tincture of the English leaves should be given to contract the heart muscle, and the infusion to increase the flow of urine. The keynote for the administration of digitalis: relaxation and dilatation, weakness, cyanosis, with a slow pulse increased on exertion. This remedy is a two-edged sword and must be carefully watched at all times.—*Journal of Therapeutics and Dietetics.*

Independence of mind, freedom from slavish respect to the taste and opinion of others, next to goodness of heart, will best insure our happiness in the conduct of life.—H. HOOKER.

THE ECLECTIC MEDICAL JOURNAL

A Monthly Journal of Eclectic Medicine and Surgery.

TWO DOLLARS PER ANNUM.

Official Journal Ohio State Eclectic Medical Association

JOHN K. SCUDDER, M.D., MANAGING EDITOR.

EDITORS.

W. E. BLOYER.	H. W. FELTER.	W. N. MUNDY.	R. L. THOMAS.
W. B. CHURCH.	K. O. FOLTZ.	L. E. RUSSELL.	L. WATKINS.
JOHN FEARN.	J. U. LLOYD.	A. F. STEPHENS.	H. T. WEBSTER.

Published by THE SCUDDER BROTHERS COMPANY, 1009 Plum Street, Cincinnati, to whom all communications and remittances should be sent.

Articles on any medical subject are solicited, which will usually be published the month following their receipt. One hundred reprints of articles of four or more pages, or one dozen copies of the Journal, will be forwarded free if the request is made when the article is submitted. The editor disclaims any responsibility for the views of contributors.

Discontinuances and Renewals.—The publishers must be notified by mail and all arrearages paid when you want your Journal stopped. If you want it stopped at the expiration of any fixed period, kindly notify us in advance.

IDLE SPECULATIONS.

Doubtless physicians of the older régime will bear the writer out in the assertion that appendicitis is a disease which has occurred with frequency only within the past twenty or twenty-five years. In more ancient times, say thirty or more years ago, the affection was comparatively unknown. The writer practiced medicine for thirteen years prior to 1882, and did a large general practice during much of that time, with the singular experience, compared with present-day occurrences, of meeting but a single case of appendicitis during all that time, and it was the only one he heard of.

This case, which was met during consultation between two country practitioners with little surgical knowledge and experience, recovered without any knifing. The pus worked its own way through the tissues, opened in the groin spontaneously, as the patient would not consent to any meddling except the application of poultices and the internal administration of sedatives. He remained in bed something over six weeks, and resumed the occupation of farmer upon recovery. He remained well after that for several years, if he is not well to-day. In these times he would have been railroaded to a hospital, *nolens volens*, and might have come out feet foremost. The idea of treating such a case by radical measures was unthought of at that time. It was probably about the year 1876.

But what a change has occurred within the past twenty-five years! Appendicitis is now one of our most common fatal diseases, and a source of great revenue to the operating surgeon. It is safe to assert that more deaths occur from it than from almost any other disease except tuberculosis. We do not pretend to refer to any vital statistics, but there is no doubt that mortuary reports are very much swelled every year from this affliction.

Undoubtedly, many fatal cases are due to the injudicious application of the knife by surgical tyros, but somehow it is difficult to deny that genuine cases of the disease occur with alarming frequency. How do we account for it? Certainly the increase of such cases during latter times cannot be due to any climatic change, nor to any new mode of living. It is doubtful that it depends upon any new microbe, for microbes have been with us always if they are with us at all, though then we were not as well acquainted with them as now. That a new microbe of appendicitis has appeared in modern times, however, would seem a preposterous proposition.

Nor is the claim that our surgeons have become better diagnosticians accountable. Had this affection been so common as now in earlier times it would have been recognized. The truth is, that it is comparatively a new disease; that is, so far as its frequency is concerned. The medical world would not have overlooked it for centuries if it had been such a common affection.

One fact is patent, and that is, the prevalence of appendicitis came into notice contemporaneously with the coal tar products. Can it be that these agents set up a latent poisoning of the mucosa of the cecal region which ultimately results in suppurative inflammation in the cecum and its appendix?

It seems as though this might be a pertinent question, considering the relationship. The actual cause of appendicitis has not yet been satisfactorily settled. Bacteriologists have found several different forms of minute organisms about such foci of inflammation, but nothing which might not be found in any other ulceration of the lower bowel, and which might not be a sequence, rather than a cause. It is hardly to be believed that these organisms have begun any new tricks in recent years.

The use of coal tar products has been too common within the appendicial epoch. It has doubtless caused many collapses from cardiac insufficiency; has it not caused other troubles quite as serious? The suggestion might be worthy of consideration and further study. Observation and inquiry on the subject might be worth while.

The writer would not like to be quoted as making the assertion that the many cases of appendicitis occurring nowadays are blamable to the action of the coal tar products. This would be too aggressive altogether, considering his knowledge in the premises. However, his personal observation enables him to assert that the prevalence of appendicitis at the present time is not due to advanced discrimination on the part of the profession.

He is confident that it was once a very rare disease. It is no discovery due to professional acumen, but an unfortunate condition which has forced itself upon us in modern time. About the time of its advent another unfortunate disease came upon us—the coal-tar-habit. WEBSTER.

SEPTIC INFECTION OF THE HAND.

Owing to the many exposures to accidents, both deep and superficial, the fingers and hand are quite liable to injuries, which are followed by cellulitis or blood poisoning; from traumatic conditions, often neglected, the injured field is seldom sterile enough to resist infection.

When an infected hand is presentd for surgical care, the first duty is to direct a thorough cleansing of the hand and forearm, which can be accomplished by the use of turpentine with a scrub brush, followed by a thorough immersion of the hand in a strong hot soap-suds water, allowing the hand to remain in this bath until it looks almost parboiled.

The hand is then cleansed with gasoline, using a swab of antiseptic gauze. The finger nails are thoroughly cleansed and trimmed, and the hand again washed in soap-suds water made from the tincture of green soap or from the original soft soap found in nearly every country home. The wound is then rinsed with 98 per cent. alcohol, and is then in a fairly good condition to receive surgical attention.

If a puncture wound, it should be first freely incised and the thick skin shaven down to the quick, cauterized with pure carbolic acid before commencing the deep and liberal incisions for the proper drainage of burrowing pus.

Injuries to the *little finger* and *thumb* are much more dangerous than are the same injuries to the other digits or hand, and this is because the synovial sheaths of the flexor muscles do not terminate at the distal end of the metacarpal bones, but extend upward under the annular ligament, and the pus disseminates into the tissues that offer little resistance, and the blood poisoning continues on up the arm infecting the axillary glands.

If this were all there might not be so much danger of cellulitis of the hand, for we have to reckon with the destruction by inflammatory exudates in the sheaths and delicate structures of the fingers and hand, which too often are rendered permanently useless by a lack of proper drainage, to say nothing of the dangers to life and limb.

Let the hand be held by an assistant for a few minutes high above the head; this will make the hand and arm quite anemic. The Esmarch bandage may now be applied, using care in its winding not to drive pus on beyond its localized field. When the deltoid muscle is reached, several tightly drawn folds of the bandage will constrict the blood vessels, so that the field to be operated on will be practically bloodless.

The surgeon should make liberal incisions above the wrist, in the forearm, if the pus has burrowed in this region. The incisions I would advise prior to the openings on the hand and fingers, as the operating field is more dangerous, to injuries by the knife, and is just at this moment the most bloodless.

If the openings in the fingers, hand and forearm have been freely made and proper drainage secured, there will be less damage to the hand than by trusting partly to the good offices of nature.

RUSSELL.

PRIMITIVE PROPERTIES OF PROTOPLASM.

The primitive forms of life, especially the unicellular entities, are almost wholly composed of undifferentiated protoplasm. The vital properties possessed by these simple cellular organisms are called fundamental because they are equally manifested by both the animal and vegetable cell. In fact, it is difficult to detect any difference between the simple forms of animal and vegetable life, and, at times, we are unable to determine with which we are dealing, although in the higher forms of either differentiation is readily made. The primary properties of portoplasm are few and simply manifested in unicellular organisms, but although thus elementary at first, they by combination and elaboration. reach great complexity in the higher animal.

Irritability, or power of response to stimulus, is a physical characteristic of protoplasm. The one-celled being will respond to various stimuli, by movement of the cell as a whole or of some part of its structure, the extent of the movement depending upon the nature and character of the stimulus.

This is a simple experiment, yet here we have the basis of the nervous system in man and all the nerve functions, those that confer upon us a knowledge of our own existence and the existence of things around us, are due to the irritability of nerve cells; the whole neuronic apparatus of man depends for its manifestations upon the power of response to stimuli. When neurons cease to respond, intelligence and power of movement are gone. . In the nervous system we have one fundamental property of protoplasm developed to the complete subordination or exclusion of all the rest.

How wonderfully this property is magnified in man when compared to the undifferentiated mass of protoplasm composing lower
entities. All the possibilities of the future being are locked in the
cell. There is no perceptible difference between the ovum of a dog
and that of the human being, and yet the great differences are there
latent and undeveloped.

All those complicated processes which in man are called digestion,
absorption, secretion, excretion and nutrition are expressed by the
term metabolism, and are present in the unicellular organism in an
elementary form. When the floating cell comes in contact with a
foreign substance in its media, it surrounds the object by infolding it
with pseudopodia, and, after having absorbed that which was suitable
for its structure, unfolds and floats away, or, in other words, excretes
that which was unfit for pabulum. This simple casting off or withdrawing from effete matter is an example of excretion which is carried on in the human body by more complicated processes through
skin, kidneys, lungs and intestines.

Two forces are continually at work in the cell—assimilation and
disassimilation, building up and tearing down. These, plain and uncomplicated in the unicellular organism, are more intricate although
of the same nature in higher animals. Nothing is added to the higher
animal that is not foreshadowed in the simplest form of life. Growth
is also a primitive and inseparable property of cell life. Living things
grow by addition from the interior; the application of food to the
external surface of the body does not increase its growth or sustain
its life.

All pabulum must enter the cell body and growth occurs from the
multiplication of cells. Decay is constant while renewal is just as constant, and the body lives and grows not because it resists destructive
influences, but from its power to replace that which was destroyed.
But all living bodies have a limit to growth and life and death is a
physiological process. Reproduction, a fundamental property of protoplasm, is a very simple process in the primitive cell, and consists
of the division of one cell into two, which may occur either by fission
or by budding from the parent cell. In the human animal the result
is similar, for where there was but one two are found. In the higher
animals the reproductive function requires more time and is more
complicated and usually attended with trouble and pain, but ultimately,
as in the unicellular forms, there is a division of the individual.

The power of spontaneous movement is characteristic of animal
life. Vegetable protoplasm does not possess this function to any great
extent, and the tree or the blade of grass remain stationary. The
ability to move about and to change location is shown in the undiffer-

entiated protoplasm of the leucocyte and in many unicellular organisms. It is largely developed in man.   WATKINS.

OVER-STIMULATION OF THE KIDNEYS.

Several weeks ago I was consulted by one of our merchants whose health seemed to be failing and he did not know why.

Examination showed eyes dull, skin dry and dirty, tongue pale and lightly coated, bowels sluggish, urine pale and very abundant, appetite poor, weak and beginning to be emaciated. A few weeks before he had felt a little malaise and a friend had advised him to get a patent kidney remedy. He got it and took it for awhile; besides increasing his trouble, he noticed he began to pass very large quantities of urine.

Evidently the remedy he had taken was a powerful renal hydrogogue. He passed an abnormal amount of pale urine, but the solid contents of the urine were retained, so that he was being poisoned from retention of the urinary solids. Hence the muddy eyes, dirty skin, failing health and strength. And hence the swollen joints and pain in the fingers.

Treatment.—The patent medicine was stopped. The kidneys were soothed. The stomach was gently stimulated, an electric light bath, with gentle massage, following same. In a short time the change in his general appearance was remarkable. His appetite improved, his skin and eyes cleared up. He felt like a new man. He paid his bill and went on his way rejoicing. And what pleased him especially—he had taken but very little medicine.   FEARN.

QUESTION.

"Are you sure the sick man wanted me?" Ans. "He didn't mention your name, but he's screamin' for some one that'll put him out of his misery, and I thought of you right away."—*Houston Post.*

An answer of this character is liable to diminish rather than increase the bump of egotism of the physician, but it is too often a fair example of the reply received when called or consulted professionally. Often it is intended as a compliment, probably always is, but the wording is anything but complimentary. Who is to blame for the usual estimate of the average physician? There is no profession requiring so much judgment and ability as the medical profession. It means in many instances the restoration of health, or a lingering illness and probably death if the physician is not capable. Why do so many persons visit the corner drug store when they are ailing?

Why do people buy and take the patent nostrums offered by the druggist? Surely there must be some reason for this, and the reason is easily found if one will investigate a little the prescriptions and advice of the average doctor.

Baby is troubled with constipation; the fond mother goes to the family physician, who often makes no examination, but tells her to go to the drug store, or perchance writes a prescription for some well-known and advertised patent medicine. A man may be afflicted with rheumatism, and the same method is taken. Some member of the family has a cough; the directions are to go to the drug store and get some advertised cough compound, or some equally as well advertised oil emulsion. Some confiding patient goes to the doctor with a catarrhal condition of the nose or throat. No careful examination is made, but the victim is told to go to the drug store and get "So-and-so" catarrh "balm," "specific" or "cure."

These illustrations are not "pipe-dreams" but facts. I have heard professors advise, and while behind the prescription counter have seen prescriptions written by legally qualified and reputable physicians for these nostrums. These same individuals decried the use of so-called patent medicines, but instead of using their own faculties for diagnosis and treatment, were content with the professed symptomatology and compound of the nostrum manufacturer whose literature is in the family almanac, or the interesting articles written by Doc. Credulous, extolling pale enemas for pink people, have created much excitement in the medical profession.

Certain compounds are of value, but only when intelligently prescribed. These are not vaunted as cure-alls, but it is a well-known fact that in some conditions a combination of drugs will do better work than a so-called single remedy. However, there is a vast difference between a secret nostrum and a compound manufactured for a definite purpose by a reliable firm. The former is for the purpose of supplying the lazy doctor or credulous public; the latter for putting in palatable form a drug or combination of drugs for a definite condition determined by experience and prescribed only after a careful investigation of the patient. In this case there is no question.

FOLTZ.

THE OHIO SOCIETY.

The forty-fourth annual meeting of the Ohio State Eclectic Medical Association will be held in the Algonquin Hotel, Dayton, O., commencing at 10 A.M., Tuesday, May 5, 1908, and closing on May 7. The Executive Committee has arranged for a three days' session.

As soon as the meeting closed last year at Cleveland, the Executive

Committee began to plan and work for this year's meeting. After such a splendid program and meeting as was held at Cleveland, we knew we must work or fall below the high mark set at that meeting.

The Executive Committee met early in the year and appointed the Section officers, who were urged and commenced at once to secure essayists, and after these officers had completed their labors at a subsequent meeting the Executive Committee departed somewhat from the usual rule and appointed some one to open the discussion on each paper. We urge your attendance and hope you will come prepared to take an active part in these discussions. We are led to believe from the letters received from the men over the State that this will be the largest convention ever held by the Eclectics of Ohio, and we hope to make it the most profitable.

You will observe by the program that there will be work from the time the gavel calls us to order until its final fall for adjournment until 1909. Any physician who cannot learn enough in the three days' session, with papers and discussions like these will be, to pay in dollars and cents in his next year's work, is not a progressive Eclectic.

On Tuesday evening the local committee have arranged a fine musical program, to be followed by a collation. On Wednesday evening a symposium will be held, having for its subject, "Tuberculosis." At this time Dr. Chas. O. Probst, Secretary of the State Board of Health, will address us on "Tuberculosis from the Standpoint of the State," and Dr. B. F. Lyle, of Cincinnati, on "The Modern Conception of Consumption and Its Treatment." Dr. Lyle has made a considerable study of consumption and has charge of the Branch Hospital of Cincinnati. Dr. Otto Juettner will talk on "The Physical Treatment of Tuberculosis." These lectures alone are worth all the time spent in the attendance on the meeting. They are worth a trip across the State. These men are *experts* in their work.

There are many places of interest in and about Dayton that your family will enjoy. It is a beautiful city and essentially a city of homes. Bring your wives and sweethearts, your grown-up sons and daughters, your babies and Teddy Bears and all have an outing, and go home refreshed with renewed energy and pleasant memories. Come meet your old acquaintances, classmates, and renew friendships.

The Algonquin Hotel is centrally located, first class in every particular, and all meetings will be held in the hotel. The rates are from $2.50 to $4.00 per day, American plan, and the management have thrown open the house to us for the occasion. It is only a few minutes' walk from the depot. Visiting physicians from neighboring States will be welcomed. Come, let us make this a *Red Letter Day for Ohio Eclecticism.*"   A. S. McKitrick, M.D., *President.*

COLLEGE STATISTICS.

The following is an accurate record of the graduates of the Eclectic Medical Institute and their registrations for the class of 1907 :

Number of graduates 81
Thirty registered on examination in 12 States 85
Number who have not applied 1
Number failed 1

	Arkansas.	California.	Florida.	Illinois.	Indiana.	Iowa.	Kentucky.	Minnesota.	Ohio.	Pennsylvania.	Tennessee.	Texas.	W. Virginia.	Total.
Passed.	1	2	2	8	2	1	1	...	1	4	1	2	8	85
Failed.	..	...	...	.,.	...	...	...	1	.8	...	...	...	...	1

This makes the revised schedule for the years 1900 to 1907, both inclusive, eight years:

Total number of graduates 240
Ninety-five registered on diploma in States 108
One hundred and seventy-one on examination in States 186
Number not applied for registration 8
Failed after one or more trials 10

TABLE—REGISTRATION BY STATES.

STATES.	On Diploma.	Examination.	Failed.	Total.
Alabama	...	1	...	1
Arkansas	...	4	...	4
California	1	8	1	5
Colorado	2	1	...	8
Florida	...	4	...	4
Georgia	...	· 2	...	2
Illinois	...	15	...	15
Indiana	...	28	8	81
Iowa	...	1	.1	2
Kansas	1	5	...	6
Kentucky	14	8	1	28
Massachusetts	...	1	...	1
Michigan	2	1	...	8
Minnesota	...	...	1 ·	1
Missouri	2	4	...	6
Nebraska	1	...	...	1
New York	...	· 4	...	4
Ohio	80	89	8	122
Oklahoma	8	1	...	4
Oregon	...	8	1	4
Pennsylvania	...	27	...	27
Tennessee	...	2	· ...	2
Texas	1	9	...	10
Washington	...	1	...	1
West Virginia	...	22	...	22
Wyoming	1	...	...	1
Total	108	186	10	805

The above record shows 186 passing out of 195 applicants, a failure of 5 per cent., several passing on a subsequent examination.

SECRETARIES AND ECLECTICS ON STATE BOARDS.

Alabama—W. H. Sanders, Secretary, Montgomery.
Arizona—Ancil Martin, Secretary, Phœnix.
Arkansas—A. J. Widener, Secretary Ecl. Board, Little Rock.
California—J. Park Dougall, Ecl., Douglas Bldg., Los Angeles.
Colorado—S. D. Van Meter, Secretary, 1723 Tremont Street, Denver.
Connecticut—John W. Fyfe, Ecl., Saugatuck, and T. S. Hodge, Torrington.
Delaware—J. H. Wilson, Secretary, Dover.
District of Columbia—Eclectic Board, President E. B. Benson, 824 Fifth Avenue, N. E. Washington.
Florida—S. F. Smith, Secretary Ecl. Board, Leesburg.
Georgia—M. T. Johnson, Ecl., Lawrenceville, and C. H. Field, Marietta.
Idaho—J. L. Conant, Jr., Secretary, Genesee. R. Truitt, Ecl., Cottonwood.
Illinois—J. A. Egan, Secretary, Springfield. W. R. Schussler, Ecl., Orland.
Indiana—W. T. Gott, Secretary, 120 State House, Indianapolis. M. S. Canfield, Ecl., Frankfort.
Iowa—L. A. Thomas, Secretary, Des Moines. A. C. Moerke, Ecl., Burlington.
Kansas—D. P. Cook, Secretary, Clay Centre. Ecls., W. F. Flack, Longton, and F. P. Hatfield, Grenola.
Kentucky—J. N. McCormack, Se., Bowling Green. G. T. Fuller, Ecl., Mayfield.
Louisiana—F. A. LaRue, Secretary, 211 Camp Street, New Orleans.
Maine—W. J. Maybury, Secretary, Saco.
Maryland—J. M. Scott, Secretary, Hagerstown.
Massachusetts—E. B. Harvey, Secretary, State House, Boston. C. Edwin Miles, Ecl., Boston Highlands.
Michigan—B. D. Harrison, Secretary, 205 Whitney Bldg., Detroit. Ecls. Wm. Bell, Belding, and H. C. Maynard, Hartford.
Minnesota—W. S. Fullerton, Secretary, St. Paul.
Mississippi—J. F. Hunter, Secretary, Jackson.
Missouri—J. A. B. Adcock, Secretary, Warrensburg. Ecl., Ira W. Upshaw, 5015 Shaw Avenue, St. Louis.
Montana—W. C. Riddell, Helena, Secretary.
Nebraska—E. J. Sward, Secretary, Oakland. Ecl., W. T. Johnson, Pawnee City.
Nevada—S. L. Lee, Secretary, Carson City.
New Hampshire—Secretary Ecl. Board, W. H. True, Laconia.
New Jersey—J. W. Bennett, Sec., Long Branch. Ecl., D. P. Borden, Patterson.
New Mexico—J. A. Massie, Secretary, Santa Fe.
New York—C. F. Wheelock, Regents Dept., Albany. Ecl., Lee Smith, Buffalo.
North Carolina—G. T. Sikes, Secretary, Grissom.
North Dakota—H. M. Wheeler, Secretary, Grand Fork.
Ohio—Geo. H. Matson, Secretary, Columbus. Ecl., S. M. Sherman, 224 Twentieth Street, Columbus.
Oklahoma—J. W. Baker, Secretary, Enid. Ecl.,E. G. Sharp, Guthrie.
Oregon—B. E. Miller, Secretary, Portland. Ecl., H. E. Curry, Baker City.
Pennsylvania—C. L. Johnstonbaugh, Pres. Ecl. Board, Bethlehem, and W. H. Blake, Philadelphia.
Rhode Island—G. T. Swarts, Secretary, Providence.
South Carolina—W. N. Lester, Secretary, Columbia.
South Dakota—H. E. McNutt, Secretary, Aberdeen. Ecl., H. S. Graves, Hurley.
Tennessee—T. J. Happel, Secretary, Trenton. Ecl., W. H. Halbert, Nashville.
Texas—G. B Foscue, Secretary, Waco. Ecls., M. E. Daniel, Honey Grove; J. P. Rice, Alpine.
Utah—R. W. Fisher, Secretary, Salt Lake City. Ecl., C. L. Olsen, 932 E. Fifth Street, Salt Lake City.
Vermont—P. L. Templeton, Secretary Ecl. Board, Montpelier.
Virginia—R. S. Martin, Secretary, Stuart.
Washington—C. W. Sharples, Secretary, Seattle. Ecl., J. S. Hoxsey, Spangel.
West Virginia—H. A. Barbee, Secretary, Point Pleasant.
Wisconsin—Ecl., J. V. Stevens, Jefferson, Secretary.
Wyoming—S. B. Miller, Secretary, Laramie.

* No reciprocity recognized by these States. Applicants for registration should correspond with either the Secretary or Eclectic member mentioned above, regarding the particulars of either examination or reciprocity.

THE ECLECTIC MEDICAL JOURNAL

ESTABLISHED 1836.

| Vol. LXVIII. | CINCINNATI, JUNE, 1908. | No. 6. |

Original Communications.

VARIOLA: SYMPTOMATOLOGY AND DIAGNOSIS.*

H. J. SHELLEY, M.D., MIDDLETOWN, N. Y.

In a brief paper on the diagnosis and symptomatology of variola I can give you nothing that is new. Though I have had the pleasure of seeing more cases during my professional career than the average physician, I do not come before you thinking that I am an expert. The time I shall consume in telling you a few points on diagnosis will be brief, but if I were to start to tell you what I don't know I would rival the celebrated essay, "Harris on Gonorrhea." What I have to say is largely from my own observations, but I have also drawn from prominent writers. If you have never seen a case of variola, when you get a case that seems at all suspicious, remember the sign seen at many railroad crossings—"Stop, Look and Listen!"

That variola has been confounded with almost every known disease, including measles, scarlet fever, chickenpox, impetigo contagiosa, cerebro-spinal meningitis, typhus fever, syphilis and penumonia, you all know, but to bring this down to local conditions I will speak of a few of the mistakes in diagnosis that have come before the Middletown Board of Health. The disease most commonly met with, and in many ways closely resembling variola, is varicella. Errors in diagnosis between the two are common, and in epidemics furnish the most cases for controversy between the local physicians and the health authorities.

A serious case of mistaking varicella for variola occurred in New Orleans when a man was sent to the Isolation Hospital suffering from what was diagnosed variola, but which proved to be varicella. While there he contracted a typical case of variola, from which he died.

Among the many features of variola to be mentioned, the tempera-

---

* Read before the Medical Society, County of Orange.

ture drop is almost pathognomonic. This I wish to make especially prominent, for in my mind it is a symptom of great diagnostic value, and affords an almost sure guide at a comparatively early stage. In variola the temperature rises rapidly, and even in mild cases reaches 103° or 104°, when on the appearance of the eruption it drops to normal within a few hours, where it may remain until the close of the case. This drop in temperature on the appearance of the eruption occurs in no other eruptive disease, and when this does occur it should be well considered.

The prodromal symptoms of variola compared with varicella are very marked. In variola the prodromes are so marked as to be suspicious. We have the head- and backache, the backache so intense that the patient will often say that they are going to break in two; the fever, in which delirium occurs in some cases; the eruption appearing in fauces, roof of mouth and on forehead in order named; appearing also on body, soles of feet and palms of the hands; the drop in temperature, are as near typical as any pathological picture we meet.

The varicella cases, as a rule, have no prodromes; the eruption appearing first on body, followed by fever and constitutional symptoms, show a picture diametrically opposite from the variola case.

After the eruption has appeared it is well to remember that the lesion of varicella is a distinct vesicle containing a clear, watery fluid, more profuse on body, especially on back, and rarely on plantar surfaces of hands or feet. The lesions appear in successive crops, so that it is not uncommon to see cases in all stages to desquamation. The varicella is soft to the touch, not umbilicated except by desquamation beginning in the center; the contents can be easily evacuated by a single puncture; crusts form in from two to four days after the appearance of the vesicles.

These, briefly, are some of the prominent diagnostic points between variola and varicella. Yet the attention of the Board of Health was called to a case of variola with typical symptoms, including the eruption, which had been treated as varicella for several days.

Measles is another disease which was confounded with variola, and caused the city much trouble and expense. While it would appear that there is nothing in common between the two, in some cases of variola there appears an early rash that causes the error in diagnosis. Take the history of the case; measles has a longer period of incubation, as a rule, but to prove the exception we have just discharged a case with a period of incubation of twenty-one days. The prodromes of measles more closely resemble a cold, with shivering rather than a chill, sneezing. injection of conjunctiva, running at nose, with cough—in fact, most marked catarrhal symptoms. The eruption appears about the third, fourth or fifth day, with no fall in temperature. It has no tendency to become vesicular, and only slightly papular, and does not possess the shot-like feeling so typical of the early papular stage of variola. Finally, when a measles-like rash does occur in the early stages of variola it disappears in about twenty-four hours, leaving no stain, while in measles it lasts a number of days. Again, while we have the temperature drop in variola, which is pathognomonic, so in measles we have Koplik spots.

Strange as it may seem, syphilis plays an important part in the diagnosis of variola, and in our recent outbreak most of the cases were infected from a pronounced case of variola being diagnosed as syphilis. Next to varicella, syphilis with a pustular syphiloderm is a nut for the diagnostician to crack. The eruption of syphilis may be preceded by fever, pain and aching, but does not have the well-marked prodromal symptoms of variola. Here, as in other eruptive diseases, we do not get the temperature drop, nor does the patient appear very ill. Even in the so-called variola form of syphilide the history of the case settles all doubts.

Not long since a case of variola came under the care of the Board of Health that was being treated for pneumonia. Simply a case of not "Stop, Look and Listen!"

In passing we mention Cuban itch only to say that variola under that name is just as contagious as when called smallpox, and is so recognized by the health authorities.

In closing, a casual glance at the symptoms of a typical case may not be amiss. In variola the period of incubation will vary from seven to twenty-eight days, according as the opsonic index is high or low, the average time being twelve days. The onset is sudden, beginning with a chill, possibly more than one, followed by pains in head, back and muscular system generally. At this time there is usually gastric and intestinal irritation, with vomiting and diarrhea. The pulse is rapid and full, the temperature reaching 103° or 104°; in many cases delirium occurs during this stage. To sum the case up, we have seemingly a case of grippe with gastro-intestinal irritation. The patient looks sick and is sick, and we have before us a pathological picture which once seen is not easily forgotten.

It is during this stage that in a small percentage of cases (13 per cent., according to Osler) that we get the initial rash that sometimes resembles measles in a macular-like eruption, again in a diffused redness like scarlet fever, and occasionally being elevated, resembling urticaria. This rash, whatever form it assumes, usually appears on the inner side of the thighs, near the axilla, lower portion of the abdomen, and sometimes on the extensor surfaces of knees and elbows. This comparatively small percentage of cases are the ones where, if "Stop, Look and Listen!" is not closely followed, a diagnosis of measles, scarlet fever or hives is made.

At this point it is well to withhold your diagnosis for twenty-four to thirty-six hours, unless you are sure of your case. The true variola eruption is usually seen on the third day at the edge of the hair and about the forehead. It also appears about the mouth, anterior surface of the forearm and about the fauces. The strong diagnostic point in the case occurs at this time; the temperature, which has been high, drops to normal in a few hours. It is well to reiterate that this drop in temperature occurs in no other eruptive disease. The patient who had been in agony from pain and fever is now, as the majority will express it, "feeling good." The lesions spread over the whole body in twenty-four to seventy-two hours, and at times might be mistaken for measles.

About the fourth or fifth day the eruption becomes papular, with the shotty feeling as the finger is passed along the surface; the papules becoming vesicles in twenty-four to thirty-six hours. About the eighth day the vesicles have become pustules, with a slight depression in the center. The secondary fever occurs at this time, with many of the symptoms of the first stage, especially the delirium. While I have never seen it in print, I believe the secondary fever comes from absorption, and can be aborted or modified by treatment and cleanliness.

Desquamation sets in after four or five days from their appearance (thirteenth to fourteenth of disease), and the pustules begin to dry up; the scabs fall off a few days later.

The terms discrete and confluent are used to compare the degree of severity. Hemorrhagic smallpox, or purpura variolosa, is almost always fatal. Complications occur in severe cases involving respiratory, digestive, circulatory and nervous systems; also the joints, skin, urinary apparatus and organs of special senses. This, expressed in a few words, is a résumé of a typical case of variola.

In conclusion, during a smallpox epidemic the cases of grippe with an eruption, the drop in temperature or any eruption with a fall in temperature on appearance of eruption, the patient feeling better, it is smallpox 999 times out of 1,000.

PULSATILLA.—Indigestion with sensation of a foreign body lodged beneath the sternum. Also melancholia with fear of impending danger. Patient feels better in the open air.—*Journal of Therapeutics and Dietetics.*

HYSTERIA.

THEODORE D. ADLERMAN, M.D., BROOKLYN, N. Y.

Hysteria can perhaps better be defined as a disordered condition of the nervous system, due in some cases to disturbances of the uterus, and in others to various causes, such as want of sleep, disordered digestion, mental shocks, indolence, high living, sedentary habits, hereditary predisposition; to nervous degeneration, pregnancy, and grave diseases of the uterus, especially of its appendages.

Nervous disturbances which are commonly attributed to gynecologic lesions are in most cases instances of true hysteria or hystero-neurasthenia.

We can also consider hysteria as a psychic disease, and it can, and does, assert itself as a disturbance of certain organs or regions of the body, without any demonstrable lesions being present, or, if present, no connection can be traced or established between the two conditions.

All and each of the above-mentioned causes may act and react in any given case; in fact, it is very seldom possible to assign a particular cause in a particular instance, and we can therefore also say that hysteria consists of an instability of all the nervous and reflex centers throughout the body, and that hereditary predisposition to nerve instability can be asserted as the most prolific cause, and that it is more common in females than in males.

Females of an irritable and nervous nature are more subject to it, and the paroxysms occur oftener, about the period of menstruation, than at any other time. Hysteria is very frequent in girls between the ages of twelve to fifteen; in women on the cessation of the menstrual flow.

Among women, occupation (or shall I rather say want of occupation) is a prominent cause. In dealing with hysteria, therefore, we have to do with a disease which, although marked by very peculiar characteristics and prominent symptoms, yet possesses no anatomical seat.

The depressing effects of almost any disease may be directly productive of hysteria. Excessive discharges and exhausting diseases frequently give rise to attacks of hysteria, which can even occur during convalescence, and are renewed subsequently upon the slightest cause.

The diagnosis of hysteria should not be based on any symptom alone; it must depend on the general psychic and nervous condition of the organism.

The symptoms are often extremely diverse; the patient may appear in all other respects quite healthy, or may be slightly nervous and irritable; there may be some 'mental excitement, violent outbursts of alternate laughter and weeping, and in some cases even convulsions.

The patient sometimes complains of a very peculiar ringing in the ears, a sinking sensation, and a marked feeling as if a few sharp nails or insects were creeping all over her body, especially over the head.

On the other hand, we sometimes have a complete loss of sensation in different parts of the body, which, however, does not last long, and is followed by a hysterical (characteristic in itself) pain in the region of the spine.

All of the above-described sensations for the most part disappear suddenly, leaving the patient in a somewhat exhausted condition.

I have seen cases where the patient commences crying and laughing, and in a few seconds it is followed by tearing out of hair, and then an imploring of all present for sympathy, and then an involuntary flow of urine.

The special senses of taste, sight and hearing may be affected, and in some cases temporarily obliterated.

In a few cases hysteria will pass into absolute insanity. When hysterical convulsions occur they can be easily determined from epileptic by observing that in the former there is no frothing at the mouth, no protrusion of the tongue or biting of it, and after the paroxysm is over the patient recovers the usual state, and does not fall into sleep, as in epilepsy.

You will also find that in women who develop hysteria their menses commenced unusually late, and menstruation is inclined to be tardy and weak, an indication of defective physical development, to which can also be attributed the predisposition to hysteria. Dysmennorrhea is nearly always present.

The treatment of hysteria is peculiar; it must be distinct according to each case, and no general rules can be laid down. And here I want to say that in no other disease can experimentation with drugs, without reference to previous therapeutic applicability, be more completely justified than in hysteria, and if all would only try and study the peculiar forms of hysteria and do a little experimenting and report results obtained, an efficient treatment would soon result.

In the general treatment of hysteria attention must be paid to such special symptoms as arise. The diet should be nutritious and of easy digestion. If the bowels are costive and the paroxysm of long duration, purgative injections and baths should be given daily. The submission of the patient to the best moral influence is very important.

If the patient is anemic, give the arsenates of quinine, iron and strychnine in small doses thrice daily. Zinc valerianate, tr. valerian ammon., the bromides, hyosciamine, tr. lobeliæ, capsicum, comp. spts. lavender, asafetida, musk—all these remedies come in handy in their respective places, and, as I said before, no general rules can be laid down. Each case must be studied by itself. I am now experimenting with fluid extract of salix nigra with fair results, but "am not as yet prepared" fully to state its influence and value in hysteria. I will also mention here that as an after-treatment climate seems to be an important factor in hysteria, and the tonic climate of Maine is especially suitable. High altitudes should be avoided for prolonged residence.

NERVOUS DYSPEPSIA.*

A. Swartzwelder, M.D., Cleveland, O.

Of all diseases of the digestive tract, this is becoming one of the most prevalent, especially in our large cities under the nervous strain of business, with men burning both ends of the candle at once.

The first manifestations of trouble are only a slight nervousness and belching of gas after meals, but the disease develops gradually until a larger number of symptoms are apparent.

When a case of indigestion places himself under our care the first thing to be done is to arrive at the cause of the disease before we dare give any treatment. To know the cause is absolutely necessary to treat the case scientifically.

If it is a lady, inquire carefully into her female life by careful examination for reflexes, as a diseased uterus or ovaries many times sets up aggravating stomach trouble. Observe also if there is disease of the bladder or kidneys. Probe for secret vices in young single girls or boys, and sexual excesses in the adult. Inquire also carefully concerning piles or chronic constipation. In the male observe if the prepuce is normal, if case ever masturbated or indulges in coitus to excess.

In the female observe the character of menstruation, hard or easy, as wrongs here may cause serious difficulties of reflex origin in stomach and bowels.

Another remote cause of trouble is polypi in the nose or growth upon abdominal organs, such as tumors.

Each case must have our most careful attention that we may ascertain whether the lesion is reflex or exists in the stomach alone.

* Read before the Northeastern Ohio Eclectic Medical Society.

Inquiry must.be made into the habits of the parents, if of neurotic temperament, as nervous parents usually beget like offspring.

If upon examination of the stomach we find it normal in size, meal digesting in a normal time but with raising of gas with sour belching, we must look for some reflex cause, as it invariably exists. This class of cases is largely found in brain workers of both sexes, especially those who keep their minds active during meals or read a newspaper, swiftly bolting the food, washing it down with much liquid. No organ can long withstand such usage and a breakdown must come.

The disease at the first is not a grave one, yet as it continues fastens itself forever upon the patient until there is a marked disturbance of the mucous membrane lining the stomach, as well as a change in the gastric secretions, causing those acid, sour belchings and vomitings as well as headache, constipation, heart-burn, nervousness, weakness and loss of flesh.

If this condition long exists, look out for graver manifestations to manifest themselves from the continual formation of acid gas, such as neuralgia, rheumatism or chronic headache every week to two weeks, when the measure of wrong living is full to overflowing.

After arriving at a true diagnosis we have three main conditions to correct:

1. If reflexes exist, correct them if possible.

2. If wrong living, such as sweet meats, liquors or overloading stomach, too much liquid at meals, this must be stopped to cause a cure.

3. Your medicine must be of such a nature as to alter the action of the digestive secretions. In other words, regulate stomach, intestinal, pancreatic and liver secretions to do their normal work, for when one organ suffers they all suffer together. Therefore, in wrongs of the stomach look for weakness all the way down the digestive tract.

No diet for all cases can be outlined; each must use what agrees with his case. On general principles I would advise no fried stuffs or greasy foods. No coffee, sweet meats or warm bread. Meats, as a rule, oppose a cure. Second-day bread and zwieback always are the best for these cases. Use second-day graham, rye or whole wheat bread in preference to white breads.

Advise no liquids from one-half hour before meal to two hours thereafter, as digestive juices will be diluted and weakened. Liquids not allowed at meals will also cause slower eating and far better mastication of the food, as well as smaller amount satisfying the patient's appetite.

Upon the first visit of your patient get his confidence, assuring him you can cure his case if he follows your advice and outlined treatment. After choosing an easily digested diet, assure him he can digest the same, getting his mind off his stomach and troubles. Advise good cheer, pleasure and outdoor life and exercise.

Remembering your case is largely of a nervous origin, get the happiest mental condition possible, as less mental strain, freedom from worry and excitement is half the battle in all these cases.

Next, pay strict attention to his habits of eating, absolutely insisting on thorough mastication of all foods, as a cure is impossible if he bolts his food. Forbid any night eating or eating between meals. Absolutely forbid banqueting, sweetmeats and soda water while you are treating the case.

Remember, above all things, these cases have an insane desire for the most indigestible kinds of food; therefore you must conquer these evil habits if you will win success in their cure.

If you succeed in getting these happy conditions, the medical treatment will be much easier for you, as well as gratifying to your patients.

Medical Treatment.—One of the first medical aids to a cure is to change the action of the perverted secretions of the stomach, liver, pancreas and intestines, bringing them back to a healthy action. To accomplish this you must formulate a tablet or pill which will gently stimulate glandular action as near like nature as possible; correct hyperacidity, and soothe the nervous system, which is also at fault. To treat these cases, as well as all digestive wrongs successfully, such a regulator is absolutely necessary.

Your next medicament must be given to upbuild the weakened nervous system, and such remedies as phosphates, hypophosphites, carbonate of iron, kali phos., or phosphoric acid, can be used to great advantage.

If your case also lacks natural hydrochloric acid, indicated by the sleek, red tongue, brown or dry, with constipation, you should prescribe the dilute acid, ten to fifteen drops, well diluted, after meals, repeated in an hour or two hours if necessary.

Should the tongue show violet, carmine or clear red color, with tendency to diarrhea, use dilute nitric acid, three drops every three hours.

For the soothing and cure of the sensitive mucous membrane nothing is equal to hydrastis in some form, which is also a nervine, allaying irritation of the nerve endings as well as the structures of the nerves.

If excessive hyperacidity exists one to two hours after meal, bicarbonate or sulphite of soda must be used to correct fermentation.

For your nervous, irritable cases, with marked belching, nothing excels nux vomica as a gentle stimulator and nerve builder.

Paw-paw is also of great assistance in these cases, acting in an acid or alkaline medium, and deserves investigation.

Many cases are distressed two to three hours after eating, showing poor action in pancreas. Here pancreatin is indicated.

Watch for undigested fats in the bowel discharges to confirm your diagnosis of poor pancreatic action.

Some cases do well on ingluvin, especially if there is a tendency to nausea or vomiting.

Other remedies deserving our attention are gentian, columbo, wahoo and charcoal.

Study each case carefully, suiting your medicine to the needs of each patient.

AUTO-INTOXICATION—A REPLY.

V. A. Baker, M.D., Adrian, Mich.

A concise article in the April number of The Eclectic Medical Journal, page 244-5, on "Auto-Intoxication," is so practical, instructive and, withal, in order, as the *craze*, so to speak, is so overwrought that it is time a little thought and sense be expended in consideration of the subject.

"Nothing," says the article, "is more characteristic of many enterprising physicians than their readiness to accept new remedies and procedures in advance of complete demonstration of their efficacy." How much of real value the paragraph contains! We are too apt to jump at conclusions. It may be compared to a presidential campaign—we shout ourselves hoarse—*i.e.*, the rank and file do—for their respective candidates, but to-morrow, as the flight of time goes, it is all forgotten, and we are ready to follow in the wake of others who lead.

If we are well up in the physiology of the digestive tract we will note that intestinal digestion is perpetuated in an alkaline medium, stomach digestion in acid self-regulating medium.

I had recently a case under care that had been treated by stomach and intestinal lavage on the premise that auto-intoxication was the cause of what proved to be hectic fever from incipient consumption.

The treatment had been carried so far that the case became exhausted more and more daily. This treatment had been operative in Cleveland until the patient was dismissed and sent home to die.

A diet suited to the condition of the patient, whose digestion was reduced to a minimum, he being unable to take any but the blandest of fluids, a condition that developed since treatment by lavage.

This gentleman stated that he had never been troubled with painful digestion until after being subjected to treatment for auto-intoxication.

He had venous congestion of liver, scant urinal action, obstinate constipation, hectic every afternoon lasting several hours, succeeded by chilliness that did not leave him until middle of forenoon.

I ordered rest in bed and about three teaspoonfuls of Horlick's Malted Milk three hours apart. No medicine was given him. The third day I commenced giving, additional, a small quantity of peptonized milk. Fever gradually abated, as did the chills that had followed the fever, and in ten days patient up and dressed, fever and chills gone, and he gradually returned to a normal diet. This patient had been so thoroughly deluged with water that gastro-intestinal secretion had been neutralized and checked. *He was made too clean.*

The case under consideration is now riding on horseback several hours daily, the bowels and urinary apparatus are in fair order, and I expect with care he may prolong his life many years. The only medicine he is taking is Scott's emulsion of cod-liver oil, which, with a generous diet, he takes without pain.

So, with my friend Church, I fully agree that "putrefaction is not so common in the intestinal canal as many suppose." The subject of Professor Church's article and the terse way it is stated will, if considered, bear study to a fuller understanding generally.

The article I intended for your journal—Obscure Stomach Maladies—I omit for now, as I have written quite at length on Dr. Church's article.

A REMARKABLE DIET FOR A TWO-YEAR-OLD.

J. H. Forrest, M.D., Marion, Ind.

May 1, was consulted regarding a child that had eaten some prunes. The mother was considerably worried, said the child had secured a dish of prunes from the table while she was out of the room and had eaten the whole dish full, seeds and all.

The child was a large, healthy one, and I advised the mother to wait until morning and see first what nature would do for the child and let me know the result. Next morning the mother telephoned the child had passed nine large prune seeds, one large pearl button, and three smaller pearl buttons. She could account for the seeds, but had no idea when or how he had secured the buttons. The child had apparently suffered no inconvenience or injury whatever.

MEDICO-LEGAL.

E. S. McKee, M.D., Cincinnati.

Deaths from Anesthetics at Guy's Hospital.

Thirty-nine deaths have occurred under an anesthetic at Guy's Hospital during the past six and a half years. At the last coroner's inquest, which occurred in January, a committee was appointed to thoroughly investigate the whole question. In the last case the anesthetic administered was the A. C. E. mixture, and occurred in a boy fourteen years of age after a mastoid operation of one hour and a half's duration. Dr. Theodore Fisher, a specialist in pathology, who was called by the coroner to make a post-mortem, said that death was due to the anesthetic primarily, and respiratory failure, followed by sudden heart failure, and that was probably caused by the child's being predisposed to a sudden death owing to the state of the thymus gland. The jury rendered a verdict of "Death from misadventure," and added that in their opinion the anesthetic was properly administered and was necessary.

Death of Dr. Danziger.

Dr. Leo Danziger, of Cincinnati, born 1871, graduated Medical College of Ohio, 1892, member of the Cincinnati Academy of Medicine and the Ohio State Medical Society, was shot and killed while at the bedside of a patient recently. The patient was a young girl fourteen years of age. A criminal abortion had been performed on her and the doctor was called in and found her in a critical condition. The girl had been brought to Cincinnati by her uncle, who was with her. He was extremely anxious about the girl and had words with the doctor about his treatment. He had asked other doctors to supersede him in the treatment, but they had refused to do so. The extreme anxiety of the uncle was explained by developments which proved that he was the author of the girl's trouble. This was evidently known to the doctor, and either to put him out of the way and hide his crime or from some words the hot-headed mountaineer whipped out his ever-ready weapon and shot the doctor dead.

Ready Revolver—Dead Doctor.

The writer remembers in his boyhood seeing the *Police Gazette* once. There was a picture of a doctor in his overcoat and silk hat with a woman in his arms just turning to put her in bed. A man, her husband, enters the door suddenly, and seeing the position of the parties whips out a revolver and shoots the doctor dead. The doctor had been sent for to see the sick woman and found her alone and unconscious on the floor. He at once addressed himself to placing her in bed. The husband, who had been absent and did not know of his wife being ill, returned unexpectedly with the tragic result. This is not alone an instance of the danger to which doctors are subject, but also the danger of being always prepared to commit murder. If that man had not been armed thirty seconds would have been sufficient to have cleared up the matter. The picture made a lasting impression on me, and it is a wonder that I ever studied medicine.

Danger from Designing Women.

Contagious diseases, bad weather, night riders and highwaymen do not seem to be the greatest dangers with which doctors have to contend. Women, designing, malicious women, either disgraced, about to be, or desiring to be. A reputable Detroit doctor recently had an experience to make one shudder. He was called once to see a woman he had never seen before. He found her suffering from a slight cold, for which he prescribed and left. A week later she was taken to the hospital suffering from an abortion. Death imminent, the last sacrament having been administered, the prosecuting attorney and his stenographer being present, she made a dying declaration that the doctor had committed an abortion on her. She did not die. A month later the case came to trial, and instead of her ante-mortem statement the woman herself was on the stand. On severe cross-examination she admitted that the doctor knew nothing at all about her condition, nor had he committed an abortion on her. She said she thought that she would be sent to prison if she did not blame some one else for the abortion. We should have ample laws making it a crime to solicit an abortion and to better protect physicians from blackmail. Surely, the crime is as great as to solicit or offer a bribe. It seems customary among women who have abortions performed upon them, if they willingly or by force accuse some one, to accuse a doctor who did not do it or the one, by preference, who refused to do it.

"Accidental" Abortion.

A point of considerable interest is raised by a correspondent in the *British Medical Journal*. He was called to attend the unmarried housemaid of a patient. The maid was losing blood profusely per vaginam. The condition present was found to be a two months' incomplete abortion. The medical attendant was first amused, then staggered, by the housemaid saying that as she considered the miscarriage due to overwork for her mistress she considered the mistress responsible for her illness and expenses attached thereto. At first sight this seems the height·of impudence, but is it really so? The normal end of pregnancy is full-time delivery. Abortion is abnormal and accidental. This "accident" occurs while in service and prevents the girl from working. Few would be willing to prognosticate the action of a jury if the girl's mistress is sued, especially if the weight of evidence goes to show that the abortion was due directly to her work. If she can prove that it was due to this she might be able to hold her mistress liable. Of the two evils, it would be much better for her to blame the mistress than the master.

JONATHAN ROBERTS PADDOCK, M.D.

HARVEY WICKES FELTER, M.D., CINCINNATI.

Jonathan Roberts Paddock, M.D., was the son of James and Grace Paddock. Many of his ancestors on both sides were distinguished in law, literature and medicine. He was born near Cromwell, Conn., November 19, 1803, and died of paralysis of the heart at his home in Maysville, Ky., June 7, 1878, aged seventy-five years.

Of his early education little is known, but it must have been good; for he entered Union College at Schenectady, N. Y., of which he was a graduate, under the eminent Dr. Nott. In 1830 he was one of the founders and a professor in the Reformed Medical College of Worthington, having been, previous to this time, a professor in the Worthington College (literary). He remained with the medical college all its life.

Dr. Paddock was a very skillful physician, being learned in all the different schools of medicine and a scholar of extraordinary attainments, reading Greek and Latin with great ease, and taking pleasure in his classical studies to the very latest period of his life. With all his learning, skill and eminence, he was very modest and retiring in his disposition. Dignified, yet affable and pleasant in conversation, amiable and charitable to all the poor in his practice, he constituted a noble and elevated character, and was an

JONATHAN ROBERTS PADDOCK, M.D.

ornament to the community in which he lived. Dr. Paddock was a competent chemist and splendid botanist, able to name all the plants and trees of the State by sight.

He was a resident of Maysville, Ky., about thirty-four years, about twenty of which he was engaged in active practice. During the last fourteen years he was an invalid, and confined his practice to his office work.

He was twice married; first to Caroline, daughter of Captain Thomas Stowe, of Upper Houses, Conn., by whom he had two children; his second wife was Julia, daughter of A. Bristol, of Worthington, by whom he had two daughters.

In the college, Dr. Paddock taught Chemistry and Pharmacy and Botany and Materia Medica.

His remains were interred in St. John's Churchyard at Worthington, his modest sandstone monument bearing this simple inscription: "A kind and learned gentleman."

Seton Hospital Reports.

L. E. RUSSELL, M.D., SURGEON.

Case 121.—Mr. G. S., presented to the clinic by Professor Spencer, on account of a hernia which had been injected with paraffine.

Before we classify the hernia in the inguinal canal we must first ascertain if the course of the hernia has been external, or on the outer or iliac side of the deep epigastric artery; if so, we call it external or oblique inguinal hernia; this form obtains much more frequently than the other, while internal or direct inguinal hernia does not follow the direct course of the cord, but protrudes through the abdominal wall on the inner or pubic side of epigastric artery.

In oblique inguinal hernia the intestine escapes from the abdominal cavity through the internal ring, taking with it a pouch of peritoneum, which we designate as the hernial sac. The hernia passes along in front of the cord and makes exit at the external ring, and when it descends into the scrotum we give it the name of scrotal hernia. This form of hernia passes in front of the cord and vessels, and on account of adhesions very seldom extends below the testicle.

In incarceration of the gut the seat is generally at the external ring, though occasionally at the internal ring.

We speak of a hernia as reducible or irreducible, and also give another classification, as when the irreducible becomes constricted, and prevents the passage of gas, or the contents of the bowels. When this condition exists there is no relief except by surgical interference, and if the gut has been long strangulated it is better surgery to not attempt to force back the gut and sac, as there is danger of rupture of the intestine, or a pushing of the incarcerated intestine in its sac back into the abdomen with the intestine locked.

Let us now make an incision over this protruding mass. We come upon quite an amount of paraffine injected into the hernial sac, and it has caught and now holds the omentum and gut in the sac irreducible.

The fault with this operation and this method of operating is that the hernia has not been properly reduced before injecting the paraffine into the hernial sac, and this has imprisoned the contents of the sac. I can readily see how this method of operating might occasionally be of value, as it has the appearance of being bloodless and "without the use of the knife or ligature," and this is "catchy" with some people.

In this case all the paraffine must be turned out and the thickened walls of the sac removed before we attempt to loosen the omentum or the intestine.

We shall ligate quite a quantity of the omentum, excise, and dispense with it, as it is more than useless. The intestine will now easily return to the abdominal cavity.

In the completion of the operation the cord and vessels are raised and given a new bed, the old one sutured to prevent a recurring hernia. Different methods have been described by different operators, and they have in turn been given a mark of distinction by naming the operation after the said operator.

As a matter of fact, the same operator very seldom performs exactly the same method, though each may, in a general way, almost do the same act.

What we want is, first, a complete opening of the hernial sac and reduction of its contents; second, removal of the long strips of omentum, if long incarcerated; third, an obliteration of the sac and suturing together of the pillars, walls or retaining parts of the abdomen.

There is comparatively little danger in the open surgical way of doing a herniotomy.

CAPSICUM is a pure stimulant. In nervous depression, given in small doses, it is very sustaining. Capsicum and strychnia are valuare able heart sustainers when indicated.—*Journal of Therapeutics and Dietetics.*

CROUP.—One teaspoonful of acetic emetic tincture in one-half glass of water; teaspoonful every fifteen minutes will cure spasmodic croup.—*Journal of Therapeutics and Dietetics.*

ECLECTIC MEDICAL INSTITUTE.

A Portion of the Sixty-fourth Annual Announcement.

Board of Trustees

HON. AARON McNEILL, President.
ROLLA L. THOMAS, M.D., Vice-President.*
JOHN K. SCUDDER, M.D., Secretary.*
PAUL R. SCUDDER, D.D.S., Treasurer.

WM. P. BEST, M.D.,*	S. M. SHERMAN, M.D.,*
N. ASHLEY LLOYD,	C. GORDON NEFF,
LeROY BROOKS,	JOHN T. ROUSE,
JEROME P. MARVIN, M.D.,*	JOHN URI LLOYD, Phr. M.,
HENRY DURY,	CLYDE P. JOHNSON,

L. H. BLAKEMORE.

Faculty†

JOHN URI LLOYD, Phr. M., cor. Court and Plum Sts., Cincinnati.
Emeritus Professor of Chemistry and Pharmacy.

BISHOP McMILLEN, M.D., - - - - - - Shepard, O.
Emeritus Professor of Mental and Nervous Diseases.

ROLLA L. THOMAS, M.D., - - 792 E. McMillen St., Cincinnati.
Professor of the Principles and Practice of Medicine; Dean of the Faculty.

WILLIAM E. BLOYER, M.D., - - "The Lancaster," Cincinnati.
Professor of Materia Medica and Therapeutics.

JOHN K. SCUDDER, M.D., - - - 1009 Plum St., Cincinnati.
Secretary of the Faculty; Instructor in Latin.

LYMAN WATKINS, M.D., - - - - - Blanchester, O.
Professor of Pathology and Physiology.

HARVEY W. FELTER, M.D., cor. Chase and Pitt Sts., Cincinnati.
Professor of Medical History.

L. E. RUSSELL, M.D., - - - - "The Groton," Cincinnati.
Professor of Clinical Surgery and Operative Gynecology.

JOHN R. SPENCER, M.D., - - - 952 W. Eighth St., Cincinnati.
Professor of Obstetrics.

* Representing Alumni.
† Arranged in order of seniority of appointment.

KENT O. FOLTZ, M.D., - - 105 Odd Fellows Bldg., Cincinnati.
Professor of Didactic and Clinical Ophthalmology, Otology, Rhinology and Laryngology.

CHARLES GREGORY SMITH, M.D., 224 Dorchester Ave., Cincinnati.
Professor of Chemistry.

HERBERT E. SLOAN, M.D., - - - - - - Cincinnati.
Professor of Didactic Surgery.

WILLIAM N. MUNDY, M.D., - - - - - - Forest, O.
Professor of Diseases of Children.

THOMAS BOWLES, M.D., - - - - - - Harrison, O.
Professor of Diseases of Women.

BYRON VAN HORN, M.D., - - - - Oakley, Cincinnati.
Professor of Anatomy.

WILLIAM L. DICKSON, LL.D., 703 Union Trust Building, Cincinnati.
Lecturer on Medical Jurisprudence.

JOHN L. PAYNE, M.D., - - - 918 W. Eighth St., Cincinnati.
Lecturer on Hygiene and Demonstrator of Histology, Pathology and Bacteriology.

WILBUR E. POSTLE, M.D., - - - - - Shepard, O.
Lecturer on Mental and Nervous Diseases.

EDWIN R. FREEMAN, M.D., - Seventh and John Sts., Cincinnati.
Lecturer and Clinical Instructor on Skin and Venereal Diseases.

J. STEWART HAGEN, M.D., - - 1506 Harrison Ave., Cincinnati.
Lecturer and Clinical Instructor on Surgery and Gynecology.

J. CORLISS EVANS, M.D., - - 2948 Colerain Ave., Cincinnati.
Lecturer and Clinical Instructor on Physical Diagnosis.

OTTO JUETTNER, M.D., - - - - 628 Elm St., Cincinnati.
Lecturer and Clinical Instructor on Electro-Therapeutics.

LOUIS C. WOTTRING, M.D., - Richmond and Linn Sts., Cincinnati.
Lecturer and Clinical Instructor on Medicine.

VICTOR P. WILSON, M.D., - - 1612 Western Ave., Cincinnati.
Clinical Instructor on Diseases of Women, Children and Dermatology.

CHARLES S. AMIDON, M.D., - - - - - Cincinnati.
Lecturer and Clinical Instructor on Diseases of the Eye, Ear, Nose and Throat.

𝕳𝖎𝖘𝖙𝖔𝖗𝖎𝖈𝖆𝖑*

THE ECLECTIC MEDICAL INSTITUTE was the direct outgrowth of a reform medical movement inaugurated in New York City in 1827 by Dr. Wooster Beach.

This remarkable man, who is generally conceded to have been the founder of *American Eclecticism*, has been characterized by a prominent surgeon of the opposite faith "as one of the really great men of his day."

He established the United States Infirmary in 1825, and the Reformed Medical College in 1830.

Later the national organization, of which Beach was President, included such distinguished men as Morrow, Jones and King.

The Reformed Medical College was inaugurated at Worthington, Ohio, in 1830. This institution was better known as *Worthington College*, and was the predecessor of the Eclectic Medical Institute.

Among the faculty were John J. Steele, Thomas Vaughn Morrow, I. G. Jones, J. R. Paddock, J. L. Riddell, T. E. Mason and J. B. Day.

The Worthington Infirmary was opened for clinical instruction in 1837. In 1836, Professor Morrow wrote, "There are now in different sections of the United States about 200 regularly educated scientific medical reformers." The term *botanical* reformers was usually employed, although they had no professional connection with the followers of Samuel Thomson.

The Worthington College was closed in 1839 and reopened in Cincinnati in 1843 as the Reformed Medical School of Cincinnati.

After heroic efforts, and overcoming strong opposition, the *Eclectic Medical Institute* was chartered by special act of the Legislature of Ohio on March 10, 1845. Thus was the intolerant and illiberal spirit of medical monopoly of that date most signally rebuked. The interests of the Eclectics had been intrusted to the watchful care of Colonel Kilbourne.

---

* We are indebted to Felter's "History of the Eclectic Medical Institute" for portions of this material.

Success now attended the efforts of the friends of medical reform. The *Western Medical Reformer* announced the passage of the bill "erecting the Reformed Medical School into a college, with the title *Eclectic Medical Institute*. Our College will be strictly what its name implies—Eclectic."

The first faculty embraced Beach, Hill, Morrow, Cox, Jones, Oliver and Baldridge.

A new college building was erected on the corner of Court and Plum Streets, and was opened November 7, 1846.

The lectures of the Commercial (now City) Hospital were opened to all students in the fall of 1846.

In this year Joseph Rodes Buchanan entered the faculty. In 1849 a homeopathic department was established, presided over by Prof. Storm Rosa, M.D.

This continued during one college year only. The faculty of the Memphis Institute came to Cincinnati in 1851, adding Robert S. Newton, W. Byrd Powell, Zoeth Freeman, J. Milton Sanders and John King.

Later, Hoyt, Cleveland, Sherwood and Sanders were added. In 1856 John Milton Scudder and Edwin Freeman were elected to the teaching staff.

J. F. Judge and Andrew Jackson Howe were added in 1859. Up to August, 1859, the Institute had graduated 851 students.

All of the above-mentioned men were leaders and active members in medical reform, and were authors of many textbooks.

On November 20, 1869, the college building was partially destroyed by fire, and on October 15, 1871, a new building adjoining the old building, on Plum Street, was opened for use, on a lot 38 x 90, four stories high, of Ohio free stone. Over three hundred physicians were present at the dedication of this building.

About this time John Milton Scudder announced his well-known theory of Specific Medication, which is now the leading tenet of the Eclectic theory of practice.

The faculty now embraced the following distinguished names: King, Locke, Scudder, Howe, two Freemans, Judge and Marvin.

Up to this time the College had enrolled 4,785 students and 1,575 graduates.

In 1874 John Allard Jeancon and in 1878 John Uri Lloyd were added to the faculty. Women were again admitted as students on the same terms as men.

From 1887 to 1893 Rolla L. Thomas, William E. Bloyer, Lyman Watkins, Robert C. Wintermute and Harvey W. Felter joined the teaching force.

In 1889 the Exposition Universelle of Paris awarded the College a diploma and silver medal for an educational exhibit of text-books and catalogues.

The later additions to the faculty in the last fifteen years are well known and need not be enumerated.

In 1901 the College affiliated with the Seton Hospital, conducted by the Sisters of Charity, at Eighth and Cutter Streets. In 1907 the latter purchased the former Presbyterian Hospital buildings at Sixth, Mound and Kenyon Avenues.

The three buildings are well equipped and modern in every respect, and contain sixty beds in wards and private rooms.

A daily *Dispensary* is conducted by the College instructors in the first floor of the McDonald Surgical Building, at 625 Kenyon Avenue.

The Trustees of the College have purchased a large lot at 630 W. Sixth Street adjoining the Seton Hospital on the west, on which, in the near future, it is inteded to erect a modern college building.

It will probably be five stories in height, and the first floor will contain a students' room, lavatory, store-room and janitor's living rooms.

The second floor, a large lecture-room, offices and library.

The third floor, well equipped laboratories of physiology, histology, pathology and bacteriology.

The fourth floor, anatomical and surgical amphitheatre, museum, and an operating-amphitheatre, to be connected with the Seton Hospital by a covered bridge.

The fifth floor will contain well-lighted anatomical and chemical laboratories.

Up to 1908 the Eclectic Medical Institute has enrolled 12,881 matriculates and graduated 3,942 physicians, over 2,000 of whom are in active and lucrative practice in various States.

In the United States there are now eight Eclectic colleges, ten medical journals, thirty State and one National Medical Society, and numerous local and district organizations.

During the past eighty years more than sixty medical books on various subjects have been written by Eclectic teachers, many of which have become standard works of study and reference.

Eclectics believe in the curative action of remedies in kindly doses. They believe in the specific action of drugs properly administered. We teach the student how to practice successfully the most effective, pleasant form of therapy extant. We find it impossible to supply numbers of localities asking for graduates of the Eclectic Medical Institute.

Eclecticism, as a system of medical practice, is just completing its eighty-fourth year. It is no longer an experiment, but an established and potent factor in our scientific and social world, and as likely to be permanent as any other doctrine now held in the whole realm of art and science. This system, at the present time, has over eight thousand practitioners in the United States; and they are as widely known and highly distinguished for their learning and skill as are other physicians in this and other countries. They are filling positions of honor in colleges, hospitals and societies, in literature, on sanitary boards, and other governmental relations, equally with their fellows of other schools. The constantly growing popularity of the new system of medicine, and the ever-increasing influence of its practitioners in all governmental and social relations, seem to make the Eclectic profession of medicine one of the most inviting and prominent avenues open to those whose physical, moral and intellectual qualifications fit them for its duties and responsibilities.

Announcement

SESSION 1908-1909

NOTE.—These regulations refer particularly to new students and graduates of the years 1909, 1910, 1911 and 1912.

Matriculation.—The Eclectic Medical Institute is open for matriculation to well-qualified young men and women who have attained the age of seventeen.

This College does not solicit the matriculation of negro students, believing that they can be better educated in institutions devoted exclusively to their race.

The Sixty-fourth Annual Session.—The sixty-fourth annual session of the Eclectic Medical Institute will begin on Monday, September 14, 1908, and continue thirty-two weeks, until April 28, 1909.

Entrance Examination.—Entrance examinations for students who cannot procure the credentials as mentioned on page 22 under the heading of Regulations, are held at various dates, under the authority of the several State boards of medical registration.

No examination embracing less than the following will be accepted from any one:

REQUIRED.—Orthography, geography, English grammar and composition, history and constitution of the United States, arithmetic, including the metric system and mensuration, algebra to quadratics, Latin (grammar and Cæsar, bk. 1), elementary physics.

In addition to the above studies, two or more must be certified to, the two to be chosen from the following:

ELECTIVES.—General history, one year, or English history, or history of Greece and Rome; English literature, one year; rhetoric, one year; German, one year; French, one year; Latin (Cæsar, Virgil or Cicero), second year's work; physiology, one year; chemistry, one year; botany, one year; zoology, one year; physical geography, one year; plane trigonometry, one year.

Medical examinations to determine the standing of students who have attended elsewhere, and for removing conditions of first, second or third-year students, will be held by the respective professors before October 1.

Students who have attended two or three sessions elsewhere

will be examined in Anatomy, Chemistry, Physiology, Principles of Medicine, Hygiene, and Materia Medica. Students passing a majority of these subjects will be entitled to enter, and make up the deficiencies in additon to the regular year's work. *Pass grades* will be accepted from certain accredited medical colleges.

Graduates of accredited medical colleges will be admitted to the Senior Year without examination.

Term Examinations.—Throughout the entire course daily examinations or quizzes are held by the professors, thus aiding the student's memory and assuring his continued advancement. The Freshman, Sophomore, Junior and Senior examinations will be held in writing, beginning April 19, and at no other time. Candidates for graduation can be examined only at this time.

No Private Quiz Classes.—All the instruction in this College is given in the regular lectures and regular every-day quizzes. No private classes for which students must pay an additional fee are allowed. There are no special courses to add to the student's expense. In many colleges the extras are said to approach the cost of regular tuition.

Reading Medicine.—It is our experience that the sooner the student attends his first course of lectures the better he will read medicine in the physician's office. In the college he learns how to study and what to study, and will usually make as much progress in one session as in three years of ordinary reading. Our best students are those who commence with a course of lectures, and continue their attendance session after session until graduation. Some very successful physicians received their entire education in the College, without any office instruction.

It is quite advisable for students to take a short course of study under a preceptor at home, or medical reading without the help of a physician, and they are earnestly advised to confine themselves to the following text-books:

1. Chemistry—*Simon's Medical Chemistry.*
2. Physiology—elementary parts, circulation, respiration, etc. —*Kirke's Handbook of Physiology.*
3. Osteology and General Anatomy—*Gray.*
4. Specific Diagnosis and Specific Medication—*Scudder.*
5. Materia Medica—*Locke or Ellingwood.*

State Laws.—With but two exceptions, each matriculate must study medicine four years, and take four annual courses of lectures of at least seven months each, and graduate, and also undergo an examination before a State Board.

Our diplomas are recognized and are everywhere on an equality with those of any college in the United States.

FEES.*

Each year's tuition.........................$90 00
All laboratory courses...................... Free
Matriculation, demonstrator's fees, dissecting material, and graduation or examination fees are included in the above.

Post-graduate instruction, per month, $15.00.

The fees are cash in all cases.

No scholarships are sold.

Hospital Instruction.—Students have two hours of clinical instruction daily in the Cincinnati Hospital. In addition to this there will be clinical instruction two hours in the new Seton Hospital Dispensary daily upon diseases of the eye, ear, nose and throat, diseases of the skin, medical and surgical diseases of women and children, general surgery and medicine, physical diagnosis and electro-therapeutics.

Facilities for the care of surgical patients have been provided, and operations will be performed before the class. Physicians will recollect that all medical treatment before the class is free of charge, and that in surgical cases the charge will only be sufficient to cover the necessary attendance after operation.

The new Seton Hospital buildings, formerly the Presbyterian Hospital, are located on Sixth Street and Kenyon Avenue, west of Mound Street, cost over $200,000, and are owned and operated by the Sisters of Charity.

The Eclectic Medical Institute has been affiliated with the Seton Hospital for seven years and has *exclusive* control of the *clinical* facilities and the out-door dispensary. In the operating-room clinical cases are brought exclusively before students of our College, thus affording us an excellent opportunity to demonstrate the many advantages of Eclectic medication and the exactness of our surgeons. Operations before the class take place Wednesdays and Saturdays throughout the College year, and at other times by appointment.

The three Seton Hospital buildings are heated by steam, have hydraulic elevators and all the modern equipment. They have hard-wood floors and open plumbing, and most excellent sanitary arrangements, insuring good accommodations for patients. All classes of cases are taken, barring, of course, conta-

---

* Under no circumstances are fees returnable. Single session tickets are not transferable. Students can, however, make up lost time in any future session without extra charge.

gious diseases. There are three wards and thirty-five rooms in the Hospital. The cost of room, board and nursing ranges from $7.00 to $21.00 per week.

A limited number of charity patients will be taken. The medical and surgical service furnished by the various members of the faculty of this College is absolutely free where the patients contribute in a clinical way to our classes.

Information regarding rooms and board can be secured by

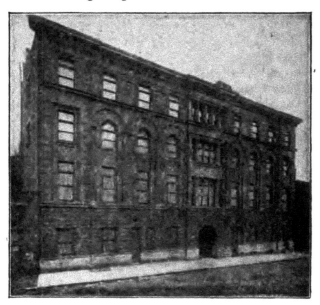

The New Seton Hospital (McDonald Building, facing Bathgate Park).

addressing John K. Scudder, M.D., 1009 Plum Street, Cincinnati.

Internes.—Four students are selected each year by competitive examination, from the Junior class of this college only, to serve as internes during their Senior year, at the Seton Hospital. Two are on duty the first half of the College term; the others after the holidays. These positions are highly prized and much sought after. The following have served heretofore:

1901-1902.—G. H. Knapp, C. G. Patterson, Susan R. Cooper, A. O. Barclay.

1902-1903.—W. F. Weikal, C. W. Beaman, A. J. Kemper, P. A. Kemper.

1903-1904.—G. D. Callihan, P. E. Decatur, J. G. Sherman, C. P. Krohn.

1904-1905.—G. E. Dash, C. M. L. Wolf, Wm. A. Ellsworth, C. J. Otto.

1905-1906.—M. F. Bettencourt, A. T. Rank, C. L. Hudson, D. E. Bronson.

1906-1907.—Nellie Van Horn, D. E. Rausch, A. C. Jenner, J. C. Shafer.

1907-1908.—C. C. Hamilton, E. W. Horswell, C. C. McCaffery, G. W. Sauter.

TO OUR ALUMNI.

The strength of the College is largely in its alumni—their interests and that of the College are one. A strong and active alumnal influence is and always has been an invaluable asset to this College, while the growth and prosperity of the latter adds not a little to the pleasure and success of her graduates. May we not confidently appeal to our two thousand alumni for their help in maintaining the fair name and in promoting the success of the Eclectic Medical Institute?

We have recently been told by a student now in attendance, who took two years of his course elsewhere, that he thought if the advantages of the Eclectic Medical Institute were more widely known, we would have many additional students. We must look to our Alumni to make the advantages of the College known. You are, of course, making them known by your work and your standing in the profession, but will you not make a special effort to explain to your friends, as opportunity presents, the facilities, the teaching, the educational standards, the rank, and the *esprit de corps* of your Alma Mater? We trust that you may share with us the hope that our classes shall steadily increase in size, and that the day is not far distant when our laboratories and chairs of didactic teaching shall be endowed, and grounds and buildings added to meet increasing requirements.

We shall welcome your counsel in reference to the needs and possibilities of the College. It is not too much to hope that within the near future our Alumni may interest their benevolently inclined patrons in the cause of medical science, and that by their benefactions, and those of our Alumni themselves, the College shall be enabled to render much greater service to medical education and humanity.

We hope our graduates will, whenever opportunity presents, visit the recitations and clinics; it will cheer your old instructors, encourage the students, and strengthen the bonds of mutual interest which unite us.

Library.—The College has a working library of five hundred volumes. Books can be kept for one week for reference. Students can also consult the City Hospital, the Public and Lloyd Libraries. The latter is located but a few doors from the College, and its priceless collection is housed in a beautiful building newly constructed specially for library purposes. It comprises the largest and most complete collection of books and pamphlets

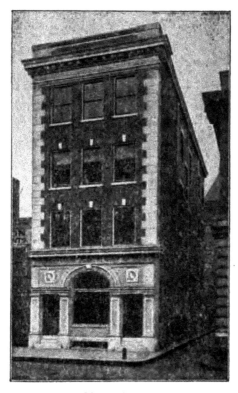

Lloyd Library.

devoted to botany, pharmacy, general and pharmaceutical chemistry and materia medica in the world. Its Eclecticana is the most extensive extant. An herbarium represents all parts of the world, and comprises upward of thirty thousand species, in bound volumes.

This library contains between 15,000 and 20,000 volumes and pamphlets, and is the creation of John Uri Lloyd, scientist and litterateur, and Curtis Gates Lloyd, botanist and mycologist. It is incorporated, is free to the public, and is pledged to be donated intact to science.

Y. M. C. A—The college department of the Young Men's Christian Association meets once a week in the College, at which speakers of public note address the meeting. All students are eligible to membership. New students are especially invited. A bureau of information for assisting new students in procuring rooms, etc., can be found at the College. There will be a committee of students at the College during the week previous to the opening of the session, to aid new students in securing suitable rooms, boarding, etc. This committee will arrange to meet students at the railroad depots, if the time of arrival is sent to the President of the Y. M. C. A., Mr. A. M. Uphouse, 1009 Plum Street.

Boarding.—We take special pains to select boarding in private boarding houses, where students will have all the comforts of a home, and at the same time have a quiet room in which to pursue their studies. Board and room can be had at from $3.00 to $5.00 per week. To accommodate those of limited means, rooms can be procured in which students can board themselves, bringing their expenses below $3.00 per week. Those who intend to pursue this latter course will do well to write two or three weeks in advance, and bring sufficient quantity of bed-covering.

Information.—Students arriving by railroad will do well to take the omnibus ticket, and have their baggage taken immediately to the College building, Court and Plum Streets, where they will get all necessary information in regard to board and matriculation.

Letters to students must be addressed, "Care of Eclectic Medical Institute, No. 1009 Plum Street." But money packages by express, and letters containing valuables, should be addressed to the care of John K. Scudder, M.D., thus preventing trouble in identification and danger of loss. Arrangements have been made with the City Hall Bank to receive on deposit the money of students. The attention of the student is particularly called to this paragraph, as it may save much trouble, if not actual loss.

For further information address—

JOHN K. SCUDDER, M.D., Secretary,

1009 Plum Street, Cincinnati, O.

Long Distance Telephone, Canal 2062.

𝕽𝖊𝖌𝖚𝖑𝖆𝖙𝖎𝖔𝖓𝖘

Requirements of Entrance—Certificate of Study.—For matriculation the Faculty requires:

1. A certificate of good moral character.

2. Diploma of graduation from (*a*) a four years graded high school, or (*b*) normal school, or (*c*) seminary, or (*d*) literary or scientific college, or (*e*) university, or (*f*) evidence of having passed the matriculation examination to a recognized literary or scientific college, or (*g*) a medical student's certificate secured by examination from a State medical board.[1]

---

1 OHIO.—Matriculates who will be applicants for registration in the State of Ohio must possess:—a diploma from a reputable college granting the degree of A.B., B.S., or equivalent degree; a diploma from a normal school, high school or seminary, legally constituted, issued after four years of study; a teacher's permanent or life certificate; a medical student's certificate issued upon examination by a State board; or a student's certificate of examination for admission to the Freshman class of a reputable literary or scientific college. These credentials must be presented to Professor Harris, at Walnut Hills, prior to September 26.

Or a certificate of having passed an examination conducted under the direction of State Board of Medical Registration and Examination of Ohio, by certified examiners, none of whom shall be either directly or indirectly connected with a medical college.

This latter examination will be held by Professor Harris, September 27 and 28, for Cincinnati students. Fee, $2.00. The examination will embrace: Foreign language—two years of the Latin language—English literature, composition and rhetoric. History—United States history and civics, with reference to the constitutional phases of American history. Mathematics—algebra through equations and plane geometry. Science—botany or zoology, physiography or chemistry, and physics. Further particulars will be sent on request.

NEW YORK.—A Regents' medical students' certificate, granted on forty-eight counts. Particulars from Regents' office, Albany, N. Y.

PENNSYLVANIA.—(*a*) High school, normal school, seminary or literary college diploma. (*b*) Certificate of examination in ten branches under seal of principal or county superintendent. Or (*c*) Entrance examination before State Board in Pittsburg or Philadelphia.

Required.—Orthography, geography, English grammar and composition, history and constitution of the United States, arithmetic including the metric system and mensuration, algebra to quadratics, Latin (grammar and Cæsar bk. 1), elementary physics.

(In addition to the above studies, two more must be certified to; the two to be chosen from the following.)

Electives.—General history, one year, or English history, or history of Greece and Rome; English literature, one year; rhetoric, one year; German, one year; French, one year; Latin (Cæsar, Virgil or Cicero), second year's work; physiology, one year; chemistry, one year; botany, one year; zoology, one year; physical geography, one year; plane geometry, one year.

INDIANA.—(*a*) High school, normal, or college diploma. Or (*b*) an

3. No Faculty entrance examinations are held and no credentials except those authorized by the various State medical boards are accepted. Students are urged to perfect their credentials in advance of matriculation.

Students MUST comply with the· State Board requirements of the State in which they wish to practice.

Students who have attended one annual session at an accredited medical college, are admitted as second-year students.

Students who have attended two annual sessions elsewhere are admitted to the third-year course on credentials. Graduates of accredited medical colleges are admitted to the fourth year without examination.

For Graduation.—Students applying for graduation must be' at least twenty-one years of age, must have read medicine four years, and attended four annual sessions of not less than thirty-two weeks each, the last of which, at least, must have been in this college.[1]

Time of reading includes college attendance. All students must have taken the chemical, histological, pathological, and bacteriological laboratory courses, attended the clinical lectures in the Cincinnati Hospital during one session, the college clinics during at least two sessions, have dissected at least half a cadaver, and taken the practical course in obstetrics and surgery. The candidate must notify the dean six weeks prior to the end of the session of his intention to take the final examinations, must submit an original thesis on some subject pertaining to medicine (embracing from ten to forty pages of thesis paper), must have previously paid all fees, and must pass satisfactorily the term as well as the final examinations.[2]

The judgment of the Faculty upon the fitness of candidates is based on their knowledge of their general attendance, industry, character and general habits, as well as upon the results of their final examinations.

A rejected candidate may be re-examined at the discretion of the Faculty, after having attended a half or full additional session. Each graduate, at the close of the session, will be required to attend the Commencement Exercises, and personally receive his diploma. No honorary diplomas are issued by the Eclectic Medical Institute.

---

entrance examination in ten high school branches before Secretary W. S. Gott, 120 State Capitol, Indianapolis, September 1, 1908.

KENTUCKY.—High school, normal or college diploma, or an examination at Louisville in ten subjects.

MICHIGAN.—High school, normal or college diploma, or an examination at Detroit, Grand Rapids, Hillsdale, or Bay City, in ten branches of a high school course.

1 To constitute a full term or session the absence should not exceed one month in the aggregate.

2 Students who have matriculated here in years· past cannot, under any circumstances, claim graduation under requirements then in force.

Order of Exercises—1908-9

FIRST YEAR—Freshman Class.

Hours.	Monday.	Tuesday.	Wednesday.	Thursday.	Friday.	Saturday.
7:30 a.m	Chemistry.	Anatomy.	Chemistry.	Anatomy.	Chemistry.	Anatomy.
8:45 a.m 9:45 a.m	Dissections, Histological and Chemical Laboratory, in rotation, in Sections.					
1 p.m		Physiology.			Physiology.	
3 p.m	Mat. Med.	Mat. Med.	Hygiene.	Mat. Med.	Mat. Med.	
4 p.m	Hygiene.					

SECOND YEAR—Sophomore Class.

Hours.	Monday.	Tuesday.	Wednesday.	Thursday.	Friday.	Saturday.
7:30 a.m	Chemistry.	Anatomy.	Chemistry.	Anatomy	Chemistry.	Anatomy.
8:45 a.m 9:45 a.m	City Hospital, Dissections, Pathological and Bacteriological Laboratory in rotation, in Sections.					
10:45 a.m	Prin. Med.					
1 p.m		Physiology.	Phys. Diag.		Physiology.	
3 p.m	Mat. Med.	Mat. Med.	Hygiene.	Mat. Med.	Mat. Med.	.
4 p.m	Hygiene.				Phys. Diag.	

THIRD YEAR—Junior Class.

Hours.	Monday.	Tuesday.	Wednesday.	Thursday.	Friday.	Saturday.
8:45 a.m	Lecture. Eye & Ear.	Set. Clinic or Hospital.	Set. Clinic or Hospital.	Set. Clinic or Hospital.	Set. Clinic or Hospital.	Lecture. Nose & Th
9:45 a.m	Set. Clinic or Hospital.					Set. Clinic or Hospital.
10:45 a.m	Dis. Wom.	' Practice.	Oper. Gyn.	Practice.	Practice.	Oper. Gyn
11:45 a.m	Principles.	Obstetrics.		Obstetrics.	Obstetrics.	
2 p.m	Elec. Ther.	Pathology.	Phys. Diag.	Y.M.C.A.	Pathology.	
3 p.m.	Surgery.	Surgery.	Surgery.	Surgery.		
4 p.m.					Phys. Diag.	

FOURTH YEAR—Senior Class.

Hours.	Monday.	Tuesday.	Wednesday.	Thursday.	Friday.	Saturday.
8:45 a.m	Lecture. Eye & Ear.	Clinics.	Clinics.	Clinics.	Clinics.	Lecture Nose & Th
9:45 a.m	Clinics.	Clinics.	Clinics.	Clinics.	Clinics.	Clinics.
10:45 a.m	Lecture. Women.	Practice.	Clinics. Hospital.	Practice.	Practice.	Oper. Gyn
11:45 a.m		Obstetrics.	Oper. Gyn.	Obstetrics.	Obstetrics.	
2 p.m	Elec. Ther.	Pathology.			Y.M.C.A.	Pathology.	
3 p.m	Surgery.	Surgery.	Surgery.	Surgery.		

Time of Special Lectures, Diseases of Children, Medical Jurisprudence, and Neurology will be announced later.

PROCEEDINGS OF THE

Ohio State Eclectic Medical Association.

W. N. MUNDY, M.D., EDITOR.

The Ohio State Eclectic Medical Association convened, pursuant to adjournment, in its forty-fourth annual session at Dayton, Ohio (Headquarters, Algonquin Hotel), May 5, 1908, at 10 A.M., and was called to order by the President, Austin S. McKitrick, of Kenton, Ohio; opened with prayer offered by Rev. W. A. Hale, of Dayton.

An Address of Welcome was delivered by Mr. Ezra Kuhns, President of the City Council of Dayton, which was responded to upon behalf of the Association by John J. Sutter, of Bluffton.

Roll-call of the officers resulted as follows:

OFFICERS.
President, Austin S. McKitrick, present.
First Vice-President, Harry D. Todd, present.
Second Vice-President, W. F. Lehr, present.
Recording Secretary, William N. Mundy, present.
Corresponding Secretary, John L. Payne, present.
Treasurer, S. M. Sherman, present.

Reading of the minutes being next in order, John J. Sutter moved that same be dispensed with and that the minutes as edited by the Secretary, W. N. Mundy, in THE ECLECTIC MEDICAL JOURNAL, be adopted; seconded by W. T. Gemmill and carried.

The President appointed the Committee on Registration as follows: J. D. Dodge, U. O. Jones, H. C. Duke, C. E. Stadler, and John L. Payne, Corresponding Secretary.

The Treasurer read his report, as follows:

TREASURER'S REPORT.
May 9, 1907—Received from R. B. Taylor, Treasurer....$372 65
June 24—Received from J. J. Sutter, left from banquet... 1 50
March 30, 1908—Received from Lloyd Bros.—Contribution. 15 00
Received dues to date................................. 155 10—$544 25
July 3, 1907—Paid Scudder Bros. Co.—Subscriptions to
   JOURNAL 69 75
January 6, 1908—Paid Scudder Bros. Co.—Subscriptions to
   JOURNAL 107 60
March 14—Paid Scudder Bros. Co.—Subscriptions to
   JOURNAL 98 05
August 1, 1907—Paid J. L. Payne, Secretary, Postage and
   Stationery 15 00
September 11—Paid J. L. Payne, Secretary, Postage and
   Printing 14 75
December 14—Paid J. L. Payne, Secretary, Postage and
   Stationery 24 32
April 21, 1908—Paid J. L. Payne, Secretary, Postage and
   rent of typewriter................................. 35 46
April 16—Paid St. Louis Button Co., Badges............. 24 00
April 16—Postage and express for Treasurer's use....... 10 40— 399 33

Balance on hand, May 5, 1908................................$144 92

W. N. MUNDY: I move that the report be accepted and referred to the Finance Committee. Motion seconded by W. T. Gemmill and carried.

JOHN K. SCUDDER: I move that we proceed to the consideration of the amendment of Article 3, that was proposed a year ago, so that the Treasurer will be in a position to go ahead and take the annual dues.

LYMAN WATKINS seconded Dr. Scudder's motion.

W. N. MUNDY, Recording Secretary, read the proposed amendment, as follows:

AMENDMENT.

"An amendment was proposed in 1907 to be voted on at this meeting to change the initiation fee from $3.00 to $3.50, and the annual dues from $2.00 to $2.50."

JOHN K. SCUDDER: I wish to ask if the Committee on Organization is not correct in receiving applications for membership, which they have done in the past month or six weeks, on the basis of the present initiation fee of three dollars. These particular applications, perhaps a dozen of them, are all based on the present initiation fee. As I understand the matter, this would refer to the initiation fees a year from to-day, but it would raise the dues that are payable to-day. Otherwise these men, who have made applications in the last six weeks, would be laboring under a disadvantage.

JOHN J. SUTTER: I believe if a person has made an application prior to the passage of this Article, he comes under the old law, or old rule. I was under the impression that this second clause of the amendment had in that every member of the State Association is entitled to THE ECLECTIC MEDICAL JOURNAL.

LYMAN WATKINS: It is so stated on the program.

JOHN K. SCUDDER: That is a matter of contract. That is not in the Constitution. The contract is between the officers of the Association, representing the Association as its agents, and the publishers.

JOHN J. SUTTER: Then that may only last one year?

W. N. MUNDY: Yes, sir. It is for the Association to say how long this contract shall last. It was simply a contract. If the Association sees fit, at any time, to abrogate this contract, it is their privilege to do so, as I understand it. I will say that my understanding is that three dollars is the initiation fee until this resolution is adopted, and it could not be retroactive. Asking those who have already applied to pay three dollars and a half would be making it retroactive. I have accepted three dollars.

W. T. GEMMILL: The old law is undoubtedly in force until we actually vote on this new amendment. After that, if it is passed, we will abide by whatever the Association does. All that made applications for membership into this Association prior to the passing of this amendment, will come under the old rule and pay three dollars, but after the passing of this amendment, they will pay three dollars and a half.

S. M. SHERMAN, Treasurer: I have been going on the other theory, that they would not be members until they were elected and then that they would come under the new arrangement. I have accepted three dollars and a half from some. If this amendment is adopted, they will all come under that, it seems to me.

R. L. THOMAS: This is a little unfortunate, and discriminates against the doctor who comes up here to join the society this afternoon and has to pay three dollars and a half, when the man that has sent in three dollars gets in for three dollars. It rather puts a premium on the man that stays at home and sends three dollars. If it were not for the fact that the Treasurer cannot accept the dues until it is decided, I would think the best thing to do would be to act on the last day, and that will let everybody in this year at three dollars, but that leaves out the dues. I presume we will have to pass it and put every one under the necessity of paying the extra fifty cents. It is hardly fair, but it is about the only way we can do.

S. M. SHERMAN: I have only received three or four that way that have sent the three dollars and a half. I can refund the half dollar, if necessary.

W. N. MUNDY: In reply to Dr. Thomas, I want to say that the Committee on Organization has thoroughly canvassed the State. Every Eclectic in the State of Ohio has received one or two petitions, —not letters, but petitions,—with blank application, to join this organization, when they can get in for three dollars.

R. L. THOMAS: I know, and I have got three dollars from a man. He is at home. Some one comes in this afternoon and has to pay three dollars and a half.

W. N. MUNDY: He ought not to delay. Don't you know that there is an "accepted time?"

The question was called for, and upon being put, it was carried.

The President appointed the Credential Committee as follows: John K. Scudder, B. K. Jones, O. P. McHenry.

A. S. McKITRICK, President: Have we any committees to report at this time? Any communications?

JOHN K. SCUDDER: The Committee on Organization will have a report, but we prefer to wait until to-morrow morning, at the business session, rather than to report to-day, because there will be more members here; and we have some important matters of organization and legislation to bring up.

PRESIDENT: Is there any new business to come before the Association? If not we will proceed to section work.

The Association then proceeded to Section I—Ophthalmology, Otology and Laryngology.

SECTION I—OPHTHALMOLOGY, OTOLOGY AND LARYNGOLOGY.

J. J. Sutter, Chairman, presiding.

T. D. Hollingsworth submitted a paper on "Tonsillitis," which was read by W. N. Mundy. Discussed by R. L. Thomas, W. T. Gemmill, A. S. Stemler, C. M. Neldon, W. N. Mundy, J. D. Smith, W. H. Swisher, Lyman Watkins, O. P. McHenry, E. R. Freeman, K. O. Foltz, J. D. Dodge.

K. O. Foltz talked upon the subject of "Specific Indications in Eye Diseases," in lieu of submitting a paper. Discussed by Lyman Watkins, W. T. Gemmill, E. R. Freeman and K. O. Foltz.

J. P. Harbert read a paper entitled "Penetrating Wounds of the Eye." Discussed by K. O. Foltz, W. N. Mundy, A. E. Ballmer, J. P. Harbert and E. R. Freeman. Section closed.

After Section I arose, the President resumed the chair and appointed the following committees:

Press Committee: W. N. Mundy, J. P. Harbert, F. J. Wuist.

Committee on Surgical Clinics: L. E. Russell, W. T. Gemmill, W. K. Mock.

Committee on Medical Clinics: R. L. Thomas, A. S. Stemler, J. D. Smith.

Committee on Eye and Ear Clinics: J. P. Harbert, K. O. Foltz, J. J. Sutter.

PRESIDENT: What is the further pleasure of the Association?

W. T. GEMMILL: I move that we adjourn to two o'clock. Motion seconded and carried. Adjournment to 2 P.M.

Tuesday, May 5, 2 P.M., the Association was called to order by W. K. Mock, who introduced Austin S. McKitrick, President of the Association, who then delivered the President's Annual Address (to be printed later).

The President then took the chair and called for any business that should come before the Association. There being none, Section II, Pathology and Practice, was taken up.

SECTION II—PATHOLOGY AND PRACTICE. .

E. A. Ballmer, presiding.

The subject of "Pneumonia" was discussed by E. R. Freeman and C. E. Stadler.

P. E. Decatur, Chairman, coming in at this time, was called to the chair and presided during the remainder of the section.

A paper on "Erysipelas," by P. E. Decatur, was read by W. N. Mundy. Discussed by S. Schiller, J. P. Dice, W. K. Mock, W. N. Mundy, E. A. Ballmer, J. J. Sutter, G. E. Starner.

A paper on "Bronchitis" was read by W. H. Graham. Discussed by W. S. Turner, E. Florence Stir Smith, and E. R. Freeman.

Upon motion by J. J. Sutter, seconded by W. N. Mundy, the subject of "Appendicitis" was taken up for discussion, which was opened by A. S. McKitrick, followed by L. E. Russell and W. T. Gemmill. Section closed.

At the close of Section II, the President resumed the chair.

W. K. Mock moved that, inasmuch as Lyman Watkins was present and would leave this evening, he be asked to read at this time his paper entitled "Are Drugs Ever Useful," and that W. S. Turner read his paper entitled "Faith in Medicine."

W. S. Turner submitted his paper by title.

Lyman Watkins then read a paper entitled "Are Drugs Ever Useful?" Discussed by W. S. Turner, K. O. Foltz, D. H. Welling, M. H. Hennell, L. E. Russell, J. D. Dodge, and Lyman Watkins.

The President called for the reports from Committees on Clinics. R. L. Thomas, of the Committee on Medical Clinics, reported three cases (reports of which, with discussion, will be given later); W. T. Gemmill, of the Committee on Surgical Clinics, reported one case (report of which, with discussion, will be given later); J. P. Harbert, of the Committee on Eye and Ear Clinics, reported no cases brought before the Committee.

PRESIDENT: We are ready now to hear the report of the Committee on Credentials.

JOHN K. SCUDDER made the report of the Committee on Credentials as follows:

REPORT OF COMMITTEE ON CREDENTIALS.

We, your Committee on Credentials, beg leave to recommend the following for membership:

G. L. Tinker, New Philadelphia,
L. Boulware, Midland City,
J. D. Johnson, Wharton,
J. F. Galley, Cincinnati,
Joseph B. Barker, Piqua,
Edwin E. Myers, New Madison,
N. P. Hunter, N. Lewisburg,
J. Corliss Evans, Cincinnati,
Joseph F. Berry, Cincinnati,
G. W. Lyle, Scio,
Harry G. Blain, Chicago Junction,
W. A. Fahl, Mt. Blanchard,
J. L. McHenry, Hamilton,
J. H. Fritz, West Alexandria,

Albert H. Nesbitt, Hamilton,
N. Hull, Blandensburg,
P. Henry O'Hara, Lewisburg,
J. R. McCally, Dayton,
Charles J. Otto, Dayton,
W. J. Newcomer, Dayton.
W. F. Carson, Berlin Centre,
Will J. Prince, Piqua,
J. W. Strosnider, R. F. D., Houston.
P. A. Kemper, Germantown,
W. H. Ambrose,
E. G. Beckwith,
S. D. Logan, Middletown.

J. K. SCUDDER,
B. K. JONES,
O. P. McHENRY,
Committee.

W. T. GEMMILL moved that same be accepted and the gentlemen mentioned be elected to membership. Seconded by Dr. Ambrose Motion carried.

The President appointed Committees as follows:

Auditing Committee: R. L. Thomas, S. Schiller, G. E. Starner.

Committee on Necrology: W. S. Turner, P. E. Decatur, E. M. Wright.

Committee on Nominations: W. K. Mock, A. E. Ballmer, R. L. Thomas.

It was moved by John L. Payne, and seconded by several, that the Association adjourn to meet at eight o'clock in social session. Motion carried, and the Association adjourned to eight o'clock.

Tuesday, May 5, 8:15 P.M., a reception was held in the Sun Parlor of the Algonquin Hotel, and a most interesting program was carried out, consisting of vocal and orchestral music, with reading.

Wednesday, May 6, 9 A.M., the Association was called to order by President McKitrick. Unfinished business, new business, reports of committees and communications were called for.

JOHN K. SCUDDER: I have a bill here from the Lancet-Clinic Publishing Company for printing one thousand programs for 1908 meeting, $14.00.

PRESIDENT: The bill will be referred to the Auditing Committee.

JOHN K. SCUDDER: Are you ready for the report of the Committee on Organization and Legislation?

PRESIDENT: We will hear it.

JOHN K. SCUDDER thereupon read the report of the Committee on Organization and Legislation, as follows:

REPORT OF THE COMMITTEE ON ORGANIZATION AND LEGISLATION.

Your Committee appointed two years ago has been actively at work. We have subdivided the State into ten districts, each in charge of a member. We have prepared an accurate list of members and non-members by counties, and have sent out several appeals for new members, with favorable replies in some cases.

Our active membership approximates 250, and we ought to have 400 at the very least to do good work. If our individual members will only take occasion to bring the advantages of society membership to the attention of others in their county they can materially assist us. If it were more generally known that our annual dues of $2.50 includes a copy of THE ECLECTIC MEDICAL JOURNAL and later several years of the Transactions in bound volume, our membership would increase. There are possibly fifty in the State who have allowed their membership to lapse; they should be urged to reinstate.

A few months ago your Committee was invited to co-operate with a similar Committee from the Ohio State Medical Society and the Ohio Homeopathic Association, looking towards securing a number of physicians of various political and medical faith to stand as candidates for the next Legislature. The result of this move is not apparent at the present time, but your Committee was of the opinion that our interests must be well taken care of in the event of the possible appointment of county health officers under a proposed law.

Your Committee, with the aid of sub-committees in fifty-seven counties, will guard your interest against any adverse medical legislation at the next session of the Legislature.

Dr. F. F. Demuth, of Cecil, Paulding County, has been of assistance to us. He is strongly of the opinion that with a combined effort he may be able to secure various appointments for our medical men in State institutions.

The question of the choice of a medical man as candidate for the national Senate must necessarily be left to the individual views of each member.

Respectfully submitted,

JOHN K. SCUDDER, *Chairman.*

J. P. HARBERT: I move that the report be accepted and the Committee continued. Seconded by Dr. Postle. Motion carried.

President appointed the Advisory Committee as follows: W. N. Mundy, Recording Secretary, Chairman; John J. Sutter, Northwestern Society; J. D. Dodge, Northeastern Society; J. P. Harbert, Central Society; R. B. Taylor, Ohio Central Society; J. L. Payne, Cincinnati Society; J. D. Smith, Dayton Society.

PRESIDENT: What is the further pleasure of the society?

JOHN K. SCUDDER: Dr. Mundy ought to have a communication from the Secretary of the National in regard to closer affiliation and the payment of two dollars.

W. N. MUNDY: I have not received it. He failed to send it.

JOHN K. SCUDDER: I presume the Secretary had a communication from Dr. Wm. P. Best, Secretary of the National, asking this Association as to whether they would view with favor an arrangement by which this Association would become auxiliary to the National and every member of this society would become a member of the National Association on the payment of two dollars additional dues per year. In other words, if such a plan is worked out, as the National officers have now outlined, they are trying to make arrangements with the majority of the State societies—such societies as would consent to make the arrangement—that the State societies should collect two dollars from each member in the State society, and that would make him a member of the National Association, so that his annual dues to the National would be two dollars instead of five dollars, as at present, and that every member of the State society would be a member of the National. I am not prepared to argue this point, one way or the other. It is a big problem. It is a question in my mind whether the National will have sufficient information at their meeting at Kansas City this year, to justify them in coming to any decision as to the advisability of it. There are about 2,350 members of the various State societies and less than 500 members of the National Association. The question is whether these 2,350 members will care sufficiently for membership in the National to consent to the plan for the payment of the additional two dollars dues. In some societies, like Arkansas, the annual dues are only a dollar. In this State it is two dollars and a half. The Indiana annual dues have heretofore been only one dollar and the initiation fee is five dollars. It is a question whether they would care to enter into an arrangement to pay the additional two dollars.

I believe it was decided last year, in California, to ask the various societies for an expression of opinion as to whether they would consider the plan feasible or not. It is nothing against the society if it declines to accede to the plan. Personally, I doubt very much whether the plan is feasible unless the National will go into the publishing business and publish their Transactions in the shape of a monthly bulletin and furnish this to the members, similar to the *Journal of the American Medical Association*. If they would do that, they might produce something that would be sufficiently attractive to justify the States in increasing their dues to the extent of two dollars, thereby gaining National membership for their members.

DR. R. L. THOMAS: This is a matter in which I think we are all vitally interested, and while I concede that we are not in a position to take definite action as to whether or not we shall affiliate with the National Association, I believe we ought to have some expression that we would consider it with favor, or something of that kind, not any definite action, because this is going to come up before the National Association at the next meeting and it is a matter in which every Eclectic in the United States, I think, is vitally interested.

The idea of a school having 2,350 State members and less than 500 in the National! I am sure that the burden of the two dollars extra will not stand in the way of the members, and I believe—of course, this is all theoretical—I believe they will soon take steps to publish their transactions monthly, in place of in one volume, and it will serve as a monthly journal, which will more than repay the member who pays his two dollars. Yet, at the same time, we are not in a position to act definitely. Such an expression of opinion would not mean that we affiliate. Ohio, of course, leads the world, and we ought to lead in this matter of States affiliating with the National.

J. P. HARBERT: This matter should be referred to the Advisory Committee, and they should bring in a report.

PRESIDENT: It is referred to the Advisory Committee for report.

DR. SCUDDER inquired as to the status of the Advisory Committee.

W. N. MUNDY: In answer to Dr. Scudder, I will say that you will find that in the report of Dr. Harbert, Secretary, there is a resolution that—

The President shall appoint an Advisory Committee, consisting of one member from among the officers of the Association, and one from each auxiliary society, to which committee all resolutions, reports, propositions and suggestions, as well as all matters others than medical and scientific subjects, shall be presented in writing and referred without debate thereon, and no discussion shall be had on the floor of the Association upon any subject so referable except upon the report of said Committee.

The Association thereupon took up the work of Section IV.

SECTION IV—MISCELLANEOUS.

J. K. SCUDDER, Chairman, presiding.

A paper entitled "Treatment of Pulmonary Tuberculosis," by M. H. Hennel, was read by J. K. Scudder. Discussion by J. K. Scudder, M. H. Hennel, E. R. Freeman, L. E. Russell, B. K. Jones, Ivadell Rogers, R. L. Thomas, R. B. Taylor, D. H. Welling, Wm. Phillips, and M. H. Hennel.

J. D. Dodge read a paper entitled "The Medical Profession and Purity." Discussed by J. H. Huntley, E. Florence Stir Smith, W. B. Church, T. E. Griffiths, J. S. Hagen, G. E. Starner and J. D. Dodge.

Dr. Hensley read a paper entitled "Advancement of Medical Practice and Medicines." No discussion.

William Phillips read a paper on "Tuberculosis." Discussed.

Section closed.

The President urged every one to be prompt in attendance at one o'clock. The Recording Secretary urged every one to register. W. K. Mock made an announcement of the evening's program, "Symposium on Tuberculosis." The Association adjourned to one o'clock.

Wednesday, May 6, 1:20 P.M., meeting was called to order with President McKitrick in the chair. Reports of committees called for, uone responded, and the Association went into the work of Section V.

SECTION V—SURGERY.

J. F. Wuist, Chairman, presiding.

August Rhu read a paper on "Abdominal Adhesions." Discussed by B. K. Jones and J. H. Huntley.

J. H. Huntley read a paper on "Pathology and Treatment of Chronic Joint Diseases." Discussed by O. P. McHenry, W. B. Church, C. W. Russell, J. H. Huntley and E. R. Freeman.

L. E. Russell submitted by title a paper entitled "Late Surgical Ideas." Discussed by L. E. Russell, J. S. Hagen, J. R. Spencer.

Section closed.

SECTION VI—SPECIAL DIAGNOSIS AND MEDICATION.

J. D. Dodge, Chairman, presiding.

J. L. Payne submitted by title a paper on the subject of the "Practical Use of the Microscope."

G. E. Starner read a paper entitled "H. M. C. Compound in General Practice." Discussed by J. R. Spencer, W. N. Mundy, R. B. Taylor, C. W. Russell, H. D. Todd, E. Florence Stir Smith, J. P.

Harbert, J. A. Shirack, M. H. Hennell, S. M. Sherman, W. T. Gemmill, S. W. Mattox, B. K. Jones.

R. L. Thomas submitted his paper, "Care in Diagnosis," by title. Section closed.

W. N. Mundy read communications from Prof. John Uri Lloyd and Bishop McMillen, M.D., sending their best wishes and regrets at being unable to attend this meeting.

PRESIDENT: The appeal to Professor Lloyd to go to Nebraska this year was exceptionally strong. It is a critical time with them, and they needed him. Although we would like to have him with us, I felt that his duty was with them and not with us. The suggestion in Dr. McMillen's letter should be referred to the Advisory Committee.

W. N. Mundy: As you are aware, there is in session at Columbus the Ohio Medical Association; in Louisville, Ky., the Kentucky Eclectic Medical Association; in Lincoln, Neb., the Nebraska Eclectic Medical Association; and in Wheeling, W. Va., the West Virginia Medical Association; and I move that congratulatory telegrams be sent to the several meetings.

The Association then took up the work of Section VII.

SECTION VII—OBSTETRICS AND GYNECOLOGY.

J. Stewart Hagen, Chairman, presiding.

J. R. Spencer read a paper entitled "Perineal Support During Labor." Discussed by R. V. Dickey, S. M. Sherman, E. R. Freeman, W. H. Ambrose, W. K. Mock, S. Schiller, B. K. Jones, L. E. Russell, A. E. Ballmer, R. W. Sharp, J. D. Dodge, W. B. Church, R. B. Taylor and J. R. Spencer.

A paper entitled "Anesthetics in Obstetrics" was submitted by title by A. W. Hobby.

A paper entitled "Miscarriage and Abortion" was submitted by title by J. F. Conrad.

A paper on "Gynecological Surgery," by J. S. Hagen, was submitted by title.

A paper on "Placenta Previa," by W. H. Ambrose, was submitted by title.

A paper entitled "Obstetrics" was submitted by R. W. Sharp.

SECTION VIII—MATERIA MEDICA AND THERAPEUTICS.

J. D. Smith, Chairman, presiding.

M. M. Brubaker submitted by title a paper on "Asclepias Tuberosa."

C. W. Beaman submitted by title a paper on "Yellow Mercuric Oxide."

H. E. Dwyer read a paper on "Crataegus Oxycanthus." Discussed by J. D. Dodge, J. F. Conrad, S. Schiller, H. E. Dwyer.

A paper by E. E. Bechtel on "Avena" was submitted by title.

A paper by T. D. Hollingsworth on "Sticta" was submitted by title.

A paper by J. D. Smith on "Pilocarpus" was submitted by title.

Section closed.

W. N. MUNDY: I am requested to ask the physicians of Mercer, Darke, Preble, Montgomery, Green, Clark, Champaign, Shelby and Miami Counties to remain in this room after the adjournment of the Association.

DR. McKITRICK: I suggest that we be prompt in our attendance at eight o'clock to-night. If there is nothing further a motion to adjourn is in order.

Motion to adjourn was made by A. W. Hobby, seconded by J. L. Hensley, and carried.

Wednesday, May 5, 8 P.M., the meeting was called to order by President McKitrick, for the "Symposium on Tuberculosis."

A. S. McKITRICK: I am sure that we have an intellectual treat for you this evening in the program that will be presented, and I have the pleasure of introducing to you Dr. C. O. Probst, Secretary of the State Board of Health, who will address you on "Tuberculosis from the Standpoint of the State."

C. O. PROBST: In the first place, I want to express my sense of the honor that you have shown me in inviting me here to talk to you on the subject of tuberculosis; and also wish to say that I am extremely pleased to see, by your program, the space that you have given this subject of tuberculosis. The title of my paper, perhaps, does not quite cover what I have prepared to say to you. I have a short paper, descriptive of the methods that will be followed with our new State sanatorium, which is under construction at Mount Vernon, and which I thought would be of interest to you, considering the sanatorium and also the hospital as relating to the prevention, as well as the cure, of tuberculosis.

(Dr. Probst then read his paper, which will be published in the JOURNAL.)

DR. McKITRICK: "Modern Conception of Consumption and its Treatment" will be presented by B. F. Lyle, who has charge of the Tuberculosis Branch of the Cincinnati Hospital.

B. F. LYLE: This is such an extensive subject, that I have not attempted to cover it, but hope that the discussion, which will follow, will bring out the points in the treatment of the disease.

(Paper will be published later.)

DR. McKITRICK: "Physical Treatment of Tuberculosis" will be

treated by Otto Juettner, of Cincinnati, who needs no introduction to this Association.

(Dr. Juettner then read his paper, which will also be published.)

DR. McKITRICK: I am sure we are under great obligations to these gentlemen for their instructive lectures which we have listened to this evening, and I voice the sentiment of the Association, I am sure, when I express the thanks of the Association to them for their presence with us this evening.

J. K. SCUDDER: I move that we extend a formal vote of thanks to Drs. Probst, Lyle and Juettner for their kind consideration in consenting to come and address us this evening, and that we ask their permission to publish their excellent papers in our Transactions.

There were a number of seconds to the above motion, which was unanimously carried by a rising vote.

DR. McKITRICK: If there is nothing further to come before the Association, we will stand adjourned.

Thursday, May 6, 9 A.M., meeting called to order, with President McKitrick in the chair.

J. P. HARBERT: The Committee on Eye and Ear Clinics have an opportunity to report one case referred to them.

(Report of case to be given later.)

Report of the Auditing Committee was read by S. Schiller, as follows:

REPORT OF AUDITING COMMITTEE.

To O. S. E. M. Association: DAYTON, O., May 7, 1908.
We, the undersigned Auditing Committee, have this day examined the books and vouchers of S. M. Sherman, and find the same correct. R. L. THOMAS,
                                              G. E. STARNER,
                                              S. SCHILLER.

It was moved by Dr. Mock, seconded by Dr. Gemmill, that the report of the Auditing Committee be accepted. Motion carried.

The Committee on Necrology reported the following deaths during the year: Drs. J. M. Crismore, of Helena, and Dr. W. O. C. Harding, of Elmwood Place. Suitable biographical sketches will be prepared for publication in the Transactions.

W. N. Mundy read the report of the Advisory Committee as follows:

REPORT OF ADVISORY COMMITTEE.

We beg to recommend that this Association view with favor the proposed movement looking toward a closer affiliation with the National Association, and are heartily in favor of any feasible action in that line.

We recommend that the name of J. M. Crismore, of Helena, be placed on the Roll of Honor for the year 1908. Respectfully submitted,
                    W. N. MUNDY, Chairman,   R. B. TAYLOR,
                    J. J. SUTTER,   J. L. PAYNE,
                    J. D. DODGE,   J. D. SMITH.
                    J. P. HARBERT,

Adopted.

PRESIDENT: Are there any other reports of committees?

J. D. DODGE: Mr. President, I don't know what the Resolution Committee has seen fit to do, but I have a resolution that I wish to offer here, one that I am very anxious to have passed by this Convention, which I will read:

WHEREAS, There exists a general ignorance among the youth of the land regarding sexual physiology and hygiene and the evil effects of venereal vices and diseases which is resulting in widespread disease, and contributing to race deterioration; therefore, be it

Resolved, By the Ohio State Eclectic Medical Association, in convention assembled, that we recommend a general diffusion of sex knowledge among the young by means of a plan of instruction in the public schools of the State.

Resolved, That we request the Ohio State Board of Health to take such action as is necessary to establish such education.

Resolved, That a copy of these resolutions be sent to the Ohio State Board of Health and that a copy be furnished the press for publication.

DR. McKITRICK: I think that, as that is a resolution, it would properly go to the Advisory Committee, or be carried over for next year.

Remarks having been called for, J. D. Dodge said: I advocate the passage of this resolution for several reasons: First, because of the immense importance of the subject; second, because it is generally admitted that this subject should be thoroughly taught in the home, by the parents, and that they do not do so, as a rule. The teaching of the subject in colleges is advocated by some of the leading physicians of this country and many leading laymen. I believe it would be an honor to this Association to pass such a resolution; to say that this was the first medical convention in the United States and in the world to pass such a resolution, and I believe it will contribute more than any other one thing to the elevation of the people of this country and of the world as the influence spreads."

S. SCHILLER: I would like to say a word on this subject. I am heartily in accord with the purpose aimed at by this resolution; but it would be taking a step by this Association, that I think we ought to consider pretty carefully. While the object to be attained is commendable, there is a question in my mind whether it is practicable at this time. How will it be taught in the public schools? By whom? Are our teachers in the public schools capable of imparting this delicate knowledge to the children, the boys and girls? A large majority of our school teachers are ladies, young women, and I doubt very seriously whether many of them are familiar with this subject and are capable of teaching it in the proper way. It is a very delicate thing, and I would not like to see this Association pledge itself to anything that would be absurd or impossible at this time. I think it might be a good thing for us to consider this matter for some time before taking decisive action.

R. V. Dickey: I am sorry to say that I am not in accord with the resolution whatever. It seems to me too precipitate. In the second place, the public schools are loaded down now with the various courses of instruction, lectures and so on,. until they have almost eliminated the old-fashioned school. They keep talking on different branches until there is practically no time for the child to study. If you do not believe it to be too precipitate, do a little missionary work of your own and you will find where you are. I think it would be much better if one would put a resolution before this society, to strengthen quarantine against such diseases to such an extent that the man or woman who contracts such disease would be quarantined. This would be more to the point than to put this in the public schools.

A. W. Hobby: It seems to me that the proper place for the teaching of this subject is in the home. This sort of thing is being promulgated by some of the leading magazines, especially the *Ladies Home Journal*.

W. N. Mundy: I feel like Dr. Schiller, that it is a delicate thing. A large majority of our teachers are ladies. For them to teach these matters to boys in the high school is a delicate matter. If this teaching could be done by men teachers it would be a different thing. We teach physiology and this branch could be incorporated into physiology.

W. T. Gemmill: I believe that this is a subject that ought to receive careful attention before we act on it, and I move that it be laid on the table until next year. Carried.

There being no further business, the work of

SECTION IX—MENTAL AND NERVOUS DISEASES,

was taken up, Dr. R. V. Dickey presiding.

C. W. Holzmuller submitted by title a paper on "Neurasthenia."

W. E. Postle submitted by title a paper on "Hysteria."

R. V. Dickey read a paper on "Epilepsy." Discussed by W. N. Mundy, S. Schiller, J. F. Conrad and R. V. Dickey.

Bishop McMillen, "The Insane Who Get Well," by title.

Section closed.

The President resumed the chair and called for the report of the Nominating Committee, which was read by the Recording Secretary.

The Association thereupon proceded to the election of officers. J. P. Harbert was elected President by acclamation.

The Secretary read the names presented for Vice-President. Ballots were prepared, A. W. Hobby and J. D. Southard appointed tellers, and the Association instructed to vote for two names, the one receiving the largest number of votes to be First Vice-President, the one receiving the next largest number of votes to be Second Vice-President.

During the counting of the ballots, J. K. Scudder moved the adoption of the usual resolution that the sum of ten dollars be paid to each of the Secretaries and to the Treasurer for their services during the past year. Carried.

The tellers reported the result of the vote taken for Vice-Presidents to be as follows: J. F. Wuist 29, G. W. Deem 19, C. E. Stadler 14. The President declared Dr. Wuist elected First Vice-President; G. W. Deem, Second Vice-President.

W. N. Mundy was elected Recording Secretary by acclamation.

J. L. Payne was elected Corresponding Secretary by acclamation.

Dr. Sherman was elected Treasurer by acclamation.

The President appointed W. T. Gemmill to present and introduce the incoming officers.

PRESIDENT: Nominations for the place of next meeting are in order.

B. K. JONES: Cincinnati.

J. L. HENSLEY: I have the honor to nominate "Greater Marion."

S. W. MATTOX: I would like to second that nomination. I want to say that Dr. Hensley has asked for this for ten or eleven years and I believe that we should honor his request at this meeting.

W. N. MUNDY: I have some letters from Springfield—from the Springfield Commercial Club. Dr. Russell also asked that the matter be presented. The older members of the Association will remember that we had many pleasant meetings in Springfield in times past. We have not been there for a number of years. It is centrally located, and I present to your consideration the city of Springfield. I nominate Springfield.

B. K. JONES: I nominated Cincinnati awhile ago.

W. E. POSTLE: I would like to second the nomination of Cincinnati. I believe it would be a good thing for this Association to go back to Cincinnati once more for the State meeting and to meet there Commencement week. It will be the means of getting a great many in who come to the Commencement exercises and the annual banquet of the alumni; it would be a good thing for the Association to get together once more at the College; it would bring more people from all over the State. I think it is just the thing to take it to Cincinnati next year. (Cheers.)

PRESIDENT: Are there any other nominations? If not, prepare your ballots.

The tellers reported the result of the ballot to be: Cincinnati 26, Springfield 5, Marion 3.

DR. MUNDY: I move that we make the election of Cincinnati unanimous. Motion was seconded and carried.

The Committee on Resolutions, consisting of John K. Scudder, J. D. Dodge and R. C. Van Buren, presented the following report:

REPORT OF THE COMMITTEE ON RESOLUTIONS.

Resolved, That a vote of thanks be tendered the retiring officers for the'r earnest efforts in making this meeting the most successful in years; to the members of the Dayton Eclectic Medical Society for our courteous reception; to the Vice Mayor and citizens of the city; to the press of Dayton for well-prepared reports of our meeting; to the exhibiting pharmacists and book dealers for their instructive exihibts, to the Algonquin Hotel for the use of the Sun Parlor and Exhibition Rooms; and finally, to Drs. Probst, Lyle and Juettner for their excellent addresses on "Tuberculosis," which proved so instructive and interesting. This one feature of our Dayton meeting stamps it as a progressive move and was alone worth the trip here.

> J. K. SCUDDER, *Chairman*,
> J. D. DODGE,
> R. C. VAN BUREN.

A. W. HOBBY moved the adoption of the resolution. Dr. B. K. Jones seconded the motion. Carried.

PRESIDENT: If there is nothing further, I will ask W. T. Gemmill to present the new officers.

Each newly elected officer made appropriate remarks.

DR. MCKITRICK: This has been one of the pleasantest years since I have been in the profession; through my year's work there has not been one discordant note. No one has ever had more loyal support; there has been no more loyal set of officers or loyal members since the beginning of the Association than in the past year. We sent out letters asking for suggestions and received many valuable suggestions for this meeting. It has not been due, altogether, to the officers' work that this meeting has been a success; it has been because the members have been willing to work. When you go home if you will begin immediately to select your subjects and prepare your papers there is no reason why we should not have a much bigger meeting next year than we have had this. I want to thank you for the support you have given me. And I assure you, Dr. Harbert, that it is a great pleasure to me to turn this Association over to you, as its executive officer, for a man with your ability and loyalty to the cause bespeaks an excellent meeting next year. I present you with the gavel.

DR. HARBERT: I certainly thank you for your kind words. I could ask nothing more than to be able to preside over as successful a meeting as you have been privileged to preside over. I desire the undivided support of the entire Association, and if they are as loyal to me as they have been to you, I assure you that we will have a successful meeting next year.

Upon motion of R. V. Dickey, the Association adjourned.

Periscope.

Thuja Occidentalis.

In these busy days, when every general practitioner feels the need of therapeutic agents from which he may expect definite results, when, if he holds his patients, he must satisfy them that they are receiving at least a return for their money, the mention of a remedy, be it old or new, that has proven successful in the hands of those who have had occasion to use it, in a large per cent. of cases should be of interest to us all.

There seems to be a diversity of opinion among the profession as to which is the more desirable practice to cultivate, the office or bedside. Then again there is a doubt in the minds of many regarding the problem of using and dispensing one's own remedies, in the office or in general practice. To those who favor office procedure, and lean towards minor operative measures, there is probably no remedy that has a wider range of usefulness than thuja, or, as it is more often called, arbor vitæ. There certainly is none that can produce such *satisfactory results*, attended with *so little danger* to the patient, as this one.

This agent is no new arrival, and the fact that it has contributed to the alleviation of over two centuries of suffering humanity is not at all to its discredit. Introduced into England in 1600, and into America a hundred years later, it has merited the esteem of all "pathies." Although it is now considered an Eclectic remedy, it was not adopted by that branch of the profession until both homeopathic and allopathic practitioners had tested its virtues and included it in their list of approved remedies.

This evergreen coniferous American tree, from twenty to fifty feet high, grows on rocky banks of rivers and in low swamps, from Pennsylvania northward, and is used in many places as a hedge plant.

Like most remedies of this kind that have come into use through their *own intrinsic value,* its use was at first empirical. It remained so, practically, until 1862, when through an editorial by Dr. Scudder, Dr. Dickey took it up and made some investigations along scientific lines. It was not until twenty years later, however, that this valuable remedy received the recognition that was its due. It was then that Professor Howe became interested in it, and through his thorough investigations and warm commendations the drug was firmly established in the class to which it belongs.

Through this investigator the active principles were definitely established and placed in the hands of the general practitioner in the form of a specific tincture, in which form it is best exhbited to-day. There is an aqueous form manufacured that is for use in cases that do not tolerate alcohol, but this form does not seem to fully represent the true activity of the drug and is not in as much demand as the former.

Regarding the properties of this drug no words can be found more expressive than those of Professor Felter. He says that "Thuja has become one of the most important remedies employed in practice, both for its internal and local effects. Specifically it acts upon the vascular, cutaneous and mucous tissues, stimulating them to normal activity, and in cases of flabby vessels, exciting them to contraction, and in cases of cutaneous over-activity, restraining hypertrophies and excrescences. Furthermore it is a decided antiseptic. It will deaden and repress fungous granulations, and may be applied to 'proud flesh' and ingrown nails with considerable success. It has a marked influence upon such chronic granulations as those of trachoma and epithelioma, and is a věry useful remedy in bed sores, sloughing wounds, fistulous openings, and to overcome the stench of senile and other forms of gangrene. Few mild agents have a greater reputation for the destruction of the various kinds of papillomata and for condylomata about the nates. It does not cure all cases, but is best adapted where there is softness and foul exudations. It cures many, though not all, cases of genital and venereal warts. It may be applied full strength to the surface or hypodermically. It is a valuable remedy in fissure of the anus. It is valuable in checking hemorrhage from malignant growths, hemorrhoids and bleeding moles, and has been of inestimable value in cases of 'bleeders.' In this case it has been applied after the extraction of teeth. It is of great service in nasal hemorrhage and for incised wounds. By the use of a compress, the full strength thuja has been the means of saving the lives of many children suffering from umbilical hemorrhage occurring ten to fifteen days after birth. Professor Howe and many others testify to its efficiency in the treatment of bulging nevi, or 'mother's mark.' Ballington reports the cure of a child in three weeks' treatment from birth, with compresses of specific thuja."

It is in cases of hydrocele and hernia that this agent seems to fill a long-felt want. No single remedy seems to have given the universal success with so little discomfort in the cure of these very distressing conditions.

The use of the drug in these conditions is not absolutely painless, but the discomfort to the patient is so slight, as compared with that attending the use of the mixtures generally advised, that it is practically so. Then it is absolutely non-toxic, and the method of its use is very simple.

The technique used most successfully by the writer in treating hydrocele is as follows: Dilute one part of specific thuja (Lloyd's) with five parts of water in a test-tube, and with an alcohol lamp bring the mixture to a boil. Now take a "pen filler" (a large dropper holding about two drachms), and, after boiling it, fill it with the solution and place in readiness for instillation.

Now tap the distended sac of the tunica vaginalis and, after all the liquid has escaped that it is possible to obtain, instill two drachms of thuja solution through the cannula, and carefully knead the tissues so as to bring the solution in contact with every part of the sac. Some pain may or may not ensue, and of course there will be some swelling, after the subsidence of which, in about a week's time, if the work has been carefully done, there will be a very perceptible evidence of the formation of tissue, showing the influence of thuja. It may be necessary to tap the sac again as a small amount of serous fluid will be in evidence in the sac even after the tissue formation has begun, and, as this will not at all be changed into tissue, it is a good idea to remove it, but it is not necessary to repeat the instillation, only in a small per cent. of the cases. The patient is not inconvenienced in his occupation at all, and it generally takes about a week for the swelling to subside, and after that it is but a question of time when the adhesions will contract down so as to very materially reduce the former size of the hydrocele. It will not return to normal size, but will be very much smaller than it was before treatment.

In hernia the solution may be the same, or full strength may be used, and the method will of course differ according to whether we are dealing with a direct or indirect case. The fluid should be delivered so as to cause a formation of tissue just across the hernia, and prevent it from advancing farther. These cases require a longer time, and more careful treatment than the hydrocele. In the case of hernia, after each instillation, which should be given about once a week, the truss should be well adjusted and this should be worn for six weeks and possibly more. The most satisfactory results are obtained when it is possible to have the patient off his feet for a week or ten days after the first treatment. After this he may follow his usual occupation, unless it is of such a nature that it will aggravate his trouble, in which case give him the alternative of either resting or changing his occupation.

Many other cases might be mentioned in which this valuable agent has proven its versatile utility, both in external and internal administration. The scope of this article will hardly admit of it, however, and with a few suggestions for the relief of nasal conditions and incontience of urine in cases of senile prostate, the writer will leave the subject for the consideration of such of the readers as care to prove the efficiency of this valuable remedy by trial.

For nasal polypus put a few drops of specific tincture of thuja on a piece of surgeon's lint and lay this on a sixteen candle-power electric light. Adjust the light so that the vapor from the solution can be well inhaled, together with the heat and light, and the results will please any one who cares to try it.

In incontinence dilute three drachms of specific tincture with four ounces of water and administer a teaspoonful every three or four hours and the results will be most satisfactory.—C. E. BUCK, in *Journal of Therapeutics and Dietetics.*

Nihilism and the Use of Drugs.

Before the Medical Society of New York, Abraham Jacobi delivered an address with the above title. The reader will find it published in *The New York State Journal of Medicine* for February. Had we the space we should publish this address in full, but must content ourselves with the following notes from it:

"The question as to the value of drugs in the treatment of the sick has been recently answered contradictorily by flippant arrogance and by men of honorable ambition and great genius." Founded on the French school of pathology, the Vienna school of medicine was established seventy years ago by Rokitansky, who claimed that pathological anatomy was the essence and sum total of medicine, and Skoda cared for the physical diagnosis of an organic anomaly but not for the patient. It was all care, but no cure was seriously tried. In Vienna the ideal patient was he who was satisfied with being auscultated and percussed by Skoda and autopsied by Rokitansky.

The callously scientific atmosphere of Vienna spread far and wide. Dietl, in 1851, said: "Our practical work does not compare with the amount of our knowledge. Our ancestors laid much stress upon their success in the treatment of the sick, we on the results of our investigations. Our tendency is purely scientific. The physician should be judged by the extent of his knowledge and not by the extent of his cures. So long as there are successful physicians, so long are there no scientific physicians. Our power is in knowledge, not in deeds."

Under the influence of this icy atmosphere Oliver Wendell Holmes made his outbreak, which has since been repeated and re-echoed far and wide. Holmes was not a pharmacologist or a practician of medicine. Many have repeated the quotation, believing they thus ranked with Holmes by imitating the grave mistakes of his scurrilous and sarcastic mood, and with Astley Cooper, who is quoted by Holmes on account of his remark that more harm than good is done by medication. "If he be correct, the only and the simple thing to be done by me and by you is to omit the harm and do all the good we can, and are expected to do, by medication and otherwise." However, Holmes also expressed himself as follows: "It is not of the slightest interest to the patient to know whether three or three and a quarter cubic inches of his lungs are hepatized. He wants something to relieve his pain, to mitigate his anguish or dyspnea or bring back motion and sensibility to the dead limb."

Dr. Jacobi then proceeds to discuss Osler's most recent outbreak, which led the *Evening Post* to say of it: "Here we have three trump cards placed squarely in the hands of the barefoot, sunshine, barleywater and other cures, the new-thought health givers, and the sufferers from various forms of religious mania." Dr. Jacobi says that what he read in Osler's crisp sentences was: (1) Be critical of the pharmacopeia as of everything else. (2) He is the best doctor who knows the worth and the worthlessness of medicine. (3) Study your fellow men and fellow women, and learn to serve them. Therapy means service." He adds, "I wish he had said that."

Dr. Jacobi goes on to say a good word for polypharmacy, objecting to the dictum that compound prescriptions are rarely desirable. He says: "The inexperienced and lazy should rather be admonished to learn how to find indications, and how to write a compound prescription when it is demanded, after his college has, like some others, neglected its duty to teach him. He should know the indications for the selections of drugs, as he is expected to know the rules for ordering diet, water, electricity, heat, cold and massage, aye, even the placebos of consolation and hope. Surely I prefer them to the prediction of an imminent fatal termination, according to the dictates of our aggressively brilliant Richard (Cabot) the Lion-hearted of a neighboring State. Unless the practician knows and does all that, he drives his patients to the manufacturer, the proprietary-medicine vendor, the Christian scientist and the rest of the quacks."

In the discussion of this topic he shows his own practical ignorance of precise medication. For instance he says: "There is no ground for the pedantic demand that two medicines with similar action should not be prescribed together. Even though all your pharmacists were of perfect knowledge and accuracy, on the shelves of the very best of them drugs are liable to lose their efficacy. That is why I recommend and frequently practice the combination of such drugs as digitalis, strophanthus and adonis." Apparently he does not appreciate the difference in the indications between digitalis, strophanthus and adonis. The idea of giving a single drug to meet a single indication seems to have entirely escaped him. We may give any number of drugs at one time, if they can be so administered as not to interfere with each other, provided there is an indication present for each of the drugs given.—*American Journal of Clinical Medicine*.

Sir Frederick Treves' Estimate of the Japanese.

Sir Frederick Treves, the eminent British surgeon, in a speech at the dinner of the Japan Society in London, the other evening, spoke enthusiastically of the medical and surgical skill of the Japanese. He said that anybody desirous of seeing the last thing, the most ingenious thing, and yet the simplest thing in the equipment of war, must go to Japan. Many of the problems which concern European armies, and have been to a large extent a terror of war in European countries, the Japanese were solving or had solved. British troops, he said, enter a war with many determinations. One is 10 per cent. of sick. It is what they are accustomed to expect, and they get it. The Japanese are quite content with 1 per cent. of sick, and they get it. It was a question of ambition, perhaps, he said, but one which might well be imitated. Proceeding, the speaker said he was convinced that Japan not many years hence would provide one of the most remarkable schools of surgery that the world has ever seen. "You will understand why," he continued; "there is the infinite patience of the people, their infinite tenderness. Kinder, more sympathetic people do not exist. Then comes one very important factor, at least, in the making of a surgeon: they have no nervous system. Nerves is an untranslatable term in the Japanese language. I am confident that we shall find in the islands of Japan, not many years hence, one of the most curious, interesting and progressive schools of medicine that this world has seen.—*Med. Review of Reviews*.

Bright's Disease and the Strenuous Life.

T. L. Macdonald, M.D. (*American Medicine*, June 3, 1905), in a paper concerning the nerve strain of official life at Washington and the bodily excesses attendant upon excessive eating and drinking as causative factors of nephritis, concludes with the following summary:

Unemployed food products become toxic irritants and menace the structural integrity of the kidneys.

Man is an organism built around an eliminative system; when that is abnormal he cannot be normal.

When the balance between ingestion, metabolism and elimination is absent, danger is present.

Apparently nutritional excess is the germ of nephritis.

Mental activity and physical quiescence aid in its production.

Carking care and the corrosive influence of worry and mental strain render prominent aid in producing it.

It is prone to attack the intellectual and the anxious.

Alcohol, while affording it encouragement, has been given a too conspicuous place as a causative agent.

It is an extremely insidious disease, and is often well advanced when discovered.

It is so far-reaching that its first noticeable effects may be visited upon organs and tissues remote from the original disease.

The conditions which lead to it are quite amenable to correction if efforts are made sufficiently early.

It occurs somewhat frequently at the nation's capital because the congregation of eminent public men means a concentration of worries, wealth and official feasting.—*Med. Review of Reviews.*

Pass It Along.

THE COLLEGE PRESIDENT.

Such rawness in a student is a shame.
But lack of preparation is to blame.

THE HIGH SCHOOL PRINCIPAL.

Good heavens! what crudity! The boy's a fool.
The fault, of course, is with the grammar school.

THE GRAMMAR PRINCIPAL.

Would that from such a dunce I might be spared!
They send them up to me so unprepared.

THE PRIMARY PRINCIPAL.

Poor Kindergarten blockhead! And they call
That "preparation!" Worse than none at all.

THE KINDERGARTEN TEACHER.

Never such lack of training did I see.
What sort of person can the mother be?

THE MOTHER.

You stupid child! But then, you're not to blame;
Your father's family are all the same.

THE PHILOSOPHER.

Shall father in his folks' defense be heard?
No! Let the mother have the final word.

—*Puck.*

THE ECLECTIC MEDICAL JOURNAL

A Monthly Journal of Eclectic Medicine and Surgery.

TWO DOLLARS PER ANNUM.

Official Journal Ohio State Eclectic Medical Association

JOHN K. SCUDDER, M.D., MANAGING EDITOR.

EDITORS.

W. E. BLOYER.	H. W. FELTER.	W. N. MUNDY.	R. L. THOMAS.
W. B. CHURCH.	K. O. FOLTZ.	L. E. RUSSELL.	L. WATKINS.
JOHN FEARN.	J. U. LLOYD.	A. F. STEPHENS.	H. T. WEBSTER.

Published by THE SCUDDER BROTHERS COMPANY, 1009 Plum Street, Cincinnati, to whom all communications and remittances should be sent.

Articles on any medical subject are solicited, which will usually be published the month following their receipt. One hundred reprints of articles of four or more pages, or one dozen copies of the Journal, will be forwarded free if the request is made when the article is submitted. The editor disclaims any responsibility for the views of contributors.

Discontinuances and Renewals.—The publishers must be notified by mail and all arrearages paid when you want your Journal stopped. If you want it stopped at the expiration of any fixed period, kindly notify us in advance.

FACULTY CHANGES AND ADDITIONS.

A portion of the new announcement is reprinted in this issue. We hope that our readers will look over it carefully, particularly the sections referring to entrance requirements for new matriculates.

The following additions have ben made in the Faculty list:

Herbert E. Sloan, A.B., M.D., formerly of Clarksburg, W. Va., has been appointed Professor of Didactic Surgery, *vice* Dr. Church, resigned. Dr. Sloan graduated from Marietta College in 1895 and the Eclectic Medical Institute in 1898. He has been on the staff of the Clarksburg Hospital for seven years, and is well fitted by post-graduate instruction and general experience in surgery to fill creditably this important position.

J. Corliss Evans, M.D., Physical Diagnosis.

W. E. Postle, M.D., has been chosen Lecturer on Mental and Nervous Diseases.

E. R. Freeman, M.D., Lecturer and Clinical Instructor on Skin and Venereal Diseases.

Louis C. Wottring, M.D., Lecturer on Clinical Medicine.

Victor P. Wilson, M.D., Clinical Lecturer on Diseases of Women, Children and Dermatology.

The staff of "Special Lecturers" will be reorganized, and we expect to have fortnightly addresses on various medical topics, open to all students and local physicians on alternate Wednesdays. These will embrace addresses and lectures by Drs. W. P. Best, C. G. Winter,

J. P. Harbert, F. Ellingwood, E. J. Farnum, A. F. Stephens, E. R. Waterhouse, B. K. Jones, A. S. McKitrick, O. A. Palmer, F. O. Williams, and others.

PROPRIETARY REMEDIES.

There seems to be a hue and cry in certain directions against some proprietary remedies.

The Council of Pharmacy of the A. M. A., part of the self-constituted *clique* of the Chicago Octopus, has attempted to draw the inference that all pharmaceuticals which have not been presented to their scrutiny are consequently more or less worthless.

When one takes into consideration the fact that over 60 per cent. of the remedies that have passed the Council are patented synthetics made in Germany, and that a score of prominent manufacturers in this country have not presented their preparations for alleged inspection, one might well seek for a reason.

In a paper presented to the A. M. A. in Boston, in 1906, Dr. Thomas F. Reilly said:

"It seems to me that the chief reason for the use of the proprietaries is not that they contain any wonderful medicinal agent or combination of agents, but that they do present disagreeable tasting medicines, of more or less value, in palatable form."

To this the May *Gleaner* adds:

"That we know of proprietary preparations not at all secret, to which many years of study have been applied, and concerning which thousands of dollars have been spent in experimentation for the purpose, as the doctor states, of rendering them palatable, effective, permanent, and convenient. It goes without argument that every reputable manufacturing pharmacist in America who has a distinctive position as the maker of some preparation that has acquired a national reputation, has attained this conspicuity by the aforenamed methods, and we congratulate Dr. Reilly in that he has caught a fact that many earnest persons overlook either intentionally or unintentionally.

"It might be asked, what could induce a person to attack *intentionally* an elegant and effective preparation that appears under the name of a manufacturing pharmacist, who presents it as a definite compound, without any secrecy whatever as concerns its medicinal constituents, or even as concerns its one constituent, and who has perhaps given years of labor and study to its evolution? To this it may be replied that the world is full of pirates, and that some perfectly honest men have been made to fork the chestnuts out of the fire for a pirate, and that if these pirates can get the working formulas that have been established by a series of expensive experimentation, they have accomplished a very important feature in the line of piracy. Hence, one of the methods that has been adopted by them is that of attempting force in such a way as to compel a dis-

coverer or an evolver, in self-defense, to publish his working formulas
for the benefit of the pirates."

Why does a physician specify Squibb's *Chloroform*, Lloyd's *Hydrastis*, P. D. & Co.'s *Adrenalin*, Mulford's *Antitoxin*, or Hayden's
Viburnum, or any one of a hundred valuable proprietaries advertised
in this or other journals.

It is *because* he wants a preparation true to name and label and
made by a manufacturer of known ability.

The physician leaves the *making* of the preparation to the manufacturer; the latter allows the former to determine its *therapeutic*
position.   SCUDDER.

BUBONIC PLAGUE IN CALIFORNIA.

The situation at the "seat of war" reminds us of the nursery
rhyme of olden days: "Big cry and ·little wool anyhow, as Farmer
Jones said when he sheared his old sow." Oakland is appropriating
twenty thousand dollars per month to the catching and poisoning of
rats, and no one can, be found who has seen or even heard of an
authentic case of plague within the city limits or in the suburbs. The
only case of mortality occurring under the notice of the writer is
the demise of a valuable (to the owner) bull dog, which partook too
freely of poisoned "dope" promiscuously spread about by the poison
brigade.

It would be amusing to watch the excitement, from a distance,
caused by this bugaboo, were it not for the outrage upon the pockets
of an already tax-ridden people. The writer has taken pains, within
the past few months, to interview every physician he has met upon
the subject, and not one has seen a case which resembled plague in
the least respect. In spite of this fact, many autopsies have been
enforced, and much bacteriological research has been prosecuted, in
the vain endeavor to find something tangible to found the "scare"
upon.

A few physicians who are reaping a harvest by conducting autopsies at fifteen dollars each, and government officials who are drawing
salaries from Uncle Sam and dictating taxation to the City Council,
are the ones who intimidate susceptible readers with the story of the
"Three Black Crows."

If anybody who reads this is hesitating about visiting the Golden
State on account of the plague epidemic, let him take heart from
the experience of the writer, who has lived here twenty-six years, in
the midst of the plague's alarums, and has never yet met a case of
the kind, nor seen anyone else who has. The whole matter is largely,

apparently, one of disordered imagination. The disease ought, properly, to be diagnosed as "Ratiphobia."   WEBSTER.

VEHICLES FOR MEDICINES.

There is no universal vehicle for medicines, and yet with many writers, they seem to use little but water. In my own practice I find it well to vary the vehicles according to the case in hand. Care and thought on these lines makes the medicine often pleasanter, and not less effective.

If you can renew your medicine every day it makes quite a difference, but if you see your patient once in two days, then from five to sixty drops of medicine in four ounces of water gets very vapid in two days.

Some years ago, feeling the want of a vehicle for children's medicine that should have keeping and therapeutic power in it, I formulated borated asepsin solution. This had quite a wide use; it could be used in sprays for the throat, or it could be used internally with advantage in gastro-intestinal conditions, adding nux, chamomilla or any other indicated remedy.

In other cases of stomach and bowel trouble, especially when there is marked acidity, what better vehicle could be found than glyconda?

In many cases the keeping power of the medicine as well as its usefulness can be increased by adding to the mixture chloroform water. In cases of bowel trouble where I am prescribing bismuth, etc., I find aqua cinnamon instead of plain water or syrup is a great improvement. It sweetens and sedates.

Syrups I rarely use, but glycerine, 25 per cent., added to the water makes a splendid addition and a good vehicle. There is one vehicle I do not like; it looks nice to many people, it tastes nice, but I don't want it in mine. That is simple elixir. There is altogether too much alcohol in it. I have heard a patient say when taking medicine where elixir was the vehicle, "Doctor, that medicine goes to my head every time I take a dose."

Berberis is a bitter dose, but it tastes better and acts better when glycerine is added to the mixture, say spec. berb. aqua, oz. i.; glycerine, oz. i.; aqua to oz. iv. M. Sig. Dr. i. four times a day. Try glycerine in your prescriptions where you are using juglans, cin., collinsonia, etc. I don't care what anyone says to the contrary, I know the medicine acts better and I know it tastes better.

I saw a case of serious heart trouble some time ago. A good Eclectic was prescribing the right heart medicine, but that prescription needed what the old writers used to call a *corroborant*. She needed a stimulant and I added to that prescription about ten drops of aromatic spirits of ammonia to each dose, and it did well.

A few weeks ago, in a case of counsel, the consultant wanted to give teaspoonful doses of Warburg's tincture. I had never used the remedy because it had too many ingredients in it, but the doctor was very insistent that the remedy should be given. In five or six days the dumb ague was improving, but the patient's stomach was the seat of a good deal of distress. I wanted to cut out the medicine, but it was insisted we must persevere for a while. I then changed the vehicle and instead of giving the medicine in plain water we compromised on having the water well sweetened with sugar. After this there was no more trouble with pain in the stomach. The medicine was taken with good effect.

Study your cases and give the medicine in each case in the proper vehicle. FEARN.

INTESTINAL DIGESTION.

Of late years intestinal digestion has assumed an importance not formerly accorded to it. The stomach was regarded as the chief organ of digestion, and all other processes of food solution were considered of secondary importance. But more recent investigations have shown that the gastric organ occupies a secondary position in food reduction, and that its chief function is solution and preparation of food for more thorough digestive processes in the small intestine, especially the duodenum.

In the duodenum food is subjected to the action of bile, the pancreatic fluid and the intestinal juices proper, or the succus entericus. While we have but two digestive enzymes secreted by the gastric glands, pepsin and hydrochloric acid, in the small intestine we have trypsin, amylopsin, steapsin and rennin from the pancreas, bilin from the liver, and a diastatic and a proteid ferment in the succus entericus.

Trypsin is a more powerful proteolytic ferment than pepsin, and exerts its activities in an alkaline medium. The proteids which have escaped the action of pepsin are finally and completely digested by trypsin. Amylopsin digests carbohydrates, ferment converting them into maltose and dextrose. This ferment, while of the same nature as ptyalin, is more effective, for it not only acts upon cooked starch, but also upon raw starch, digesting the cellulose envelope of the granulose cells. Gums and gelatins are converted into sugar by amylopsin. Steapsin or ptyalin acts upon fats, and, with the assistance of the bile, emulsifies or saponifies all fatty matters of the food, thus preparing them for absorption. Digestive processes in the small intestine occupy from six to twelve hours, and normally it requires from thirty-six to forty-eight hours for substances to pass the intestinal tract. The secretion from Brunner's glands and from the crypts of Lieberkuhn is diastatic in function, acting upon carbohydrates.

Carbohydrates are digested in the mouth and in the small and large intestine, but not in the stomach, while proteids are digested in the stomach and duodenum, the entire alimentary tract being active in the solution of food. A harmonious relation of all parts of the nutritive canal is essential for the welfare of the body. Complete and normal digestion cannot be accomplished when pathological conditions exist in any part of the organ. A comprehensive view of the process of digestion as a whole is necessary for successful and intelligent treatment. WATKINS.

Commencement Exercises.

The sixty-third annual Commencement Exercises of the Eclectic Medical Institute were held at the Scottish Rite Cathedral, 417 Broadway, Wednesday evening, April 29, 1908, at eight o'clock. The following program was rendered:

1. MUSIC—March, "The Mascot of the Troop," - - *Herbert.*
2. INVOCATION, - - - - - - Rev. Henry C. Jameson.
3. MUSIC—Overture, "Bridal Rose," - - - - - *Lavelle.*
4. DEAN'S REPORT, - - - - Prof. Rolla L. Thomas, M.D.
5. MUSIC—Waltz, "The Red Mill," - - - - - *Herbert.*
6. CONFERRING DEGREES, - - - - Hon. Aaron McNeill, President Board of Trustees.
7. MUSIC—Cornet Solo, Selected, - - - Mr. Charles Joseph.
8. ADDRESS, - - - - - - Hon. Howard C. Hollister.
9. MUSIC—Selection, "The Time, The Place, The Girl," - *Howard.*
10. BENEDICTION, - - - - -, Rev. Henry C. Jameson.
11. MUSIC—March, Dedicated to the "E. M. I." - - - *Hofer.*

Hofer's Orchestra.

The following is a list of the graduates: Julius Emil Bach, Theodore Barnes, Adam P. Basinger, Jesse W. Bowers, James F. Burgin, W. Kirt Dyer, Fred Herman Finlaw, Lewis T. Franklin, Curtis C. Hamilton, Earl W. Horswell, George W. Martin, Charles C. McCaffrey, Mark M. Moran, D. Edward Morgan, Herman F. Pohlmeyer, Benjamin F. Preston, George F. Sauter, Clinton T. Saylor, William H. H. Shrock, William Seitz, Daniel S. Strong, Elmer E. Watson, Firman M. Wurtsbaugh.

Notice.

It has always been the policy of this journal to insist on a prompt payment of the subscription, believing that if a thing was worth having it was worth paying for. Consequently we have not been a very great sufferer from a long delinquent list. There are some, however, that we have carried along, and have always been perfectly willing to do so, when there was any excuse for it. The Post Office Department, however, has made a ruling that prevents our carrying an unpaid subscription on our books longer than four months. If we do this we will have to charge our patrons for the extra postage that it will take, or else cut them off altogether. We do not want to lose a single one of our subscribers. We believe that it is just as easy to pay for the subscription at the beginning of the time as at the end, and thus save the subscriber the annoyance of repeated bills and ourselves a large amount of postage. Therefore, *all you delinquents,* please send your subscription to us in June or July. This is the *limit.*

Mundy's Diseases of Children.

Prof. William N. Mundy has revised his work on "The Eclectic Practice in Diseases of Children." It will be issued in an enlarged form and well illustrated, and will be ready for delivery in September. It has been rearranged and brought up to date in every respect. Advance orders will be taken now on receipt of $2.50. After publication the price will be $3.00. We quote the following notice:

"The treatment is essentially Eclectic, the therapy being based largely on the author's personal experience in practice. When vegetable remedies are named, as aconite, ipecac, rhus tox., etc., the specific medicines are understood, these preparations being the only plant liquids Eclectics use in their practice. This work will be found a valuable one in children's diseases, and all physicians, regardless of *pathy,* should thoroughly read same."—*Medical Brief.*

NATIONAL *Kansas City, Mo. June 17-20, 1908*

The Eclectic Medical Journal

ESTABLISHED 1836.

Vol. LXVIII.   CINCINNATI, JULY, 1908.   No. 7.

Original Communications.

MEDICINE AND PHARMACY IN REVOLT.

John Uri Lloyd, M.D., Cincinnati.

Readers of THE ECLECTIC MEDICAL JOURNAL will remember that from the very beginning of the synthetic craze until the present, Eclectic authorities have protested against the theoretical therapeutic invasion attempted by modern synthetic chemistry. First, it was a little cloud that arose in the direction of Germany, ushered in, practically, by the discovery of a method of making salicylic acid from carbolic acid. Notwithstanding the possibility of the presence of injurious by-products, the world was soon flooded with artificial salicylic acid made by patented processes that could be employed only in Germany.

Quickly following this entering wedge, came, successively, other products, not such as were old in name and familiar in quality, but new in structure and absolutely untried in medicine or in pharmacy. Ushered into existence were these products, as a rule, under the authority of laboratory experimenters, who practiced on frogs and dogs and rabbits and such.

University professors, interested more or less in the distribution and production of these legions of substances, united their efforts to displace well-known and tried remedies by what were too often untried monstrosities. To give even the names of the materials so enthusiastically forced upon the world and so artfully advocated, even in the editorial pages of staid medical journals, would fill volumes.

Let us now repeat the thought expressed in our opening sentence. The leaders in Eclecticism, and thoughtful practitioners of Eclecticism, alone, met this invasion in a manner that was both dignified and effective. Refusing to give up old and tried remedies, they maintained their position as therapeutic expounders of the axiom, "Hold fast that which is good."

It is a lamentable thought, but, nevertheless, a reflection that must come to thousands of physicians of the dominant school who reflect over the death of this or that person, who, had their physician followed methods established, and used remedies known, might have recovered. This burden of weight, fortunately, does not rest upon the Eclectic profession.

It seemed as though the dominant school would never awaken to confronting conditions, and yet, as the years passed, it was evident that the time must come when their leaders would rebel against the host of synthetic monstrosities hurled into their ranks. The day has probably arrived when this weight of untried and questionable medicaments will be unloaded from the profession and from pharmacy.

Already the leaders in the dominant school are questioningly criticising both the materials and the methods by which these materials are forced into conspicuity. Let us, with this thought in mind, reproduce a leading editorial in the current number of the *American Druggist and Pharmaceutical Record*, that indicates how that thoughtful, independent and unconcerned editor reviews the past, the present and the future of the problem that, fortunately for the Eclectic profession, was foreseen in its very beginning, and is not with them a problem.

"Everywhere there are signs of a revolt against the cult of the synthetic. We in America have suffered long in silence from the invasions of the robber barons of modern synthetic chemistry, with their cohorts of new and wonderful organic compounds—the latest sure cures for the various diseases of the human corpus. The neglect of the older remedies has become notorious. It would seem as if the modern physician was ashamed to be found using any of the old-fashioned drugs or combinations of drugs, when a new and more expensive novelty might be employed instead. The note of revolt against the subserviency of medicine to the manufacturers of chemical compounds has been sounded recently by the pharmacists of Germany, the home of the synthetic, who protest with good reason against the increasing expense to which they are put by the multiplication of new remedies and the necessity for burdening their already overloaded shelves with the ounces, quarter-ounces and drachms of substances which may be called for once in quantities of a grain or more, never afterward be ordered, the place of the marvelous compound of to-day being taken by the equally wonderful discovery of to-morrow."

But this is not all the dominant school has to contend with, and here again the Eclectic has wisely refrained from falling into the net of the faddist. The animal extract men have arisen as a swarm to usurp the place of the physician. In the very beginning of this animal extract craze we called attention to the fact that it was much like paralleling the methods of medieval pharmacy in Europe. Turn to the pharmacopeias of the olden time, and see how less scientific, if any, were the repulsive animal substances then administered than are those even now advocated as standing upon the pinnacle of modern therapy in the dominant school.   True, the advocates of these animal remedies of the present day disclaim any connection with the empiricists, as they call them, of two hundred years ago; but the question may be asked, were not the men two hundred years ago as sure that they were scientifically exact as are the men who practice "under authority" to-day?   And is it not self-evident to the man who thinks that long before two hundred years have passed the theories of the animal extract man of to-day will repose beside the empiricism of the animal drug man of two hundred years ago, and be looked upon as twin curiosities in the progress of medicine and pharmacy?

Again we note in the leading editorial of the *American Druggist* a cry of alarm, and it pleases us to note that the awakening seems to be coming sooner than it did in the case of the heart depressants and other untried synthetics.

"As always happens when the pendulum has swung too far in one direction, the return swing is likely to be violent.   One can trace in the increasing attention which is being paid to the treatment of diseases by the administration of the substance of animal organs, a return to the practices of savage tribes and the ignorant Chinese.   Of course, we have refined on these practices, and employ more elegant means of administering the animal extracts, but the principle is there.   In England careful students of medicine are expressing alarm over the present-day neglect of certain of the old and well-tried medicines, and articles are appearing in the medical journals counseling the younger generation of medical practitioners not to neglect the old-fashioned remedies, many of which are intrinsically valuable and worthy of at least the same study which is paid to the products of the chemical factories.   The work of the various local pharmaceutical associations in efforts to familiarize medical men with the preparations of the Pharmacopeia and the National Formulary are bearing fruit in this country, and the propaganda movement, so called, is really a development of the growing feeling against the domination of the manufacturers of synthetics, who are able, apparently, to cast a spell over a large portion of the medical profession, with the mere proclamation that their products are 'definite chemical compounds.'   It is becoming more evident day by day that this claim has been overworked, and that therapeutists are beginning to recognize this fact, and are growing weary of being constantly importuned to try one new compound after another on the say-so of chemists."

LACHESIS.

Herbert T. Webster, M.D., Oakland, Cal.

The following article recently appeared as New York correspondence in the San Francisco *Bulletin:*

"A Brazilian lance-head viper, the deadliest snake known, traversed New York's streets last night, had a ride in a subway train, and was exhibited to a crowd of admiring scientists. It is the first snake of the species the city has ever had the honor to entertain.

"To-morrow at the Bronx Zoo the snake's deadly poison will be extracted from its fangs, for it was for this purpose that the reptile was imported from its native jungle on the upper reaches of the Amazon River.

"The poison of the lance-head is a valuable drug, used in cases of mental disease and insanity. So minute are the particles employed as medicine that no new supply has been received in New York for eighteen years. There is still plenty left in the hands of a prominent chemist in the city, but physicians believe that it has deteriorated and have demanded a new supply.

"The head of the house instructed his agent in Brazil to secure a healthy specimen of the snake. After much trouble, for the natives are much afraid of the lance-head, one was secured and transported to the coast. The new troubles began. The Portuguese sailors on ships sailing north from Brazil ports declined to serve as shipmen with the snake, and while the agent was attempting to secure its transportation, it died.

"Months passed before another could be captured, and again the sailors objected. After trying every ship making the northward run without success, the agent gave up the attempt and had the snake killed.

"But the demand was stronger than ever, and the captain of one of the ships running to New York agreed to bring the snake up in his cabin without letting the sailors know that it was on board. In this manner the snake arrived in New York a few days ago, and after passing the customs authorities was taken to the Bronx Zoo, where it remained until last night, when it was brought downtown by Dr. E. W. Runyon and exhibited at a meeting of the Academy of Pathological Science. Dr. Runyan carried the snake in a glass-sided box under his arm, riding downtown and back to the Zoo in subway trains.

"A number of prominent scientists, including Raymond L. Dittmar, curator of the reptile house at the Zoo, will assist at the operation of removing the poison from the snake. There will be enough secured from the one reptile, Dr. Runyan says, to fill the requirements of the physicians of America for fifty years. The removal of the poison weakens the snake, and it is not believed that it will long survive the operation."

The *lachesis trigonocephalus* belongs to the rattlesnake family, but differs from *crotalus horridus* in having the tail terminating in a spine instead of a rattle, and in having a head covered with scales and not with plates. It is a native of the warm countries of South America, where it is the most dreaded of venomous serpents. It is usually seen coiled up, with keen glaring eyes, watching for prey, on which it darts with the swiftness of an arrow, after which it again coils itself up, to watch and wait quietly until the death struggle of its victim is over. It is so predatory that it will attack man, even when not molested.

The poison of this reptile was introduced to the Homeopathic profession by Constantin Hering, one of the shining lights in the early history of that school. It has its history, and that history is interwoven with the biography of Dr. Hering. Dr. Constantin Hering was educated at Leipsic, under old-school tutelage. He must have been endowed with marked versatility, for he was soon employed to prepare a book confuting Homeopathy. Entering upon the task with enthusiasm, he soon became impressed with some of its truths, and after reading Hahnemann's works he became a convert, sought out the author, and became his personal friend and follower. After serving as instructor in an institution at Dresden for a time, he was appointed by the King of Saxony to go to Dutch Guiana, a country bordering on Brazil, to make botanical and zoölogical collections. At Paramaribo, the capital of that country, he established himself in practice, and there became much interested in an investigation into cures for the bites of venomous serpents and hydrophobia. It is not strange that he should then have begun the study of serpent poisons along Hahnemannian lines.

In 1833 he went to Philadelphia, where he assisted in establishing the first Homeopathic college in the world, and in 1837 he published a work entitled "Effects of Snake Poison." Since then lachesis has been more or less prominent among Homeopathic remedies.

Many claims are made for the therapeutic possibilities of this agent. It resembles echinacea much in some ways, and has been employed by Homeopaths in various conditions of toxemia with excellent success, according to their statements.

Taking the provings of this remedy, as well as its clinical records as a basis, lachesis possesses two distinct characters of action. One of these may be termed hematic or blood properties, and the other neurotic or nerve properties.

The first of these properties allies it very closely with baptisia and echinacea, and it has been accredited with the cure of many cases of desperate character, such as traumatic gangrene, malignant erysipelas, malignant diphtheria and scarlatina, yellow fever, malignant pustule, etc. From my personal experience I am inclined to believe that it has been overestimated in this direction, though I admit that I have given it but limited trial, since echinacea came in soon after my first acquaintance with it, and I have given that remedy preference over all others in such conditions.

In the year 1881 or 1882 an endemic of diphtheria attacked several families in the northern part of Atwater Township, Ohio, and proved rapidly fatal to both children and adults. Whole families were swept away, numerous physicians in the vicinity failing to arrest its course in the least. The only family in the neighborhood that escaped unscathed was one which was attended by a young Homeopathic physician located near. If I remember correctly, the family consisted of several persons, and no fatality occurred, though all were attacked before the infection ceased its influence. The physician informed me not long afterward, in referring to the cases, that lachesis was his main reliance in treating them. I had no reason to doubt his word, as the information was voluntary, and as I was in no sense a professional rival.

Dr. Carroll Dunham, in his work on materia medica, describes the effects of this remedy in his own case, which was a remarkable one. While assisting in an autopsy where a woman had died of puerperal peritonitis, he received a dissecting wound on the index finger of the left hand. Within a week very serious symptoms had developed. The finger, hand and arm had become enormously swollen, a hard red line extended from the wrist to the axilla, the axillary glands were enlarged, and the entire left side was partially paralyzed. Constitutional symptoms were extreme prostration, low muttering delirium at night, and other typhoid manifestations. The pain was intense, and deep abscesses were forming under the tissues of the finger and hand. The neighborhood afforded no Homeopathic physician, and Allopathic surgeons advised opium and calomel [year 1850], but rendered a very discouraging prognosis. The patient finally determined to trust the issue to lachesis, and refused all other drugs. Five days of lachesis, first dose on the third day of illness, banished all constitutional symptoms, though recovery of the finger was delayed some time longer.

The same writer describes another case still more striking. A little girl of nine years, who the year before had suffered a severe attack of scarlet fever and been left delicate and deaf, came down with measles. The rash appeared on the 6th inst., and on the 8th a discharge from the ears, which had begun with the appearance of the rash, ceased, and the rash disappeared. She immediately became prostrated, was seized with wild delirium, high fever, great thirst, and pungent heat of skin. The doctor saw her twenty-four hours later, during which time she had lain in alternate stupor and delirium, completely irrational. The pulse was soft and wavy, hardly to be counted; respiration moaning, rapid and whistling; pupils widely dilated; urine scanty; breath putrescent, and countenance cadaverous. A dose of lachesis, 30th, was ordered every two hours, also strong beef-tea. The first dose was given about eleven in the morning, and when the medical attendant called at six in the evening he found the patient sitting supported in an arm chair, playing with some toys, rational, temperature normal, skin moist and natural, eyes normal, and convalescence apparently established. The child recovered without more medicine. The writer remarks: "This change from apparent impending death to established convalescence within the space of seven hours was very impressive and even startling."

The same author states that in 1853 an epidemic of what was called "malignant pustule" occurred in Brooklyn. It was characterized by a furuncular formation which appeared generally upon the lower lip, with severe pain. An erysipelatous areola usually surrounded the pustule. Extreme prostration speedily followed the appearance of the eruption, vigorous persons being reduced to complete prostration within from twenty-four to thirty-six hours. Allopathic physicians treated these cases with nitrate of silver cauterization and usual constitutional treatment, probably calomel and opium. Every case coming under Dr. Dunham's observation so treated died within twenty-four hours after cauterization. Eight cases treated by himself with lachesis, and this was the only remedy he employed, recovered speedily.

Hughes suggests this remedy in malignant erysipelas, but I have recently had an experience with it in this line which was not very satisfactory. About the middle of February of the present year I was called at three o'clock one morning to visit an old patron, a maiden lady of about forty-three years, who had been suffering excruciating pain in her thumb all night. The afternoon before she had noticed pain in the part and found a small pimple at the radial side of the thumb of the right hand, which showed a purulent apex. She pricked this with a clean needle and squeezed the pimple, but failed to express any pus, or relieve the pain. Her suffering increased from then on, and she finally decided that she could not wait until morning before calling for medical aid. There was little or no swelling in the thumb, and my first impression was that it was a case of periostitis with pus formation on the bone. I therefore administered chloroform and pushed a sterilized sharp-pointed bistoury down to the bone, hoping thus to relieve tension and abate the pain. The little opening was padded with absorbent cotton saturated with specific echinacea, and echinacea was administered internally.

Within four hours I was called again, with the information that the patient was worse than ever. I now administered a fourth-grain of morphine, to be repeated every four hours, and continued former treatment. The next day I found the entire hand much swollen, all the deep tissues being apparently involved, as the swollen part was very firm and unyielding upon pressure. The point of opening was reddened and angry, and a watery fluid was discharging. The pain was increasing. On the second day a reddened streak of lymphatics could readily be traced from the wrist along the inner side of the arm nearly to the axilla. The swelling also was involving the entire arm, and the pain was almost unbearable. The opening on the thumb was becoming gaping, dark and sloughy. Temperature about 102° F. I now pronounced the case erysipelas, for the time had come when a diagnosis was necessary in order to satisfy friends. Lachesis was added to the list of remedies, as echinacea had not thus far seemed of much use. The local application had been bandages wrung out of tepid water, but ichthyol in olive oil was substituted at the suggestion of a trained nurse now in attendance, with the hope that it might assist in relieving the pain, which was increasing hourly. On the third day all symptoms were aggravated. The arm was swollen to the axilla, full, hard and tense, the patient was very much exhausted from loss of rest, the pain was increasing and the initial point of attack was black and sloughy. In the afternoon I received a summons to make a second visit, and found that a sister desired the presence of an "eminent consultant" from San Francisco, in order to determine whether everything possible was being done. The consultant was called, met and interviewed. He was divided in opinion as to whether it was a case of erysipelas or malignant edema, but was fixed in opinion as to the proper treatment—ten grains of quinine every four hours, and twenty drops of tincture of muriate of iron every two hours with hypodermics of morphine. The treatment was accordingly changed, but within a few hours vomiting of everything taken began. The patient could not retain as much as a teaspoonful of water. The friends and family now decided that it would be best for me to return to my own method of medication, and I administered minute doses of aconite and rhus to relieve the gastric irritability for a few hours, and returned to echinacea and lachesis, in alternation. A strange feature of the case was that the tongue manifested little abnormal appearance throughout.

By the sixth day the arm was enormously swollen, livid, covered with watery blebs and gangrenous patches, and almost insensible to touch, but extremely painful. The only relief from pain was that afforded by large and frequent hypodermic injections of morphine.

The treatment, for want of a better one, was continued, but septicemia set in on the afternoon of the sixth day, the patient became wildly delirious, though rational up to that time, and died on the morning of the seventh day. Temperature, at its highest, reached 103° F.

I have just signed the death certificate of a youth of sixteen who died from cerebro-spinal meningitis. The case came into my hands one week after he had been given up by two of the leading physicians of this city. He was in a comatose condition when I found him, and apparently paralyzed in all the extremities. He could breathe regularly and swallow with difficulty, and moan at times, but did not speak, and seemed entirely oblivious to all surroundings. On echinacea he improved until he could speak, swallow well, and move his extremities, but when strength began to return clonic convulsions of all the muscles set in, alternated with tonic spasms of the back, with opisthotonos. Three relapses occurred during a period of a little more than four weeks, the last one carrying him off. Purple spots, ecchymoses, appeared along the spine and upon different portions of the body during my experience with the case, and as that is a prominent indication for lachesis, that remedy was alternated with echinacea during the last fortnight of treatment.

And now I will relate some of my successes with the remedy. My first experience with it was during the winter of 1880-81. I was treating a case of pneumonia in an elderly lady—past seventy—of delicate constitution. Her children did not expect her to survive the attack, but the case progressed favorably for several days, until it seemed as though the acme had been passed and that convalescence would soon follow. One evening, however, I found her much prostrated, breathing faintly, with the pulse almost entirely gone. What could be found was feeble and tremulous, so rapid and indistinct as to prevent counting, though it seemed to be about 160 per minute. I concluded that the end had come, but decided, remembering what Hughes says of lachesis and tremulous action of the heart, to give it a trial. I left some powders of the drug without any hope of success, and returned the following day expecting to find crape on the door. To my surprise, I found her convalescing, with a regular pulse, less than 100, and all other symptoms improved. She was well a few days afterward, and remained well for several years.

The same winter I encountered a case of stubborn and racking cough in a man about middle age. He was a robust farmer, and did not seem very sick, but the cough would not "down." I treated the case for a fortnight without impressing it in the least, and became discouraged. Little signs of local irritation could be found in the bronchial tubes or pulmonary alveoli, but the cough was explosive and rasping, aggravated at night from the cold air, and very much provoked by dust when the wife did any sweeping. It was evidently a case of irritability of the pneumogastric branches, and I finally "tumbled" to lachesis. I had a very small quantity of the remedy on hand, about nine small powders, if I remember correctly, but these cured the cough, and it did not return.

About five years ago a boy of five years was brought to me in a go-cart from San Francisco who was a cripple from post-diphtheritic paralysis. A younger child, a little girl, had succumbed to diphtheria, and the boy had nearly died with it, but finally survived, in this condition. They had been treated with antitoxin and allopathic remedies, *secundum artem*. The paralysis had continued for about five months, in spite of electricity and strychnia. There was complete paralysis of the lower extremities, and deglutition and phonation were much impaired. The child was peevish and babyish, though the parents informed me that before his illness he was a self-assertive and cheerful boy. Enough lachesis to last a fortnight was furnished him, with instruction to return when it was gone. When brought back great improvement was reported. The boy could swallow well and speech was nearly normal. Also, the boy could stand on his feet without help for a short time, and made frequent efforts to do so without prompting. In another fortnight he had entirely recovered, and afterward remained well. The parents became patients of mine, so I see him occasionally. He is a strong, healthy child, full of romp and mischief.

Lachesis specifically influences the pneumogastric nerve, and is applicable to any case where any of its branches require normal functionating power. Irritable and paralytic states both respond favorably to its action. Diphtheria, in which death is liable to occur from cardiac paralysis, demands it. Aphonia and irritative laryngeal cough responds to it when due to disturbance of the par vagum. Paralysis of the laryngeal and pharyngeal muscles find in it the best remedy. Cardiac insufficiency, due to impaired nervous stimulus, calls for lachesis. It also acts on the peripheral extremities of the motor nerves, and it is thus applicable to paralysis from peripheral neuritis after inflammatory action has subsided.

It is doubtful that it excels, if it is capable of equaling, the influence of echinacea in putrefactive conditions. However, it is not likely that we have been able to obtain the best quality of the remedy in past years, as a new supply is to be had only at long intervals, on account of difficulty in obtaining it. It is worthy of investigation.

The lowest attenuation obtainable at pharmacists is the 6x. I usually carry this to the 7th by trituration. Homeopaths often use it in much higher attenuations. Dunham employed the 30th and 200th. It is probable that in his time (the 1850's and 1860's) the remedy was more potent than now, on account of being more recent. It may prove potent in toxemia, when the recent drug is employed.

EFFECT OF ASHEVILLE CLIMATE UPON TUBERCULOSIS.

M. H. HENNEL, M.D., ASHEVILLE, N. C.

To the late Dr. Alfred L. Loomis belongs the credit of first pointing out to the medical world the effects of climatology upon pulmonary tuberculosis and the benefits to be derived from high, dry altitudes in these cases. Experience has taught us that the results are not so much due to the altitude but to climate, as the percentage of cures obtained at medium elevations where the climatological conditions are favorable are greater than those obtained in higher and in lower altitudes. True, many cases derive benefit at some of our sea-coast resorts, while others have the disease arrested in our high altitudes, six or eight thousand feet, but statistics go to prove that a greater per cent. of cases have the disease arrested and remain cured at altitudes of medium elevation.

The physician, in selecting a location and climate for his tuberculous patients, should take into consideration not only the climate but the location, scenery, social surroundings, cost of living, railroad accommodations, distance from home, etc., as it is too frequently the case that climatic advantages are neutralized by homesickness, poor food, poor water, social incompatibility and monotonous surroundings. The principal climatological conditions to be thought of in these cases are pure, dry air with just sufficient rainfall to lay the dust, with not too great extremes between sunlight and shade, daylight and dark and summer and winter. This insures the greatest number of days of sunlight in which the patient may live out of doors in the open air.

Asheville comes as near filling all these requirements as any other health resort in America. The thousands of people that have come here and regained their health verify this statement. It is a city of about twenty thousand inhabitants situated upon an elevated plateau between the Blue Ridge and Smoky Mountains in western North Carolina. It has an altitude of about twenty-two hundred and fifty feet. It is surrounded on all sides by numerous peaks many of which have a height of from four to six thousand feet. The currents of air are thus robbed of a great deal of their moisture in passing over these mountain ranges and are impregnated with the purifying fragrance of the pine and balsam which cover many of the mountains from base to summit. Geographically its latitude is too far south for a prolonged low drop of mercury during the winter and its altitude prevents the hot depressing effects of the solar rays during the summer. Thus, it can be seen that we have a fairly even temperature throughout the year. Malaria is a thing unheard of here except among those who have it when they come, and then it is not long until it is eradicated from the system.

Asheville is a modern, up-to-date city. It enjoys nearly all the privileges of the larger cities and many others which they do not enjoy. It can truly be called "The Land of the Sky." Its many miles of paved streets, its excellent street car system, its public buildings, its large up-to-date stores, its many beautiful residences and palatial homes in connection with its beautiful scenery, invigorating air and equitable climate bespeak its many advantages. It can thus be seen that the monotony found in so many health resorts does not enter as a factor here.

The water supply is one of the best in America. The city purchased ten thousand acres on the south side of Mt. Mitchell, the highest mountain of the entire Appalachian system. This forest has never been despoiled by the woodman's axe and is carefully guarded. No trespassing, in fact, nothing is allowed upon it that would contaminate its mountain streams which are fed by hundreds of springs with the best water that Mother Nature can afford. This water is conveyed to Asheville, a distance of seventeen miles, through two large pipes to reservoirs, from whence the city receives its supply. The casual observer is impressed with its clear sparkling appearance, its purity and its cool refreshing taste.

Good board and room can be had at from six to fifteen dollars per week. Cheaper board can be obtained, but it is not adapted for the sick as they need special foods and attention.

Asheville, being centrally located, upon the main branch of the Southern Railroad, can be easily reached from all parts of the United States. Patients coming here from the Eastern, Central, and Southern States are not far from home; hence, should they become seriously ill and their friends wish to visit them or should they become homesick they can make a short visit home and not be tired out and exhausted and not be at the expense of travel that a single trip to one of the more distant resorts would cost.

It can be seen from what has already been said that this is an ideal climate for the treatment of pulmonary tuberculosis. If all cases of pulmonary tuberculosis could be sent here during their earliest recognizable incipiency, with the climatic conditions that exist and with proper hygienic, dietetic and specific treatment, in a very large per cent. of cases the disease could be arrested and cured. The great drawback in too many cases is that they are kept at home and treated until the disease is far advanced or until there is no hope of recovery and then are sent—somewhere to die. *Don't do it!*

THE TRUE ACTION OF CAULOPHYLLUM (BLUE COHOSH).

ELI G. JONES, M.D., BURLINGTON, N. J.

Ten drops of the tincture caulophyllum once an hour in a little water is one of our best remedies for hiccough. In chorea of young girls from *irregular* periods it is the remedy, and it should be given in the third decimal trituration—two grains once in three hours. In young girls, when the menses do not appear and they are restless, have headache, cold hands and feet, and are cross and irritable, the blue cohosh is the remedy in the form of leontin (Lloyd), fifteen drops in a little water once in three hours. It has never failed me in such cases.

For the prevention of premature labor there is no remedy that can compare with caulophyllum. In such cases it is best to use the first decimal dilution of the tincture as it is more agreeable to the patient— five drops once in two hours.

In delayed labor with rigid os and spasmodic pains, the patient worn out with fatigue, give ten drops of the tincture caulophyllum once in a half hour.

It is better adapted to chronic rheumatism than cimicifuga, the latter being better for the acute form. In dysmenorrhea (rheumatic), or when the pains are irregular and spasmodic like labor pains, and the sufferer screams aloud with the severe pain, and in hemorrhage after confinement with pain from back to pubes, caulophyllum is indicated. In such cases ten drops of the tincture caulophyllum should be given every half hour. It will "cause firm contractions and arrest the flooding."

In after pains it is a reliable remedy and should be given the first decimal dilution, a teaspoonful in a cup of water, teaspoonful given every half hour.

In rheumatism of the wrist and fingers it is the best remedy that we have, especially where the pains are worse at night.

It is a remedy that should be studied carefully, and if given when indicated is a remedy to be depended upon.

LEPTOMENINGITIS.*

GEO. T. FULLER, MAYFIELD, KY.

It is not the purpose of this paper to discuss meningitis in all its forms, but to limit the discussion principally to leptomeningitis (inflammation of the pia and arachnoid membranes of the brain). This condition, so far as my observation goes, is never idiopathic or spontaneous, but when present is always the result of some previous malady. I am firm in the conviction that this malady is in all cases secondary—aside from trauma, always metastatic and always of septic origin, whether from bacteria or their ferments I will neither affirm or deny, although individually I am inclined to accept this theory of its origin.

The primary lesion, or the malady upon which the disease under discussion depends, is not always clear and pronounced; it is often obscure or masked, but a searching investigation will almost always result in the discovery of the antecedent trouble. Affections of the ear are, probably, one of the most fruitful sources of leptomeningitis; chronic suppurative inflammation of the tympanic cavity, or suppurative otitis media, more frequently lead to meningeal inflammation than any other aural trouble. Under the conditions named there is likely to be caries of the roof of the vault, where the bone is exceedingly thin, and in some cases congenitally wanting, leaving the meninges exposed, an easy prey to the septic material generated in that locality, or the avenue of infection may be along the sheaths of the auditory or facial nerves or through the mastoid cells. The infectious and exanthematous diseases are, also, a fruitful source of the trouble, such as pneumonia, pyemia, septicemia, empyema, acute articular rheumatism, endocarditis, typhoid fever, entero-colitis, smallpox, measles, and especially scarlet fever (aside from ear disease). Trauma is also one of the causes, but will not be considered in this paper, as are also syphilis and tuberculosis. When a meningitis results from either of the last mentioned diseases it is usually easily traced and is almost invariably fatal under any kind of treatment, while that resulting from the other causes mentioned is always serious, yet not necessarily fatal, if the proper therapeutic measures are vigorously and properly applied. We see the trouble in children oftener than in adults, and it develops in the course of some of the troubles mentioned above. For convenience I have divided this disease into four stages, viz., initial, inflammatory, congestive (or stage of pressure) and paralytic. The first, or initial stage, is short, and may pass unnoticed into the second,

* Read before the Kentucky Eclectic Medical Association, 1905.

or inflammatory stage; the initial symptom is nausea, or vomiting; sometimes the vomiting is violent and may continue up to the third stage, but is usually less marked after the initial stage and often changes to a kind of regurgitation of a greenish yellow material from the duodenum; following this nausea, or vomiting, in a few hours there is a slight chill, or cold stage, followed by febrile reaction—the beginning of the second, or inflammatory stage. A peculiarity of this fever is its temperature curve, sometimes remitting as many as four times in twenty-four hours. The chief symptom of the second stage is developed almost simultaneously with the febrile reaction from the cold stage, viz., extreme pain in the head with its accompanying phenomena, rolling the head from side to side, restlessness, pulling the hair, squinting the eyes, contracting the corrugator muscles, face flushed, pupils contracted, sometimes hyperesthesia to the extent that they shrink from being touched or handled by the nurse or attendants; irritated by noise to the extent that it often causes spasms. The bowels during this stage are almost invariably constipated, and the secretion from the skin and kidneys scant; in the latter part of this stage the muscles of the neck, on one or both sides, become stiff, or may be contracted and rigid, drawing the head either to one side or slightly backward, in which position it remains fixed. The pulse in this stage is not so frequent as the temperature (which often reaches 105° F. or more) and other conditions would indicate.

If not relieved during the first or second stages the patient passes into the third stage, or stage of pressure; the transition from the second to the third stage takes place gradually; in fact, there is a period of uncertain duration, which might not inaptly be called the mixed stage, in which the symptoms of irritation still linger and the symptoms of pressure manifest themselves; paroxysms of pain, extreme restlessness, irritability and delirium are succeeded by a period of drowsiness, or stupor, from which they arouse to another paroxysm of pain, restlessness, etc. These phenomena may alternate a few times, the paroxysms of pain and restlessness are less marked each time, while those of pressure become more pronounced until the patient sinks into a profound stupor, from which it is difficult to arouse him; if you succeed in arousing him it will be to stare at you vacantly, through half open lids, to again lapse into his former condition. The most characteristic symptom of this, the third stage, when fully developed, is a complete loss of consciousness; in this stage of complete insensibility he occasionally moves and shrieks out wildly; the pupils are now dilated, the muscles of the neck rigid, the respiration slow, bowels constipated, secretions from kidneys and skin still scant, temperature falls sometimes below normal. This third stage is the antipode of the second, or preceding stage, and is the result of that inflammation, which causes exudates—both plastic and serous—on the pia and into the ventricles of the brain, this exudate being the cause, in a mechanical way, of the change of symptoms noticed In the third stage —a semi-paralytic condition of the nerve centers from mechanical pressure.

If still not controlled the fourth stage, or stage of paralysis, supervenes. From twelve to thirty-six hours before death some of the characteristic symptoms of the third stage undergo a marked change; there is now a complete comatose condition, and the patient is utterly irresponsive to external irritations; there are no movements, the muscles of the neck relax, involuntary discharge from the bowels and kidneys, accelerated pulse-rate, elevated temperature—sometimes 108° F.—profuse sweating, then complete paralysis and death ends the scene.

I have described the different stages of this trouble somewhat at length that we might get a clearer idea of the conditions present in each stage, so that we may be able to more intelligently apply our therapeutic measures and change them as the conditions change to accurately fit the case.

It is hardly necessary to outline a treatment for the first, or initial stage, as you are rarely ever positively certain of the condition until the development of symptoms announcing what I have denominated the second stage. What are the actual conditions now? Irritation, hyperemia, if not actual inflammation of the meninges under consideration and in the region named, with a septic condition of the blood added, a blood poisoning, if you please. What is the object of our treatment in this stage? To promptly arrest or at least reduce the irritation or inflammation, and neutralize as quickly and as far as possible the septic condition of the blood. As the actual pathological conditions are always the same and differ only in degree practically the same treatment is suited to all cases in the inflammatory stage. I put them on the following combination: Specific gelsemium, drachms from one to three; specific lupulin, drachms from two to six; bromide of sodium, drachms from two to four; water, a sufficient quantity to make four ounces and direct a teaspoonful every two hours. I have tried these remedies singly and in combination, and I find they act better in the combination named above. I push this unless the symptoms yield to the mild physiological effect of the gelsemium—slight ptosis. With this you not only limit the blood supply to the already overcharged membranes, but you soothe the nervous system as well. For the depraved or septic condition of the blood I prescribe echafolta, in from five to thirty-drop doses every three or four hours in water; it not only neutralizes the poison *per se,* but arouses the entire glandular system, especially the skin, kidneys, liver and bowels, and gives you all the elimination necessary, if given in sufficient doses.

This line of treatment, if vigorously applied, will, in most instances, arrest the trouble and you will have no third stage, or, if it does not entirely abort it, it will so modify the inflammation that there will be but slight exudation and consequently a mild third stage. If, from any reason, your case should develop the third stage, or you be called to a patient in that stage, give them specific belladonna, from four to eight drops; iodide of potash, from two to four drachms; water sufficient for four ounces, and direct a teaspoonful every two hours. The belladonna stimulates the capillaries, in which the blood is almost at a standstill, to more active work, giving a better circulation, and facilitates the removal of plastic exudate that is being dissolved by the iodide of potash. Keep up the echafolta, adding to it an equal amount of distilled apocynum, which promptly eliminates the serous exudate, the combined treatment removing both the serous and plastic exudate, thereby relieving the pressure and restoring your patient.

BENJAMIN FRANKLIN JOHNSON, M.D.

HARVEY WICKES FELTER, M.D., CINCINNATI.

Benjamin Franklin Johnson, M.D., son of Governor Joseph Johnson, of Bridgeport, W. Va., twice governor of Virginia, and the only

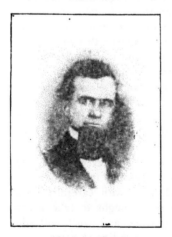

BENJAMIN FRANKLIN JOHNSON, M.D.

governor of that State chosen "from a county west of the Alleghenies," was born at Bridgeport, W. Va., June 8, 1816, and died at Columbus, O., August 19, 1855. He graduated from the Worthington Medical School in 1837, his diploma bearing the names of Kilbourne, Morrow, Paddock, Mason, and I. G. Jones. He subsequently became a professor in his alma mater, and remained with the college throughout its days of adversity. He practiced at Worthington and Columbus, and in 1840 was married to Miss Emily Griswold, of the former place. During 1853-4 he was physician to the Ohio State Penitentiary. His grandson, Hon.

Newton L. Gilbert, is now lieutenant-governor of Indiana. Dr. Johnson is buried in old St. John's Churchyard at Worthington.

Ohio State Eclectic Medical Association.

Proceedings of the Forty-fourth Annual Session.

W. N. MUNDY, M.D., EDITOR.

PRESIDENT'S ADDRESS.

A. S. McKITRICK, M.D., KENTON, O.

Ladies and Gentlemen of the Ohio State Eclectic Medical Society:

I take this opportunity to express thanks for the honor you have conferred on me in electing me President of this Association. I also want to thank you for your loyal support and help in preparing the program which will be presented. I also take this opportunity to thank the other officers anl local committee whose faithful and painstaking efforts have made this meeting possible. No set of men could have been more faithful, capable and willing than they have been.

For the second time in our history we meet in the beautiful city of Dayton. When we met here in 1875 we were in knickerbockers, just ten years old, but with the hope and animation of youth. At that meeting were such men as Scudder, King, Howe and Freeman—men with keen intellects and courage to be in the despised minority in order to develop a better system of medicine than was known at that time. They were like emigrants who, with teams and wagons and families, turned their backs on the comforts and quietness of their homes and went out on the boundless prairies and across the sandy deserts, underwent privation and hardships and encountered dangers, that they might make new and better homes for their children and lay the foundation for the more splendid civilization, with the rich and fertile farms and beautiful homes of to-day, connected by telephone, telegraph, trolley and train. Those same children accept the luxuries and advantages of this wonderful civilization with scarcely a thought of the toil and hardship and even bloodshed that had made the transformation possible. So we accept the modern methods and improvements and marvelous accomplishments of modern medicine and surgery with scarcely a thought of the difficulties with which these men had to contend.

With this large attendance assembled here, with carefully prepared papers and discussions, every one of us ought to take away something valuable that he will use in his practice, and which will add to his usefulness as well as to his standing and prestige at home.

The time has come when our patrons demand that we attend medical conventions and take post-graduate courses and keep abreast of the times. The doctor who cannot afford to attend the Association this year can less afford it next year, because his competitor, who attended this year, will, on account of his increased knowledge and superior skill, have acquired some of his patrons. You are selling brains, and the better quality you offer the more you will receive.

The Eclectic school glories in its past success and growth, but we must not forget that our good brethren, the Regulars and Homeopaths, have not stood still, but have also made marvelous growth.

While we have been carefully watching the action of drugs and studying their specific effect, our brethren have been investigating in the laboratory and elsewhere and have succeeded in discovering the cause of and the way to prevent yellow fever, malaria, typhus fever, to decrease tuberculosis and to rob diphtheria of its terrors. All these are given us freely; in fact, we are agreed upon everything except the important thing of administration of drugs. In that we have blazed the way, and many of our regular brethren are taking advantage of our pure drugs and specific or definite way of using them; we bid them godspeed.

We need have no fear of assimilation or of being the lamb in the lion's stomach. Until we use all the good things the old school have discovered for us, and until they use our specific medication and all the rest of the good things that we have discovered for them, when that time comes, we will be like two mighty rivers, which unite and mingle their waters and flow on as one stream out into the mighty ocean of truth. In the meantime, let us go on perfecting our system and improving it, not imagining that it all has been finished for us. Every Eclectic physician should, by hard work and application, become one of the leaders in his profession in the community in which he practices, but in order to do this he must work, work, work.

The time has come when an educated and discriminating public demands much of its physician, and insists that he deal honestly with his patrons and tells them the truth. If they have tuberculosis they want to know it, and you should tell them so. If you do not know what the matter is, they have a right to know it and you should tell them that you do not. They will not be satisfied with your telling them, instead, how much sleep you have lost, nor how many patients you have turned away for lack of time, nor how many thousand operations you have performed without a death, nor how many failures your competitors have made, but they will demand that you continue to be a student and keep in intelligent touch with the progress of the times, and that with sincere frankness you give them a "square deal."

If we are to continue our existence as a separate school of medicine, we have not only to digest and assimilate the best things from all sources, for which we should cheerfully give credit, but we must go on and investigate new drugs, add to our knowledge of old ones, and be really specialists in therapeutics.

Among our needs is that of more complete organization. We have about eight hundred Eclectics in this State. We ought to have several more societies, and a much larger membership in the State society. Is it not possible, by our next meeting, to have five hundred members?

We are glad to note the improvement in our colleges throughout the land, and especially the great improvements at the E. M. I. in Cincinnati. They have under their control one of the best equipped hospitals in the Middle West, a corps of specialists in the various departments equal to the best in the country, and the promise of a magnificent building in the near future.

We also have men in various parts of the State who are connected with first-class hospitals, and doing credit to themselves and to the cause.

We have met the highest standard of education that has been adopted, but we must guard well our interest, and see that we have a fair deal in educational and legislative matters. Some who have asked for a high standard have tried to evade the issue to their own advantage by having their literary and medical courses overlap and thereby gain a year.

We should insist on reciprocity, so that any qualified M.D. can change his location to any place under the flag that he may choose.

We, as a school, should be leaders in sanitation; should support the efforts being made to furnish the people with pure food and milk; should insist that our public schools be made safe from fire and provided with sufficient light and adequate ventilation. We should lend our support to laws preventing injurious child labor. We should stamp the Rose Local Option Bill with the seal of our approval, lend our votes and influence to abolishing the saloon from our several communities, and insist upon the after-enforcement of the law. We should be in the front rank in preventive medicine. Jenner paved the way in 1798; by thorough vaccination, the greatest scourge of mankind, if not banished, has been chained, and thousands of lives saved. The Pasteur treatment for rabies, antitoxin in diphtheria, the discovery that yellow fever and malaria were caused by certain species of mosquitoes, have led to the lessening of these diseases and the saving of many lives, as illustrated in the two last mentioned diseases in Havana and the Canal Zone.

There is ample room for further discoveries and improvement as long as the list of incurable diseases remains as large as it is. We will be the first to sing the praises of him who will prevent cancer, and we hope to see the day when scarlet fever and measles will be as much of a reproach to the victim as itch or the parasite that, seen on a lady's bonnet, called forth the immortal verse of Burns. And we will hail the day when the surgeon's scalpel will have been largely displaced by yet undiscovered remedies and electrical currents more potent than the X-ray.

Eclectics should all be optimists when they think upon the changes that have been brought about in the three-quarters of a century of our existence, and realize that the changes that have been wrought are as nothing in importance to those that are to come.

The medical profession has progressed as all other departments of human knowledge have done. Science has delved in the earth and brought forth her hidden wealth of treasure, has tunnelled mountains and bridged streams to give rapid modes of travel and transportation, and has harnessed the invisible ether to secure instant communication of thought. Nations have changed from the rule of tyrants to self-government. Even religion and theories of religion have changed. If the clergy have not entirely extinguished the fires of the underworld, they have modified the climate to about that of the average summer resort. And in no point of human activity has a point been reached where there will not continue to be improvement.

Let every Eclectic do the best that is in him, and try to find ways and means to cure, or, better still, prevent infectious diseases, and blindness, and to decrease the number of helpless cripples, and to lessen the death-rate of childhood, and transmission from parent to child of diseases that are no less than crimes.

These and much more await our doing. Let us go forward with love and enthusiasm for our work and profession, and with hope for the future.

SECTION I.

OPHTHALMOLOGY, OTOLOGY AND LARYNGOLOGY.

J. J. Sutter, M.D., *Chairman*...........................Bluffton.
U. O. Jones, M.D., *Vice-Chairman*................West Jefferson.
Ralph B. Taylor, M.D., *Secretary*....................Columbus.

SPECIFIC INDICATIONS IN EYE DISEASES.

Kent O. Foltz, M.D., Cincinnati.

I had intended to write a short article on "Specific Indications in Eye Diseases," but have been prevented.

I will speak now of a few of the indications, also of the use of drugs that may be of benefit. I am not going to take up the more serious lesions of the eye.

There is a very frequent condition of conjunctivitis, especially in the spring and fall, in which there is an excessive watery secretion, tears running over the cheeks. They do not even redden the skin, but are extremely annoying, because the eyes are simply swimming in tears all the time. In this condition distillate of hamamelis, both locally and internally, is good. Locally I generally use about twenty to thirty drops, or half a drachm to about four drachms, and in making the four-drachm mixture boracic acid solution is used. This is dropped into the eye every one or two hours. Internally we use from one to two drachms of distilled hamamelis to four ounces of water, and that is given every one or two hours. Usually within twelve hours, and frequently in less time than that, the excessive secretion is very much diminished and the patient is fairly comfortable.

That is the specific indication for hamamelis.

As a local application, to protect the skin, especially where it is very much excoriated, I found in the majority of instances that the ointment of eucalyptus, about five to ten drops to half a drachm of white vaseline, gives better results than either the plain vaseline or any other preparation I have tried.

In a conjunctivitis in which there is muco-purulent discharge (and that we find quite frequently where there is some infection), I use a combination of hydrastis (Lloyd's) and calenduline.

The calendula, I will speak of that next. Unless it is properly prepared it is going to do mischief. It should be the non-alcoholic preparation. If you mix that and allow it to stand any length of time, it throws of a heavy precipitate of peculiar appearance, and it has to be filtered. It also is liable to undergo some changes that I have not been able to determine, and it is better to have it stand for some little time before using, and filtering occasionally, especially in warm weather.

Now there is one purulent type that we have. I had two cases in the clinics recently. One ophthalmia neonatorum, the other gonorrheal ophthalmia. When I saw the case later the cornea had entirely sloughed off. In the case of ophthalmia neonatorum the left eye was pretty near gone, and the right eye looked as though it was going to go. That I only treated once. Dr. Wottring took care of it the balance of the time. He was at the clinics every day and I was not. He used a solution of ten grains nitrate of silver in the eye, after thoroughly cleansing it. The baby was pretty young, and he did not bother with internal medication.

In ulceration of the cornea, in suppurative conditions, if the ulceration is near the periphery of the cornea, nearly always you will have hyaloid or sclerotic complications. You may have both, and in order to draw the iris away from the periphery you will have to use eserine, and in order to keep down the iritic complications you will have to use atropine; use it once or twice a day, perhaps two or three times a day.

Then there's iritis. Whenever you have a contracted pupil, a zone of redness around the cornea, complete or nearly complete, intense pain, burns at night or in damp weather, you have got most unfavorable iritis. And there's only one specific for that, and that is the mydriatics, and my preference is the old-fashioned atropine sulphate; that I use entirely. I tried others and I never had a case where there were idiosyncrasies that I couldn't use it. That's the specific indication.

Now if adhesions have formed before you see the case, you sometimes can break them down by the alternate use of atropine and eserine internally. In those cases the specific indication, to me, where there are any adhesions, is jaborandi and bryonia, usually in combination. I get better results from the two combined than I do from either one singly. I have occasion to use them very frequently.

Acute dacryocystitis comes very frequently in general practice. The patient complains of tears running over the cheeks, swelling in the corner of the inner canthus, and the pain is excruciating, almost always in an acute case. If you will examine the nose you will find that the inferior turbinate is very large, and by using a tampon of cotton saturated with glycerine, a large tampon, that is to be introduced in the nasal cavity, you will deplete that condition and in a majority of cases may be the sac, and the patient will get relief in a very short time. Sometimes it may be necessary to repeat the tampon, but frequently one application will give relief inside of half an hour. If it does not, I would repeat it.

Now there's another specific indication in eye diseases that I have found of value. In the different diseases where there is considerable pain, a neuralgic pain, pain of iritis, either post-operative or simple iritis, where the pain is excruciating, and that is salts. Move the bowels thoroughly, and you will get quicker results from a good big dose of saline cathartic than from a hypodermic of morphine.

DISCUSSION.

DR. W. T. GEMMILL: Just a few words in regard to iritis. As to the two particular symptoms that should lead the physician to be able to make a diagnosis of inflammation of the eye, one is the intense pain —Dr. Foltz says the neuralgic pain in the supra-orbital region. The other is the rosy zone that makes its appearance around the margin of the cornea. With that rosy zone, and with that intense pain, you ought to be able to make a diagnosis of iritis. Of course, the earlier the treatment is applied, the less trouble you are going to have later on, but keeping the pupil fully dilated will avoid things that make no end of trouble later on, and oftentimes impair the vision for life. In those cases I generally use atropine, and use it sufficiently to keep up extensive dilatation, and keep the iris away from the margin of the lens, if possible.

EYE-STRAIN AND OTHER FACTORS THAT PRODUCE HEADACHE.

C. A. Moore, M.D., Youngstown, O.

Specialists are thought to be narrow in their views; that they only see things through the eyes of their specialty, which is often true. I would say, however, that this applies only to those who have never practiced general medicine.

It is well known that a very large number of headaches are caused by anomalies of refraction, and that the proper adjustment of lenses will cure them. If, however, we meet with patients in whom we find hypermetropia, myopia, astigmatism, simple or compound, regular or irregular, or mixed, we examine the conditions of the eye muscles, we prescribe the proper lens, but we only partially relieve them. Why? Because there are other factors in the production of the case which cannot be corrected by the use of glasses or any treatment directed to the eyes.

Oculists look with disgust at the advertisements which we see in the daily papers. In them so-called opticians, who sign themselves Dr. So-and-so, optometrists, neurologists, etc., claim to cure nearly every ailment in the decalogue by the use of glasses alone. Among their ailments are: Staring, jerking, blinking, catarrh, failing memory, epilepsy, sleeplessness, sour stomach, fetid breath, heart and lung troubles, indigestion, constipation, piles, female disorders, sallow complexion, ill-temper, suicidal tendencies, pterygium, and so on *ad infinitum*. Such claims as these can only do harm by causing the physician to look at it all with disgust and distrust, as well as the intelligent men and women of the laity, and cause doubt of the entire. business. As a consequence, the sufferers of refractive anomalies do not always get the relief they should.

It is a fact proven many, many times a day, that the examination of the eyes, especially in the young, where there is indicated trouble, such as headaches, nervous conditions, etc., should be most carefully done and always under the influence of a mydriatic, unless contra-indicated. This is very seldom the case, and the mydriatic does good instead of harm in these cases, as they relax the accommodation and thus force rest for the eyes. This often does as much good as the glasses found necessary.

It is necessary for the oculist and the physician to work hand in hand in these cases of headache, which, to say the least, are a great torture to humanity, and in nearly all cases can get relief and often permanent relief by a combination in the treatment of the case by properly fitted glasses and the internal treatment of the functional wrong of the organ or organs. . Whilst the oculist who has had experience in the practice of medicine recognizes the conditions and possibly can prescribe for them as well as the family physician, he should refer the case back to the physician for treatment, with a written or oral finding of the case by himself. I think it is also proper for the family physician to advise the patient to go to the oculist instead of some vender of spectacles. He should insist that they go to such instead of the other class of men mentioned.

I find, after many years of experience in this work, that it is best in nearly all cases of headache that come to the oculist, and especially those that the family physicians have exhausted their resources upon, to use a mydriatic for making examination, unless it be contraindicated. Either homatropine, which usually answers the purpose and does not entail the loss of so much time, when time is an object to the patient, the eyes usually becoming normal two or three days after its use, whilst with atropine mydriasis will last for ten or more days. When thorough relaxation is desired atropine is the better of the two.

I find that anomalies of refraction or eye-strain increase the symptoms of a number of diseases, and that by a proper correction of such cases much good will result. I do not find that these same anomalies of refraction cause all these conditions as advertisers would lead people to believe. Some good authorities claim that the ocular element of mixed headaches are 40 per cent.; fully 50 per cent. of all functional headaches are affections mostly functional to the eyes. The site of the ocular headaches in the order of frequency are: (1) supra-orbital; (2) deep orbital; (3) fronto-occipital; and (4) temporal.

The exciting causes are those tasks which require the use of accommodation and convergence, such as reading, writing, drawing, painting, typewriting, etc. The characteristics of ocular headaches are almost always accompanied by signs and symptoms easily referred to the eyes, such as running together of letters, reddening of the sclera, burning and itching of the lids. The forms of headache which are most apt to simulate ocular headaches are the supra-nasal pain of nasal disease, supra-orbital malarial neuralgia, and the so-called nervous headaches. It is of great importance that such exciting causes as insomnia, dyspepsia, and the over-indulgence in tobacco, alcohol and coffee be removed.

Now, in conclusion, I wish to say to the physician that he should not pass too lightly over these complaints of headaches, as they are of importance if not of any real danger to the party afflicted. They have more confidence in him as a family physician if he can relieve them, or be the first to advise them to go to the oculist. The other cases of headache not due to eye-strain or anomalies of refraction should be left to the care of the physician.

------*------

TONSILLITIS.

T. D. HOLLINGSWORTH, M.D., AKRON, O.

The tonsils are adenoid structures, closely resembling Peyer's patches, but instead of having flattened surfaces the lymphoid tissue in the tonsils is folded upon itself, forming from fifteen to twenty quite deep depressions—the tonsillar crypts. The surface of the tonsils and crypts are lined with epithelial cells. The tissue is bounded by a fibrous capsule. The ducts of numerous mucous glands open into the crypts. The tonsils exude a viscid secretion which lubricates the food as it passes them in the second part of the act of deglutition.

Under normal conditions the tonsils take no part in absorption from the mouth, but when the epithelium is removed or weakened they absorb with great rapidity any poison the mouth may contain. Such poisons are taken up by the lymphatics, and through them reach the general circulation.

Tonsillitis is subdivided into:

1. Acute catarrhal—an inflammation of the mucous membrane covering the surface of the tonsils, and is usually associated with pharyngitis.

2. Follicular—an inflammation of the mucous membrane covering the surface and extending to the mucous lining of the tonsillar crypts.

3. Acute suppurative—an inflammation of the parenchyma of the tonsil, with a tendency to abscess formation.

Some authors give further subdivisions, but the one given is sufficient for all practical purposes.

Follicular tonsillitis occurs more frequently than the other varieties. The most susceptible period to follicular tonsillitis is between the ages of ten and twenty-five years. Those having a rheumatic history seem more prone to the disease than others. Exposure to wet and cold is an exciting cause, with bad hygienic surroundings.

Tonsillitis is undoubtedly contagious, and it is well to isolate the patient in order to not infect other members of the family.

The prognosis is favorable and the disease runs a short course, but there is a great deal of suffering in severe cases, and as the disease yields readily to specific medication, there is no excuse for letting the disease run its course without interference.

There are few drugs indicated in tonsillitis. Aconite or veratrum, as indicated by the pulse or temperature, should be given at the onset of the disease. Belladonna may be given with the aconite when indicated, although I do not find the belladonna indication often. Phytolacca and baptisia in combination may be given in alternation with the aconite or veratrum. These remedies with podophyllin trit. for the yellow-coated tongue so often seen in tonsillitis will meet the indications for treatment in the greater part of the cases. Another remedy of value, when there is lymphatic involvement, is calcaria flour. Tr. guaiac is regarded by some physicians as a specific for suppurative tonsillitis. Spraying the throat with specific aconite in water, as recommended by Professor Scudder, will abort many cases of quinsy. Gargles, as a rule, do very little good. They may be of value in giving the patient something to do, but they do not reach the diseased surfaces many times. The internal treatment alone is usually sufficient.

DISCUSSION.

DR. J. J. SUTTER: Dr. Todd, who was to open this discussion is not present. The subject is open for discussion, and I hope that all of you will take an active part in it and discuss the many interesting features in the paper. I will ask Dr. Thomas to make a few remarks on tonsillitis.

DR. R. L. THOMAS: I would like to call attention to one remedy that is mentioned rather slightingly, or of not much use. It is the remedy that I usually *do* use in tonsillitis, and that is belladonna. I believe if there is any one remedy that will correct or prevent the suppurative process, or will abort tonsillitis, it is belladonna. You take that tonsil when it has that unpleasant looking redness, angry, fiery-looking redness, and use your belladonna every twenty or thirty or sixty minutes for the first few hours and you will not have any suppurative tonsillitis. I agree with the rest of the paper as to treatment.

DR. W. T. GEMMILL: I presume that there is no other disease that every physician has to meet as much as we have these forms of throat trouble, especially tonsillitis; and people are anxious to get rid of them just as quickly as possible. We have remedies that will abort many of these troubles very early, if the proper remedy is selected to meet the condition. If you are called early to see a case of tonsillitis and you find a congested condition existing there, like Dr. Thomas speaks of, that will indicate belladonna; but it is only used early in the case. After the congested condition disappears, the inflammation disappears, you will have to resort to aconite and veratrum. Veratrum is good where the pus collection results in a great majority of cases. Phytolacca is used later, after the disease has existed long enough that the little polyp is filled up with adhesive matter, and after a certain length of time decomposes, and then again if glandular trouble follows —in those cases you will find phytolacca will meet the conditions promptly. Belladonna, aconite, veratrum and phytolacca will meet the great majority of cases.

Dr. A. S. Stemler: I wish to speak of one thing. Peroxide of · hydrogen is one of those things that may be used, and it will frequently reach the spot where you have those little ulcerations in the throat. Cleanse the mouth good and thoroughly, and follow it up with hamamelis and glycerine and it does a lot of good.

Dr. W. H. Swisher: I have been a sufferer from tonsillitis for a great many years, and I find that it is good to take fifteen to twenty grains of quinine in about three hours. And then, as a wash, I have used boracic acid and glycerine and chloride of potash with splendid results, especially in follicular tonsillitis.

Dr. Lyman Watkins: I do not know what tonsillitis is, hardly. It seems to me that there is a difference between tonsillitis and quinsy; I don't know whether there is or not, but I am confused on these things. I do not know how to treat names very well. I quit treating names a long time ago. I treat conditions. When a man asks me what the treatment is for quinsy, I don't know how to answer him. I want to know the conditions; I want to know the temperature; first look at the throat, whether it is bluish, or whether it is bright red; I want to know the color of the throat; and then after I know a great many things about it, if that's quinsy, I know what quinsy is; but sometimes I look in the throat and find neither dark red nor bright red, but kind of cheesy looking deposits around about; and that's another condition. Then I go to work to treat that condition; I don't care whether you call it quinsy or tonsillitis or sore throat. I would like to know of all these gentlemen who have spoken of tonsillitis and treating tonsillitis, if they make a practice of treating names or treating patients. Then I would like to know the condition of the throat that phytolacca will cure; or the condition of the throat that aconite will cure, or echinacea will cure. I would like to know those things, · for we must treat the condition and not the name.

Dr. J. D. Dodge: Dr. Watkins has said that we should treat the condition. It seems to me that there is an infinity of methods of treating and an infinity of conditions, an infinity of differences in patients, and we cannot expect to find many limited treatments that will fit all cases. In my estimation, there is where the Eclectic has the best ground of any of the three schools of physicians. Now, I know from practical experience that gargles are acceptable to some patients while they are not to others. I know from practical experience that swabs, if properly used, are of amazing benefit in many cases. Since I attended lectures at the old institution I have never thought that there was the extremest benefit in these statements that we must never do so and so, because of the wonderful difference in the cases that we get. I believe that probably every physician here has a different class of patients from any other, and we have to learn our patients and their conditions and learn to treat them the best way we can. So I believe it is best for us to express ourselves as we feel, but I don't believe that we ought to feel that any one doctor's experience is a governor for any other doctor in a very large measure.

TREATMENT OF NASAL CATARRH.

G. M. Deem, M.D., Columbus, O.

It has been said that more than 90 per cent. of the American people are afflicted with catarrh in some form. While I cannot vouch for the truth of that statement, there is no doubt that it is a very common disease.

The term catarrh literally means inflammation of a mucous membrane, and the term "nasal catarrh" has such a wide scope that one could not hope to do justice to the whole subject in a short paper, so what I shall have to say will be mostly along the line of treatment.

Nasal catarrh is, for convenience, divided into two grand divisions, acute and chronic, and each of these is subdivided into several varieties.

Acute catarrh is usually the result of taking cold, or neglecting an ordinary cold. The chronic form is the result of repeated attacks of the acute.

Before undertaking to treat a case of catarrh the physician should make a careful examination of the nasal cavity, throat, etc., and familiarize himself with all the conditions present.

He should be able to answer to his entire satisfaction the following questions:

Is this a case of catarrh? Is it acute or chronic? Are the membranes congested? Is the congestion active or passive? Is there hypertrophy or atrophy? Are the turbinated bodies in a healthy condition? Is there deflection of or spurs on the septum? Are the Eustachian tubes affected? Are there ulcers anywhere on the membranes? If so, are they syphilitic?

To make a satisfactory examination, several specula and throat mirrors are needed. A good reflector is also a necessity. One with a headband, worn on the forehead, is preferable, as it leaves both hands free to manipulate the instruments. A small electric globe with a reflector back of it, and attached to a headband, is a very desirable outfit.

After analyzing the case as above indicated the question of treatment will not be difficult. What are the indications for treatment in this particular case. Do the membranes need stimulating or sedating? Should the secretion be stimulated or retarded? Does this particular ulcer need an astringent or a cauterizing agent?

The treatment of catarrh should be both local and general. I do not think it necessary to detail the general treatment when speaking to a body of Eclectic physicians. The remedy is to be chosen by specific indications with which all Eclectics are familiar. I will only mention a few remedies that I often find useful. They are aconite, belladonna, rhus, gelsemium, opium, phytolacca, echinacea, etc.

Local remedies are more important, especially in chronic cases. These may be used with an atomizer, nebulizer, nasal douche, a swab or camel's hair brush. Those of a volatile nature can be used very nicely by means of Dr. True's inhaler.

The physician who does much nose and throat work will need a compressed air tank and several atomizers and nebulizers.

First cleanse the membranes with some alkaline solution, using the atomizer or nasal douche. For this purpose we may use a Seiler tablet dissolved in two ounces of water, Dobell's solution, or soda bicarb., or common salt. After cleansing the membranes with one of the above solutions, apply the proper remedy thoroughly to all parts of the cavity. This is best done with a nebulizer.

In acute catarrh, where the membranes are dry and much burning in the nostrils, spray with a solution of boric acid containing two grains of cocaine to the ounce. If we have the burning, but instead of dryness we have a profuse watery discharge, use an astringent, say, tannic acid, gr. i, hydrastin, gr. i; aqua, oz. i, and give internally belladonna, gtts. v; tr. opii, gtts. xx; water, oz. iv; teaspoonful every hour. If the membranes are congested and swollen, spray with a solution of adrenalin chloride. If the discharge is thick and ropy use carbolic acid, gum camphor, aa., xv; liquid vaseline, oz. i, with a nebulizer.

In chronic rhinitis it is well to administer for some time one or more of those remedies usually classed as alteratives, such as iodine, mercury, phytolacca, iris, echinacea, etc. The local remedies are selected by the indications in each case. If the discharge is thin, the membranes not much swollen, use oil eucalyptus, dr. i; tr. iodine, dr. ss; liquid vaseline, oz. i, with a nebulizer. If the odor is bad, a little carbolic acid, or gr. i, potassium permanganate may be added to each ounce of the above. If the discharge is thick or purulent, menthol, camphor, aa., grs. x; tr. benzoin, oz. i. Hydrogen peroxide is also good in these cases.

If there is ulceration, with formation of dry scabs, the carbolic acid and camphor mentioned above will be found useful If this should fail to heal the ulcers, they should be touched with a very little pure carbolic acid.

The most troublesome cases of catarrh, and the most rebellious to treatment, are those cases in which much thickening of the tissues or hypertrophy has occurred, known as hypertrophic rhinitis. Here we have not only a thickening of the membranes, but an infiltration of the submucous and cellular tissues as well. New connective tissue is formed, and the walls of the sinuses are abnormally thickened. The membranes become more sensitive to atmospheric changes, and the least exposure causes a sudden engorgement, which often results in complete stenosis for a time. Thick fetid mucus accumulates in the post-nasal cavities, causing the patient to hawk till they are drawn into the throat and expectorated. The turbinated bodies are usually most affected, but no part of the nasal cavity is exempt, not even the septum.

If seen early, before much infiltration has taken place, the proper application of local remedies combined with internal alteratives may effect a complete cure, but in old, long-standing cases very little can be done with medicines.

Several forms of treatment have been advised by different authors, all more or less of a surgical nature, and intended to destroy a portion of the tissues, such as cauterizing with nitric or acetic acid or with galvanic cautery, removing a portion of the hypertrophied tissue either with knife or scissors, or with the wire hook. I have tried most of these methods with more or less success, usually less. Most cases were improved, but few were cured.

Professor Neiswanger, of Chicago, recommends electricity, not for its cautery but for its phoric and electrolytic effect. A twisted copper wire is used for an electrode, covered with absorbent cotton, wet with adrenalin. This is passed into the nasal cavity and connected to the positive pole of a galvanic battery. The negative may be on the back of the neck or even held in the hand. A current strength of about five milliamperes is used for ten minutes, and repeated two or three times a week. I have treated several cases in this way with entire satisfaction both to myself and patient. The results so far have pleased me very much, and I shall continue to use it in this way till I find something better.

The next form I shall mention is even more stubborn and rebellious to treatment, though not so distressing to the patient. I refer to atrophic rhinitis. In this disease we have almost the opposite condition. The tissues are contracted and dry, and often covered with dry scales which mature and fall off, only to be followed by another crop. Burning and smarting are often troublesome, but the most distressing symptom to the patient is the unusual fetor of the breath, which is very noticeable to the patient. The membranes are usually dry and often crack and bleed. The tissues are more or less contracted, and the cavity is usually enlarged, so breathing is not much interfered with.

The indications for treatment are to soften the membranes and stimulate secretion.

First cleanse the cavity carefully with the following wash: Soda biborate, ammonium chloride, aa., grs. xxx; potassium permanganate, grs. x; water, Oi. Use with an atomizer or nasal douche. Follow this with menthol, grs. v; glycerine, extract hamamelis, aa., oz. ss. Use with a nebulizer. Listerine is also good.

While treating a case of hypertrophic rhinitis recently with positive galvanism, and thinking of the polar effect, it occurred to me that as the negative pole attracted the oxygen and alkalies, dilated vessels, produced hyperemia, softened the membranes, and stimulated secretions, it should be good in these cases, and I resolved to try it when opportunity offered.

I have had only one case since, but the effect of negative galvanism in that case was so prompt and so marked that I am anxious to try it in other cases. The first treatment produced decided improvement, and after four treatments the membranes appeared nearly normal, secretion was established, the odor nearly gone.

The patient declared he was well and needed no further treatment, and I could not persuade him to continue treatment. I heard through a mutual friend, about three months later, that he still thought he was well. I shall surely use the same means on my next case. If any of you have the means and the opportunity I wish you would try this treatment and report.

I used a No. 18 copper wire, doubled and twisted together, and one end attached to the conducting cord. On the other end I wound a wad of absorbent cotton, large enough to fill the nasal cavity. This was wet with a solution of potassium iodide, grs. x to water oz. i, passed into the nose and attached to the negative side of my wall plate. A current of five milliamperes was used for fifteen minutes in each nostril. The first treatment caused some sneezing, but not much after that.

With this treatment we got the softening and stimulating effect of the negative pole, and the germicidal and alterative effect of the iodine which seems to fill all the indications for treatment.

PENETRATING WOUNDS OF THE EYEBALL.

J. P. HARBERT, M.D., BELLEFONTAINE, O.

Wounds of the cornea are the most common, in my experience, of all injuries to the eyeball. These may vary in extent from a simple disturbance of the superficial epithelium to a perforating cut which comprehends the entire thickness of the cornea. Infection and ulceration may follow a superficial wound leaving the vision much impaired on account of resulting opacity. Penetrating wounds of the cornea made by a clean instrument may cause no serious complications provided no deeper structures are injured, the aqueous humor being quickly replaced and the irritation rapidly subsiding. However, even slight injuries inflicted with an unclean instrument may be followed by a corneal ulcer or by an abscess which may result disastrously on account of sloughing or panophthalmitis. The cases in which the traumatic agent penetrates through the anterior capsule of the lens, allowing the aqueous humor to come in contact with the lens substance, will be followed by traumatic cataract, more or less complete; portions of the opaque lens fibers may be seen in the anterior chamber. These may be entirely absorbed, or, by accumulating rapidly at the iris angle, may interfere with filtration and give rise to acute glaucoma, or by continued pressure produce irido-cyclitis.

Prolapse of the iris into the wound is not infrequent, and also of the vitreous in cases where the wound is near the sclero-corneal margin. Septic agents penetrating into the vitreous are especially dangerous, generally producing a purulent intra-ocular process. Wounds of the sclero-corneal margin are also especially dangerous on account of the injury to the ciliary body and resulting sympathetic processes, and on account of the frequency of complication with prolapse. Foreign bodies may lodge in the sclera or the scleral coat may be perforated; if the wound extends to the choroid, vitreous, or retina, the danger is increased. Occasionally the injury is so serious that the eye is lost at once, while in other cases an insidious inflammation results which destroys the sight. The lens may be dislocated after a penetrating wound, being forced out of its position or from the eye together with the vitreous and iris.

Injuries to the eye with retention of the traumatic agent are of frequent occurrence and may give rise to very serious inflammatory processes. These are usually produced by a very small body traveling at a high rate of speed, and do not produce a large or gaping wound. Large bodies lacerate the globe more extensively, inflicting a large wound, through which they may be withdrawn or escape spontaneously. Slowly moving bodies do not penetrate the globe as a rule, and produce injuries by contusion or concussion. Small chips of steel and iron, or fragments of stone and glass are the most common foreign bodies finding their way into the eye. Copper is more dangerous as it gives rise to severe irritation by its chemical reaction, producing purulent inflammation and should be removed speedily. When the foreign body cannot be detected, its course may be traced by the evidence of injury produced in its path. In cases of prolapse of the iris the foreign body is not usually retained, for the wound must be large, and this allows the foreign agent to escape with the aqueous and iris.

The diagnosis will depend on the objective manifestations, the history of the injury, and the subjective symptoms. Oblique illumination will materially aid in the location of small corneal wounds; a drop of 2 per cent. solution of fluorescin will produce a green stain whenever the corneal epithelium is absent and will assist in locating small abrasions of the cornea.

The treatment will vary with each case and will depend on the severity of the injury. In perforating scleral wounds, the conjunctiva may be sutured, after thorough disinfection, and a pressure-bandage applied in order that the eye may have a complete rest. If the iris has prolapsed the protruding portion should be snipped off with scissors. In case of a retained foreign body, the treatment will consist in its removal, though exhaustive attempts to remove small bodies which have penetrated the globe are to be discouraged. In fact, their removal may be impossible and our treatment must be limited to the complications that arise, keeping the patient under observation.

Because of the tendency to sink and come in contact with the uvea, early extraction of freely movable bodies is advisable. The magnet may be used in case the foreign body is steel or iron. Operative interference should be deferred when the site of the foreign body cannot be determined and the eye remains quiescent, or when it is fixed in the coats of the eye so that it may become encapsulated. If a foreign body is suspected and cannot be located by the ordinary methods, the magnet or X-ray may be used. In all cases where the foreign body is still in the globe, our treatment should be to preserve as long as possible the function of the eye and next its form; deferring enucleation until progressive inflammation or danger of sympathetic inflammation make it imperative.

In cases where it is evident that the eye is lost at once on account of serious injury, enucleation is to be advised; this procedure simplifies the recovery very materially, doing away with long and painful suffering, to say nothing of the dangers of sympathetic inflammation.

CASE 1.—Mr. S., while shearing a recalcitrant sheep, had the point of the shears kicked into his right eye, penetrating into the vitreous. Enucleation on the tenth day with perfect recovery and no disturbance of fellow-eye.

CASE 2.—Master Y. was shot in the right eye with an arrow. The case was first seen by me five months after the injury, at which time both eyes were hopelessly blind, sympathetic inflammation having destroyed the left eye.

CASE 3.—Mr. H., machinist, was struck in the right eye in the ciliary region by a needle-like piece of steel, one-eighth of an inch long, which was removed about one hour after the injury, and, contrary to our expectations, the patient had a smooth recovery.

CASE 4.—Mr. W., a wearer of spectacles, was struck by a flying body which broke the right lens of his spectacles, driving a triangular piece of glass through the cornea, and extending posteriorly into the vitreous. Enucleation with satisfactory result.

DISCUSSION.

DR. K. O. FOLTZ: This is a subject that is of interest to the general practitioner, particularly the cases of sheep-shearing and of persons who are trimming hedges or grubbing out blackberry bushes, work of that character being frequent in the country. It has been my misfortune to see a great many cases where an eye has been injured by a thorn or branch striking the eye and penetrating the cornea near the sclero-corneal margin, the ciliary region being the recognized danger zone. In these cases, as a general thing, I have found enucleation was advisable. However, if they are seen soon, before much inflammatory action has occurred, and the ulceration of the tissue is not too great, there is a chance of saving the eye, and then I give the victim the benefit of the doubt. There is no necessity for immediate enucleation, where the vitreous has not been allowed to escape.

A piece of glass of some size entering the eye, entering the anterior chamber and passing through the globe, calls for immediate removal; but in these other cases it is just as well, for a few days, to go on the expectant plan, and I make it a rule in those cases to put them immediately on atropine, cleansing the eye thoroughly, keeping the pupil dilated, and keeping down inflammation of the iris.

Last fall there was a boy brought to my office, about two hours after an injury had been received, in which a piece of steel had been driven through the lower lid. An examination showed conclusively that it entered the eyeball, as the vitreous was filled with blood. As near as I could determine it had passed just back of the ciliary region. The first idea was immediate removal of the eye. The doctor who brought the case in thought that would have to be done. I advised waiting a few days because there was a chance. I put the boy under treatment for about ten days. The vitreous had cleared; the blood had cleared, so we could get a view, and we found there was lesion in the retina. An X-ray was made and the steel located in the sclero-coat, in the posterior portion of the eye.

On an examination of the normal eye, I found it was about two diameters imperfect, making the eyeball short, and the small piece of steel had passed clear through and was located in the orbital tissue. The child has vision, or had when I last saw him, which was a number of months ago, of not quite two-thirds, twenty-thirtieths, lacking a few letters on the line. Probably his vision is as good as it was before the injury.

Where eyes have been injured, by a thorn or a branch of blackberry or anything of that kind, I, myself, have been unable to save those eyes, where it penetrated the cornea. In a few days, if the eye does not show any sign of improvement, I advise enucleation. It saves the patient time and worry and pain, but I always give a few days time.

Dr. W. N. Mundy: The great danger in penetrating wounds of the eye, to my mind, is delay in sending them to the specialist. That eye might be saved. General practitioners (and I am speaking from the standpoint of a general practitioner) are too apt, because one eye looks well, to delay it until it is too late to even save the good eye, the uninjured eye; and as a result we have a sympathetic trouble and a total loss of vision.

Enucleation does not always save the other eye. Nor does enucleation always bar a sympathetic ophthalmia that results in total blindness. I think the most dangerous thing is these penetrating wounds of the eye, especially in the sclero-corneal margin.

Dr. A. E. Ballmer: Allow me a word, not on this subject particularly, but Dr. Mundy opened up the way a little, and others have mentioned it, and that is that the general practitioner sometimes neglects these cases too long. I don't wait very long. If I meet with something that I am not sure of, I hustle the patient off to the specialist, and I do not think it is a mark of ignorance to say to your patients that you do not know how to handle their case, that that belongs to the specialist.

Dr. J. P. Harbert: I think that prompt enucleation sometimes simplifies matters very much, instead of allowing the tissues to slough. Your patient is going to suffer if you wait two or three weeks.

I had a case under observation that was blind in the right eye, resulting from an attack of whooping cough some seven years ago. There was no external manifestation of the injury. Probably the general practitioner would have difficulty in diagnosing this case and would not have known what to do. After some three or four months the other eye, the left eye, began to pain, the right eye had never pained in the least, but the left eye became very painful, a deep-seated, boring pain along the course of the nerve to the base of the brain. This case had been the rounds of several specialists in different States, and at last was advised to have the blind eye, the right eye, enucleated, with the hope that the pain in the other eye would cease and that she would be well. She is a young lady by this time, eighteen or nineteen years old, and she consented rather reluctantly to this ordeal in order that she might get relief from this distressing pain, which kept up day and night and disturbed her general condition exceedingly. So this right eye was removed, with the result that the left eye still continues to pain to this day. She has had no relief whatever from that awful pain in that left eye, although she has been refracted by specialists everywhere, including myself, and that eye still pains.

So I think that when you advise enucleation, it is well to qualify your prognosis and pave the way for disappointment.

Periscope.

The Prophylactic Value of Normal Marriage.

Taking part in a most interesting and suggestive symposium in the *Medical News* on the question of the social evils of the day, Dr. Andrew H. Smith points out that the ideal preventive against these evils is to be found in normal marriage. He defines normal marriage as the union between a man and woman, both in sexual health, prompted in the first instance by the natural inclination of the two sexes one to the other, and determined in each particular case by the presence in each person of qualities which excite the admiration, esteem and affection of the other. Normal marriage must have a physical, or if you choose a physiological, basis in the sexual instinct. A platonic affection, no matter how deep or strong, could never result in a normal union, nor could a union dictated by policy alone ever be other than abnormal.

Dr. Smith believes in the education of young persons of either sex normal marriage should be presented as the natural prospect before them, as the thing that more than anything else will bring them happiness—the thing absolutely most important in their lives; a thing most solemn, most sacred, a thing that is to determine their earthly destinies and to influence their posterity for all generations. Particularly should this be impressed upon the young man, and his mind should be imbued with high ideals in connection with the subject.

He should be reminded that some time he will ask for the hand of a young woman in whom he will expect absolute purity—purity in thought, purity in word, purity in deed; that every chivalric sentiment should revolt at the thought of laying at her feet a life less pure than that he expects of her, that as he would smite to the earth one who would question her stainlessness, so he would challenge his own heart as her stainless knight, and pass judgment upon himself if he did not meet the ordeal.

The young should be taught that the man who would sell himself for money or the woman who would sell herself for a title has hopelessly degraded the higher nature, and is shut out from the aristocracy of self-respect.

Normal marriage could thus be made to cast its light before; and the youth trained in chivalric ideas would keep himself pure for the, as yet, unknown mistress of his heart. Purity of thought carries with it physical purity, and to this he would be the father stimulated by regard for posterity, to whom he would wish to transmit not only untainted blood, but also unsullied traditions. In this he would only

be following at a distance the Japanese, who, in worshiping his ancestors, realizes that he in turn is to be worshiped by those who come
after him, and deems that death by his own hand is the only expiation
that can avert a stain upon the succession if he prove unworthy.

The fact of normal marriage being such a protecting influence is
a powerful argument for early marriage. The sooner a young man
comes under its ægis, the more likely he will be to pass through early
manhood unsullied. But early marriage is often impracticable, and
in such cases the writer earnestly advocates early engagements. How
a young man is carried safely through university life, including perhaps a period of residence among the corrupting influences of European capitals, simply because of a pure attachment for a pure maiden
who trusts him, anyone who has had the opportunity to observe, or has
perhaps himself experienced, need not be told. And if there is anything on earth that heaven smiles upon, it is an influence like this.

Dr. Smith then considers the other kind of marriage, the abnormal.
As the one we have just been considering is physiological, this is
essentially pathological. Very often the physical basis is wanting on
one side or the other, or if present, exists in a perverted and perhaps
a repulsive form. Very often it has gone down in the general wreck
which his disease has left. At the best, it is not supplemented by any
personal qualities that attract the respective parties to each other. The
only end in view is a sordid one, based upon the expectation by each
of material or social advantage to be gained at the expense of the
other. This expectation is commonly disappointed, and the yoke
which it was thought might be endurable becomes day by day more
irksome, and at last is thrown off entirely. Indifference is now ex-
changed for animosity, and not infrequently disregard for public
criticism opens the way to the gratification of every passing fancy
until nothing but a moral and social wreck remains. True, if there
is money it may buy divorce and perhaps buy another partner. It
may also pre-empt a place in the ranks of the gilded nastiness known
as the fast set, and thus the maleficient influence is reinforced.

This kind of marriage is perhaps as potent for evil as is the other
for good. It were far better for public morals if the parties to it
remained single, and stood before the world for what they were,
rather than that they should degrade the noblest of human relations
to the meanest of human ends.

And now a word especially for mothers. The young girl should
be taught by her mother the dignity and sanctity of normal marriage,
and the degradation and the physical danger of abnormal marriage.
As to the latter point it should be explained to her that innocent wives
by thousands receive from infected husbands diseases of a well-nigh

incurable character, that not only make their lives permanently wretched, but will descend inevitably to any children they may bear. Let her be taught to distrust a man who talks flippantly about marriage, or whose bearing toward the opposite sex is other than that of respectful deference. Romantic young women are apt to see an embodiment of chivalry in any good-looking man who seeks their acquaintance, and they should be made to promise not to allow themselves to become in the slightest degree interested in any man without the knowledge of their parents.

Upon the first sign that a man has singled out their daughter for special attention that man should be required to desist from his attentions until he shall have satisfied the father as to his freedom from venereal taint. An attempt to evade this issue should be accepted as a confession of guilt, and the turpitude of such evasion should be brought home to the daughter's consciousness. If the girl has previously had the matter presented to her in the abstract she can be depended upon to act wisely when the concrete illustration is put before her, whereas, without such previous teaching, her course could not be predicted.

Normal marriage is the strongest influence that exists as a preventive of immorality and of the diseased conditions growing out of immorality. But it is only when it is broadly differentiated from marriage in general, and placed in contrast with abnormal marriage that we fully appreciate its prophylactic value.

The Good and Ill Effects of Cold Baths.

Dr. Robert Wallace, in *London Opinion*, reviews the alleged merits and demerits of the cold bath, so that persons who are likely to derive benefit from cold bathing may be encouraged to make a beginning, or to persevere with it; and those whom the practice is likely to injure may be warned in time against its harmful effects. Considering that no two persons are constituted exactly alike, differing as they do even in the trivial detail of finger prints, it is easy to understand that the practice of the cold bath must have different effects on different people.

As a general rule, the cold bath is beneficial to the robust, to young men, and to men in the prime of life; it is, however, injurious to children, whose normal growth and development cold, in any form, interferes with, while it is generally unsuitable for early childhood, for women, for the aged, and for the delicate. Since, however, there are individual exceptions to every general rule, each adult is able to discover the suitability or unsuitability of the cold bath to his or her individual constitution by giving it a trial. The first effect experienced on taking a cold bath—*i.e.*, a bath in which the water is below the temperature of 70°—is, of course, a sensation of cold, with a gasp or two for breath, and perhaps slight shivering. There is, in a word, a certain degree of shock to the system.

As a result of this shock to the nerves (for such in reality it is) the skin becomes pale and shrunken, due to the driving out of the blood from the minute vessels in the skin, owing to their sudden contraction from cold, the papillæ of the skin become distinct, giving rise to a roughness of the integument commonly called "gooseskin," the cutaneous exhalations are checked, and the senses dulled; there is depression of the entire nervous system, and the pulse falls as much as ten or twenty beats a minute if the water is very cold.

So far the action of the bath has been distinctly sedative. And now, if the bath be continued for more than two or three minutes, there is a diminution in the cutaneous temperature. If, however, the bath is left, in the case of one with whom it agrees, a different set of symptoms follows; a glowing sensation soon sets in, with increased circulation in the capillaries of the skin. This process is known as the reaction, and is an almost certain indication that the bath has agreed with the subject, and that the practice of cold bathing is likely to be of benefit to him.

In the case of the weakly and delicate, on the other hand, a mild glow is perhaps established only after some delay, or, indeed, may be said to be scarcely established at all, while the primary sensation of the chill, and the ensuing condition of nervous depression, may persist so long as to be distinctly harmful. In such cases the fingers and toes of the bather may be numbed and shrunken, and the cutaneous surface may remain blue for a long time afterward. Persons who suffer in this way are not, and in all probability never will be, fit subjects for the cold tub. Injudicious and over enthusiastic friends sometimes encourage the unfit to persevere in the use of cold water, in the hope that they will become accustomed to its rigors, and so derive ultimate benefit, but such a course can be productive of nothing but mischief.

The best as well as most convenient time to take the cold bath is, of course, in the morning before breakfast. But even in this respect the personal equation has to be taken into account and there are those who dare not venture into cold water until they have had a cup of coffee and a biscuit, or it may be even a light breakfast. In any case cold bathing should not be indulged in after the system has been fatigued by exercise. And cold baths should be particularly avoided at all times by sufferers from weak, fatty hearts, or a tendency to apoplexy. Persons suffering from varicose veins should not take baths which are cold—the serpentine in winter, for example. Such baths are also likely to be injurious to persons liable to congestion of any of the internal organs.

The Colloidal Form of the Casein of Milk.

It is becoming more and more apparent that the successful feeding of cow's milk to infants and invalids is dependent, in largest measure, upon the physical condition of its casein. Until recently it has been assumed that the casein was in solution, but the researches of Hammarsten and others have clearly shown that such is not the case. Casein is present in milk as calcium-casein, and is in suspension in a colloidal or jelly-like form. This is proved by the fact that if the milk be filtered through porous clay, the caseinous matter does not pass through like the other albuminoids, which are in true solution.

When chemical modifiers are used with milk the physical condition of the casein is changed. Such a change is objectionable for a number of reasons. The colloidal casein in milk serves several functions. First, it keeps the fatty globules of milk in a state of emulsion, and second, it presents a form of food that requires work for the digestion. Naturally, when chemical modifiers are used with milk, its physical form is disorganized, and coming in contact with the gastric juice, the casein is precipitated in more or less tough and cheesy curds that are most difficult of digestion. Not only this, but the fatty globules being no longer surrounded by colloidal material, tend to coalesce, form masses of fat, and cause fatty indigestion.

When, however, mechanical modifiers are used with milk, such as the cereals contained in Eskay's food, the insoluble or gelatinizable starch of the cereals takes the place of the colloidal form of the casein in the milk, and not only prevents the coalescing of the fat, but also mechanically breaks up the casein into fine flakes (instead of tough and cheesy curds) that are most easily digested.

It is for these reasons, chiefly, that Eskay's Food is of such supreme value as a milk modifier. It does not change the chemical character of the milk, but it adds a colloidal material in the form of gelatinizable starch, that takes the place of the colloidal casein, when the latter is disorganized or decomposed by the gastric juice, and performs the same physical functions, thereby minimizing the possibility of fatty indigestion, and making proteid digestion most easy.—*Exchange.*

TRUE ANGINA PECTORIS.—B. W. Richardson gave amyl nitrite, three minims in a dram each of glycerine and water, to be taken in water in the course of an hour.—*Denver Med. Times.*

THE ECLECTIC MEDICAL JOURNAL

A Monthly Journal of Eclectic Medicine and Surgery.

TWO DOLLARS PER ANNUM.

Official Journal Ohio State Eclectic Medical Association

JOHN K. SCUDDER, M.D., MANAGING EDITOR.

EDITORS.

W. E. BLOYER.	H. W. FELTER.	W. N. MUNDY.	R. L. THOMAS.
W. B. CHURCH.	K. O. FOLTZ.	L. E. RUSSELL.	L. WATKINS.
JOHN FEARN.	J. U. LLOYD.	A. F. STEPHENS.	H. T. WEBSTER.

Published by THE SCUDDER BROTHERS COMPANY, 1009 Plum Street, Cincinnati, to whom all communications and remittances should be sent.

Articles on any medical subject are solicited, which will usually be published the month following their receipt. One hundred reprints of articles of four or more pages, or one dozen copies of the Journal, will be forwarded free if the request is made when the article is submitted. The editor disclaims any responsibility for the views of contributors.

DEATH OF DR. KENT O. FOLTZ.

Dr. Kent Oscanyan Foltz, foremost as an Eclectic ophthalmologist and aurist, died at the Seton Hospital, Cincinnati, June 6, 1908. Not in good health for several years, an operation upon the nasal passages, complicated by acute nephritis, hastened the end. Dr. Foltz was born in Lafayette, Medina County, Ohio, February 16, 1857. His father, Dr. Wm. K. Foltz, was one of the best known Eclectic physicians in the State. In 1898 he removed to Cincinnati, having been called to the chair of Didactic and Clinical Ophthalmology, Otology, Rhinology and Laryngology in his alma mater—the Eclectic Medical Institute. Dr. Foltz was a member of the National and several State societies, and in 1891-2 was President of the Ohio Eclectic Medical Association. He was also one of the associate editors of this JOURNAL. He enriched Eclectic medical literature by two valuable text-books, "Manual of Eye Diseases" (1900) and "Manual of Diseases of the Nose, Throat and Ear" (1906).

In the death of Dr. Foltz the Eclectic school of medicine loses one of her most loyal and gifted physicians. Painstaking, thorough, a splendid operator and clinical instructor, he will be sadly missed by the students who were so fortunate as to have benefited by his teachings. He was a strong specific medicationist and was the first to bring this feature prominently into his specialty. His friendship was of the solid and lasting kind that will long remain with his associates a "fragrant memory." His optimism was unbounded, and a keen sense of humor made him a most enjoyable companion. A more extended biography will appear in a later issue of the JOURNAL.

SUMMER DISPENSING.

As the hot season approaches the question of employing substances to preserve medicines dispensed in water becomes of interest to us. The Eclectic doctor is partial to water-dispensed medicines, and in most instances believes that he gets the best and promptest results from them. A certain quantity of alcohol will, of course, preserve them fairly well, and where weak tinctures containing considerable alcohol are used the medicines keep in good condition. But usually it is not desirable to employ so much alcohol, especially in medicines for children, nor in those in whom we do not desire to arouse a smothered craving for alcoholics. Eclectic specific medicines are concentrated, and so little of them is required for each prescription that a very small quantity of alcohol is thus dispensed. The simple elixir, elegant as it is, has caused some opposition on account of the great amount of alcohol administered in dispensing it. Water-dispensed specific medicines, on account of lack of much alcohol, do not keep well at any time, and spoil quickly in hot weather if to be kept more than two days, hence the necessity of some preserving substance both harmless and compatible, and, if possible, one that is also an indicated substance.

When there are indications for an acid, hydrochloric acid forms a good preservative agent. We frequently so administer strychnine, nux vomica or quinine. When fermentive changes are liable to occur, as are actually taking place in the digestive tract, glycerine forms a good anti-fermentative and preservative, and may be liberally used. Besides, in dispensing such agents as iris, macrotys, and particularly rhus aromatica, it forms a means of suspension superior to water alone, as well as serving to preserve the medicine from changes. Cough medicines can be put up with a considerable quantity of glycerine, and usually with benefit to the case in hand. In throat troubles, with a tendency to dryness, as little glycerine as possible should be employed. Glycerine forms an excellent addition when such lotions as of boric acid and salicylic acid are to be applied to the cutaneous surfaces.

The aromatic oils are sometimes useful in preserving medicines, and we frequently use in preference specific cinnamon. This is not only preservative, but is both pleasant and antiseptic, and is carminative. In certain bowel disorders a weakly alcoholic essence of cloves is very useful when added to the indicated remedy.

When pain or cough are prominent symptoms choloroform water affords an excellent anodyne and preservative. It is warming and not unpleasant unless used too strong. A few drops of chloroform are sufficient to preserve a four ounce mixture. Where medicines to be dispensed in water are prepared every day no preservative should be used, and in both instances—with or without preservatives—the medicine should be kept cool, preferably on ice.	FELTER.

LATHYRISM.

Lathyrus is a genus of plants related to the pea family (legumes), the seeds of which, unlike the garden pea, contain latent poisonous properties. In past times, in various parts of Europe, the seeds of different members of this genus have been ground and incorporated into the flour from which bread was made and employed as human food. It has thus proven an insidious poison, the noxious element acting specifically on the spinal cord, finally, though almost imperceptibly, producing organic disease of that part when long continued. Transverse myelitis, with ultimate sclerosis, finally results. This condition is variously designated as lathyrism, lathyrismus, and lupinosis.

The fact of this poisonous influence became so patent in the seventeenth century that the authorities of Wurtemberg, in order to prevent widespread disease, interdicted its cultivation as a food. Spastic paraplegia, characterized by stiffness and dragging of the lower extremities when walking, with exaggerated tendon reflexes and sensory disturbances, appears after its protracted use. The upper extremities are seldom involved. Complete paraplegia marks extreme cases. It is strange, considering the premises, that the Homeopaths have not investigated this agent as a remedy in diseases of the cord.

A member of this family is the lathyrus odoratus, or sweet pea, a plant quite popular for ornamental and other esthetic purposes. It is a native of the far East, Europe and Asia, but is cultivated in many parts of the world on account of its handsome and fragrant blossoms. It flourishes exceptionally well in California, the soil and climate rendering it easily cultivated, and during the spring and summer it is a prime favorite among cut flowers with many. A bouquet of sweet pea blossoms on the dining-table adds zest and pleasure to the partaker of choice viands on account of their beauty and fragrance.

However, it seems as though they ought hardly be considered a safe edible, yet we are informed that it is becoming the fashion to appropriate them as a salad. Whether their protracted use will eventually result in "wobbly" legs, more permanent than those occasioned by the popular "dago red," generally known as California claret, remains to be seen. If the seeds cause spastic paralysis, what may the flowers of the fresh plant not do? Some of our San Francisco "bloods" imagine they constitute a relish of the proper and exalted sort, and are making use of them for that purpose.

These thoughts are inspired by an article recently appearing in the San Francisco *Call,* which we will reproduce. It is not at all likely the originators and followers of this delicate fad realize that they may be standing on slippery places. The initiated will hardly follow recklessly in their train.

"Have you tried it, the sweet-pea salad? It is the very latest in table delicacies. Powers extraordinary are said to reside in its fragrant petals. To various colors are ascribed widely different virtues. The white, these gourmands tell, act with the appetizing magic of a Martini cocktail. The red is better than a seltzer sour when you feel that way. To the mixed and mottled variety there are no end of potencies assigned.

"The relish has already found its way into favor in the big downtown hotels. A party of four sat in the grill of the St. Francis Hotel yesterday afternoon and excited the wonder and amazement of the whole room by unconcernedly munching the blossoms from their green stems. They were Joseph Abbott, Frank Hazel, Samuel Whitney and J. Edward Kramer. Three first of this quartette are prominent in racing circles and the last is a well-known mining man with interests in Arizona and Mexico.

"Abbott deserves the honor of introducing it in the St. Francis. It was new to Kramer. In fact, he was astounded when Abbott, reaching to the silver receptacle in the center of the table, withdrew a few of the choicest flowers, sprinkled them with salt and a slight spraying of pepper, and began to eat them. To his bewildering inquiries Abbott merely made answer: 'You eat parsley, don't you? You eat celery and lettuce and all that sort of things? Sweet peas are the most delicious relish ever concocted by an imported chef.'

"Kramer was nettled for awhile, but as Abbott was joined by Whitney and Hazel he also began to pick out a few choice blossoms, sprinkle them with salt and pepper, and partake thereof."

Possibly this was a bluff on the part of Abbott, in order to hoax Kramer. It may all have been a joke which ye reporter made avail of in order to provide his paper with a little sensational news. The avidity of such ilk to grab at trifles in order to create sensationalism is not altogether unknown.

Possibly the latherus odoratus is devoid of the poisonous principle contained in several of its relatives, but the element seems to be pretty well distributed through the family. The seeds of three varieties, latherus cicera, latherus sativus, and latherus clymenum, are powerfully imbued with it, and it would thus seem as though the poisonous trait might be a family failing. It is true that individuals of the same family of plants often vary much in their properties, and it is to be hoped, if this is to become a fad, that sweet-pea blossoms are harmless. However, if the custom prevails we shall get a good proving of sweet-pea blossoms, and a few of the simpletons may not get about quite so lively in time to come.   WEBSTER.

INTESTINAL INTOXICATION.

Auto-intoxication and auto-infection from the gastro-intestinal tract may arise either from disorders of secretion, absorption or elimination. Auto-intoxication may be acute when large quantities of toxic material are rapidly produced by abnormal digestive changes, or more gradual when the toxins are formed in small quantities but continuously and are constantly passing into the blood stream. They are then disseminated throughout the body and produce chronic pathological disturbances.

Under the head of causes of intestinal infection may be classed ptomaines arising from decaying proteid material such as milk, cheese, oysters, fish, sausage and various kinds of meat, and the results of bacterial activity. These poisons, whether derived from proteids, carbohydrates, hydrocarbons or from germ proliferation, by their absorption, give rise to a number of disorders in the various tissues and organs. Symptoms resulting from infection of the central nervous system are of frequent occurrence. These are headache, dizziness, dullness and insomnia. They are easily recognized and readily relieved by a thorough cleansing and disinfection of the gastro-intestinal tract. But it sometimes happens that the symptoms arising from auto-infection are more serious, and there may be delirium, convulsions, paralyses or mental disturbances of a serious nature, all dependent upon an unclean alimentary canal.

Many cases of inveterate skin disease can be directly traced to intestinal auto-infection. Thus erythema, urticaria, bronzing, icterus, and some forms of acne and eczema resist treatment until intestinal disinfection. Vomiting and diarrhea occur as an effort of nature to eliminate toxic substances, and constipation with eructations and anorexia are frequently due to their retention.

That urinary disorders arise from the absorption of intestinal ptomaines is now established beyond doubt, and many cases of albuminuria and diabetes date their inception from this cause. Disordered metabolism, beginning in the organs of digestion, produce irritating substances which, by their absorption, affect the renal organs, and later cause serious constitutional derangements.

A large number of diseases of the human body are caused or influenced by intestinal auto-infection, and this condition must be recognized and dealt with before a cure can be accomplished. Only recently has the action of morbid ferments or bacterial toxines derived from the intestinal tract been recognized as an important factor in the causation of systemic diseases.   WATKINS.

A PRECISE STUDY OF INDICATIONS.

In the consideration of specific indications, we are apt to' be too narrow, and to lay down as exact rules, suggestions that in some cases would be misleading. A writer in the *National Transactions* says that in determining the indications for drugs, the physician must not stop at mere surface indications, he must be a profound student of physiology and pathology. All red tongues do not indicate acids, a bright red, narrow, pointed tongue points to an irritation of the alimentary tract, which would be increased by the use of an acid. The red, pointed tongue, covered with a grayish white coat, points to an accompanying inflammation, the treatment of which would promptly change the tongue appearances. The broad, deep red, smooth tongue, in low grades of fever, suggests sepsis and will be benefited by acids, especially those of an antiseptic character.

All white tongues, on the contrary, do not indicate alkalies. A white tongue due to anemia is white because it is pale, and there may be present at the same time a necessity for iron or nux vomica, or other bitter tonics with the best of nutrition. A broad, pale, heavily coated tongue in acute disease is the result of fermentation in the stomach or bowels; this is corrected by the sulphite or phosphate of sodium. If the coating is very white and moist, and covers the tongue uniformly, there is usually present extreme acidity, and until this is corrected other remedies are of but little avail. Sometimes a single dose of thirty grains of sodium or magnesium bicarbonate will change the whole condition by neutralizing the excess of acidity.

Aconite is indicated when the pulse is small, hard and rapid, but the rapid, small, feeble pulse present in protracted fevers, or after a shock, must not be treated with aconite. An active, circulatory stimulant must be used and persisted in. Aconite given under these circumstances will increase the conditions present and would be decidedly unsafe. These statements will illustrate the necessity of considering all specific indication with reference to any possible indications which might resemble them, but which would appear under different conditions, in order that the exact indication be met only with its correctly indicated remedy. ELLINGWOOD.

SULPHIDE OF CALCIUM.

·The keynote for its use is *its power for preventing and arresting suppuration*.

In inflammation threatening to end in suppuration it will avert the formation of pus. After the pus has really formed, its action is still more pronounced. Then it not only hastens maturation, but diminishes and circumscribes the inflammation, promotes the passage of pus to the surface, and the evacuation of the abscess.

If you are looking for facts to prove these statements administer the one-tenth grain of sulphide of calcium every hour or two in some of your cases of tonsillitis when there is a tendency to form deep-seated abscesses in these glands, and watch the results. Compare these with what you have obtained before with other means. Take also some deep-seated abscess on other portions of the body and treat with the same sized dose and see how much quicker relief is procured. In both boils and carbuncles this remedy will yield excellent results. The one-tenth grain given every one, two or three hours will prevent the formation of fresh boils and also lessen the inflamamtion and reduce the area of those already existing. When the skin is not broken and the slow-separating core not yet exposed, the sulphide of calcium will often convert the boil into an abscess, so that on bursting, pus is freely discharged and the wound at once heals; or if the center of the hardened swollen tissues is not yet dead, the pustule dries up, the inflammation subsides, and a hard knot is left which disappears in a few days without the formation of a core, and without any discharge. The effect of this remedy is equally conspicuous in mammary abscesses, although in rare instances they appear temporarily to increase the pain—a fact which seems sometimes to hold good with respect to boils, though, as a rule, the pain is speedily mitigated.

The good effects of sulphide of calcium are often observed in certain scrofulous sores not uncommonly seen in young children. They will readily yield to its use.

It may be urged that it is difficult to imagine how this remedy can produce effects so different and apparently opposite as the dispersion of inflammation in one case and the expulsion of pus in another; poultices, however, and hot fomentations both subdue inflammation and prevent suppuration, and in other cases considerably hasten the evacuation of pus.   HOWES.

————————

THE *Medical Era,* of St. Louis, Mo., will issue its annual series of gastro-intestinal editions during July and August. In these two issues will be published between forty and fifty original papers of the largest practical worth, covering every phase of diseases of the gastro-intestinal canal. Sample copies will be supplied readers of this journal.

————————

INTESTINAL CATARRH.—Hare gives full doses (five to twenty grains) of sodium bicarbonate by the mouth and uses iodoform suppositories.—*Denver Med. Times.*

The Eclectic Medical Journal

ESTABLISHED 1836.

Vol. LXVIII.   CINCINNATI, AUGUST, 1908.   No. 8.

Ohio Society—Section on Tuberculosis.

TUBERCULOSIS.

Wm. Phillips, M.D., Jackson, O.

The great question that confronts the medical profession to-day is, what can be done to stay the ravages of tuberculosis? The last census report shows that in 1900 there were 1,039,094 deaths from all causes. Of this number, 111,059 are classed as consumption, 105,971 as pneumonia, 20,223 as bronchitis.

I have no doubt that many cases classed as pneumonia and bronchitis were in reality tuberculosis. Some of our best observers place the total number of deaths from tuberculosis in the United States at this time as being over 200,000 annually.

The fact that so many die of tuberculosis invests the etiology of the disease with the utmost importance. The inhabitatnts of the extreme north and south appear to be free from attacks of tuberculosis, otherwise it is common to all sections of the world. It is more prevalent in densely populated districts and among those employed in dark, ill-ventilated shops and factories. Persons that dwell in crowded tenement-houses, where sunlight and pure air never reach the occupants, coupled with poor food and filth, soon provide a suitable soil for the growth of tuberculosis.

Strictly speaking, tuberculosis may affect any organ or part of the body. I wish to confine myself in this paper to the consideration of its manifestation in the lungs, which is known as phthisis pulmonalis. This disease, characterized as it is by cough, with a purulent expectoration, emaciation, and decay of the lungs, has been recognized for centuries under the general name of consumption.

Schonlein, in 1839, used the term "tuberculosis" to indicate a definite diseased condition.

The investigations of Bayle, Laennec, Virchow and others up to 1865 prepared the way for further research. Villeman at this time made the discovery that tuberculosis could be communicated to animals by inoculation. The infectious character of the disease has been gaining in the minds of close observers up to the present, and is now almost universal. The discovery of Koch, in 1882, of the tubercle bacillus has settled the question in the minds of the majority as to the cause of tuberculosis. The constant presence in any lesion of these peculiar rod-shaped bodies is now considered conclusive evidence of its tubercular character. Many believe, however, that the bacillus is not the cause of tuberculosis, but only present in the sputum, etc., as a result of the progress of the disease.

The manner of entrance of the bacillus and mode of infection is supposed to be as follows: The sputum containing the bacilli, becoming dried and broken up, is carried in the air to the lungs, and if deposited in a ·fertile spot grow and multiply rapidly.

The favorable site considered by close observers is the infra-clavicular region, but many eminent physicians believe that the posterior margin is the part earliest affected, also the interlobar septa between the upper and middle lobe on the right, and the upper and lower lobe on the left. "Says one authority, in order to detect fine crepitant râles in this location we must have the patient place his hand on the opposite shoulder, and raise his elbow high in the air, which will carry the scapula out of the way and leave a clear space between it and the vertebræ. Crepitant râles and moisture in this location indicate pulmonary tuberculosis ninety-nine times out of a hundred." I have noticed that many cases have occasional twinges of pain, sharp and stitching in character, at the lower posterior margin of the lungs, upon taking a deep and prolonged breath, with a tied-down feeling and a tendency to cough.

The temperature in the morning may be normal or subnormal, while in the afternoon and evening the thermometer shows a slight elevation in temperature. In the early period of the disease sweats at night may be the first symptoms noticed by the patient. Some weakness may be experienced, but the appetite is fairly good, and the patient as yet has little or no cough. Often a hemorrhage seems to mark the onset. I am led to believe that the latter symptom should not be disregarded. It is the early symptoms that are the most important to the physician, as his success depends largely on his ability to arrive at an early diagnosis in order to cure the disease. It is too late to make a diagnosis from the sputum by the microscope to be of any benefit to the patient, who has coughed some time prior to the peculiar yellow, greenish-yellow or grayish-yellow expectoration containing the rod-shaped bacillus.

I find in the majority of cases physicians are too careless in making examinations. A look at the tongue, a few questions and the dismissal of the patient with a bottle of cough syrup has been of too frequent occurrence for the good of the patient. Remember that the patient's life is at stake, and your duty is to make a thorough examination of the case.

In acute miliary tuberculosis the attack is sudden and virulent. The patient is in apparent health, and while engaged at his ordinary avocation is stricken with symptoms similar in many respects to those of typhoid fever. The morning temperature may be normal or subnormal in miliary tuberculosis, while in typhoid it does not reach normal until the beginning of convalescence. The rapid decline in strength and flesh, the dyspnea and lack of oxygen evidenced by the patient's demand for breath, which seems to be out of all proportion to the physical condition of the lungs, as shown upon auscultation and percussion.

I here introduce a clipping from an article in *Clinical Medicine,* by J. J. Herrick, M.D., which may throw some light on these cases.

"It has always been a problem in physiology how it was that the blood, in passing through the lungs, gave up carbon dioxide and took up oxygen. As an explanation the well-known tendency of gases to diffuse was advanced; here, however, we have a condition unfavorable for diffusion. The oxygen in this case has to overcome a higher tension on entering the blood, and would naturally be taken in very small quantities, if at all. There must, therefore, be in the blood some highly oxidizable substance with which the oxygen eagerly unites. There is evidence that this substance is the suprarenal secretion, since the removal of the suprarenal gland destroys the power of the blood to take up oxygen, as is evidenced by air hunger, cyanosis and all the symptoms of suffocation."

May there not be in these cases a lack of secretion on the part of suprarenal glands?

Predisposition.—At one time it was a popular belief that consumption in many instances was inherited. The general opinion of physicians at the present time is, that parents transmit to their children certain bodily defects, which prove a fertile field for the development of disease. I have taken some time in the investigation of persons where a number of the members of the same family have died of lung trouble. I found one or all of the following conditions prevailing—first, deficient lung capacity, upon actual test showing, in many instances, from fifty to one hundred cubic inches. The chest is flattened, with depression in the infraclavicular regions, shoulders thrown forward, with an inclination of chest walls to collapse and bend forward; such individuals never walk or sit erect, but have a tendency to stoop forward, until the chest walls become fixed and practically immobile. Such persons are preferred subjects for tuberculosis. Second, the skin is defective and presents the following appearance—thin, relaxed, transparent, cold, bluish and lacking in capillary circulation. Such individuals perspire easily and are very susceptible to changes in temperature; in fact, they seem to be continually taking cold. Another characteristic condition is where the skin is dry, scaly, wrinkled and drawn tightly like parchment, totally unfit to do the work of the skin as an eliminating organ. I am thoroughly convinced that the skin plays a greater part in the production of consumption than is generally supposed.

Defects in the digestive system will forever play an important rôle in the development of tuberculosis, as well as in many other diseases. Strong, healthy digestive organs will insure immunity against the inroads of the bacillus. Food products thrown into the blood which have undergone imperfect change in the digestive process are not the proper materials to repair and build up a body of the greatest resistance to disease. On the other. hand, it is quite likely that it is there tubercles have their beginning.

I have no doubt whatever but the state of the mind has often an influence in inviting an attack of tuberculosis. The person that persistently holds the thought that they will die at some time of tuberculosis, because other members of the family have died of the disease, will quite likely, by reason of the worry and anxiety, ultimately die of the disease. This class should have encouragement to make proper effort to throw off such preconceived ideas, and impress them with the fact that if they will make persistent effort at deep breathing they need have no fears of tuberculosis. I have in mind a girl with a strong predisposition to tuberculosis. Several of the family had died of the disease, consequently she was sure she would die of consumption. This girl has gained in lung capacity in the past six years from 90 cubic inches to 175 cubic inches and is in perfect health at this time.

Prevention of Tuberculosis.—The province of the physician is thought to be by many the cure of disease only. The real work of the physician ought to be the prevention of disease. In no instance is the result of such effort shown more effectively than in tuberculosis. Children are born into the world weak and defective in certain organs or parts. After years of observation and careful examination of children and adults, I am led to believe the defect is oftener of the lungs than any other. A law of mechanics is that a machine is no stronger than its weakest point. The fact that so many die from tuberculosis, pneumonia and bronchitis is strong evidence that the weakest part of mankind is the lungs. Out of 1,500 persons, 600 females, 900 males, whom I have tested with Paul von Boeckmann's pneumauxetor, only one female showed a capacity of more than 200 cubic inches, and two males were able to register more than 300 cubic inches. The majority of males fall below 250 and females 160 cubic inches. The average of over 5,000 young women at Oberlin, Wellesley and the University of Nebraska was 152 2-3 cubic inches.

The home and public school are the proper places to begin instructions in deep breathing. The first instructions to children should be how to keep healthy. Parents and teachers often, in their eagerness to develop the mental, lose sight of the physical condition of the child. I have known children kept at their tasks continually, cramming the head with book knowledge, so that by the time they were through school they were physical and nervous wrecks, upon whom tuberculosis or other diseases fastened their relentless grip, and death ended the short life of the victim. The importance of physical development is receiving attention in all the schools. The daily drill in deep breathing and lung gymnastics will accomplish much in the prevention of tuberculosis. We must begin with the children and give them better hygienic surroundings. Educate them how to grow strong bodies, not mere athletes, developed on certain lines, for it is well known that many noted athletes have died of tuberculosis, showing that a strong body without large lung capacity is not an absolute safeguard against tuberculosis.

Living in the open air and sunshine as much as possible every day helps develop a robust constitution, that is proof against tuberculosis. Especial attention must be given the skin, to keep it in the best possible condition to do its work of elimination, by proper bathing, massage, and sun or light baths direct to the skin. Good food, well prepared and properly digested, is essential to life and health. Poor digestion has much to do with the development of tuberculosis.

Children or others should never sleep in the same room with a consumptive. Neither should a room be occupied which has been occupied by a consumptive without first thorough disinfection. All clothing worn by a consumptive should be thoroughly renovated or burned; the same rule holds good in regard to bed-clothing. All sputum from consumptives should be caught in paper cups and burned.

In concluding this section of my paper I must say that I am sure it is possible, even when there is a strong predisposition to consumption, to grow strong lungs by the foregoing methods mentioned in this paper. I stand before you as an example of what continuous effort will do even where there is seeming insurmountable obstacles. My mother, two brothers and one sister died of tuberculosis. Why did they die? Because thirty-five years ago little was known about the prevention or cure of tuberculosis. I have been making the fight for more than thirty years, with stronger lungs each year, and feel sure that I shall not die of tuberculosis.

Pennell, the famous wrestler; Professor Dowd and Professor Winship, the well-known physical culturists; Dempsey and Peter Jackson, the great pugilists; Kennedy, the man who lifted 4,000 pounds a few years ago at Madison Square Garden; Nick Murphy, the world's greatest pedestrian—all died of consumption.

Climate.—The effect of climate on the cure of tuberculosis is greatly overestimated. I am sure that if we will make the most of our environment and give our patients the attention they deserve we will meet with success.

Prognosis.—Numerous sanitariums in various parts of the country claim that it is possible to cure 75 per cent. of the incipient cases, arrest the disease in 25 per cent. of the second-stage cases, and prolong the life of at least 10 per cent. of those in the third or last stage of the disease. In general practice the showing is not as good. The difficulty is in getting the case early and impressing the patient with the gravity of the disease so as to follow out a systematized method or methods of treatment. The second stage cases are rarely, if ever, permanently cured; many cases are arrested, when the patient ceases to make the fight and ultimately dies of the disease.

Treatment.—In the successful treatment of tuberculosis three things must claim the attention of the physician, viz., pure air, sunlight and good food. Strange that pure air, so essential to life, is looked upon by many as a deadly foe which must be kept out of the home, and into which they fear to go lest they take cold. Patients with diseased lungs are shallow breathers, hence enough oxygen is not taken into the lungs to aerate the blood. I find all these patients need a daily drill in deep breathing and lung gymnastics. It is not enough to tell the patient to breathe deeply, as very rarely they follow such advice. Some method of accurately measuring the amount of air taken into the lungs is a great stimulus to the patient to make greater effort. The pneumauxetor of Prof. P. Von Boeckmann is the instrument I use.

The sleeping-room of the patient should have abundant air through open windows, or, better still, sleep in a tent, with open sides in the summer and an opening at the top in winter.

Sunlight, so essential to vegetable growth, is no less so to animal life. The patient must spend much time in the sunshine. In the winter season in our climate in cloudy weather I would recommend the use of the arc light. In many cases we have pleurisy as a complication, or the onset dates back to a pleurisy with effusion or pleuritic adhesion. In all these cases the local use of a strong arc light is a successful method of treatment. The general use of the light to the entire body improves the capillary circulation and changes the aspect of the skin from a dry, scaly, atonic condition to a normal state. It also acts as a tonic, increasing metabolism and relieving internal congestions. I am using the Helios lamp made by Frank S. Betz & Co., which is easy to operate and has shown splendid results in my hands in the treatment of tuberculosis.

Food is the foundation of life, digestion and assimilation the condition of existence. No system of diet is suitable to all cases; in fact, each case is a law unto himself or herself. Milk and cream agree with some, while others cannot use them. Eggs, raw or cooked, raw beef or cooked rare, pork, fish, fowl, game, olive oil, butter, fruits, vegetables and nuts constitute a list of articles of diet best suited to cases of tuberculosis. The stomach must not be overloaded with food that cannot be digested. I have never seen any permanent results from forced feeding. Quite frequently, where the digestion is feeble, pepsin or papain can be administered with benefit. I get good results by using the juice expressed from raw vegetables, also beef juice obtained by boiling a nice piece of steak, then put into a grinder and press, and you get the greater part of the nutriment in the expressed juice.

The remedies that are of benefit in treating tuberculosis are limited in number. When the appetite is poor I have found nothing better than the elixir glycerophosphates comp., containing sodinm, calcium, manganese, iron, quinine and strychnine, giving it in teaspoonful doses every four hours. The syrup of hypophosphites, containing the same as the glycerophosphates, is much used. For chills I have found nothing better than the following: Tinct. of alstonia constricta, gtt. v to x, three times a day; or agaricin, 1-10 grain four times a day.

Olive oil is a remedy of benefit as well as a food. Its action is on mucous membrane and aids expectoration where there is extreme dryness. The dose is one to two tablespoonfuls every four to six hours.

Guaiacol carbonate is the remedy where there is high fever with rapid decline in flesh and strength. Expectoration is streaked with blood. Dose, one to five grains every three hours.

Creasote is the most abused remedy in the materia medica. It seems to be the sheet anchor of the dominant school, and the more serious the case the larger the dose. I have learned of cases taking as high as 120 drops every three hours until the patient dies, which invariably takes place. I believe it acts well in some cases in doses of gtts. ii to gtts. x every three hours, when there is diarrhea with gastro-intestinal catarrh. The cough is usually troublesome, and some means for combating it must be employed. I instruct my patients to use the will to control the cough as much as possible. A cough is a constant source of aggravation to all diseases of the lungs, and should not be encouraged by the patient. Codeine in one-eighth to one-fourth grain doses at bed time will usually control the cough.

Heroin is also valuable in doses of one-tenth grain every three hours. Ichthyol is of much benefit where the larynx is involved; it may be given in doses of gtts. ij to v every three hours. Where there is aphonia with hoarse croupal cough, the following formula used in a nebulizer is of great benefit: Ichthyol, oil stillingia, aa., oz. ss; tinct. benzoin, oz. j; alcohol, oz. ij. M.

I think it is an excellent plan to have the patient visit the office daily and take the treatment with the nebulizer. It gives the patient something to do, and the physician can give instructions in deep breathing. The treatments are curative in their effect and cannot interfere with other treatment.

Where the stomach is weak and digestion feeble I. get good results by administering tablets containing papain gr. 1, hydrastin sulph. gr. 1-10. If there is diarrhea, bismuth subnitrate, grs. v, may be added to the above with much benefit.

In conclusion, let me urge upon every physician that you make a careful study of your case. In so far as possible remove every obstacle that stands in the way of curing your patient. Do not undertake to treat a patient with uberculosis if you have made up your mind that the disease is incurable. Many cases get well after having been told by their physician that they could not get well. They had the good sense to try some one else or trust to nature, with a determination to get well.

I have seen cases get well when it seemed impossible. Let us then push forward with courage and confidence, that success may crown our efforts.

THE MODERN CONCEPTION OF TUBERCULOSIS AND ITS TREATMENT.

B. F. Lyle, M.D., Cincinnati.
Superintendent Tuberculosis Branch, Cincinnati Hospital.

So constantly do we find the lymphatics involved in tuberculosis that we may maintain it is a disease primarily of this system. This frequency of involvement is not due to any particular susceptibility, but to the fact that as the scavengers of the body and the agents for the transmission of the nutritive elements the lymphatics first come into intimate relations with the tubercle bacilli.

Tuberculous meningitis being found three times as frequently as the pulmonary form of the disease in infants, gives support to the contention of Von Behring that tuberculosis is contracted early in life by way of the intestinal tract, which at that time is deficient in the protective epithelial coats of the mucous membrane that are found later.

The fact that a large proportion of our cattle have tuberculosis, that the milk is frequently infected, that children suffer from those forms of disease that would be due to dissemination through the blood current by way of the thoracic duct, gives credibility to the theory.

The frequency of general tuberculosis, of tuberculosis of the meninges, intestines and mesenteric glands, is corroborative evidence. Holt found post-mortem evidences of tuberculosis of the lymphatic glands in a majority of children who had died of diphtheria. Northrup found the bronchial glands caseous in every one of 125 autopsies held upon tuberculous children in the Foundlings' Home. While we may regard this as evidence incriminating the lymphatics, it really shows that they have not attained the functional perfection of maturer life.

From the fifth to the fifteenth years is the period when tuberculosis is least in evidence. This is the time when the nutritive processes are most active, when the digestive and assimilative functions are not hampered by organic disease, the restraints and enervating influences of industrial and business life, or intemperance and other excesses. This exemption is due to the ability of the organism to inhibit or destroy the causative agents, and not because the sources of infection are removed.

Naegele tells us all individuals over thirty years of age are infected with tuberculosis, 96 per cent. of those between nineteen and thirty have it, that it is present in 50 per cent. of those between thirteen and nineteen, in 33 per cent. between five and thirteen, and 17 per cent. between one and five years of age.

With these statistics in mind, when we contemplate the fact that but one-seventh of the people die from the disease, we can appreciate the inherent prohibitive power mankind possesses.

Were we to rest content with these figures our purpose would not be advanced, for they do not indicate the startling fact that it is during the time of active mature life tuberculosis claims its victims, and not one-seventh, but one-third of those who fall in the age period between fifteen and fifty die of tuberculosis.

The reports in Cincinnati do not vary much from those of other places, and here we find that while the deaths from tuberculosis are only 4 per cent. of the whole in persons under fifteen, they constitute over 30 per cent. in those between fifteen and nineteen; 41 per cent. in the years twenty to twenty-nine; 33 per cent. between thirty and thirty-nine, and 22 per cent. in the fifth decade.

These figures would not be appropriate in connection with a paper dealing with the treatment of consumption did they not illustrate the influence of predisposing factors in the causation of death, and prove the soil a very essential factor in the etiology of the disease. In truth, we would be amply rewarded were we to delve still further into these figures, for we would be shown the pernicious influences of crowded and unsanitary homes and workshops, improper environment, dusty and sedentary occupations, overwork, poor food and improper cooking, poverty, ignorance, intemperance and vice.

In the majority of cases it is by way of the lymphatics the infection occurs in the lungs, and the liability to contract the disease depends upon the condition of the mucous membranes of the respiratory tract and the functional capacity of its lymphatics. If catarrhal conditions are present, the inflamed and swollen mucous membranes offer a favorable nidus for the reception of the germs, and in a small proportion of cases even a local tuberculous process may be inaugurated. In the vast majority of instances, however, the lymphatics take up the germs, destroy them, retain them, or transmit them to the lymph nodes, where they may be destroyed or remain latent until some infection such as measles, whooping-cough, typhoid fever, influenza or pneumonia causes their inflammation and injury, when the tubercle germs are enabled to renew their activity and pass on to more vital structures.

You are all doubtless familiar with instances of consumption following immediately in the wake of the diseases just mentioned. In the nodes the bacilli are usually harmless, but when they regain the lymphatics or are taken into the blood current the results of their activity are noticed in the peri-vascular or peri-bronchial lymph spaces, the vesicular walls or in close proximity to the pleura. The effort on the part of the tissues to destroy the germ leads to an inflammatory exudation about it, resulting in the so-called miliary tubercle. If the resisting power is sufficient the germ is destroyed and the exudation absorbed or converted into fibrous tissue. If this does not occur, the toxins eliminated by the germ cause a coagulation necrosis of the exudation and contiguous infiltrated tissues and a caseous mass results.

It is well for us to bear in mind that the processes occur primarily in the lung parenchyma and not in the bronchial tubes, although the small tubes may soon become involved and filled with the inflammatory exudation.

You can readily appreciate that until the tuberculous masses caseate and the calibre of the bronchial tubes is reached, no indication of tuberculosis will be shown by an examination of the sputum. This period, during which the tuberculous process is technically called "closed," is of variable length, and is accompanied by physical signs and symptoms that make the diagnosis positive. If proper treatment is now inaugurated a cure will result in the majority of cases. If the diagnosis is delayed until the microscope shows the presence of bacilli in the sputum, much valuable time is lost and the prospects of cure greatly compromised because of the mixed infection that occurs from the presence of pus-formers, influenza bacilli and pneumococci.

Physicians have not yet awakened to the fact that much of the mortality from tuberculosis is due to their lack of appreciation of the importance of early signs; for the disease is not heralded by pronounced symptoms, but is as insidious, stealthy and uncompromising in its approach as a thief in the night.

A slight lassitude, with or without loss of weight, coming on without apparent cause; inability to perform accustomed tasks without fatigue and dyspnea; possibly a slight cough in the morning and evening; a pulse more rapid than normal and a temperature slightly raised early in the afternoon, or after slight exertion, may be all that is presented besides a light dullness on percussion and prolonged expiratory sounds over a small area of an upper lobe. Possibly in addition to these physical signs a slight click may be produced by coughing. Never forget to have the patient cough, as this slight click may verify your suspicions. If in doubt still, use the thermometer and try the pulse daily. The temperature is more apt to be raised early in the afternoon than at other times of the day, but there is no definite time in the after part of the day when it may be expected.

When the diagnosis is made, immediately inaugurate measures for the cure of the patient. Approach the task confidently, for tuberculosis is curable in 85 per cent. of early cases, and the establishment of improved nutrition and its concomitant blessings the method. First take the patient into your confidence, frankly but hopefully tell him his condition, outline the treatment and endeavor to secure his cooperation, for without it a favorable result is hardly to be expected.

Have the courage of your convictions; do not suggest a cold, or bronchitis, or thin blood; but call it early consumption. If the patient is dissatisfied and goes to one less honest, the triumph of the latter will be short-lived, and you will have the satisfaction of a clear conscience, and the knowledge that the patient lacked intelligence enough to carry out the necessary measures to cure him.

If the patient is ready and willing to make the fight, the first step will be the choice of a battle ground. Shall it be away or at home? In the great majority of cases financial reasons dictate the home treatment, and I believe it will be only a short time until professional experience will also decide in its favor. The suitable climate is where the air is pure and invigorating and one can live out of doors. So long, however, as we live under the delusion that climate alone constitutes the only effective measure of combating consumption, our efforts will lack enthusiasm and our results be unsatisfactory. Frequently we hear sunshine, fresh air and good food heralded by the unsophisticated as the trinity that, unaided, can bring back the bloom of youth to the sallow cheek. Like all half-truths, this belief is apt to lead to disaster. Possible results will never be obtained until it is recognized by the profession that the physician himself is the chief factor in obtaining a favorable outcome.

What is the practice of the majority of physicians to-day after making a diagnosis of incipient consumption? The patient is left in entire or partial ignorance of his true condition, told to live out of doors as much as possible, eat good food, exercise moderately, and drop into the physician's office when anything goes wrong. He does this for a few weeks, when Neighbor Grundy recommends a positive cure, and the reign of the doctor is over.

If our clients were as intelligent on the subject of tuberculosis as they are about the treatment of typhoid fever or pneumonia, the physician who gives such advice would soon be relegated to obscurity. Can you imagine a physician retaining control of his patient if, after making a diagnosis of either of these diseases, he were to say that as they were self-limited treatment is of but little use, and if anything went wrong he was to be called?

It is not the province of the physician any more in tuberculosis than in typhoid fever or pneumonia to try to stem adverse conditions, but by careful attention to anticipate their possibility and by proper medication and advice prevent them.

Before beginning treatment the individual should be made to recognize that the cure of the disease will require many months of patient, careful adherence to all orders, and that the progress of the disease cannot be gauged by the favorable results early obtained from improved conditions. He must also be instructed to report to the physician no less than three times a week.

The first question asked is about the advisability of continuing work. When he is the breadwinner it is difficult to answer. Complete freedom from the necessity of all occupation is best, imperative if the disease has progressed beyond the incipient stage. If this is impracticable, the hours should be shortened as much as possible, and complete rest enjoined while away from work. If considerable muscular effort is demanded or the shop is dark, damp or dusty, lighter work under favorable conditions must be secured. It must be accepted that absolute quietness is essential, and any digression can be permitted only when the disease is not active. This will be indicated by the temperature and pulse. A temperature above 100° or a pulse above 100 during rest makes quiet imperative. When the former ranges between 99° and 100° or the latter is above 90, care should be exercised, and if effort is accompanied by a considerable rise of temperature or acceleration of pulse, it should be curtailed or entirely abandoned. Exercise when the disease is active increases the inflammation about the areas involved and thus extends the trouble.

Investigation has also shown that the opsonic index presents a continuous negative phase in such cases, probably caused by the liberation of toxins into the general circulation. The conditions generated are very similar to those following the injection of a test dose of tuberculin.

We should always endeavor to limit excessive inflammatory exudation and infiltration of contiguous tissue in order that a conservative fibrosis be established.

I shall not consume your time with the details of methods of securing sunshine, fresh air and good food. They are imperatively necessary. Shacks are to be preferred to tents, because they are dry, more cheerful and can be better ventilated. If they cannot be secured, a porch can be arranged to answer the purpose, or even a structure erected upon the roof. In their absence a window tent will fulfill the indications fairly well.

The patient must be enjoined to breathe fresh air at all times, the fact being emphasized that the air in the house can never be as good as that out of doors. Living outside does not mean that the patient should be cold; woolen clothing and blankets should be thick and abundant, and comfort insured by hot water bottles or other devices for heating.

Careful attention must be given the dietary. Food must be plain, abundant and properly cooked and served. Crisp bacon and good butter are preferable to cod liver oil. Whisky, wines and other forms of alcohol have no place; the journey is a long one, and a goad increases the exhaustion.

Breakfast should consist of fruits (oranges, bananas, small fruits, cooked apples), bacon, broiled steak or lamb chops, toast, coffee and milk. Eggs prepared in various ways may also be given.

Luncheon at 11 A.M. and 4 P.M. Cold meats, raw eggs prepared with various disguises, crackers, cocoa or chocolate, milk, lemonade or orangeade.

Dinner should be served at mid-day, and the patient enjoined to lie down for one or two hours after. It should consist of soup, fish or oysters, roast fowl, lamb or beef, two vegetables, a salad and a simple dessert.

Supper should not be substantial—cold meats, broiled chops, cereals, potatoes, rice, stewed fruit, bread, tea, coffee and milk.

At night when the patient is restless or coughs, a glass of hot milk sipped slowly enables him to secure rest.

I shall not trespass further upon your time and patience by indicating the medicinal treatment of the disease. Medicines still play an important rôle in assisting to correct the anemia, quieting the cough, helping the weak digestive functions, and promoting the welfare of the patient in many ways.

Local treatment is almost as important. The application of mild antiseptics and anodynes to the nose, throat and larynx relieve congested conditions, promote proper breathing, lessen expectoration, and quiet cough. Counter-irritants to the chest relieve pain and promote absorption of inflammatory exudations, and plasters properly applied cause relief in pleurisy by fixing the chest wall.

I wish again to bring to your attention the important position the physician occupies in the treatment of tuberculosis, and I crave your indulgence if I transgress by asking you to avail yourselves at all times of the services of three eminent old-school physicians—Doctor Diet, Doctor Quiet, and Hope in the person of Doctor Merryman.

TREATMENT OF PULMONARY TUBERCULOSIS,

M. H. HENNEL, M.D., ASHEVILLE, N. C.

As about one-seventh of the deaths produced by disease in the United States are caused either directly or indirectly by tuberculosis, it behooves us to devote our most careful attention to its prevention and cure. It is the most universal disease known, occurring in all countries, at all times and seasons and among all races. The discovery of Koch in 1881 of the tubercle bacillus probably marks one of the greatest epochs in medical science. It definitely establishes the germ origin of tuberculosis. It proves the limitations of its infectiousness from man to man by means of sputum, the fallacy of heredity, the positiveness of the tuberculin test in man and beast, and the possibility of prophylaxis. That tuberculosis is a curable disease cannot be denied. Statistics made from post-mortems have proven that a large per cent. of all adults have had the disease without their knowledge of having had it. Naegele, in his statistics made from five hundred cases at autopsy, says recognizable tuberculosis lesions were found in 98 per cent. The significance of this in showing the ability of the human body to resist the disease is very important, and it definitely proves that tuberculosis is *controllable, arrestable* and *curable*. One of the great drawbacks in the past has been the lack, and, in many cases the negligibility, in making an early diagnosis and the instituting of proper treatment, before the ravages of the disease have so impaired the system as to make an arrest and cure impossible. It is surprising to know the number of patients that are sent to our different health resorts annually, that are told by their physicians that they have just a slight bronchial affection and that their lungs are somewhat weak; that what they need is a change of climate, live out of doors, breathe the fresh air, eat good nutritious foods and take plenty of out-door exercise; when the true facts of the case are, they are in the advanced stage of consumption. A cure is impossible, and an arrestment of the disease is questionable and very remote. When the general practitioner—that is, the family physician—shall recognize the importance of an early diagnosis, and will act at once and will institute such changes in the patient's mode of living, his surroundings, climate and treatment, to prevent the further ravages of the disease, then tuberculosis will be looked upon as one of the most curable of chronic diseases. But so long as early suspected cases are allowed to drift along in an indifferent manner, living in surroundings polluted with tuberculous germs, coughing and expectorating indiscriminately, endangering everybody with whom they come in contact, just so long will the present high mortality be maintained.

Knowing the prevalence of this disease, the physician should ever be on his guard, ready to detect it, if possible, in its earliest incipiency. Should any doubt exist the tuberculin test should be used. If properly administered, it is perfectly safe, and can be relied upon as a diagnostic agent. The physician should have a plain, candid talk with his patient. He should tell him that he has tuberculosis or consumption; that these cases, when not too far advanced, are arrestable and curable, but that a cure largely depends upon the patient himself. If he wishes to get well he must make a business of it. Many of the things he has done in the past, he may have to give up. He will have to avoid indiscretions and lead a model life. Unless he is willing to do that, the chances of a cure are against him. Having gotten the patient's consent, treatment may be outlined and adapted to the particular case in hand.

There are two lines of treatment that have met with a fair degree of success in this disease, viz., the hygienic dietetic treatment and the specific or tuberculin treatment. The former should be applied in all cases, but with the latter there may be certain conditions that may contraindicate its use—hence, great care should be exercised in selecting tuberculin cases. The ideal surroundings and conditions for a patient, whether in a sanatorium, in a boarding-house or in his own home, are as follows: His quarters should be free from dust, properly sheltered from inclement weather, but admit of many hours daily in the open air, if very ill, lying upon a cot or reclining chair. His bedroom must be well ventilated, the windows being let down from the top, but drafts should be avoided. A room with a southern and western exposure is to be preferred, as this insures the greatest amount of light and sunshine. It should be uncarpeted, free from hangings, and kept scrupulously clean. The bed should be well furnished. It should have a good cotton, felt or hair mattress. The cover should not be too heavy, but warm. During the winter small woolen blankets are indispensable. All sputum should be collected in paper inset cups or pocket cuspidors and burned daily or oftener if necessary, thus obviating all danger of infection. If the patient's means will permit, a change of climate may be advised, as a change of air, scenery, diet, water and social surroundings, when properly selected, all have a tonic or upbuilding effect. The chief requisites in selecting a climate for the tuberculous are pure dry air with sufficient rainfall only to lay the dust, thus insuring the greatest number of days of sunshine, and a temperature which does not vary too much or too suddenly between day and night; sunlight and shade, so that the patient can live out of doors the greater portion of his time.

Diet.—Diet is one of the most important factors in the treatment. This is a wasting disease. If we wish to stay its progress and cure the patient, we must see that the supply of nutrition taken up by the system is greater than that consumed by the ravages of the disease, or our battle is lost. This necessitates taking an extra supply of properly selected foods and assimilating the same. We should select those foods that are rich in proteids and fats; are easily digested and assimilated; are not too bulky and do not form too much residue. It can be readily seen that milk, eggs and wholesome animal foods rank first among the chief articles of diet. The average patient should take from five to eight raw eggs a day, about three pints of good fresh milk, plenty of nutritious red meats, and as much other foods as are relished. This may seem like overtaxing the digestive organs, but if taken systematically, in a large per cent. of cases, it will be digested and assimilated and the patient will begin to take on flesh.

The meals should be eaten at regular intervals and a light luncheon consisting of a raw egg and a glass of milk may be served at 11 A.M., 4 P.M., and at bedtime. It is surprising how quickly the system adapts itself to this forced feeding and the relish with which it can be taken. The elimination should be carefully looked after. If the milk constipates, an occasional dose of castor oil, or some other mild laxative, should be used. The addition of a little lime-water or phosphate of soda to the milk acts admirably. When the eggs cause biliousness and intestinal trouble, this may be obviated by dropping a few drops of lemon juice or vinegar upon them before taking. The patient should be instructed to keep the teeth perfectly clean, as there is nothing that causes the tongue to become coated and the appetite impaired more quickly than to allow milk to remain upon the teeth and undergo fermentation. The teeth should also be carefully looked after, as good mastication is essential to good digestion.

Exercise and Rest.—This is a matter that must be largely governed by the condition of the patient. It is a safe rule to follow not to allow patients to exercise when their temperature reaches at any time during the day 100°, when there is active softening going on in the lung tissue, and in hemorrhagic cases so long as the sputum is tinged with blood and for forty-eight hours thereafter. Where the patient runs no temperature and where there is no active process going on in the lungs and other conditions are favorable, a certain amount of out-door exercise may be allowed, and in some instances light out-door employment may be recommended, but in no case should exercise be carried to the degree of bodily fatigue or exhaustion. When the tuberculous process in the lung is active, and the patient is running temperature, exercise is to be restricted and in nearly all cases prohibited until after fever subsides. During the day the patient should rest in a reclining position upon a cot or reclining chair in the open air, as this favors, directly and indirectly, an arrestment of the trouble. The chief aim in treatment should be to avoid as much as possible the use of drugs, and to apply rules of hygiene for the object of both local and general nutrition. Our old lauded preparations, creosote and its derivatives, cod liver oil, Fowler's solution, iron and alcohol, do not occupy the reputed places they formerly did in this disease. True, there are some cases in which they may be prescribed with benefit, but there can be no question but that their indiscriminate use in the past have been productive of more harm than good. Drugs should not be taken except when specifically indicated, and then only when absolutely necessary to meet complications that arise during the progress of the disease.

Pleurisy.—This is frequently met with in pulmonary tuberculosis.

If there is high fever, aconite and veratrum may be indicated. For the sharp lancinating pain, bryonia and asclepias may be thought of. Locally, strapping the chest, libradol and counter-irritation are beneficial.

Pulmonary Hemorrhage.—If the hemorrhage is active, atropine, morphine and nitroglycerine are among our best remedies. Strapping the chest and the application of the ice bag over the heart are beneficial. In passive hemorrhages calcium chloride, ipecac, oil of erigeron and carbo-vegetabilis may be thought of. If calcium chloride is used, it should be given in ten- or fifteen-grain doses for a few doses until the hemorrhage checks, but should not be continued too long, as its first effects are to stop the bleeding, but if continued for a long time it seems to lessen the coagulability of the blood and favor hemorrhage. Chloride of sodium or common salt is an old household remedy that acts admirably in some cases. I think it is well to advise hemorrhagic cases to carry a paper of salt in the pocket to be used in case of hemorrhage until other means, if necessary, can be procured. In all cases of pulmonary hemorrhage the patient should remain quiet in a recumbent position for forty-eight hours after all blood has disappeared from the sputum.

Cough.—As this is nature's method of throwing off the effete tubercular material from the lungs, medicine should not be used to check it unless it becomes extremely harassing, stirring up latent pleurisies, hemorrhage, etc., then some indicated remedy should be prescribed to lessen the cough till these symptoms subside. We have two coughs in pulmonary tuberculosis. The purposeful cough, one that is necessary in order to throw off the tuberculous or effete material from the lung, and the purposeless cough, a cough that is unnecessary and accomplishes nothing. The former needs no medication, as it will subside as the tuberculous condition becomes better. The latter accomplishes nothing and should be stopped. Try to determine the cause and apply such means and medication as may be necessary to stop it.

Fever.—This is a symptom produced by the absorption of toxic material, and is generally found during the active state of the disease. It comes on during the afternoon and evening, lasts for a time and then subsides. Antipyretics should not be given, as they do not remove the cause, and beyond a doubt do positive harm. If the patient's temperature goes up to 100° or above, he should be instructed to lie down and keep quiet. This will shorten the duration of the fever.

Night-sweats.—Under proper hygienic, dietetic treatment these will be greatly lessened and many times entirely arrested, but in advanced cases, where the patient is greatly weakened, medication may be used with advantage. A dose of atropine, 1-12 grain given at bedtime, or camphoric acid in ten-grain doses act nicely. Zinc oxide, aromatic sulphuric acid, and a number of other drugs may also be thought of. An alcohol rub at bedtime is beneficial. A little quinine added to the alcohol also has a tonic effect upon the skin. The patient should be instructed to get a fever thermometer and taught how to use it. The temperature should be taken every two to four hours during the day, and the same recorded in a record-book, of which I shall speak later. If he is running no temperature this is not necessary. I am aware that some physicians take exception to this, claiming that the patient taking his own temperature has a depressing effect, but clinical experience does not bear this out. In fact, the patient soon learns to know that the thermometer is his safest guide. He should be told that fever is caused by the absorption of toxic material due to some active process in the lung. That he should take no exercise when his temperature reaches 100° or above, and keep quiet in a recumbent position until the fever subsides. This will prevent his committing many indiscretions that he might otherwise commit were he not to use the thermometer.

Record-Book.—It is the duty of every physician who devotes his attention to the treatment of pulmonary tuberculosis to furnish his patient with a record-book, instruct him how to keep it and see that he does so. This enables a physician to keep a daily tab of his patient. The record-book gotten up by Dr. W. L. Dunn, of Asheville, is one of the best I have seen. It is compact, yet complete and easily kept. It is a small booklet just large enough for a month's record. It can be gotten up by any printer and is not expensive. At the end of each month the patient is instructed to turn this book over to the doctor and receive a new one. These records are filed away for future reference.

Cold Bath.—For those cases that are not too far advanced and are endowed with sufficient vitality, a cold sponge-bath over the chest and spine is beneficial. It should be taken in a warm room and followed by a brisk rubbing with a good flesh towel. It acts as a tonic and lessens the tendency to catch cold. It should not be used where the reaction following its use is not good, where the patient feels weakened and depressed after taking it.

The Specific or Tuberculin Treatment.—This was introduced by Koch in 1890, and was received with the utmost enthusiasm, but like many other great discoveries it was doomed to disappointment. This can now be easily accounted for. Being an exceptionally potent preparation it required a great deal of clinical experience and careful study in order to determine its true value. At first, it was given in doses entirely too large and to cases in which it was positively contraindicated. As a natural result, it many times produced physiological effects that were not only unpleasant but disastrous. Many of those who had used it and gotten such dire results were ready to rush into print with their condemnations, attributing all their failures to tuberculin and not to their lack of knowledge of when and how to use it. Tuberculin was soon abandoned and for a long time was considered as so dangerous that its use was looked upon as akin to malpractice. Trudeau says "that so general and bitter was its condemnation that between 1891 and 1900 it was with the utmost difficulty that he could persuade a few patients at the Adirondack Cottage Sanitarium each year to take the treatment while in the institution." However, it remained for a few faithful students to carry on the good work despite the protestations of the profession. It is gratifying to know that their efforts have been crowned with success. They have demonstrated to the world that it is not only a positive diagnostic agent, but that when indicated and given in proper medicinal doses it has a decided effect toward the arrestment and cure of the disease. Allow me to quote from Trudeau's article read before the American Congress of Tuberculosis in 1906 in which he compares 185 patients treated and 864 untreated. He says, "there have been excluded all who stayed at the sanitarium less than ninety days and all that did not have tubercle bacilli on admission. The following percentages have been calculated on the basis of an equal number of treated and untreated patients in each year.

| | Incipient. | | | Advanced. | | |
	Apparently Cured.	Disease Arrested.	Active.	Apparently Cured.	Disease Arrested.	Active.
Treated	56 p. c.	34 p. c.	10 p. c.	27 p. c.	55 p. c.	18 p.c.
Untreated ...	50 p. c.	38 p. c.	11 p. c.	6 p. c.	51 p. c.	43 p. c.

After making an allowance for the uncertainties of sputum examinations and misleading sources of error in compiling such statistics he says:

"The study of post discharge mortality would seem to promise more satisfactory and conclusive evidence. Through carelessness we may fail to find bacilli, though they may be present, and we may all differ as to whether a patient at discharge is 'apparently cured' or the disease 'arrested,' but there can be no doubt as to whether the patient be living or dead. Besides, the object of sanitarium treatment is not the condition of the patient at discharge, but the prolongation of his life, and time must be the crucial test of treatment. A comparison of 135 patients treated and 690 untreated discharged from the institution in the past fifteen years reveal the following (equal numbers of treated and untreated patients are considered; all patients that stayed less than three months, all who left the sanitarium less than one year ago, and all untraced patients have been excluded) :"

	Incipient.		Advanced.	
	Living.	Dead.	Living.	Dead.
Tuberculin treated	79 p. c.	21 p. c.	61 p. c.	39 p. c.
Untreated	63 p. c.	37 p. c.	36 p. c.	64 p. c.

Should not these statistics convince the most skeptical?

I am aware that I am treading upon dangerous ground when I advocate the use of tuberculin, as many of the members of the profession have been bitterly opposed to it. But, gentlemen, my observations and practical experience during the past three years at Asheville have convinced me of its virtues. If we believe in specific medication and in choosing the best from all sources, we must accept tuberculin. It is just as much of a specific for tuberculous conditions when indicated, as many of our old lauded preparations are for the conditions for which they are prescribed. Those wishing to acquaint themselves with some of the different tuberculins, their indications, uses and contraindications, are referred to Dr. Lawrason Brown's article in Osler's "Modern Medicine," Vol. 3. Dr. Brown has had an excellent opportunity of studying tuberculin and testing its virtues and has presented the subject in an able, concise, and scholarly manner, so that it can be readily comprehended by any student of medicine. It should, however, be borne in mind that the hygienic, dietetic treatment should not be neglected, even when the tuberculin is administered.

While much has been accomplished in the prevention and cure of this disease during the past fifteen years, yet let us not relax our energies until we have succeeded in robbing the "great white plague" of its terrors, and educating the people how to prevent it.

PHYSICAL METHODS IN THE TREATMENT OF TUBERCULOSIS.

OTTO JUETTNER, M.D., CINCINNATI.

In attempting to present to you a general résumé of the clinical possibilities of physical therapeutic methods, I could not possibly find a subject in the whole range of practical medicine that yields as good and as frequent opportunities for illustration along the lines mentioned as that of lung-consumption. Tuberculosis has for some years past claimed the lion's share of professional interest and is growing in its therapeutic and more especially in its prophylactic aspects more and more. In a sense, it has grown beyond the sphere of the practicing physician. Its rational treatment is not so much a question of therapy as it is one of sanitation. The questions involved in the proper handling of the individual patient are of small importance compared to the management of the economic problems to which the hygienic errors in the life of the human family under perverted conditions of modern existence constantly give rise, problems of habitation, of feeding, of air, of light, of cleanliness, of exercise, in fact, of all those factors upon which the healthy development of the human body depends. An animal body that is compelled to vegetate under conditions created by improper or insufficient food, foul air, scant sunlight, unclean surroundings, lack of physiological exercise, must necessarily deteriorate in its quality. Regeneration of the tissues and fluids of the body is incomplete and imperfect because of the absence or scant supply of the elements out of which and by means of which nature creates new tissues and new fluids. The body lives *on* in an auto-toxic condition, unable to rid itself of waste or supply itself with the physiological necessities of life and health. Insufficient skin activity, imperfect oxidation of the red corpuscles, retarded metabolism and general malnutrition prepare the soil upon which the tubercle bacillus grows. In the offspring that comes from the miserable stock which is bred under the wretched conditions I have referred to, the culture-bed for scavengers of the anerobic type, like the bacillus of Koch, need not be prepared. It is practically ready when the miserable specimen of the genus "homo" is put into the world. The soil upon which the destructive germ grows and thrives, and the economic conditions which prepare this soil, represent the tuberculosis problem of to-day. Ten or fifteen years ago it was the bacillus that occupied the center of the stage. To-day we assign to the bacillus *per se* but little significance. We are concerned about the natural means and weapons of defense which the normal animal body possesses and by means of which it sustains itself. Our interest to-day centers in the knowledge of the biologic elements which constitute the resisting power of the organism, or, if you please, its opsonic index. The ravages of the bacillus are in inverse ratio to the fighting quality of the organism. Increase of the one presupposes diminution of the other. This is the standpoint of the modern physio-therapeutist in connection with the therapy of tuberculosis.

If you were to ask me which of all the natural therapeutic agents I consider the most vital and most essential in the treatment and cure of consumption, I would most emphatically say light. Compared to light all else dwindles into insignificance. When I say light I practically include fresh air, because there is no such a thing as fresh air without light. Moses tells us that when the Universe in response to the will of its Creator was evolved out of eternal chaos, the first creative act was inspired by a command that emanated from the mind of the Divine Architect—Let there be light! Thus he prepared the condition which made life possible. The first and supreme command of the physician who is facing the problem of tuberculosis in one of his patients should be a repetition of those words that banished darkness and death and created light and life.

What does light mean to the animal economy? First of all, light controls the intake of oxygen and the output of carbonic acid gas. During the day the amount of oxygen which is assimilated by the human body is between 20 and 30 per cent. greater than during the night. This means that during the hours of imperfect or no illumination the retention of waste is more or less well marked. Some physiologists even consider the phenomenon of sleep as being a product of carbon dioxide retention and coincident poisoning of certain nerve centers. When the amount of light to which the body-surface is or ought to be exposed is reduced, there is at once a diminution in the manufacture of coloring matter in the blood-cells, hemoglobin. The hemoglobin of all warm-blooded animals is a biologic derivative whose extraction and deposition depends on the light of the sun. In this respect it is analogous to chlorophyll or vegetable coloring matter, which likewise is a product of solar radiation. Plants that are reared and raised in dark places are practically colorless. The human body that is deprived of its physiological amount of light, also loses its color by a gradual diminution in the coloring matter of its blood-cells. Since it is the blood coloring matter that carries the oxygen, it stands to reason that the body loses its oxygen-carrying power in proportion to the degree of reduction of its hemoglobin. Without hemoglobin to take up and carry oxygen it is worthless to attempt oxygenation. The physician who is making his patient inhale oxygen from an oxygen-tank or ozone from one of those pretentious-looking ozone-generators that are attached to static machines, is wasting his own time and that of his patient, unless the latter has had a chance to increase his capacity for oxygen. In order to accomplish this, let there be *light!* Finsen has shown us that it is principally the chemical rays of sunlight that have a characteristic affinity for oxygen. Finsen's cure of lupus by applications of actinic rays dwindles into insignificance when we think of the incomparable fitness and efficacy of these rays of light in the treatment of tuberculosis pulmonum. The true greatness of Finsen's work lies in the establishment of a scientific principle which makes sunlight, or, rather, the actinic rays of sunlight, the eternal and universal specific in the treatment of consumption. The sunbath is *the* great remedy in the management of tuberculosis. Sunlight in cases of tuberculosis is more important than air. It should be applied persistently to the nude body of the consumptive, either directly or in a solarium, or in arc-light cabinet, which, however, at best, is a poor substitute for the genuine article. I beg to emphasize that the whole body of the patient must be exposed, without the intervention of even one layer of clothing. Then only is it possible to produce the effects on metabolism, which increased excretory and respiratory skin function is capable of causing. This is the Finsen idea in its last consequences. The tendency of to-day is to divorce the tubercular patient from ill-ventilated dwellings and place him where the air is fresh and oxygen copious. Let us go one step further and divorce the consumptive from clothes of any and all sorts and expose his skin to the light. To put the patient in a pure and rich atmosphere is comparatively of little value if the patient does not possess the power of assimilating oxygen through his lungs. This power is wonderfully increased by acting upon the metabolic machinery of the whole organism through the surface of the body. Most of us are liable to forget that the skin is equal in physiological importance to any structure or organ in the body. We breathe through the skin, the output of body heat and waste products of combustion is controlled by the skin, the "tone" of the nervous system, especially the sensory system, is preserved by the impingement of actinic and luminous rays on the nerve supply of the cuticle, the oxygen-carrying power of the blood is enhanced by the pigmentation which takes place in the blood-cells in and beneath the surface. Let me make this plea on behalf of the sunbath as the necessary foundation of all rational therapy in the treatment of consumption. It is the logical beginning of physical therapy in these cases.

In connection with this subject let me add that the notorious frequency of tuberculosis in the negro is attributed to the pigment in the negro's skin, which prevents the entrance of the actinic rays and deprives the body of the negro of the germicidal effect of transillumination of this kind.

Effects similar to those of light exposures but of much less intensity are produced by certain electro-therapeutic methods. The so-called high-frequency current applied to the whole body by means of a suitably constructed cylinder in which the entire body is placed, affects the oxygen-supply and the hemoglobin-production in a very characteristic manner, as shown by the physiological experiments made by d'Arsonval. The magnetic wave-radiators which have recently been brought to the notice of the profession produce similar effects. In connection with this subject it is interesting to know that the tubercle bacillus is readily affected by these radiations of high-tension energy. A culture of tubercle bacilli is quickly rendered inert or killed by concentrated chemical rays. A high-frequency current will produce the same result after prolonged suspension of the culture in the magnetic field of an Oudin resonator.

The question of rendering the bacillary cause of the disease inactive or of destroying it entirely, suggests itself as an important step in the treatment of tuberculosis. The bacillus thrives in lungs which are badly nourished. The less fresh air and rich arterial blood find their way into any particular part of the lung, the better are the chances for rapid and prolific growth of the germ. The oxygen in the air and in the blood is the natural enemy of the bacillus. A most important therapeutic indication is, therefore, the necessity of pure oxygen-laden air. In order, however, to become a powerful therapeutic factor the air must have a chance to enter the lungs, particularly those secreted and distant portions where the bacillus has found lodgment and thrives. The tuberculous patient's respiratory movements are shallow and do not expand the lungs as they should in order to aerate the infected portions. Consequently it is of importance to adopt measures which will deepen the respiratory movements. To encourage the patients to breathe slowly ·and deeply, especially out-of-doors, is of course of great value. The effect can be many times enhanced if additional care is taken to develop the muscular cover of the chest and to render the bony framework more elastic. In suitable cases the effect of procedures of this kind is well-nigh miraculous. These therapeutic methods are classified under the head of mechano-therapy, particularly massage and Swedish movements.

In order to understand the therapeutic value of massage it is proper to acquire the manual dexterity which alone enables us to form any opinion as to the possibilities of mechanical therapeutic methods. To manipulate the muscles of the chest-wall means to increase the blood-supply, to develop them, to render them stronger and more active. This, in and of itself, means more vigorous respiration, especially if the mobility of the thorax proper has been increased. These effects should be aimed at in all cases of lung-consumption, especially during the early stages. The *modus operandi* is subject to variation owing to peculiarities of individual cases. In a general way the following suggestions will be found applicable to most cases:

The patient being placed in the dorsal decubitus the operator begins the manipulation over the costal border, gently picking up between his fingers a fold of skin and subcutaneous tissue, lifting it from the bony structures beneath and gently kneading it between his fingers. Most patients will be found to be "hide-bound," the soft tissues of the chest-wall being very tense and hard to raise. Eventually, *i.e.*, after repeated sittings, the fold of skin will come up with comparative ease. This manipulation requires all possible patience and gentleness. Lack of delicacy would be worse than worthless. Gradually the manipulation is extended over the whole chest. This form of massage may be followed by gentle stroking in a horizontal direction. Each sitting should last from fifteen to thirty minutes, to be repeated after twenty-four hours. Within a weak or two the muscles of the chest will be less tense and probably a trifle fuller. At this juncture exercise of the thorax might be begun. The operator places his flat hand over the right or left side of the patient's chest, making firm and gradually increasing pressure. The result will be a partial immobilization of a portion of the chest. If the patient is told to breathe deeply, the effect on the unengaged side of the chest will be more or less intense. The patient will expand the unengaged side of the chest more than he would without immobilization of the other side. The operator may alternately place his hand on one and the other side. He may vary the procedure by placing both hands on the lower portion of the thorax over the last three ribs, thus forcing the patient to expand the upper portions of the chest vigorously. In this way the expansive power of the chest can' be increased considerably, rendering inhalation of fresh air a therapeutic factor of prime value. In applying these mechanical methods to individual cases, much depends upon the judgment and the individualizing faculty of the physician. With proper care and judgment an immeasurable amount of good may be derived from manipulations of this kind.

In regard to the *dietetic* management of tubercular cases many physicians adhere to errors of routine and tradition. The enforcement of a rich nitrogenous regime is of doubtful propriety. Most tubercular patients live in a condition of low auto-intoxication. Their digestive and assimilative powers are greatly impaired. The night-sweats of phthisis are distinctly an effort on the part of nature to relieve a toxic condition. We can anticipate and imitate nature's method by feeding an excess of carbohydrates to prevent the formation of toxines, and by stimulating and regulating excretion, especially through the skin. The electric light bath and various hydro-therapeutic applications are useful for this purpose. A vigorous and active skin in a tubercular patient is a splendid prognostic sign. One of the best and most useful articles of diet in ordinary tubercular cases is butter-milk. It was enthusiastically recommended by Schoenlein seventy-five years ago, and I assure you it has lost none of its quality. As a regulator of skin-function in connection with the heat-output of the organism and the cutaneous exchange of gases, the sunlight, as I have already indicated, is of cardinal efficacy. In order to give it a chance to display its remarkable curative properties, it will be necessary for our patients to return to the primitive conditions of Adam and Eve, as far as clothes are concerned. Those of you who believe in the blood-making quality of iron and are in the habit of administering the latter will be interested in the statement that exposure of the patient's body to sunlight for hours after iron has been administered will enhance the effect of the ferruginous substance. By its intense oxidizing action the actinic light of the sun facilitates the change of metallic iron into blood-iron.

The relation of hydrotherapy to the treatment of consumption is so vast a subject that I cannot more than merely mention it on this occasion and reserve a more extended discussion of it until such a time when I shall again have an opportunity to appear before you in re- sponse to an invitation, provided I am again made the recipient of the distinguished honor which I have received at your hands to-day, for which I am thoroughly grateful. Physio-therapy, whose humble, yet proud champion I am, has become a part of the therapeutic resources of all progressive physicians. It does not wish to displace the achievements of the past or monopolize the whole field of clinical medicine. It wishes to add to the sum-total of our knowledge in the interests of scientific progress and for the benefit of our suffering fellow-man. To heal the sick and to comfort the afflicted, to serve the purposes of the broadest humanity, that is the one point upon which the true physicians of all schools are united. To render the best service to our suffering brother, to add your conscience as well as your knowledge to your work, to accept the good wherever you find it, to embrace the whole world in your heart and the whole truth in your brain, this is what constitutes the real physician of to-day. This is true science, true humanity, true eclecticism.

SANATORIA AND HOSPITALS FOR THE CURE AND PREVENTION OF TUBERCULOSIS.

C. O. PROBST, M.D., COLUMBUS, O.
Secretary State Board of Health.

Now that Ohio stands committed to the support of a State sanatorium, and also for county hospitals for tuberculosis, I thought it might be of interest to consider some of the questions relating to such institutions as factors in the cure and prevention of tuberculosis.

If we are to receive the greatest possible benefit from our State sanatorium it is essential that certain features of sanatorium management be closely followed.

In the beginning, I might state that the Ohio sanatorium is to be located two miles from Mt. Vernon. A beautiful tract of three hundred and fifty-five acres of land has been purchased. There is practically a virgin forest of about one hundred and twenty-five acres crowning a high, sandy hill. The building site is sheltered to the north, north-east and north-west by this hill and forest. There are two magnificent springs of pure, cold water. One of these furnishes 175,000 gallons of water a day, sufficient in itself for all purposes. There is an abundant supply of natural gas, thus doing away with all smoke. There are no nearby highways to pollute the air with dust. Most of the soil is fertile and suitable for a variety of crops.

The Administration Block, comprising practically four buildings in one, is nearing completion. The legislature appropriated $350,000 to complete the institution for one hundred beds. The sanatorium is planned to never exceed two hundred beds. If there should be a demand for a much larger institution, it will be better for several weighty reasons to build another sanatorium and separate the sexes.

When completed for two hundred beds there will be the administration block, two reception cottages, six shacks or sleeping pavilions, an infirmary, a power plant and laundry, a superintendent's residence, an employees' cottage, and, in addition, several farm buildings.

Before proceeding to discuss in some detail sanatorium management and methods, we should have clearly before us the functions of a sanatorium. It is something much more than merely a favorable place to send a few early cases of tuberculosis to be cured. Its influence both for the cure and prevention of this disease should be felt in every home in Ohio.

In the first place, the sanatorium must be made to demonstrate that tuberculosis can be cured in Ohio. I have faith that it will prove that as large a percentage of selected cases can be cured in Ohio as anywhere else. This demonstration is needed for both the profession and the laity. While there has been a remarkable change in medical opinion as regards the effects of certain climatic conditions in the cure of this disease, there remains a large number of practitioners who still act upon the assumption that the Ohio climate is not to be depended upon in applying modern methods of treatment. The laity is even more in need of being shown and convinced that the chance of cure here are as good as elsewhere.

Without going into the subject of climatology, I may say that while recognizing that a limited number of cases, for special reason may be benefited by a change to some other climate, I would maintain that in the general run of cases the fresh-air treatment will give just as good results here as elsewhere.

Looking upon the sanatorium, then, as an educational institution, and not merely for the patients who go there, but for the profession and all our people, special points in its construction and management become of great interest. You will realize at once that with this end in view it is of the utmost importance that the percentage of cures for patients sent there should be as high as possible. It was this consideration that settled the size of the institution. It is the testimony of all managers of sanatoria that the best possible results are obtainable in small institutions. In the first place, there is then possible greater individualism in treatment. This is absolutely essential in this disease, no two cases of which are likely to require exactly the same management. We all know the tendency to ruts and routine in public institutions, and this is to be avoided as far as possible in sanatoria. In the next place, only favorable cases should be received if high percentages of cure are to be obtained.

With the many thousands of cases of tuberculosis in Ohio the public will doubtless think that two hundred beds will care for a very small part of those who would go there. The experience of other sanatoria shows this not to be true. The New York sanatorium at Ray Brook, for instance, with one hundred and seventy-two beds, has had to have many of these vacant or receive unfavorable cases. The same difficulty has been met with at other institutions.

There are various reasons for this. A patient with incipient tuberculosis is still active and able to work. If the support of his family depends upon his daily wage he will seldom go to the sanatorium early in his disease unless his family can be temporarily cared for. Here, indeed, is a serious problem that must be met. The State, or organized charity, must help such a family if the bread-winner is to be saved and returned to work.

Another reason for expecting a limited number of applicants is that the sanatorium is not free. A charge of five dollars per week is to be made. This is the practice in other States, and has been found desirable as a means for securing a better class of patients. In some States this weekly charge may be paid from the county or municipal poor fund, where the patient is unable to pay. It has been thought desirable in Ohio to provide for a limited number of suitable destitute patients in another way. The board of trustees, upon the recommendation of the superintendent, are authorized to receive not to exceed 10 per cent. of the total possible number of patients for any sum *less* than five dollars that they may deem proper, after investigation. We shall doubtless find, then, as others have found, that the State sanatorium need not be a large institution if limited, as it should be, to incipient cases.

I think it will be shown that the sanatorium will have great influence in the cure of patients in Ohio who are not treated in the sanatorium. If the results are what we may expect, it will undoubtedly lead to the proper home treatment, under intelligent medical supervision, of a large number who now, by advice of physician or friend, seek a cure in other climes.

For the selection of suitable cases it is proposed to appoint a sufficient number of skilled diagnosticians in convenient localities in the State. These will make the first examination and send in their reports. If favorably acted upon, the patient may come to the sanatorium for a final examination.

The law regulating the sanatorium provides that each patient so admitted is to be accepted for a four-weeks' trial. If found to be a suitable case for sanatorium treatment at the end of this trial period, he is regularly admitted; if not, he is sent home. This is a new feature in sanatorium management, and those familiar with the uncertainties of this disease will recognize the great importance of being thus able to select cases most likely to favorably respond to sanatorium treatment. In four weeks' time this can usually be established.

In this connection we may speak of another new feature of the Ohio sanatorium adopted to fit into this plan for the selection of desirable cases. Two reception cottages are to be constructed, one for males and one for females. The patients admitted on trial will probably spend their four weeks' probation in these cottages. These are planned for either in-door or out-door sleeping. They each contain twenty-four single bedrooms opening onto a convenient veranda facing south. The outer bedroom door is wide enough to permit the bed to be rolled to this protected sleeping porch. The bedrooms are to be moderately heated, but are to be given the freest possible cross-ventilation. Each .new patient can therefore be kept indoors or out of doors according to season and individual requirements.

While possibly no harm may result from abruptly plunging a patient into out-door life with zero temperatures, any one of us, I fancy, would prefer an opportunity for acclimatization, as here provided.

At the end of the four weeks, if found advisable, the accepted patient will be sent to one of the shacks, where all must sleep out of doors at all times.

It is not only essential from all standpoints that the greatest number possible be sent home cured, as this term is generally understood, but it is also highly desirable, or even essential, if the sanatorium is to receive the proper support and does its greatest good, that a large proportion of these remain cured.

It should be stated here that the term "cured" as applied to patients who leave the sanatorium apparently well in from six to seven months, as an average stay, has been practically abandoned. Greater experience has shown that many of these carry away quiet foci of the disease which may lead to a recrudescence if the patient is placed under favorable surroundings, or leaves the sanatorium physically unfit for the work he was doing before admission.

This brings up two very interesting phases of sanatorium management. First, to find suitable employment for patients while at the sanatorium; and second, their after-care for a year or more after they leave the institution to insure a permanent cure. Neither of these problems have been satisfactorily solved.

Most patients received at a sanatorium need rest and not exercise. Where only suitable cases are received, they are in most instances capable of doing a certain amount of work, after a stay of six or eight weeks. If carefully watched, and suitable employment is provided, this may take the place of other forms of exercise and be of real benefit to the patient. The great trouble is to find continuous employment suitable for different classes of cases, and to induce patients to take advantage of this.

In meeting this problem it makes a vast difference as to the social class of the patient, especially whether he will have to make his living with his muscles or with his brain. Take a so-called working-man who performs physical labor, and keep him idle at a sanatorium for six or eight months. His muscles become soft and he is very apt to become work-shy. Send him back to his old work with his disease arrested, and he is very often unable to keep pace with his well companions who have been at it from day to day while he has been resting. He frequently breaks down, his disease breaks out of bound again, and he goes back to the sanatorium, if fortunate enough to be readmitted, or, and this is usually the case, he works as long as possible and finally completely succumbs. It is of great importance, therefore, for the working classes that they should have work for two or three months at the sanatorium before they are sent home.

Graduated work for such cases has been ingeniously provided at the Brompton Hospital Sanatorium, at Frimley, by Dr. Paterson, the superintendent. Selected, suitable cases for sanatorium treatment that come to Brompton Hospital in London are sent to their sanatorium at Frimley. They have favorable cases therefore to deal with.

In the building of paths transportation of gravel was necessary. This was carried by patients in baskets. The baskets were made of three sizes. A patient commenced with the lightest load, carried it the shortest distance, and worked only a short time. The time and distance would be gradually extended, and then he would be given the next largest basket. Finally he would carry the maximum load the maximum distance the maximum time. So he had mattocks for digging, and shovels for moving earth of three different sizes. In these and other ways he very gradually increased the amount of work done until for several weeks before leaving the sanatorium a patient would be doing about as much physical work as he would have to do when he returned home.

As observed by Dr. Paterson, if a working-man is to break down or have unfavorable symptoms develop from the amount of work he will be compelled to do to earn a living, it is infinitely better that this should happen before he leaves the sanatorium.

There is another phase of sanatorium work to be considered. Many occupations directly favor tuberculosis. To send a patient back to such an occupation with his disease arrested is to invite a return of his trouble. If it is possibe to teach such patients at the sanatorium some new and healthful occupation, this would be a great gain in the way of securing lasting cures. This will be alluded to again in speaking of the after-cure for sanatorium patients.

The commission planning the Ohio sanatorium have not been unmindful of this phase of the subject. The law to govern the institution provides that the trustees may arrange for suitable out-door labor for patients, under the direction of the medical superintendent, and may pay for such labor any sum not to exceed five dollars per week.

It was noted that a charge of five dollars per week is made for at least 90 per cent. of the patients. It thus becomes possible for patients able to labor to earn this sum for a considerable period of their stay, if suitable work can be found for them. This is an extremely important provision for the laboring classes.

The experience in sanatoria is that it is very difficult to keep such patients long enough to secure lasting results. The weekly charge is hard to meet. The family is probably in need of help. And then the patient, at the end of three months, often feels perfectly well. He has no fever, no cough, weighs more than usual, and feels strong. It is hard to make him understand that his lung trouble is still in condition to be lighted up again on small provocation. It is sometimes still harder to make his family and friends understand this. They pay him a visit and find him looking so well that they are apt to suspect he is "soldiering" if he wants to stay several months longer. If we can find suitable employment for this class and pay them for it, they are much more likely to stay the time required for the full benefits of sanatorium treatment.

The after-care of sanatorium patients is a perplexing problem. We have spoken of their going back to unfavorable occupations. They frequently must also return to unsanitary and unhygienic home surroundings, and improperly cooked or insufficient food. Much of this is unavoidable, but much could be done if these patients could be kept under intelligent, helpful supervision for a time. I believe it will be found advisable to have a State inspector to follow up these patients for a year or two after they leave the sanatorium.

Another phase of this question is that the public has been given such an unwarranted dread of tuberculosis that employers not infrequently refuse to take back a sanatorium patient, and he has great difficulty in finding another place. An intelligent State inspector would often be able to remove these unfounded prejudices.

In the after-care of sanatorium patients an open-air life is important; but so, also, is a sufficient quantity of nourishing food. He may be unable to make sufficient money to buy suitable food in some new but favorable occupation. In the choice between two evils it may be better to have him go back to his old occupation and a "full dinner pail," and depend upon giving him at night the fresh air he should have.

England has tried in a small way the plan of providing light agricultural work for patients who leave the sanatorium. In one place cottages have been set aside for the families of these men. Such a scheme has not been put upon a paying basis, and it is doubtful if it can be. These men know nothing about farming, are not able to do heavy work, and too often are inclined to shirk even light labor under such conditions.

What has been said about work at the sanatorium and after has related almost exclusively to men. There are, of course, many women who go to the sanatorium who must make their own living when they leave. Many of these have contracted the disease on account of their employment. It is easier, on the whole, to teach women than men some light, comparatively healthful, occupation that will gain them support so long as they keep strong.

This whole work problem for tuberculosis patients is a perplexing one, and is receiving more and more attention. It is allied in a general way to the greater question of finding work for the army of unemployed who are also usually more or less unfit.

As regards the cure of tuberculosis, we may say, then, that the sanatorium has two functions: To cure those who come there, and to serve as a demonstration of, and incentive for, the home cure of others.

Without giving statistics, we can say in a general way that from

50 to 75 per cent. of the patients are cured at the sanatorium, depending upon the class of cases treated and the length of time they stay in the sanatorium. That is, this per cent. of cases may be temporarily cured, by which is meant restoration of the general health and complete quiescence of local lesions. Its usefulness in the other direction—in having proper home treatment carried out in cases that would otherwise have been neglected or sent elsewhere to their detriment—from the nature of things, cannot be determined.

As to the lasting effects of sanatorium treatment, we are not yet in position to say anything definite and conclusive. Many sanatoria are of recent establishment, and the older ones failed to keep proper records of discharged patients. The results vary very greatly, according to the class of patients dealt with. A large majority of the cases moderately advanced when they enter the sanatorium are much improved when they leave, and a considerable number are able to return to work. By far the greater number of these, however, succumb to the disease in the course of a few years. With selected cases, all agree, the results are far better. A large number of these are cured and stay cured, and this is eminently true of those who are able to return to healthful occupations and surroundings.

The sanatorium as a means for the prevention of tuberculosis may be dismissed in fewer words. Each discharged patient, of course, goes home thoroughly drilled in all measures required for the prevention of infection. The educational influence of these disciples of cleanliness in their respective families and communities is worth considerable, and is added to each year. They also teach the all-important lesson of living in fresh air. Many a bedroom window is opened and kept open because of their example. This prevents the development of a certain number of cases. Visitors to the sanatorium are more or less impressed and influenced by the open-air life they see carried out there. Many people in their usual health are now building and using out-door sleeping places; and I am not sure that one of the greatest benefits that will come from sanatoria, not only as regards tuberculosis, but health in general, will not be the radical changes in housing conditions they will be largely instrumental in bringing about.

We may now turn our attention to hospitals for tuberculosis. We have, in round numbers, 6,000 people dying from pulmonary tuberculosis each year. It is usual to multiply the annual deaths by three to arrive roughly at the number of cases on hand at one time. This would give us approximately 18,000 cases in Ohio.

The sanatorium is to care for 200, and with an average stay of six months this would give us 400 cared for each year. What is to be done for the more than 17,000 other victims in our midst? The great majority must be taken care of in their homes. This can be done without great danger to others where patients are properly instructed and relatives and friends are able to provide proper care—in other words, in the upper and middle classes.

It is very different, however, with the extremely poor. They must often live in one or two rooms, huddled together to keep warm. Frequently one or more of the family is obliged to sleep with the patient. Tuberculosis is quite often the indirect cause of these unfavorable sanitary conditions. If the bread-winner is the victim he may live, but be unable to work, for a year or more. The savings, if any, are dissipated. To supply the patient with medicine and extra food other members of the household are underfed and improperly clothed. We thus have focused in such a family the two most potent factors for the propagation of tuberculosis. We have concentration of infection in badly ventilated rooms, and a weakened resistance on the part of those so exposed. It is among this class, and largely on account of such conditions, that tuberculosis chiefly prevails.

Koch attributed the great and continuous reduction of tuberculosis in England to the hospitalization of so large a number of their cases, and the consequent reduction in opportunities for infection. A recent English government report, in which this question is gone into at some length, is inclined to cast some doubt upon this. It is shown that the average time spent in hospitals by the class who seek and obtain such relief is not more than 2 or 3 per cent. of the total period during which they are presumably capable of spreading infection. Furthermore, that while England has provided probably more abundantly for the hospital care of consumptives than any other country, only a small part, after all, are so cared for. It is pointed out that the deaths from tuberculosis in England and Wales have been steadily declining, and at about the same rate of decline since 1851, and that during much of that time there were few hospitals for consumptives and no conscious effort to prevent infection, which was scarcely suspected.

No doubt better wages, with better food and housing conditions, and vastly improved sanitary conditions in general, with consequent greater national vigor, have been large factors in the reduction in tuberculosis in most parts of the civilized world. It can scarcely be doubted, however, that prevention of infection has played an important rôle, nor that the removal to hospitals of advanced and practically bed-ridden cases has exerted a great influence in such prevention. It is just at this stage of their disease that they are most liable, and when the greatest number of opportunities are present to convey infection. A few months in the hospital at this time might represent but a small per cent. of the whole time during which tubercle bacilli were present in the sputum, but this would cover, in most cases, the most dangerous period.

But even if the rôle of infection should be found to be overestimated, there would remain sufficient reason for providing suitable hospitals for the consumptive poor. As pointed out, it is this burden to the family, that must often be borne so long, that, with the poor, forces conditions upon other members of the family that are largely responsible for the development of tuberculosis. No matter whether the bacillus gains entrance to the body by inhalation or ingestion, all are agreed that poverty, overcrowding and bad hygienic surroundings so lower the vital resistance that tuberculosis and then consumption (to make a distinction) is the usual result.

Ohio has taken the second step in the prevention of tuberculosis in providing for county hospitals. A recent act provides that after January 1, 1909, it shall be unlawful to keep any inmate in any county infirmary who has pulmonary tuberculosis except in a separate, suitable building. It directs the commissioners of each county to erect a hospital for tuberculosis for such inmates, and for other residents of the county so affected. . These latter may be charged three dollars per week, if able to pay, and if not any less sum the infirmary directors choose to make it. The plans and location of such hospital are to be approved by the State Board of Health and the Board of State Charities. They are to be under the general supervision of the former board.

There is a provision in the act that any county, in lieu of building such a hospital, may send its indigent cases to some other county and pay pro rata for their keep there. As it was conceivable that some patients might refuse to leave their own county, it is further provided that unless their relatives or friends can find a suitable place for them, as determined by the State Board of Health, the probate judge of the county in which they reside may order them taken to a county hospital and there confined.

This is the opening wedge, unnoticed by many, for the forcible removal and isolation in hospitals of dangerous consumptives who have no other place where they may be safely cared for. So far as I know, it is the first compulsory isolation law for tuberculosis, although New York has been making forcible removals in some cases under general board of health regulations controlling infectious diseases.

While there may be some objections to having tuberculosis hospitals on infirmary grounds, as these will be completely separated, and run on a different scale from the infirmary, it is believed that this objection will in time disappear.

It will be seen, I think, that our State is keeping fully abreast in this great and general movement for the relief and prevention of tuberculosis. With a sanatorium for suitable cases, and numerous hospitals for that larger number that for various reasons cannot go there, Ohio has made most generous provisions for the care of this unfortunate class of her citizens. And in doing this, like in doing every good act, the benefit comes back to the State in the greater protection society will receive against this most prevalent of all the communicable diseases.

SKIMMED MILK FOR OBESITY.—Weir Mitchell reduces weight by placing the patient on a diet of skimmed milk and other fluids, gradually reducing the amount of the milk until the patient is losing about a half a pound of weight per day. During the first week or two rest in bed is enjoined, and later, for a varying period, rest in bed or on a lounge is insisted upon, while massage is used once or twice a day, and later Swedish movement. The pulse and weight are observed with care, so that if there be too rapid loss or any sign of feebleness the diet may be increased. In many such cases he allows a moderate amount of beef or chicken or oyster soup.—*Denver Med. Times.*

PRIMARY EPITHELIOMA OF THE EPIGLOTTIS.—D. B. Delavan describes this case which came under observation so early that a circular area of hyperemia one-quarter of an inch in diameter on the laryngeal surface of the epiglottis was the sole evidence of disease. Six months later a positive diagnosis could be made, and one-third of the epiglottis, including the diseased area, was removed. Nearly two years have elapsed since the operation, but there is no evidence of recurrence.—*Med. Record.*

ASPHYXIA FROM ANESTHETICS.—Hare directs to lower head and raise feet almost perpendicularly, keeping chin at a right angle to body line and pressing forward the angle of the lower jaw. Artificial respiration, by Sylvester's method, may be needed. Other measures are the intravenous injection of ammonia into the leg, and dashes of cold and hot water.—*Denver Med. Times.*

DYSPNEA OF OBSCURE ORIGIN.—The *Medical Summary* recommends fluid extract of quebracho in doses of ten to twenty minims.—*Denver Med. Times.*

CHRONIC CATARRH.*

W. N. MUNDY, M.D., FOREST, O.

This term is used to designate a chronic nasal discharge. The discharge is not the disease, but is a symptom due to a variety of pathological conditions, among which are adenoid growths of the pharynx, foreign bodies in the nose, polypi, deviations of the septum, deformities of the nasal passages and the various forms of chronic rhinitis.

Adenoid growths of the pharynx are probably the most frequent cause of a chronic nasal discharge in infants and young children. Foreign bodies in the nose should be suspected, whenever there is an abundant muco-purulent discharge, limited to one nostril. Children quite frequently push peas, beans, beads and other substances in the nose, which lodge there. The efforts of the children or mother to remove such obstructions often result in simply pushing them farther up the nose. The foreign substance soon sets up a mechanical irritation, by which pain, swelling, sneezing, and sometimes hemorrhages are produced. This is followed by a catarrhal inflammation, and in a few days by a purulent discharge. These symptoms point directly to an obstruction of the nostril.

Nasal polypi, although an infrequent cause of a nasal discharge in childhood, are nevertheless occasionally seen. The symptoms are a partial or complete closure of one or both nostrils, aggravated by every attack of acute coryza, or by the advent of damp weather. The reflex symptoms are cough, sneezing or asthma; headache, disturbances of smell, taste and hearing. The discharge is less in amount and not as purulent as when caused by a foreign body, but is of longer duration.

Chronic rhinitis is described as existing in two forms, the hypertrophic and atrophic.

Etiology.—The hypertrophic form is thought to be the result of frequently repeated attacks of acute rhinitis. It is found in children suffering from that peculiar dyscrasic condition called "lymphatism," and is usually associated with an hypertrophy of the adenoid tissue of the pharyngeal vault.

The atrophic form, known also as fetid catarrh, and of which ozena is but a type, is said to be a late stage of the hypertrophic form. Others claim it to be a primary disease, either congenital

---

* A reprint from the new revised edition of Mundy's "Diseases of Children," ready in September.

or hereditary. Syphilitic rhinitis is frequently classed as but a type of the atrophic form.

Pathology.—The characteristic changes of the hypertrophic form consist in a chronic inflammation of the nasal mucous membrane, producing an hypertrophic thickening of the mucosa. This is marked over the turbinated bodies, especially at the posterior end of the lower turbinate. The thickening of the mucous membrane increases and encroaches upon the nasal passages. In addition there is an hypersecretion of mucus. In the atrophic form the changes are a thinning or atrophy of all the structures, with enlargement of the cavities. The mucous membrane is dry and coated, with an accumulation of dried secretion and scabs. Should it be due to secondary syphilis, it is accompanied by the formation of ulcers or mucous patches. There are gummatous deposits which break down and form ulcers of the mucous membrane and deeper tissues. Periostitis and necrosis of the bones; perforation of the septum, hard or soft palate, as well as ulceration of the pharynx and soft palate, are frequently concomitant results of this form.

Symptoms.—In the hypertrophic form, there is an obstruction to nasal respiration, by reason of the hypertrophy of the turbinate bodies. The sense of smell is impaired, and there is a discharge of a thick, tenacious secretion from the nares. In these cases the secretion pours backward, and, dropping into the pharynx, is ejected by an act of hawking and expectoration.

In addition to this, there is the unpleasant nasal tone to the voice, and the occasional stopping up of the nose, compelling the child to breathe through the mouth.

Among the reflex symptoms are cough, catarrh of the larynx or bronchi, muscular spasm, giving rise at times to a spasmodic croup or asthma. From adenoid growths of the pharynx, it is differentiated by means of the rhinoscope. In infants and young children they are usually associated. Atrophic rhinitis is conspicuous by reason of the disgusting odor emanating from the nares. The scabs and crusts cause some degree of obstruction. The discharge is scanty, the sense of smell impaired or lost, and middle ear affections are common. Atrophic rhinitis is uncommon in children, except it be due to hereditary syphilis.

Diagnosis.—The diagnosis is not difficult, as the continued abundant discharge from the nose, its occasional closure, the

nasal tone of voice, and the pain and uneasy sensations in the
nose and frontal region, are very prominent.

The diagnosis and differentiation of form are made by means
of the head mirror and rhinoscope.

Prognosis.—The disease will rarely, if ever, get well without
treatment; but an appropriate general and local treatment is
necessary. Too often these patients are the subject of a routine
treatment, without any specific or special object in view. If neglected, permanent impairment of the organs of hearing, smell,
speech or respiration is often the result.

Treatment.—The general treatment will vary according to
the indications, and much care will be necessary to select the
right remedy. The possible remedies might be named, as arsenic,
iron, sodium sulphite, sulphurous acid, hamamelis, phytolacca,
Donovan's solution, potassium iodid, penthorum sedoides, and
calcium sulphide. The relaxed, atonic skin, with feeble circulation, will be benefited by arsenic; pallid skin, with blue veins,
dusky redness of mucous membranes of nose and throat, with
occasional erysipelatous flushings of skin, call for tincture of
muriate of iron; sodium sulphite, if there is eczema of the face;
sulphurous acid, if there is deep redness of mucous membranes,
with offensive discharge; hamamelis, if the tissues are full and
atonic; phytolacca, if the throat is sore, or the cervical glands
enlarged; Donovan's solution, if the bones are being involved,
the skin dirty, and especially if a syphilitic taint is suspected;
potassium iodid, if there is a broad atonic tongue, with leaden
pallor; penthorum should be used when there is fullness of the
nasal mucous membrane, abundant discharge, and spongy gums;
calcium sulphide, when the discharge is abundant and purulent.

In some cases I have employed rhus with aconite or veratrum,
with most marked benefit. The need of rhus has the usual indications: frontal headache, persistent, with burning in the eyes
or nose. The aconite is suggested by the irritable tonsils and
throat, and the veratrum by cough and mucous rattling in
bronchia.

At the same time the child should have its regular bath every
one or two days, using the alkalies when indicated, the tonic bath
if the child is anemic, or the fatty inunctions if the skin is dry
and harsh.

It is understood that should a foreign body be the cause of
the discharge, it should be removed. This can sometimes be ac-

complished by holding the free nostril closed and blowing the nose forcibly, when the child is old enough to do so. Often it is necessary to use the forceps.

Polypi are to be removed by the forceps or snare. ·My personal preference is the snare.

The treatment of adenoids has been outlined.

With young children it is somewhat difficult to make proper use of local remedies, which I prefer to administer by inhalation, or with the steam or air atomizer. In this way they can be brought into direct contact with the diseased structures. The objects of the local treatment are: first, cleanliness; second, the removal of the pathological conditions.

Cleanliness is secured by the use of an alkaline or antiseptic solution by means of the spray or atomizer. I have obtained good results from the use of a solution of potassium chlorate (gr. x. to water oz. iv.). When the discharge is purulent and offensive, we may use the solution of potassium permanganate (grs. x. to water oz. iv. to oz. viij., depending upon the condition of the mucous membrane). In place of these we have frequently used Dobell's solution, which is composed of sodium borate, sodium bicarbonate aa. dr. j., carbolic acid grs. xxx., glycerine oz. j., aqua O ij.

In young children we have used as a cleansing agent a solution of sodium bicarbonate, by means of a medicine dropper. All solutions should be used warm. After the use of the cleansing solution, the object to be attained in the hypertrophic form is the reduction of the redundant tissue. This is accomplished by the use of the snare, galvano-cautery; chromic or glacial acetic acid; astringent powders and solutions are also used. The atrophic condition is considered incurable. The object to be attained is, relieving the dryness and overcoming the odor, it being impossible to replace the atrophied tissue. ′

The crusts and scabs are best removed by using some oily solution to macerate and soften them, after which the nasal douche or spray, with an antiseptic solution, should be used.

If the discharge is very offensive, we employ the solution of salicylic acid and potassium chlorate; or, instead of this, a weak solution of carbolic acid.

Prophylactic treatment consists in preventing attacks of acute coryza, so far as possible, by the use of proper hygienic means.

𝔓eriscope.

Physicians, Persons, Contracts and Wills.

In an address before the Eclectic Medical Society of California, H. M. Owens, Professor of Medical Jurisprudence in the California Medical College (*California Medical Journal*), says:

I have been requested to prepare a paper to read before this society and in doing so I have endeavored to select subjects which will be not only instructive, but if taken home and observed by all of you there will be little if any excuse for going out of the straight and narrow path of your duty to your patients, to yourselves and to the community at large.

Physicians should be competent in all respects as such; should be men above the tongue of reproach in their community; should be leaders in all movements for the benefit of society; should be law-abiding citizens in every respect, just as much so as should the minister be, and should be respected as much as he. Under our law they should possess a license from the State Board of Medical Examiners before beginning to practice medicine. While the present State Board seems to be exceedingly rigorous in their examinations and do not impress us with the idea that they desire a greater number of physicians than there are at present, yet it is the policy of the law to encourage education, and some time we may be able to secure a State Board who will take a stand of encouraging instead of discouraging the study of medicine.

Physicians cannot testify in a civil action without the consent of their patients as to any information acquired in attending the patient which was necessary to enable the physician to prescribe or act for the patient, nor can a physician sue or collect his fee without first having received a license from the State Board of Medical Examiners. So much for the physician.

Persons and Contracts.—Under this head we will learn who cannot make contracts and under what conditions contracts can be made. Under our law, minors are males under twenty-one years and females under eighteen years of age; all other persons are adults. A minor cannot give a delegation of power, nor under the age of eighteen make a contract relating to real property or relating to personal not in his immediate possession. A minor may make any other contract than as above specified in the same manner as an adult, subject only to his power of disaffirmance under the provision of our statutes. Any contract so made may be disaffirmed by the minor himself before his majority or within a short time afterwards, and in case of his death, by his heirs or personal representatives within the same period, and if a contract be made by a minor over the age of eighteen it may be disaffirmed in like manner, upon returning the consideration. A minor cannot, however, disaffirm a contract otherwise valid, to pay a reasonable value for things necessary for his support or that of his family entered into by him when not under the control of a parent or guardian able to provide for him. This includes medical attendance. A person without understanding has no power to make a contract of any kind, but he is liable for the reasonable value of things furnished to him necessary for his support or the support of his family. Conveyances or other contracts of a person of unsound mind but not entirely without understanding, made before his incapacity has been judicially determined, is subject to recission as provided in the chapter on recission of the code of this State. After his incapacity has been judicially determined a person of unsound mind cannot make any conveyance or other contract or delegate any power nor affirm in writing until his restoration to capacity. But a certificate from the medical superintendent of the institution to which such person may have been confined, showing that such person has been discharged therefrom, cured and restored to reason, establishing a presumption of legal capacity in such persons from the time of such discharge.

Wills.—The right to dispose of one's property by will is solemnly assured by law and is a valuable incident to ownership and does not depend upon the justness, nor can courts properly permit the prejudices of the jury to set aside upon mere suspicion or that it does not conform to their ideas of what is just and proper. The parent is under obligation to provide for his minor children and if the will is made and the name of the child is not mentioned in the will the child will take as though no will was made. The uncle or aunt is under no obligation ordinarily to provide for either niece or nephew, and the failure to mention them in the will does not, under the statute, raise the presumption that they were forgotten; nor does it become absolutely necessary for the parent to leave any particular amount of property to their children; so long as they are mentioned, is all that is necessary to fulfill the requirements of the law. We have now arrived at a subject which will often be of use to a physician. Many times he is called upon to attend cases where there is to be a critical operation, and his advice is asked as to the advisability of making a will and he should have a knowledge of the manner and forms of wills and their proper execution.

An oleographic will must be entirely written, dated and signed by the testator. On the other hand, what is known as a regular will can be written by anyone, provided, however, that it is signed by the testator and subscribed to by two witnesses; for example:

SAN FRANCISCO, May 21, 1908.

I, John Jones, hereby give, devise and bequeath unto my children, share and share alike, all my property, both real and personal, whenever and wheresoever found, and I appoint my wife Jane Jones executrix of my will to serve without giving bonds.

JOHN JONES.

Witness:
JOHN DOE,
RICHARD ROE.

If a legacy is left to a witness he cannot take, under the will, and the bequest as to him is invalid. If any property is given to a charitable institution and the testator dies within thirty days such legacy is void, nor can the testator devise more than one-third of his estate to charity.

The services of a physician during the last illness is a preferred claim against the estate and should be paid out of the first monies coming into the hands of the executor. If the physician has attended at other times prior to the last illness he must present his claim to the executor for approval and allowance by the court.

The law presumes that everyone possesses a sound and disposing mind and the burden is upon the contestant to show by a preponderance of evidence that the testator was of unsound mind at the time of making the will.

Undue influence, in order to invalidate a will, must be such as in effect overpowers the testator's volition at the time of making the will.
—M. H. OWENS, LL.B., in *California Med. Journal.*

Cactus Grandiflorus.

Much is being written in medical journals at the present time concerning the various preparations of this plant. Some is of a laudatory nature, while much is derogative.

Without doubt those who cannot procure good results from its use are the ones who have been working with inferior preparations and thus cast an unjust reflection upon what is a most useful adjunct to our heart remedies. Many of the therapeutic nihilists of our day have been produced because of the *imperfectly prepared* drugs with which they endeavored to get results, and failed because the drug could not, as it was made, produce what was expected.

Cactus is another of those plants which should be used in its *green* state in order to procure reliable remedies. Probably the wrong method of manufacture is responsible for many of its failures.

Among its specific indications may be mentioned, impaired heart action, whether feeble, violent or irregular; cardiac disorder, with nervousness; precordial oppression; anxiety; apprehension of danger or death; hysteria; tobacco heart; nervous disorders with heart complications.

The effects of cactus are not merely evanescent, but lasting. The nutrition of the heart is increased, its contraction strengthened, and its irregular rhythm controlled.

Cactus spends its force upon the sympathetic nervous system and is particularly active upon the cardiac plexus.

Prof. E. M. Hale, M.D., says: "It acts upon the circular cardiac fibres, whereas digitalis acts upon all the muscular fibres of the heart. Like the latter, as a secondary effect of over-stimulation, it may induce heart failure."

One of the most advantageous fields for the successful use of cactus is in those nervous disturbances of women which are connected with the menstrual flow and are complicated with heart disorders dependent upon the nervous disarrangement.

In such cases cactus will prove a valuable adjunct to many of the remedies prescribed at these times, such as helonias, hyoscyamus, macrotys, pulsatilla, xanthoxylum. Indeed, many times the addition of the cactus to these drugs marks the result between success and failure.

Dose: Fluid extract, gtts. ij to gtts. v; specific medicine, gtts. ss. to gtts. x. It should be preferably administered in water largely diluted.—*Journal of Therapeutics and Dietetics.*

———

NUTRIENT ENEMAS.—Einhorn uses a mixture of one-half pint of milk, two eggs and fifty grams of grape-sugar. Another formula consists of three to five eggs mixed with 150 c.c. of sugar-water (30 gm. of grape-sugar dissolved in 150 c.c. of water), to which a small quantity of common table-salt is added, and the whole mixture is well beaten. One may also add a little starch solution or mucilage.—*Denver Med. Times.*

———

TREATMENT OF ANEMIAS.—For secondary types Packard recommends Fowler's solution and iron (syrup of iodide for children); good, nourishing food and abundance of fresh air. He treats the progressive pernicious form with absolute rest and careful diet; open bowels and intestinal antisepsis; inhalations of oxygen; and with arsenic well diluted, beginning with small doses and increasing up to the point of tolerance.—*Denver Med. Times.*

The Eclectic Medical Journal

A Monthly Journal of Eclectic Medicine and Surgery.
TWO DOLLARS PER ANNUM.

Official Journal Ohio State Eclectic Medical Association

JOHN K. SCUDDER, M.D., Managing Editor.

EDITORS.

W. E. BLOYER.	H. W. FELTER.	L. E. RUSSELL.	R. L. THOMAS.
W. B. CHURCH.	J. U. LLOYD.	H. E. SLOAN.	L. WATKINS.
JOHN FEARN.	W. N. MUNDY.	A. F. STEPHENS.	H. T. WEBSTER.

Published by THE SCUDDER BROTHERS COMPANY, 1009 Plum Street, Cincinnati, to whom all communications and remittances should be sent.

Articles on any medical subject are solicited, which will usually be published the month following their receipt. One hundred reprints of articles of four or more pages, or one dozen copies of the Journal, will be forwarded free if the request is made when the article is submitted. The editor disclaims any responsibility for the views of contributors.

Discontinuances and Renewals.—The publishers must be notified by mail and all arrearages paid when you want your Journal stopped. If you want it stopped at the expiration of any fixed period, kindly notify us in advance.

THE PSYCHOLOGICAL MOMENT.

Shakespeare says—

> "There is a tide in the affairs of men,
> Which, taken at the flood, leads on to fortune;
> Omitted, all the voyage of their life
> Is bound in shallows and in miseries."

This tide is the psychological period, and may come but once in a man's life, or it may be repeated several times. It is a study of much importance, and the world at large usually does not comprehend the significance of this moment, but condemns or praises according to the outcome without looking between the lines. Few there are who are capable of studying or reading between the lines, and as a consequence men are lauded or condemned by the multitude without a thought as to their merits or shortcomings in a given case.

The psychological moment may cause a man to plunge on the races, bet heavily on the turn of a card, abscond with the funds of a bank or firm, commit some crime against the laws of the country or of morality. Again, this peculiar period may make a national reputation in the line of economics, or of some discovery which will benefit the majority of the people, or it may be along the line of philanthropy. In the latter class eulogies are in order, while in the former execration only is received.

Who is qualified to act as the judge in these cases? Who can honestly say that they would have done differently under absolutely the same circumstances? We boast of our civilization, learning, etc., but really how much have we advanced over our primeval ancestors? It is true that in so far as advancement for comfort and means of communication, methods of transacting business, and along this special line of work is concerned, we have an immense advantage over our progenitors; but when it comes to the individual, the community, or the world at large, how much improvement, or rather what advancement has been made? The Christian church claims much—in fact, that it alone is the cause of the advancement in civilization. But a careful study of history reveals repression, not to use a stronger term. There is, however, a factor which is not generally credited with the advancement that has been made, and that is the psychological moment. It is not a question of church, money, or, in fact, anything which a chain of reasoning will reach, but is the fortunate or unfortunate period in one's life when the opportunity presents that the mental faculties are in perfect or imperfect working order.

Man is a peculiar animal, and his instincts are practically the same as they were centuries ago. I doubt whether they are even modified very much, but some phases are possibly under a little better control. Still, if you go deep enough, you will find the old savage instinct present. It is nature, and against nature's laws it is difficult to fight. In the majority of educated men there is an inherent recognition of the rights of others, and this is usually observed, not so much from a moral standpoint as from a sense of justice. However, in any of these men the psychological moment does and always will be an important factor. It is foolish to go to either extreme in laudation or condemnation in cases where premeditation is eliminated, but the public is very liable to become hysterical in either instance, and as a consequence injustice results.   FOLTZ.

NEW LIGHT ON DIPHTHERIA.

The Klebs-Lœffler bacillus, now generally thought to be the germ cause of diphtheria, has an associate bacillus which is distinguished by its harmlessness, and which is otherwise so like the original that the miscroscope cannot differentiate them. This non-pathogenic diphtheria bacillus may be found in the pharynx of healthy individuals and upon other parts of the body, but is eminently harmless wherever found. Consequently the microscopical diagnosis of diphtheria is rendered difficult and doubtful, and, after all, it appears that we must wait for general corroborative evidence before making an absolute diagnosis.

Stengel says that the pseudo-diphtheritic bacillus is probably not a new or different germ, but one which has lost its virulence by growth under unfavorable circumstances. Be that as it may, the discovery of this harmless microbe, which so perfectly resembles the bacillus diphtheriticus, will render more difficult the work of the various health boards, that heretofore have not hesitated to isolate individuals or entire communities in the presence of the diphtheria germ. Unnecessary hardship and financial loss have no doubt been needlessly caused by arbitrary action in some instances, and the quarantine has been unjust, although well intended.

Non-diphtheritic pseudo-membranous pharyngitis may result from various causes, and is frequently found in association with scarlatina, measles, smallpox and typhoid fever. It is impossible to distinguish between diphtheritic and non-diphtheritic pseudo-membrane except by bacteriological examination, and even then we may have but the benign brother of Klebs-Lœffler, harmless and innocuous.

The only reliable test in virulence would be to culture the suspected membrane and by injections into guinea-pigs determine the toxicity of the germ. Laboratory tests for pathogenicity, while of considerable practical utility, are not to be regarded as final, for patients have died with diphtheria with no miscroscopic evidence of the specific germ in the throat. To hold any one characteristic of this disease as predominant and unalterable is liable to lead to erroneous conclusions.

WATKINS.

GASTRO-INTESTINAL DISEASES.

As the heated season of the year approaches, troubles of this nature increase, digestive troubles arising from improper food, both of quality and quantity, being the most prolific cause. They also assume protean forms, from an acute indigestion, characterized by a sharp, but brief attack of vomiting and diarrhea, or cholera morbus, to an acute milk infection, or cholera infantum. Between these are every phase or type of gastro-enteritis and ileo-colitis.

The attempt of the Board of Health to provide a pure and clean milk for the infants of Cincinnati recalls that an impure, or a milk below a fixed standard of percentages, is not the only source of infection. An illy kept bottle, or a dirty utensil, is as frequent a cause of cholera infantum as a milk that is not up to the standard. In other words, care of the milk after its reception is fully as important as the provision of a good milk.

A neglected dyspeptic diarrhea is often the forerunner of a gastro-enteritis or ileo-colitis. Table feeding is also a prolific cause. It is a fact that we see but few bad cases of either of these conditions at the present day as compared with what we met twenty or twenty-five years ago. We cannot explain the reason, unless it be that the laity have become better informed upon the subject of infant feeding. We feel that this is the case, and that this is but a part of the triumphs of "preventive medicine," a branch of medicine which must take the laity into its confidence and partnership, and which calls for an intelligent co-operation between the profession and the laity, if it proves successful.

As we have said, a neglected dyspeptic diarrhea is usually the beginning of a gastro-enteritis or ileo-colitis. Persisting for a few days, the child becomes restless, irritable, and has an increased temperature. Vomiting ensues, the number of passages increase, and each stool is preceded by pains, evidenced by crying and fretting. The stools are watery and usually contain curds. They are often quite large and of a peculiar musty odor. Sometimes of a greater consistency and green, or turn green upon exposure to the air. The curds also vary in size, according to the diet. The stools may become small, consisting of mucus, slightly tinged with blood. These are preceded by pains, as evidenced by the fretting and crying, and attended by straining and tenesmus. Often the amount passed will be scarcely a teaspoonful. Thus we have an ileo-colitis.

Again, the vomiting and stools may be very large and watery, the first stool being attended with the greatest prostration, or even a collapse. The surface of the body is cold, the face slightly blue, eyes sunken, pulse very rapid. Each stool is attended with an increase of these symptoms, and we have a true cholera infantum or acute milk infection.

It is difficult to define the border line between the first two types of the inflammatory forms of diarrhea, either clinically or pathologically; nor is it essential for the purposes of treatment. In both types emaciation is marked and rapid, and if they become protracted in their course, marasmic conditions supervene, when the question of diet and nutrition becomes a serious problem. Intertrigo also adds to the general discomfort and distress of the little patient.

Hastily have we thus gone over this subject for the purpose of refreshing our minds upon a timely topic.

In the treatment of these cases we are guided by Eclectic principles, meeting the indications as they arise. No cut and dried prescription as an intestinal antiseptic, diarrhea or cholera infantum mixture. Attention must of necessity be given to the diet, its preparation, the care of feeding utensils—in fact, the subject of the feeding must be looked after in all its details. Often it is well to abstain from all food for a day or two, or it must be given in the blandest form. Should there be the slightest suspicion of the retention of any indigestible material in the intestines it should be removed either by an enema or oil. Often the stomach is or has been relieved by vomiting, yet stomach washing is at times indicated, but is not resorted to as a routine measure. In acute milk infection it is often well to empty both stomach and bowels, even though the child has vomited.

Internally we give the small and frequently repeated dose of aconite, when the pulse is small and frequent and there is an elevated temperature. Gelsemium or rhus tox. may be combined with this, as may be indicated by the condition of the nervous system. These are alternated with ipecac, when the tongue is elongated and pointed, when there is vomiting and the stools are acid and irritating, evidencing irritation of stomach and bowels—a dysenteric condition.

Should there be an atonic condition, as shown by the broad tongue, only slightly coated, stools frequent and large, passing without much evidences of distress and straining, we substitute the small dose of nux for the ipecac.

With tenesmus and straining, stools very small, consisting of mucus principally; sharp, colicky pains preceding the stool, very small doses of colocynth is the remedy.

Stools greenish in color, mucus and feces; child restless and uneasy all the time and wants to be carried, it is matricaria.

Vomiting persistent, tongue red and glazed, some diarrhea, but gastric symptoms predominant, liquor bismuth is the remedy.

Soda baths to allay nervous irritation, dusting powders for the intertrigo. Cleanliness and care of the napkins, clothing and person of the child. Abundance of fresh air and sunshine and a close attention to the diet until convalescence is assured count for success in the treatment.   MUNDY.

OLD ECLECTIC COMPOUNDS AND MERCURIALS.

In the infancy of specific medication antagonists and resisters of the new system criticised its advocates for using certain mixtures that had been tried so long as to have become established in Eclectic therapy and employed by the advocates of direct medication. In those days the enemies of Eclecticism seized every opportunity to disturb the efforts of the Eclectic physician, and, on the slightest occasion, spent much printer's ink in numberless attacks on the leaders of the school.

The Eclectics of old used a multitude of compounds, as needs be seen if one but consults their works on materia medica. Of these a few were not paralleled by any single drug known at that date (as true to-day as then), and were consequently adapted in specific medication. These established compounds gave the enemies of the school much needless concern.

Dr. John M. Scudder used and recommended emetic powder, stillingia liniment, neutralizing cordial, and a few others. He was the father of the compound known as Scudder's Alterative, which was, however, devised before his study of specific medication made him famous. Although he usually alternated individual remedies, he commended for convenience or otherwise in many instances the union of two or more specific remedies, as is shown in the pages of his popular work on "Specific Medication." This led the enemies of the school to attack him personally and yet illogically, for, although he assailed the prevalent hap-hazard shot-gun methods of that day, Dr. Scudder did not assert that compounds should never be employed. We have in mind one pamphlet, now in the Lloyd Library, distributed by a drug firm of physicians, in which Scudder was "shown up" by the reproduction of an editorial in which more than one remedy was commended in a prescription.

The facts are, so far as we know, representative Eclectic physicians have never proscribed legitimate drug combinations when it became necessary to associate remedies that fortify each other; or of compounds that long practice had demonstrated to carry invaluable qualities possessed by no single drug. This is shown both in Scudder's practice and by Scudder's writings, a fact intentionally overlooked by those who did not care to know the whole truth.

Although more than thirty years have passed, and by reason of the study of single remedies with definite actions, the great list of Eclectic compounds then burdening Eclectic literature has shrunk into insignificance, although a few of the celebrated representatives yet survive because no individual drug parallels them in usefulness.

As examples may be cited the three preparations Dr. Scudder found it necessary to employ. Two hundred specific medicines are now established, but we question if, in the practice of a majority of Eclectic physicians, any single plant preparation, or plant product, will take the full place of neutralizing cordial, emetic powder or stillingia liniment.

Another source of seeming concern to the enemies of the school was the fact that a few Eclectic leaders occasionally used a mercurial or other energetic that Eclecticism fought as employed by the dominant school. Here again Dr. Scudder was lampooned as being illogical, for he had been known to prescribe both Donovan's solution and Fowler's solution, each being an arsenical compound. Dr. A. J. Howe used bin-iodide of mercury, and the father of Eclecticism, Dr. John King, in his "Eclectic Dispensatory" gave place and commended a compound carrying ammoniated chloride of mercury. But the facts are, these preparations were seldom employed by Eclectics even then, and very carefully were they used or commended as concerns dosage. In the same way even calomel in one-tenth grain doses was in exceptional cases used by more than one Eclectic, an amount that in those days was not a dose to calomel doctors, although following Eclectic precedent it is now orthodox in one-tenth grain doses in the dominant school.

Whoever criticises Eclectics of the olden time for employing such energetics as these in exceptional cases needs remember that in those days the struggle was to prevent the abuse of harmful drugs, and to displace injurious remedies with those more kindly. The wonder is, not that a few such long-lauded substances were used in minute doses, but that the multitude of conglomerates and compounds then employed and the heroic drugs that cursed the materia medica that prevailed when Eclecticism was born were so soon and so effectively displaced in Eclectic pharmacy and practice.   LLOYD.

TETANUS.

The passing of another Glorious Fourth brings to mind that condition which is so frequently a sequela of the injuries incident to its celebration. The record of 1908 is not yet complete, but in 1907 seventy-three cases of tetanus were reported. Since 1903, with its 415 cases, the number has steadily decreased, due largely to a better understanding by the profession of the importance of prophylactic measures.

The researches into the etiology and pathology of this disease have been so fruitful that the extent and accuracy of our knowledge have been greatly increased. Since the discovery of the tetanus bacillus in 1884 by Nicolaier, it has been shown that it is an anaerobic bacillus found in garden earth, street dirt and the feces of some animals, whose spores are more resistant to external influences than any other bacteria, living in some instances after exposure for one hour to 212° F.; that it enters the body through some abrasion of the skin or mucous surfaces, usually by means of a punctured wound, where its growth causes no inflammatory reaction and the formation of no pus, but a toxin is produced which is so poisonous that 1-100 of a grain will kill a horse; that this toxin is carried through the lymphatics to the blood, through the blood to the endings of the motor nerves in the muscles, through these endings and the axis cylinders to the cells in the spinal ganglia, for the protoplasm of which it has a special affinity and upon which its action produces the phenomena of the disease, death resulting from the involvement of the centers of circulation and respiration in the medulla; that an antitoxin can be found in the blood of a horse after repeated injections of a non-fatal dose of toxin which, when mixed with the toxin in a test-tube, renders it harmless, or when injected in sufficient quantities into an animal after a fatal dose of toxin will prevent the development of serious symptoms, and the administration of 1,500-3,000 units of this antitoxin on the first, third, fifth and twentieth days following an injury where tetanus infection is suspected or proven is effective in preventing the development of the disease; that after the appearance of symptoms it has proven practically useless, and the mortality remains as it was before these additions to our knowledge.

The failure of serum therapy to cure tetanus is due to the inability of the antitoxin to neutralize the toxin, which is fixed in the nerve cells, where it continues to do its deadly work. To be effective, therefore, the antitoxin must be brought into contact with the toxin before it becomes fixed in these cells, hence the importance of using it as a prophylactic measure.

To make the antitoxin more effective in the cure of the disease, various expedients have been advised, such as injecting it into the branches of the brachial plexus, the sciatic, anterior crural and obturator nerves; injecting it into the subarachnoid space in the lumbar region, with or without a premeditated injury of the cauda equina; injecting it into the cervical cord and the brain itself. All these means have proven futile, and it is hard to understand why some of them are advised by leaders in our profession.

The usefulness of such other measures as the hypodermic injection of sixty to eighty grains of carbolic acid in 2 per cent. solution daily, the subdural injection of a 25 per cent. solution of magnesium sulphate, the use of eucaine or cocaine as in spinal anesthesia, and the hypodermic injection of an emulsion of brain tissue, is doubtful.

Then in the treatment of tetanus let us stick to that which is proven or to that which accords with our knowledge. The careful cleaning and draining of every wound soiled wih dirt and the enlarging and draining of punctured wounds with the use of the antitoxin when tetanus is feared will save many lives.

When the disease is present, in the absence of a specific, *treat the patient*. The antitoxin is as harmless as horse serum, and can be used, but do not expect much from it. Even at this time thorough cleansing or excising of the wound is indicated, but it does not seem necessary or right to sacrifice arms and legs unless amputation is justified by the nature of the injury. Much credit is due those men who have made some of the dark places in this disease light, and we can but deplore their failure to discover a more effective weapon with which to combat it. SLOAN.

ADJECTIVE ECLECTICS.

The medical profession contains two kinds of Eclectics. One is Eclectic because he espouses a cause which represents a distinct school of medicine, which had its origin in America, was founded on American principles, and which depends largely upon American drugs and home ideas for its existence and perpetuation. The members of this branch of medicine recognize the truth that the school needs some kind of standard to designate their position, follow a custom long ago inaugurated by the founders, and apply a name to their school— a proper name, Eclectic, with a capital initial.

Another kind may be termed "adjective eclectics." A large share of the entire medical profession are adjective eclectics, but only a comparatively small number are really Eclectics, so far as the name goes. The Allopaths and Homeopaths are adjectively eclectic. They choose the best, from all sources, according to their lights; and the Allopaths (for want of a better name) insistently declare that they are the only "true eclectics."

Let that be as it may, those who belong to our ranks and insist upon appearing in print or in any written form with the cognomen of their profession expressed with a lower case initial letter may properly be classed with them, for they can claim nothing more on their self-expressed avowal.

The adjective eclectic is not necessarily a Beach, a Morrow, a King, nor a Scudder Eclectic. He may be almost any old kind of eclectic, but he is not identified by name with the school which is peculiar on account of its origin and tenets.

Some write us down with a lower case initial because they desire to ignore or belittle us as much as possible; of course, these are our adversaries. Others may be careless or ignorant. Some of our own school seem to be endowed with a sort of superficial pedantry which inspires them to strain at a gnat and swallow a camel in order to appear orthographically and etymologically the proper caper.

They may have been informed by some self-constituted authority that the word has no correct use as a proper noun, and are in the habit of looking through the wrong end of their telescope. They may be bamboozled by ordinary proof-readers, who fail to comprehend the true inwardness of the subject, and who are likely to confound electic with electric. Eclectic is no more distinction with them than electric, and possesses no more significance. They fail to comprehend that Eclectic may be a proper noun as well as a common adjective. Dyed-in-the-wool Eclectic physicians, however, ought to know better than this, and the majority of them do, though there seem to be a few who sight through the colored glasses of the great majority.

Why the followers of the old masters, however, should foster such a delusion passes the comprehension of ordinary mortals. When we lower ourselves so much as to write us down, and our own school down with a small initial letter, it is time for us to get off the earth. Eclectic is both a proper noun and a common adjective, according as it is applied. If it is not a proper noun, why do we attempt to distinguish ourselves by the name? If we are to be just common everyday "Eclectics," let us merge, for we then possess no individuality.

WEBSTER.

THE NATIONAL.

The thirty-eighth annual convention of the National Eclectic Medical Association was held at Kansas City, Mo., June 17-20, 1908. This proved one of the most successful meetings held in several years, a hundred and seventy-six physicians being in attendance, and forty-one new members were admitted.

The mayor of Kansas City made an address of welcome, which was responded to by Dr. Mundy. After the appointment of the usual committees by President Perce, Secretary Best read his detailed annual report, which was well received, and his suggestions were later acted on by the society. Treasurer Sharp's report showed all bills paid and a good balance in the treasury.

Dr. Scudder reported for the Committee on Organization and Legislation that considerable systematic work had been done along these lines during the past year, and the same committee hopes to make further progress during the coming year.

Probably the most important work done at Kansas City was the reading of the detailed report by Dr. Mundy for the Council on Medical Education, and the action of the society in affording the Council financial assistance for the ensuing year. Dr. Mundy stated that our Council had effectually checked the Council of the A. M. A. in its self-imposed work of arbitrarily inspecting Homeopathic and Eclectic colleges, and reporting adversely to various State boards.

Active co-operation has been secured with various State examining boards, giving equal consideration and recognition to the claims of the liberal schools of medicine.

The Boards of Ohio, Michigan, Indiana, New York, Kentucky,

Idaho and Texas have invited our representative to join their committees on medical college inspection.

A combination with the Homeopathic Council for an offensive and defensive alliance has been consummated. The Council recommended that the equipment and workings of some of our medical schools be improved and modernized.

The Association voted an expenditure of $300 for the work of the Council for the ensuing year.

President Perce's address was well received, as was the special addresses of Dr. Boskowitz and Dr. Finley Ellingwood. Dr. Helbing, of St. Louis, gave a stereopticon entertainment on the second evening, followed by a banquet in the hotel.

One of the best features of the four days' session was the special address on Saturday morning by Dr. R. S. Copeland, of Ann Arbor, Mich., the President of the American Institute of Homeopathy, which met in Kansas City the week following. In a stirring address he showed the members that our two schools had very much in common, particularly in forming an alliance to protect themselves against any adverse legislation, and more particularly in furthering the study of our indigenous materia medica, which had made the new schools so strong in the line of therapeutics, and which helps them to combat the growing tendency towards therapeutic nihilism of the dominant school of medicine.

A number of very interesting papers were read and discussed, but they were hardly up to the average, either in number or quality, but part of this was due to the fact that there was comparatively little time for section work after the necessary business had been transacted.

The amendment to the Constitution was adopted providing that, commencing with the Chicago meeting in June, 1909, the treasurer of each State society should collect and pay to the treasurer of the National society an annual per capita tax of $2.00 each as annual dues, which would make every member of a State society of good standing a member of the National. Details of this new arrangement will be worked out by the Executive Committee and furnished to the officers of the State societies before their next annual meeting. The proposition to publish a quarterly or monthly bulletin was laid over.

The following officers were elected: President, John K. Scudder, Cincinnati; First Vice-President, J. T. McClanahan, Booneville. Mo.; Second Vice-President, H. Harris, New York City; Third Vice-President, J. A. McKlveen, Chariton, Iowa; Recording Secretary, W. P. Best, Indianapolis, Ind.; Corresponding Secretary, H. H. Helbing, St. Louis, Mo.; Treasurer, E. G. Sharp, Guthrie, Okla. Next meeting will be held in Chicago, June 15-18, 1909.

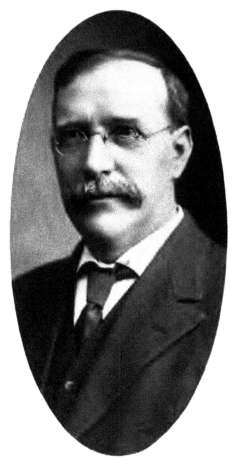

KENT OSCANYAN FOLTZ, M. D.

The Eclectic Medical Journal

ESTABLISHED 1836.

Vol. LXVIII.   CINCINNATI, SEPTEMBER, 1908.   No. 9.

Biography.

KENT O. FOLTZ, M.D.

HARVEY WICKES FELTER, M.D., CINCINNATI.

Specialism in medicine may be a feature productive of great good as well as of great harm. In the hands of the competent man it is capable of yielding the best and greatest results in both medicine and surgery. That it has been and is being greatly abused in some directions will, we believe, be generally conceded. The man fresh from the college benches may or may not make a capable and safe specialist. The chances are that he will not. On the other hand, one who has practiced general medicine, even but for a few years, is far more likely to intelligently enter the field of specialism and give both prestige and dignity to it because of the abundant experience he is capable of bringing into his new work. The Eclectic school of medicine has produced few specialists without previous training in general practice. It has been the impression among Eclectics, and well founded, we think, that he who enters at once into a specialty immediately upon graduation is handicapped and cannot with honor to himself and justice to others compete with his competitor who has seen and treated most of the maladies that afflict humanity. Hence specialties have grown slowly in our school, and her men have spent the greater part of their careers in the preparatory stage to specialism—that of general practice.

Of this class of well-prepared men came the late Prof. Kent O. Foltz. In consequence of his splendid training in medicine, in pharmacy, botany, and chemistry, and as practical optician, he brought into his specialty a wealth of knowledge that made him not only a specialist of the highest merit, but a teacher of similar power and popularity. In him was combined the skilled diagnostician, the expert operator, and not the least, and a rarity among specialists in whatever school, an accomplished and exact therapeutist. If we were to name his greatest work, we should declare it to be the elaboration and application of specific medication in diseases of his special department. It is true that many specific indications had been previously worked out as applying to eye, ear, nose and throat diseases. Prof. J. M. Scudder had noted many, and Prof. Wm. Byrd Scudder was making progress in this feature of therapy, when broken health and an untimely death took him away from it. The specific therapy in diseases of the eye and ear contributed by Professor Foltz to Professor Webster's Therapeutics brought him into prominence, and the subsequent journal articles, society papers and work, and the special monographs on his specialty made specific medication conspicuous as a part of the treatment. When we reflect that specialists in these branches run largely to operative means and optics, and little to medication, the immense advance of Professor Foltz's work in specific therapy will be the more clearly apparent and better appreciated.

Kent Oscanyan Foltz, M.D., was born in Lafayette, Medina County, Ohio, February 16, 1857. He died at the Seton Hospital in Cincinnati, June 6, 1908, following an operation upon the nasal passages. His father, Dr. William K. Foltz, was one of the pioneer and best-known Eclectic physicians in the State.

Dr. Kent O. Foltz was liberally educated. He graduated from the Ashland (Ohio) High School in 1872 and attended Buchtel College at Akron, Ohio. He early entered mercantile life, engaging in the retail drug trade, and subsequently had charge of the manufacturing department of a drug and chemical house. For a time he also worked at the optician's desk, a circumstance that made him doubly expert in his chosen specialty. Selecting medicine as his life-work, he began reading under the tutelage of his father and later matriculated in the Western Reserve Medical School of Cleveland. Being strongly inclined toward Eclectic therapy, he finished his student course at the Eclectic Medical Institute, of Cincinnati, Ohio, graduating therefrom in 1886. He at once engaged in general practice, but with a view to electing a specialty later, which he prepared for by taking special instruction on the eye, ear, nose and throat, in 1888, at the New York Post-Graduate School. This course he supplemented by another in the New York Polyclinic, in 1889. During 1890 it was his good fortune to have been asked to care for the private and institutional patients of one of the teachers connected with the Polyclinic, the Manhattan Eye and Ear Infirmary, and the Harlem Dispensary. Relinquishing this work, he again engaged in general practice for four years, after which he devoted his time and talents wholly to his specialty, in which he subsequently achieved remarkable success and a well-earned reputation for skill and good results. In recognition of his ability in his chosen field he was called to Cincinnati in 1898 to fill the chair of

Didactic and Clinical Ophthalmology, Otology, Rhinology and Laryngology in his alma mater—the Eclectic Medical Institute. Here he not only filled the chair with great credit, but built up an excellent clinic which has done much to extend the already good reputation of the school. This clinic, in order to have a wider range of surgical observation, was transferred to Seton Hospital (connected with the college) and is now one of the best clinics Cincinnati affords.

Dr. Foltz was a member of the National and several State societies. In 1891-92 he was President of the Ohio State Eclectic Medical Association. As one of the associate editors of the ECLECTIC MEDICAL JOURNAL his editorials were of a general character and his influence was always exerted for the betterment and uplifting of his profession.

Dr. Foltz was the author of two text-books of high rank, which have met with a favorable reception from practitioners of whatever creed—"Manual of Eye Diseases" (1900), and "Manual of Diseases of the Nose, Throat and Ear" (1906). He also contributed the sections of the specific therapy of the eye and ear to Prof. Herbert T. Webster's "Dynamical Therapeutics," and conducted for many years a special department on the Eye, Ear, Nose and Throat in the ECLECTIE MEDICAL JOURNAL. Dr. Foltz was an exceptionally fine botanist, able at sight to pick out almost any plant that grows in fields or forest, and was widely conversant with exotics and their culture. This love of botany was undoubtedly inherited from his mother, also a fine botanist, and the doctor developed it fully by study and observation.

Dr. Foltz was of medium stature and well-knitted frame. He had light—inclined to reddish—hair, a ruddy complexion, and a sandy mustache. His blue-gray eyes reflected clearly the merriment so strongly a part of his nature. A keen sense of humor made him one of the most enjoyable of companions. He knew and enjoyed a good story, and could tell one with effect. Dr. Foltz was a wide and critical reader. He loved art and the artistic, and appreciated good music. Choice editions of the best authors found a place in his library, and his taste in bindings was that of a connoisseur. Especially was he a deep student of psychology and criminology, and had made some important original observations concerning the relationship between visual defects and the tendency to the commission of crime. Unfortunately, only notes concerning this phase of his studies were left by him.

As a teacher Dr. Foltz was painstaking and thorough, and, though he was not a fluent lecturer, he was a splendid operator and clinical instructor. As before mentioned, specific medication was his strong forte, and he made it count for the most in his work and teaching. As a writer Dr. Foltz was concise and direct, inclined to be epigrammatic, but was never verbose. While he wrote clearly, he was seldom ornate.

He quickly detected inconsistencies in the lives and acts of others, and often saw the opportunity to score others heavily; yet he seldom gave to his articles more than a humorous vein of kindly sarcasm if such an expression may be used. Even then it was apparent between the lines that he meant to gently but effectually swing the professionally erring or inconsistent into line for the uplifting of the cause of medicine. His feelings toward men were kindly, and he let no occasion pass to do a good turn to his fellow physicians or to the school of his choice.

In matters of religion Dr. Foltz was an agnostic, and he did not hesitate to utter his convictions. For this he has been criticised, and this naturally was to be expected when the majority of people are raised to respect and to hold some existing form of religion. But, no matter what may be our personal beliefs, who in these days of enlightenment and liberality, and in view of the widely varying religious opinions, can other than comparatively condemn the honest belief of another? Dr. Foltz was a man of sterling worth, and his friendship was of the enduring and helpful kind. In the face of distractions and sorrows, and long in bodily ill-health, he maintained an unbounded optimism—an optimism that could well be emulated by all men. We can pay no better tribute to this gifted and loyal Eclectic than to reproduce the words of his friend and co-laborer, Prof. John Uri Lloyd, in the last issue of the *Gleaner:*   .

"We remember Prof. Kent O. Foltz, M.D., as an optimist who practiced optimism, not preached it. The class of the Eclectic Medical Institute well know how he suffered during the last years he was with us, and they yet will recognize the cheerfulness with which he met his duties, and the earnestness of his teaching. To us this optimism in Professor Foltz's disposition has appealed since the day of his graduation, and also previously during his course of study in the college. His father was an optimist ahead of him, and his mother was alike blessed with cheerfulness and brightness of disposition.

"We remember meeting Dr. Foltz in New York after the serious accident that befell him in Akron that so nearly put an end to his existence. We then congratulated him on the philosophical manner in which, in the very prime of life, he met a disaster that threatened to be irreparable. In our opinion, his optimism then served him well, for had he been possessed of a pessimistic spirit he would have succumbed.

"In the very midst of trials, physical and otherwise, he came to Cincinnati to meet problems, professional and otherwise, that the pessimist would never have surmounted. That he succeeded is due to the optimism that possessed him and that drew to him friends who were friends in fact and in deed."

Original Communications.

CAESAREAN SECTION—REPORT OF SEVEN CASES.

. George H. Derrick, M.D., Oakland, Cal.

I am well aware that that which I have to report will be misconstrued by many whose obstetrical experience antedates my own. There are doubtless men who have practiced medicine many years and yet have never felt called upon to make an instrumental delivery, much less a Cæsarean section. These men will argue that "Nature should take her course." It is true, however, that the course of nature frequently ends in death, and the business of the physician is to assist and direct natural processes in such a way that life may be saved. The arguments against Cæsarean section could as well be urged against appendectomy, ovariotomy, or any one of the great capital operations which are now employed to save life. In obstetrical practice we are called upon to save two, sometimes three, lives, and I take the position that any advancement of science which will lessen the dangers of maternity should be accepted as a part of twentieth century practice.

In reporting these seven cases of Cæsarean section, six of which have occurred in my own practice within the last thirty months, I wish to say that the number of maternity cases handled by me is such that I believe the percentage is no greater than would be met with in the ordinary run of practice in any part of the United States.

My first case occurred September 29, 1905. The mother, a primipara, was five feet six and one-half inches tall, weight about 130 pounds, age twenty-four. The presentation was breech, and upon the completion of dilatation hemorrhage from the placenta became profuse. She was in the maternity cottage of Fabiola Hospital, and every modern convenience was at hand for an instrumental delivery. At least one-fourth of the placenta was presenting with the breech, and no amount of manipulation could replace the prolapsed placenta or check the hemorrhage. It became apparent that something must be done at once, and I applied instruments and made every effort at delivery. This I found to be physically impossible, even had the placenta retained its normal position. I then determined upon a Cæsarean section, although I greatly feared the outcome. I had never seen the operation performed and had not the time to refresh my memory from the scanty literature on the subject as to the technique.

The patient was rushed to the operating-room, and with a realization that life was dependent upon the number of minutes employed, I delivered the child and placenta and completed the work of suturing the abdomen in nineteen minutes. I am happy to say that both mother and child left the hospital the fourteenth day, and are as well to-day as any mother and child I have ever had the privilege of attending. I have since read everything I could find on this subject, and have since been sincerely thankful that my first case occurred before I had the opportunity of reading some of the literature which is published to guide the inexperienced practitioner. I used no band or ligature to prevent hemorrhage, relying entirely upon the rapidity of the operation.

On November 7, 1906, I was called to attend Mrs. S. for her first delivery. She was thirty-four years of age, about five feet four and one-half inches tall, and of rather small pelvic development. It soon became apparent that I had to deal with a case of twins lying in transverse position, the right shoulder of the first child presenting, and after many hours of fruitless effort I determined to remove her to Fabiola Hospital and there operate. After hasty preparation I delivered two living children at 5 A.M., the work being done entirely by artificial light. The mother and both children are in excellent health to-day, and it is a source of gratification that at least this family has been made happy through one of the triumphs of modern surgery.

One month and three days later I was called to attend Mrs. H., who had already given birth to nine children. Of these, there were two pairs of twins, and in each instance labor had been very difficult, only one of the four children being saved. I diagnosed another case of twins, and determined to make an instrumental delivery if possible. After two hours of work I succeeded in delivering the first child, and believe I should have been successful with the second had not the membrane accidentally ruptured. It has been a rule of mine to prevent rupture of the second membrane until uterine contraction has set in for the second time. I have thus frequently been able to gently manipulate the child and induce the head to engage, after which the membrane may be ruptured with safety. In this case, however, the left shoulder presented, and no amount of effort on my part would change the position. I at once removed her to Fabiola Hospital and by Cæsarean section delivered a living child. The mother and both children are alive to-day and in the best of health.

On June 25, 1907, I was called to attend Mrs. D. for her first child. She was small of stature, rather poorly nourished, and thirty-two years of age. The child was of large size. The presentation was occiput left posterior. Efforts at instrumental delivery having proved futile, I removed her to Fabiola Hospital, and at 10 P.M., by the use of artificial light, made a successful delivery, the mother and child being alive and in the best of health to-day.

On August 1, 1907, I was called to attend Mrs. M. for her first child. She was twenty-two years of age, a native of Denmark, and of medium size and development. The child, however, was unusually large. The position was occiput right anterior, and appeared at first to present no unusual difficulties. She was in a sanitarium in a neighboring city, and I felt assured that little difficulty would be experienced. After twelve hours of labor, the contraction being frequently so great that I feared uterine rupture, I made an effort at instrumental delivery. It soon became apparent, however, that delivery could not be accomplished without sacrificing the life of the child. I laid the case before the authorities in the sanitarium and requested the privilege of performing a Cæsarean section. This privilege they refused, stating that inasmuch as I was an Oakland doctor they would be glad to have me remove her to an Oakland hospital, as they did not wish to injure their maternity record. No other means being open, I administered chloroform sufficient to moderately control the terrible uterine contraction, and at twelve o'clock at night began the long journey of seven miles over a miserable road to get her to a hospital where I would be permitted to operate. I am glad to say that the child was successfully delivered at 3 A.M., and the mother and child sent home the sixteenth day. They are in perfect health.

I must diverge here to say that this was the first case in which there was even a stitch abscess, all the others having healed by first intention. She had suffered from an irritable navel all her life, and the stitch which closed the incision at this point undoubtedly became infected, but presented no difficulties more than slight suppuration.

On October 4, 1907, I was called by Dr. Lyon to see Mrs. J. in her first confinement. She was of small bone but very fleshy. The heart action had led Dr. Lyon to fear that she would expire during the night. Although but twenty-one years of age, she presented one of the worst cases of varicose veins I have ever seen. The presentation was occiput left anterior. I made no effort at instrumental delivery, the doctor feeling sure that it would be unsuccessful, and might result in the death of the mother through heart lesion. She was removed to Fabiola Hospital and there successfully delivered. The child in this case has since died from natural causes, although the mother is well.

On January 27, 1908, I was called to attend Mrs. O. for her first child. She was tall and well developed, but the pelvic diameter was very small. I found cervical dilatation complete on first examination, but the condition of the vagina led me to fear the outcome. After fourteen hours of hard pain the head refused to even engage, and the vagina was too small and unyielding to permit the application of instruments. She was removed to Fabiola Hospital and delivered of a very large living child, and the twelfth day returned home, and she says she feels better than she has ever felt in her life.

I have thus delivered nine children from seven mothers, and eight of the children and all the mothers are in perfect health to-day. In the last case reported there was a slight stitch abscess at the navel, due, doubtless, to imperfect preparation. Six of the cases were in my own practice.

In conclusion, I wish to say that there is nothing about this operation that should discourage any surgeon. The patient should be thoroughly catheterized and prepared as carefully as time will permit. The incision should be carried about three inches above the navel and the same distance below. The uterine incision should be made through the anterior fundus, care being taken not to injure the child after cutting through uterine wall. The child and placenta are removed quickly and four deep stitches or sutures of chromicized gut taken into the uterus, after which the field can be carefully cleansed, intermediate stitches taken to approximate uterine walls, and the abdomen closed. The time from the first incision till the delivery of the child and placenta and the taking of the four deep stitches to control hemorrhage should not be over four minutes. After this has been done sufficient time can be taken to properly cleanse the wound and complete the operation.

In conclusion, I must express my appreciation of the timely assistance rendered by Dr. Lillian Shields, who has assisted me in nearly all these cases, and Miss Jessen, the matron of the operating-room at Fabiola Hospital, whose care has reduced septic danger to a minimum, and whose anticipation of my every want has greatly facilitated rapid work. Happy, indeed, is the surgeon whose assistants are masters of their work.

ECTOPIC PREGNANCY.

W. B. CHURCH, M.D., CINCINNATI.

Taking for granted general familiarity as to etiology, nature and varieties, the purpose of this paper is chiefly to establish points for diagnosis and treatment.

Ectopic is of Greek derivation, signifying out of place. The proper place for an impregnated ovum is the uterine cavity, but, like many other things, it sometimes fails to find its place. It then makes the best of an unfavorable environment, endeavoring to conform as far as possible to the laws of its growth and development. The spermatozoon, by virtue of its motility, is quite capable of ascending the uterine and tubal canal against the stream or wave-like movement of the cilia, which waft the ovum downward, and may and often does escape through the fimbriate extremity into the peritoneal cavity. Here it may meet and embrace its affinity. The resulting fertilized ovum may be deflected beyond the reach of the fimbriæ, and fail to secure transportation via the oviduct to the uterine cavity; subsequent development will proceed in the peritoneal cavity. It may also, when properly entered through the tubal ostium, meet with obstacles which arrest its further progress, as already intimated, and be compelled to accept wayside accommodation of a very inferior sort. If located near the cornu uteri the fetus may, in the course of development, be extruded into the uterine cavity, the placenta remaining in the tube, development going on to term. The ampulla is by far the most frequent portion of the tube in which the amputation is made. Development of the ovum causes great expansion of the tube, with thickening of its walls to correspond. It usually happens that the rapid expansion of the tube will fail to be completely compensated by increased nutrition, and on one side or the other the tubal wall gets thinner and may burst, permitting escape of the fetus, with more or less hemorrhage, into the abdominal cavity. This may or may not be accompanied by death of the fetus; it may survive and continue to develop in its new situation. In any case nature is unable to cope with the situation; without artificial aid the fetus must always perish. In some cases nature, by tedious processes of absorption, mummification and suppuration, may dispose of the products of gestation without sacrificing the mother. Surgical intervention, in pre-aseptic days, was attended with frightful mortality; with modern facilities and technique this is wholly changed. Many cases are reported of operations, instituted at the expiration of the time for normal gestation, with the result of saving both mother and child. This cannot often happen, for in the large majority of cases death of the fetus occurs long before. The prospect of survival to term, and successful delivery, is so remote that operation, as soon as diagnosis is made, is considered proper. The diagnosis is not difficult to a surgeon of experience, yet it must be admitted that fatal cases still occur without a diagnosis having been made.

A recent case treated at Seton Hospital illustrates so many characteristic features it is herewith reported.

Was called to see Mrs. R., of this city, on May 31, 1908. Messenger said she had been feeling well all day, even joining in some scuffling play with friends living in the same apartments, after which, with others, she repaired to a nearby café for supper. Before it was served she was taken with a violent cramping pain, so severe she collapsed in a faint, and had to be carried home. Reaching the bedside, the outcries and indications of agonizing pain were so extreme one-fourth grain hypodermic was given. Pains were intermittent, simulating labor, but immediately, by their severity and general diffusion, suggested something more serious than miscarriage. As soon as partial relief was secured from the morphine, an attempt was made to elicit history. Age, twenty-four; eight years ago gave birth to a still-born child; husband thought she had not been so well since. Five months ago, after menstrual irregularities extending over two or three months, had a sudden attack of very serious pains, with flooding. Besides many large clots, expelled a pinkish-colored fleshy mass, which she seemed unable to describe definitely, but was sure it was not a clot. Doctor called at the time pronounced the case a miscarriage, and prescribed medicine for internal use. Continued to have similar attacks, and menstrual irregularity at intervals of days or weeks, changing doctors without permanent relief. Then went to the City Hospital. Here she was told she had had a miscarriage with retained fragments of the placenta; was curetted, told she had no ovarian trouble, as had been intimated by other medical advisers, and after a few days, during which she was able to be up and around, was discharged as well. In less than a week thereafter the attack above described occurred, which occasioned my call. Examination revealed an oblong tumor in the left iliac region, extremely sensitive to pressure, and evidently not involving the uterus.

These data, taken in connection with the history given, made a diagnosis of extrauterine pregnancy clear. It was decided that the substance expelled with hemorrhage five months previously was a decidual cast. It was hardly questionable that it was tubal pregnancy, that rupture had taken place, with hemorrhage. While it was difficult to fix the duration, it was probably over five months. As no motion was felt, death of the fetus was to be presumed. The chief danger was stated to be from internal hemorrhage, and transfer to the hospital with immediate operation advised. This was accepted. Complicating the case was severe pleuritic pain, with coarse bronchial râles, on both sides, which developed marked bronchial pneumonia after the operation. This condition had been partly masked by the morphine found necessary to give before and after entering the hospital. Except for the danger threatened by the hemorrhage, this would have induced delay. Belief, however, that the lung affection was due to minute thrombi carried to the heart, and through the right ventricle to the lungs, made the removal of the clots, known to be in the abdomen, and almost certainly between the layers of the broad ligament, urgent. It had been possible to palpate the fetus by an examining finger in the rectum. An incision in the median line was made, and large gauze pads wrung from hot salt solution were used to dam off the general peritoneal cavity as soon as opened. Masses of coagulated blood were scooped out in handfuls. The sac was effectively walled off by adhesions of omentum and bowel. The coagula were entirely expelled by copious irrigation with normal salt solution. The nature of the case had been clearly outlined, and found to be as anticipated, an ampullar pregnancy, which had ruptured into the peritoneal cavity and between the layers of the broad ligament.

The large sausage-shaped tumor was freed of adhesions and brought outside, the ovarian vessels tied, the layers of broad ligament approximated by a continuous catgut suture, and then removed. The tube walls were much thickened and still retained a mass of placental tissue. The condition of the patient, because of the serious lung complication, did not seem to warrant any attempt to enucleate the sac, which was firmly adherent to the bowels, and to search for and remove the fetus. The edge of the sac was included in the first buried continuous suture used in closing the abdomen, gauze drainage inserted, which was probably unnecessary, and removed the next day.

The developments for the next four or five days were such as to fully justify the decision to suspend further attempts to complete the operation. Bitter complaint of pain in the chest, aggravated by violent explosive fits of coughing; great dyspnea, with a fluttering feeble pulse which could not be counted, and a temperature ranging from 102° to 103.5° F. In this emergency specific digitalis, in five-drop doses every hour, was of signal service, and the dyspnea and general distress at length overcome.

One week later she was returned to the operating-room, an incision made through Douglas cul-de-sac and the imbedded fetus, found in a mass of adhesions, removed in débris. A large fold of washed iodoform gauze inserted for drainage.

Except for the complication of bronchial pneumonia, there would at no time have been anything trying or discouraging in the course of the treatment. Even as it was she left the hospital in less than three weeks and is rapidly convalescing. I may add that the Sisters were very devoted, and Mrs. R. declares "Seton Hospital is a good place to go to."

NERVOUS DYSPEPSIA.—In nervous dyspepsia and gastralgia, says Einhorn, our main object should be systematically to increase the quantity of the food. Here milk and its derivatives (kumyss, matzoon, bonny clabber, buttermilk, cream), taken between meals, play a prominent part.—*Denver Med. Times.*

ANGOSTURA.

J. A. BURNETT, M.D., BARBER, ARK.

The synonyms for angostura are Galipea Cusparia; Galipea officinalis; Cusparia trifoliata, and Cusparia febrifuga. It is a native of northern South America and the West Indies. Angostura is the name of a town in Venezuela where this drug is obtained, hence the name "Angostura," but many authors spell it "angustura."

The constituents of this remedy are *angosturin* and several other alkaloids and glucosides.

The last edition of Potter's "Materia Medica" quotes Phillips' "Materia Medica" as to angostura being suitable in the worst forms of bilious fevers.

Lyle considers angostura of value in the treatment of intermittent, remittent and typhoid fevers, and says it influences all the secernents. Angostura deserves a thorough trial in the treatment of malaria. It could be combined with many other remedies such as gentiana, hydrastis, etc.

The following is a valuable antiperiodic compound: Fluid extract angostura, oz. j; fluid extract gentiana, fluid extract hydrastis, aa., dr. iv; simple syrup or glycerine or other suitable vehicle, q. s. ad., oz. viii. Sig.: To keep a chill off give a teaspoonful every hour until six or eight doses are taken, at other times a teaspoonful every three hours.

The liver is influenced by angostura in small doses; it is of value in bilious diarrhea, and in large doses it is of value in biliousness with constipation.

In chronic constipation with sluggish liver the following can be used: Fluid extract angostura, fluid extract cascara, aa., dr. iv; glycerine, oz. j; tinct. card. comp., dr. iv; aqua mentha pip., dr. iv. M.Sig. Dose one teaspoonful every four, six or twelve hours, as needed.

The diffusive and stimulating properties of angostura can be enhanced by combining it with such agents as capsicum, zingiber, asclepias, and amphiachyris.

The action on the mucous membrane resembles the action of myrica to some extent, also hydrastis, especially in catarrhal conditions.

In large doses angostura is emetic and cathartic, but should never be used for these purposes, as there are much better remedies. It can be combined with laxatives with good results. The general tonic influence of angostura makes it a valuable remedy in cases of debility and during convalescence from various diseases.

Lyle says: "It is an agent that may be influenced in different directions by being combined with different agents, and yet it maintains its general character of influence." Of course, this holds good more or less with all remedies, which is the secret of the extra effect obtained from compounds which many "single remedy" physicians do not seem to understand.

As angostura is a febrifuge, it can be used during fever in malaria. The stomach is influenced by angostura and dyspepsia often relieved. It is of value in diarrhea of children when the food passes through undigested, and in such cases can be combined with the elixir of lactated pepsin or used in connection with papoid.   .

Angostura is stimulant, tonic and antiperiodic. Dose of fluid extract, five drops to one drachm.

There is one good thing about angostura, and that is it is a non-toxic agent, and fatal results are not obtained from its misuse.

———————•—————

HICCOUGH—DERMATITIS?

Z. R. CHAMBERLAIN, M.D., BRADNER, O.

August 5, 1907, I was called to see Mrs. C., residing near Elgin, O., where I was located at that time. I found the patient suffering from reflex nervous hiccough, which had been coming on with increasing severity for over a year. She had undergone an exploratory operation without result or even discovering the cause of the trouble. The husband told me that nothing by "the needle" would stop the hiccough, but said he would be glad to try other means. I prescribed specific lobelia, dr. jss; specific gelsemium, dr. ss; veh. q.s. oz. iv. M. S.—One teaspoonful every five or ten minutes till thorough emesis, then small doses to relax.

When the spasm became severe, the hiccough reaching sixty to ninety times per minute, I gave chloroform by inhalation till patient fell asleep. On awakening there would be a short period of rest, followed by the hiccough as before.

This continued about four hours with no hope of relief, and then I injected one-fourth grain morphine and repeated in one hour, using chloroform as before. This ended the attack for that day. The relief was only temporary, however, and the attack would come on in from one to seven days, and each time the morphine had to be increased until one-grain doses were needed, and at one attack, which lasted seven hours, I gave one grain of morphine by hypodermic injection every hour for five hours, also one-half pound of chloroform by inhalation.

I consulted with the physicians in the near-by towns, and many sure cures were offered, as oil cajuput, codeine sulph., amyl nitrite, musk, etc., etc., but all without relief. In time I found that there had been an ovarian abscess following confinement. This discharged through the uterus at intervals of a few weeks or months.

I advised an operation, and on November 26, 1907, she was operated on at Seton Hospital by Prof. L. E. Russell. Operation revealed a pint or more of sero-pus in peritoneal cavity, also a badly diseased appendix, a sarcoma of left ovary and degeneration of right ovary. These organs were all removed and the incision closed. Patient rallied nicely and made rapid improvement and returned home three weeks later. In less than six weeks she gained twenty pounds in weight.

January 9, 1908, the hiccough returned as badly as before the operation. There was great pain and throbbing in left side, and examination revealed a tumor mass the size of a hen's egg in the ovarian region. Heat and tincture of iodine were used locally and gelsemium and lobelia internally as above, also inhalations of chloroform, and we succeeded in obtaining relief in about an hour.

A few days later the same case was repeated, only this time the swelling was in the right side. The same treatment was used with good results.

The treatment following consisted in the main of Lloyd's echafolta, and all swelling and pain passed. I removed from Elgin to Bradner, O., about March 30, and the case passed out of my hands, although my successor reported a short time since that Mrs. C. still had bad attacks of hiccough.

The next case I wish to report is, to me, an obscure case, and one which attracted much attention. This case also occurred in my practice at Elgin, O.

December 24, 1907, I was called to see a child, aged one year. She had always had perfect health, was strong and vigorous, and no hereditary tendencies to disease. Indications and diagnosis were double pneumonia. Specific treatment was used and rapid improvement followed. Five days later temperature went abruptly up to 105°, pulse 160, skin hot, flushed and dry. Prescribed specific aconite, gtt. v; specific gelsemium, gtt. x; veh. q. s. oz. iv. M. S.—One teaspoonful every one-half hour till fever abated, then less often.

The next day there were all the symptoms of measles except the odor. There had been no exposure, so no theory of measles could be established. The family asked counsel. This was held and nothing determined. Case was treated symptomatically. Five days more passed without change, except some improvement in the cough and the lungs clearing some. The tenth day the urine was partly suppressed, high color, no albumin. The skin had become dry and parched and began to scale off in flakes as large as three square inches, or even more, and as the new cuticle formed it in turn was shed as before. There was intense itching, so that the hands had to be covered to prevent injury to the skin. Prescribed specific rhus tox., gtt. v; specific apis, gtt. v; specific aconite, gtt. v; aq. q. s. oz. iv. M. S. —One teaspoonful every hour.

About the fifteenth day the glands began to swell over entire body. Consultation held again and salt water baths ordered, but stopped at once on account of their severe action on the skin. Here I began to steam the child by wrapping its naked body in flannel blankets wrung from hot salt water. This was kept up for an hour and was very pleasant to the child and beneficial to the skin. The bath was followed once daily with coal oil and once with olive oil. Now our prescription was: Specific echinacea, dr. j; specific phytolacca, dr. ss; specific aconite, gtt. v; veh. q. s. oz. iv. M. S.—One teaspoonful every hour.

Echinacea was used all through the case. Pus formed freely in the glands and became severe abscesses, and I lanced upwards of fifty of them, with a profuse flow of pus following.

February 15. The cough increased and became loose and rattling and the lungs broke down, so that by a change of position the pus would gravitate and reveal extensive cavities. February 17 the child died. There had been no regular fever or sweats, nor any hemorrhage; neither was the lung trouble prominent except at the first and last.

What ought I to have done that I did not do, and what was the real disease present?

—————·•—————

PASSIFLORA.*

J. J. MORRELL, M. D., HOPSON, KY.

The subject of this paper was suggested by the reading of a paper with the discussion of same in the transactions of the last National Eclectic Medical Association.

It is surprising that a remedy so much thought of by our school and a daily companion of a large majority of us should be called in question by some of our most prominent men.

True, a very wide range of action is claimed for it, speaking with reference to the number of diseases it is claimed to benefit, and this seems to be one objection to the remedy, while another comes a little

---

* Read before the Kentucky State Eclectic Medical Association, May, 1907.

nearer the root of the trouble and asks for a specific diagnosis calling for its use.

In the first place, I propose that the action of passiflora is confined to the nervous system. However, this is too broad a proposition to be of value as a guide to its specific use. I believe the specific use of this drug is that of a nerve equalizer, or rather pacifier, when exhibited in clonic conditions.

Let us review the suggestions of different writers on the use of this drug and add these to our own observations, and see if we are not sustained in our belief.

Take first, that trouble in which so many users of this drug depend on it exclusively, and that is convulsions of childhood—a clonic trouble.

Next, whooping-cough, a clonic trouble. I mention these because they are purely clonic in character.

Now let us see a case of typhoid fever and see when it should and when it should not be used.

Should I find my patient in a state of constant nervous excitement, eyes bright, photophobia, etc., I would not give passiflora, but gelsemium; or should I find my patient constantly rolling his head from side to side, eyes half closed, without luster, extremities cool, still I would not give passiflora, but belladonna.

My passiflora patients rest awhile and are then restless—in other words, are in a state of clonic restlessness.

Whether passiflora acts as a stimulant or a depressant to the nervous system, I cannot tell. Its office seems to me to be more that of an equalizer. For instance, I will refer to two very marked cases where it seemed to have a stimulating effect.

First, Mrs. C., advancd in years, was recovering from malaria, and in a very debilitated condition, rousing at times to talk to imaginary persons or complain of imaginary noises. I put her on passiflora and she soon became rational and convalesced nicely.

Second, my father, aged sixty-seven, recovering from an attack of bronchitis, was in much the same condition as the first case. Here, again, passiflora was the remedy used, and with prompt results.

In both these cases we seemed to get some degree of stimulation from the remedy.

For the sedative or depressing effect the remedy exerts under favorable conditions, I have only to refer back to its use in convulsions of childhood, which are generally of a sthenic character.

Ohio State Eclectic Medical Association.

Proceedings of the Forty-fourth Annual Session.

W. N. MUNDY, M.D., EDITOR.

SECTION II.

O. A. PALMER, M.D., PH.D., CLEVELAND.

P. E. Decatur, M.D., Chairman..........................Marseilles.
John W. Barry, Jr., M.D., Vice-Chairman...............Springfield.
E. A. Ballmer, M.D., Secretary...................Columbus Grove.

HYPEREMIA OF THE LIVER.

O. A. PALMER, M.D., Ph.D., CLEVELAND.

It is not an easy matter to explain the origin of hyperemia of this organ in every case, as we cannot determine the quantity of blood contained in the organ during life or in a state of hyperemia, so that we are dependent upon symptoms as the indicator of this condition. We cannot determine to what extent the different sets of vessels participate in the excessive determination of blood through the liver. As shown by Dr. Gad's demonstration, he allowed warm salt solutions to flow through the liver while it was still warm from the body of the animal. When it flowed through the portal vein alone more fluid passed through the liver than when it was allowed to enter the portal vein and the hepatic artery. This is explained possibly by the two currents opposing each other within the capillary network where they meet.

A state of hyperemia is accompanied by an increased flow of blood through the liver, and the normal and excessive flow of blood through this organ is prevented when the abdominal cavity is overfilled by food, gas, deposits of fat and feces which impede the flow of blood through the liver by exercising pressure upon this organ. An atonic condition of the blood-vessels allows them to relax and become flaccid, consequently they will become dilated and allow much more blood in the liver than should be.

It must not be forgotten that the respiratory movements are very necessary in regulating the flow of blood through the liver. Anything that prevents the normal respiratory movements causes a slowing of the flow of blood through the liver, consequently there will be an accumulation of blood in the portal and hepatic vessels.

Too frequent and copious meals is the most common cause of

hyperemia of the liver, and if this condition is accompanied by a sedentary mode of life and insufficient exercise the hyperemia, as well as difficulty in breathing, ·will be noticed, which generally impedes the power of locomotion. The use of alcohol, strong spices and coffee, as well as certain toxins developed as a result of putrefactive changes in the stomach and intestines, will lead to symptoms of indigestion and hyperemia of the liver.

As hyperemia is the first stage of changes in the structure of the liver, such as enlargement, fatty infiltration and proliferation of the connective tissues, it is important to recognize the causes of hyperemia early in order to prevent organic changes in the liver. Some affections of the heart cause hyperemia, and in organic diseases of the heart the relief of the liver· hyperemia is not possible. Injuries in the region of the liver have produced this condition. Typhoid fever and the acute exanthemata can produce these changes in the liver. One author says that hyperemia of the liver may be produced by hysteria, fright, mental excitement, as well as excessive mental effort.

The symptoms of hyperemia of the liver are rarely seen in noncomplicated form, as the varied causes are apt to produce varied symptoms. In general, they consist in the sensation of pressure and fullness in the right hypochondriac and epigastric regions, which may or may not amount to actual pain, aggravated by movement, increased breathing and change of position.

Percussion and palpation will generally reveal an enlarged liver, which will be tender and in some cases painful. All the symptoms are generally made worse by disturbed digestion, especially if there is much flatulence. If irritating food is taken in any quantity all symptoms will be increased.

Icterus may appear, which indicates a continued hyperemia, and is more manifest after an increased disturbance of the digestive organs. In certain women menstruation increases the icterus, as well as aggravating the hyperemia of the liver.

It is not an easy matter to diagnose this condition in the early stages. The condition is apt to become permanent, and frequently becomes the means of much damage before it will be discovered. In making up the diagnosis the size of the liver should be taken into consideration. In the majority of cases of abdominal plethora this condition should be looked for, and the case should be treated to remove the plethora as soon as possible.

The prognosis depends upon the presence or absence of organic changes either in the liver or any of the surrounding organs, which is illustrated by the following case:

Dr. R. B. C. was a strong burly fellow, fearless in every particular, especially when taking food he thought was for his good. He was declining for a year before the diseased conditions become fully developed. His whole expression changed from a healthy to a diseased one, causing many and varied symptoms. This diseased condition caused him to try many things and to travel quite extensively for relief, but none of the means of cure proved of any particular value to him. The disease gradually increased, bringing on conditions that were somewhat obscure.

To one not familiar with this class of cases it would be impossible to make a correct diagnosis.

But before going further I wish to speak a little more explicitly in regard to the causes of the pathological changes. There is no doubt but that derangement of the digestive organs was one of the prime factors in destroying his health. He suffered with indigestion, with all its attending symptoms, which was followed by an attack of rheumatism, which lasted some months. This rheumatic condition caused a heart lesion, which proved to be one of the main causes of hyperemia of the liver.

We must not forget that the greatest cause of obstruction to the outflow of blood from the veins of the liver is insufficiency of activity of the heart, which may be due to disease of the cardiac muscle or some valvular disease, with possibly a secondary involvement of the myocardium. Right heart lesions are especially adapted to cause stasis in the veins of the liver. Certain diseases of the lungs, such as contraction of lung tissue or atelectasis, pleuritic adhesions and empyema, may cause congestion of the liver, resulting in decided organic changes.

I take the liberty here and quote from my work on "Diseases of the Digestive Organs":

"As a rule, the changes that take place in color and consistency of the liver are not the same throughout the entire organ. Nutmeg spots may alternate with very red contracted areas. In some sections the liver cells are so atrophied that nothing will be seen but remnants of brownish pigments. The serous covering of the liver in this disease is often thickened and cloudy. The whole picture resembles the ordinary form of cirrhosis, with this difference, that in this form the distribution of the hardened areas is not uniform but very irregular."

The pleural lesions and lung involvement are apt to bring on more or less voice trouble. During the last few months of his life he suffered with aphonia. He also suffered with hydrothorax, and large quantities of effused blood were taken from the left pleural cavity.

During the last few weeks of his illness a small amount of fluid was thrown into the peritoneal cavity.

During the few months that he was with me in the sanitarium he was unable to take food to any extent, and part of the time spit it up, as he did not suffer with nausea or vomiting in the regular way, but the stomach refused to take the food and handle it. The peristaltic action of the bowels was practically destroyed. The action of the kidneys was not far from normal. He was restless and unable to sleep much without assistance. There was more or less cough, made worse by taking food. Mentally he was clear.

At death he was very much emaciated, and the post-mortem showed the conditions that I have described above. The changes in the liver seemed to be very decided and the nutmeg spots were numerous and of various sizes, leading one to believe that he might have had a cancerous disease of the liver, but, as I have already mentioned, the authorities are very accurate in their description of the difference between cancer and the pathological changes resulting from hyperemia of the liver.

A very mild form of icterus is sometimes seen in this condition, which was apparent from start to finish in his case. Authors are in doubt as to the causes of this condition, but attribute it to the retarded rhythmic movements of the liver following the slow respiratory excursion. However, this theory is not well founded.

He was unable to turn on his left side and be comfortable on account of the large accumulation in the pleural cavity. This fluid pressed upon the lung to such an extent that its size was reduced to that of an ordinary hand. The removal of the fluid from the peritoneal cavity gave him but little relief. The cavity soon refilled with the same character of fluid, which was of a dark wine color, probably containing some blood, and the pleural membrane was very much thickened. The right lung was not far from normal and the pleura was in a good condition.

There is but little temperature in these cases. The circulation is apt to vary considerable, running part of the time nearly normal, but may increase twenty or thirty beats when any of the general functions of the digestive tract are disturbed by indigestion. In the beginning of his disease his tongue was coated very much and was slow to clean, but during the time he was with me his tongue was practically clean.

Hyperemia of the liver develops slowly, and the first stages of engorgement of the organ with blood produce no symptoms until the characteristic organic changes take place. When the engorgement of the liver has caused a considerable change in the liver this condition may be discovered by palpation and percussion. The surface of the organ will be found to be smooth, tense and hard, and it may extend downward even to the umbilicus or farther, and will be noticed as a smooth hard body, sensitive to pressure. If this condition continues for a long time the liver may gradually grow smaller as a result of atrophy of the parenchyma and increase of the connective tissue.

Wagner says that where ascitic fluid is removed from the abdomen the surface of the liver may feel nodular from the fact that the blood streams into the liver as soon as the pressure within the abdomen is relieved, but owing to the structural changes that have occurred within the organ all parts of the surface are not evenly distended with blood, and hence at first irregularity of the surface of the liver will be noticed, but soon it becomes smooth.

The subjective signs of hyperemia vary considerable, owing to the rapidity of the onset of the disease. In some cases there may be considerable swelling of the liver and enlargement, while in others only a slight degree of swelling may be noticed,, with a disagreeable feeling of fullness in the epigastric region. In some cases the patient may complain of a disagreeable feeling and fullness, which will be more noticed after eating, owing to the fullness of the stomach and the hyperemia of the liver during the period of digestion, which was quite marked in his case.

Where we have considerable passive congestion in the portal system there will be marked dyspeptic and gastric disturbances and in some instances swelling of the hemorrhoidal veins. In most cases as soon as a mild form of icterus presents itself there will be a minute quantity of urobilin found in the urine, but bile pigments are not found in the urine of all these cases. Some of these cases have a combination of cyanosis and icterus, which gives us the peculiar greenish coloration of the skin.

Hyperemia of the liver is usually followed by serous exudates, edema, in some cases diminution of the flow of the urine and disturbances of respiration, but these complications do not appear with any regularity. When hyperemia of the liver does appear it will be constantly present, and when once fully developed it generally persists until death takes place, but may vary somewhat in intensity from time to time.

Another diagnostic point that it is well to mention here is that in cirrhosis of the liver the spleen takes on enlargement, but in passive hyperemia of the liver the spleen becomes indurated and not enlarged, which was the condition found in Dr. Carter's case.

Where we have ascites it is well to be careful in considering this as a positive symptom, as it may appear early or late in the disease, but as a rule it comes in the late stage of the affection, and only to a slight degree, which was the condition we found the case reported.

When he came to me his condition was beyond any remedial measures, and while the effects of the diseased condition of the liver were somewhat easy to detect, yet the real cause of his sickness and death was only cleared up in the post-mortem.

To me his case was very interesting, and caused me to spend many hours in determining the causes that would lay low such a powerful constitution. The doctor's good living habits were probably the greatest cause of the liver taking on this condition. He was quite apt to take food in season and out of season, not thinking that it was possible to derange such a powerful digestive system, but at last the great glandular organ, the liver, was forced to yield its normal action and assume a diseased condition.

GASTRIC ULCER.

Geo. W. Deem, M.D., Hilliards, O.

Ulcer of the stomach is a disease of early adult life, occurring more often in females between the ages of twenty and thirty. Men are also liable to this disease up to the age of forty, beyond which it is extremely rare.

Overwork, poor food and mental disorders are supposed to be exciting causes. It is more frequent among servant girls and among tailors and others whose occupations compel them to bend over in their work.

We often have a history of dyspepsia or of chronic gastritis which has existed for some time. Loss of appetite, a feeling of fullness in the stomach, and pyrosis with eructations are nearly always present. Pain is generally present and very severe. It is greatly increased by taking food, either immediately or a few hours afterwards. Vomiting will usually give temporary relief. There is tenderness, often localized in a small spot. Free hydrochloric acid in the stomach contents is usually present. Hematemesis is observed in about 50 per cent. of the known cases, sometimes so severe as to cause extreme pallor and weakness and to change materially the action of the heart. After one of these hemorrhages tarry blood will be found in the stools.

The ulcers that form in the mucous lining of the stomach are from one-fourth to three inches in diameter, and are sometimes very superficial and at others so deep that they cause perforation, with resulting peritonitis. It is thought that perforation occurs in 6½ per cent.

of all cases. As a result of inflammatory action adhesions sometimes form with the pancreas, the liver and the omentum.

The diagnosis of gastric or peptic ulcer is usually not difficult. The gastralgia of nervous dyspepsia usually comes on when the stomach is empty. Food will give relief. We also usually have neuralgic pains elsewhere about the body and no vomiting of blood. Dyspeptic symptoms and local sensitiveness between attacks are very rare.

We recognize hepatic colic by the sudden onset and the swelling and tenderness of the liver. If jaundice appears our diagnosis will be positive.

The gastric crises of locomotor ataxia will sometimes simulate ulcer, but when the lightning pains, the ocular symptoms and the absence of knee-jerk are noted we will have no difficulty.

In cancer of the stomach we can frequently observe the tumor, and the blood, if vomited, is not bright scarlet, but resembles coffee-grounds. The person is emaciated and nearly always past middle life.

The disease terminates in three ways—healing, perforation, and death from inanition. Some cases will heal spontaneously. A majority of your cases can be cured if you can get the patient to obey orders.

One of the most important things after an attack of hemorrhage is rest in bed. This should be insisted upon for at least one week after hemorrhage has ceased. A mild unirritating diet is essential. Milk, cornstarch, gruel, beef jelly, white of egg, and ices should form the greater part of the diet.

If the stomach is very irritable, rectal alimentation should be resorted to for several days. Milk, eggs or some of the prepared foods can be used for this purpose. Scraped raw beef is well tolerated by some after a few days. Later, rice, sago, oatmeal, arrowroot and mashed potatoes may be used.

Of the various remedies used in gastric ulcer, the most important is bismuth. Thirty grains of the subnitrate may be given three times daily. It is fortunate that this drug fails to produce constipation here as it does in other cases. If a laxative is demanded, the Carlsbad or Vichy salts will give best results. Nitrate of silver in one-sixth grain doses is used by many, but in my experience is not as satisfactory as bismuth.

If there is constant nausea, small pieces of ice, or ice-cream, may be beneficial. Opium may be needed to allay the pain. Ergot will often do good in relieving the hemorrhage. After the acute stage has subsided, a ferruginous tonic is demanded to build up the strength and restore the blood that has been sacrificed.

In the management of one of these cases the physician should be strictly honest with his patient. He should explain the nature of the disease in such a way that the patient will feel the necessity of great care, yet not become discouraged. Without the confidence and co-operation of the patient success is not assured.

ERYSIPELAS.

P. E. Decatur, M.D., Marseilles, O.

Erysipelas is an acute, contagious and infectious disease, characterized by a special inflammation of the skin due to the streptococcus erysipelatis.

It is found at all seasons of the year, but most prevalent during the cold wet months of spring. It usually occurs sporadically, but may become epidemic.

Among the predisposing causes are depressed or debilitated conditions, chronic alcoholism, Bright's disease, unsanitary surroundings, cold wet weather of the spring, wounds or abrasions, parturient women, chronic discharges. The exciting cause is the streptococcus erysipelatis.

When seen post-mortem in uncomplicated cases, there is little else than an inflammatory edema, with the cocci mostly in the lymph spaces in the zone of spreading inflammation. They may be found beyond the inflamed margin. In severe cases the swelling may be so great as to cause death of parts, with sloughing of the tissues.

There is an incubation period of three to seven days, when the disease is ushered in by a rigor of more or less severity, followed by a rapid rise of temperature to 103° or 105° F. It may start by an abrasion or injury, which becomes slightly reddened; in a few hours it swells and begins spreading, the skin being smooth, tense, shiny and edematous, pitting on pressure, turning white after pressure is removed, which gradually disappears. If of the face, the eyes swell shut and the features so swollen the patient is unrecognizable. The disease advances with redness and a ridge of swelling. The glands may be involved, blebs appear, and there will be leucocytosis. The temperature may remain very high for days, the tongue become dry, brown or coated, the pulse feeble and rapid, severe toxemia, and the patient may be delirious. In one case I had the nasal mucous membrane was involved first, with a severe swelling of the submaxillary gland; did not think of it being erysipelas till the skin of the alae became reddened, when upon careful examination found the mucous membrane involved. If there is a mixed infection we will have abscess.

Among the complications, meningitis is rare, the delirium and coma being due to fever and toxemia. Pneumonia is occasional, and may occur in a protracted case. Pleurisy seems to be more common when of the chest. Peritonitis may also occur. Pyemia is extremely rare in uncomplicated cases; it may affect the joints or may produce thrombosis.

The diagnosis is easy when of the skin, for we have the peculiar onset, the reddened, swollen, shiny hot skin, high fever and tendency to spread with the advancing ridge of swelling. Acute eczema, no fever, lack of definite border or marked swelling, intense pruritus. Erythema, no fever, swelling, nor local heat.

The prognosis in healthy adults is good. The average mortality in hospitals is about 7 per cent., in private practice, 4 per cent. (Anders). In the aged, debilitated, habitual drinkers or complicated cases, it is serious; they may die from intensity of fever or toxemia.

In the migratory form, which is more protracted, death may be due to exhaustion. When it affects the navel of the new-born it is usually fatal.

In treatment, isolate patient, especially in the hospital. The practitioner should not attend cases of confinement while caring for a case of erysipelas. After examining a patient he should sterilize the hands.

The diet should be nutritious and light.

As to drugs, there is quite a list, but we ought to study carefully the conditions and apply the drug that is indicated. I shall name a few, and will allow you to study their indications thoroughly. For local use we have tincture perchloride of iron, echafolta, ichthyol, potassium permanganate, salicylic acid and borax, sodium hypophosphite and sodium bicarbonate. For internal use, aconite, veratrum, rhus tox., gelsemium, belladonna, tincture perchloride of iron, sodium sulphite, hydrochloric acid, apis mel., baptisia, nux vom., anti-bilious physic, podophyllum, phytolacca, strychnine and quinine.

DISCUSSION.

CHAIRMAN: This paper was to have been discussed by Dr. A. P. Taylor; he is not here, and I will ask Dr. Shiller to open the discussion.

DR. S. SCHILLER: I am glad to say that I was greatly pleased with the paper as read, although the reading of it might possibly have been improved (laughter), but I mean the subject-matter of the paper. It is a plain, every-day, common-sense paper, and it is a disease that we will encounter occasionally, I presume, in practice.

Once in my forty years' experience I encountered an epidemic of erysipelas, erysipelatous fever, and the mortality was very great; I believe that the mortality was 25 to 30 per cent. of the cases. It was malignant. They became delirious. Temperature ran as high as 106°. And one case I treated died, and one case I might speak more particularly of, developed meningitis on the fourth day.

It is a disease that spreads from the starting-point. In facial erysipelas, the common variety that we meet, it starts usually about the nose, the skin of the nose, from infection no doubt. There may be just a small pimple or blister or something of that kind, that allows the germ of erysipelas to obtain entrance to the system, and from that point it spreads.

I only wish to speak about local applications. Years ago we used to paint them with iodine; it was barbarous, but the result was fairly good. I can remember, however, the agony that patients endured when we would paint that raw surface with the pure tincture of iodine, and I have done it many a time. And tincture of iron isn't much better. Now we have local remedies that I think do fully as well, if not better, than some of our modern antiseptic remedies, and I confess, with me, ichthyol is a favorite, used in about 25 per cent. ointment. The last case I treated—that is, about four or five months ago—I tried echafolta in about a 10 per cent. solution in water. I just simply wet a little piece of gauze and laid it over the face, and I think it did fully as well with that as with any other.

Erysipelas runs a definite course; in about four days it is going to be well; that is, the point where it started. It may keep on spreading, but in four days from the time it starts on the nose the nose will be well, whether you put on tincture of iodine or pure carbolic acid, or ichthyol, or echafolta, or anything else. I don't believe it is necessary to punish the patient very much with local applications. The ichthyol ointment solution is cooling, stops the burning sensation, and I like it better than carbolic acid; the odor isn't quite so offensive and it isn't so poisonous, either.

The proper treatment, as we Eclectics all know, is to treat the patients more than we do the disease; at least that is my method—without any specifics for the disease by name, not for erysipelas, not for pneumonia, nor for anything else. I treat the patient and sometimes try to forget what we call disease.

Dr. J. P. Dice: In regard to ichthyol, it is a good remedy, which every one has found out, but the odor is not good and the handling of it is often unsatisfactory. Those who wish to use it, if you will take a drachm of ichthyol and a drachm of sulphuric ether and add it to an ounce of flexible collodion, and with a hair brush brush over the diseased area once or twice in twenty-four hours, you will have a preparation of ichthyol that is nice to handle and warranted to give good color, and will give you no special discomfort or misgiving about putting on the ichthyol in some other shape, that you are not able to handle comfortably.

Dr. W. K. Mock: Among the local applications for erysipelas is one that I have not noticed mentioned, which is quite a favorite of mine, and that is an unction of boracic acid. I take boracic acid one drachm to vaseline one ounce, and make a mask for my patient. I take some cotton cloth, white, cutting a place for the nose, mouth and eyes, and I take this salve and paste it on a cloth and tie it around the face and back of the head. I have this changed every three or four hours, and as a local application I like it very much. I used. as Dr. Shiller says, the iodine and iron, and I have used ichthyol, but I believe that boracic acid used in this way beats anything else I have ever used.

DR. W. N. MUNDY: In regard to local applications in the treatment of erysipelas, one of the main points, to my mind, is the diagnosis of erysipelas. I find, at least I think so, many mistakes made in the diagnosis of erysipelas; various forms of dermatitis, erythema, are frequently called erysipelas.

Erysipelas is an acute, contagious disease, a constitutional disease, if you please, characterized by marked changes in the constitution of the patient—for instance, well-marked chill and a high fever and a general depression, with all the symptoms of toxemia.

Other varieties of dermatitis are not so marked; neither is eczema. The characteristic symptoms of eczema are the burning, itching, swelling and oozing, that oozing on the irritation of the surface. And I think that frequently many of the quick cures of erysipelas are really cures of dermatitis, for I think erysipelas is quite a serious condition. Most of the cases are a facial form. I find that aged people are prone to erysipelas, those who are depressed with age.

DR. E. A. BALLMER: I would be unfaithful to the duties imposed upon me as Secretary of this section if I did not take part in this discussion, and I want to say a word or two. I think I have as good result with a cloth wrung out of ice-cold water as with any application I have ever used.

DR. J. J. SUTTER: I have just had three cases of erysipelas about three weeks ago, and as so many drugs have been mentioned as local applications, I will add another to the list. I don't think we need any local application, but people want it, so if I have asepsin with me I make a solution of asepsin, and if not I use sulphite of soda, and keep it moist. It always seems that there is no need of any of it.

BRONCHITIS.

W. H. GRAHAM, M.D., SOUTH CHARLESTON, O.

In choosing this subject to present to you upon this occasion I have not based my choice upon any particular phase of the disease, nor do I have any new treatment to suggest. On the other hand, my idea is merely to emphasize the importance of a disease which, owing to an early diagnosis and a simple treatment, is very often neglected.

During my practice I have often been reminded of the way in which an eminent physician treated the same subject in a course of lectures delivered in Chicago. He devoted an hour on each of two days to an exhaustive discussion of bronchitis, and, believe me, the conclusion to his able address was, "Any old woman can treat it," an expression not new to us, and one which we all know is much abused.

I wish to refute that foolish conclusion to an important subject. Most authors admit that the disease bears watching in the old and in the very young, but claim that in the healthy adult home treatment suffices.

There is often nothing of a serious nature in the case we are called to treat, but too much care cannot be taken by the physician in assuring himself that this is a fact. What is bronchitis to-day is one or maybe more of half a dozen diseases to-morrow. In my own experience I find this to be true with the young as well as the old, though, of course, complications are more likely in advanced age.

Can you cite me a disease so simple in its beginning, which is so fraught with non-remedial danger as bronchitis? Measles, malaria, typhoid, scarlet fever, pneumonia, and tuberculosis lie in its wake. How many cases of the above come to us on account of a prevailing idea that "any old woman can treat bronchitis?"

Doctors, don't send your patients home to a hot lemonade or a foot-bath and hear from them next on a death-bed, where pneumonia exists or where tuberculosis has fastened its fangs. No more hopeless cases come to the physician than those arising from this neglected disease. Days of work with only alternate good and bad results, and finally failure, are the end of it all. Where you save your patient you must congratulate yourself that your competitor has not taken the case from you during its unpromising days.

One of the greatest points gained in the treatment of this minor disease is that the physician insists upon hearing from his patient. How often we say, "It's a cold; it will be over in a few days." Do not let the patient be the judge of that. Insist upon hearing from him. Large success may hinge upon so little a thing. Though a primary disease, it leaves one susceptible to a multitude of evils, and in even the lightest cases, where age and a good constitution favor the patient, there is always a likelihood of a permanent change in the mucous membrane.

Patients have come to my office on numerous occasions with serious complications arising from the neglect of bronchitis, in most of which cases it was evident that the disease had not only been regarded lightly by the patient, but by the physician himself.

DISCUSSION.

DR. W. S. TURNER: We have two varieties to consider, and in them, like every other, we treat general conditions. If there is fever, give the necessary cathartic and clean out the alimentary canal; that is one of the first items in treating the acute variety, following with whatever remedies are indicated. It may be aconite and ipecac. It may be an expectorant of squills, or something of that nature; whatever we find is indicated that we give. Of course, in chronic bronchitis there is a great variety of treatment, and I suppose if we had the experience of all the physicians here every one would have a different remedy. I have no iron-bound treatment for bronchitis; I treat my patient, and by doing that we generally bring about the results.

DR. E. FLORENCE STIR SMITH: I haven't very much to add, only that I am a great person to use local applications, because I have bronchitis myself, and there isn't anything that gives me the relief. that a good mustard plaster does. That, with aconite and ipecac, I think, would relieve many acute conditions.

APPENDICITIS.

DR. J. J. SUTTER: We have time yet, and I notice one paper on the program that has not been given, on "Appendicitis." I would like to have the question of appendicitis discussed, and I move that we take up the question of appendicitis and discuss it until time for the next section. Dr. McKittrick will open the question of appendicitis, since Dr. Gemmill is not here. Motion seconded and carried.

DISCUSSION.

DR. A. S. McKITTRICK: Dr. Sutter has taken a little advantage of these people. The doors are locked and they cannot get out very well, They will probably hear more of me than they want to.

Of course, the subject of appendicitis is a pretty good subject. Many things have been said, but probably the last word has not yet been said. There was a time a few years ago when an operation was performed for appendicitis at every stage of the game, and a good many of them were lost, and a good many of them were lost if you did not operate.

In the last few years I think the consensus of opinion of the surgical world is that if you have an absolute diagnosis made in the first twenty-four hours, that you should operate; that is, that that is the best time to operate; but if you pass the twenty-four hours, or thirty-six at the outside, that you better not operate until you either get a recovery or until you get a localized abscess, and if you use the so-called expectant treatment you will get in most of the treatments either one or the other; that is, starvation treatment, treated entirely by alimentation, leaving the bowels alone, after you empty the bowels first with a cathartic and an enema, but after that leave them alone, and leave your patient quiet, and don't bother about operating until the third or fourth day. If you operate before the third or fourth day you lose a nice percentage of your cases.

DR. L. E. RUSSELL: Operate as soon as you get security for your fees. If you have pus, drain; if you haven't pus, take away the appendix; if you have pus, let the appendix alone; get good drainage, and the inflammatory condition that has obtained in the appendix subsides and you will have no further trouble.

Appendicitis really belongs to the surgical part of the profession, instead of to the medical, although many times, if it is properly treated, the medicine man will get a good recovery, unless it has gone on to that stage where a catarrhal condition has obtained and where there is pus already formed in the appendix or sac. If you have a sac, it is really an obstruction that you must remove; it is a thorn in the flesh, and the sooner it is taken out the better for the safety of the patient and all concerned.

Many operators have many deaths because they try to do too much. They want to obtain a pathological specimen to show the friends, and the whole body turns to be a pathological specimen.

It is very much better to do a little when you have pus; simply get in and drain and allow the sac to granulate out and make a cure. There was a time when we anticipated a good deal as to *when* we should operate. The question now is as to *how much must* we operate. And if you follow it along carefully on that line, you will have success in nearly all of your cases. The pus drained, let the appendix alone; if not, you have a high inflammatory condition, some adhesions and a sac still within the zone of the appendix, take away the appendix.

Recently we had a case of a young man, working in a store, taken sick just after eating a hearty supper on Saturday evening; Sunday taken to the hospital; Monday the pain had nearly all subsided; the soreness was pretty nearly all gone; all that we had was high temperature. Made an incision down over the appendix and found a gangrene for an inch and a half of the appendix, with sac just bulging out into the abdominal cavity. In that case we removed the appendix and the patient made a nice recovery. If that case had been treated on the expectant plan we would have lost the patient. You don't want to believe, always, when the patient is entirely free from pain, that they are entirely saved. You must know your case or you will have a death in thirty-six or forty-eight hours, and you will be surprised and chagrined. I take it that the question is now not when to operate, but how much to operate.

DR. W. T. GEMMILL: From the experience I have had with appendicitis I think it is a subject upon which no surgeon is able to tell somebody else just when he must operate. You must know, from practical experience and from the conditions you see before you, what is necessary to do, and I think then the next thing is to do just as good as you can in order to relieve the trouble and save the patient's life. If you were called to see a case where the inflammatory condition has run its course, and pus has formed, and nature has walled it off around the appendix, and taken care of it and will take care of it for a certain length of time, the best plan, with the best results, is to make your incision down into this cavity and drain out your pus and let everything else alone. Whenever you attempt to hunt for that appendix, or to see how much damage has been done by the inflammatory process, you open up a door for infection, and you are going to have trouble and lose your patient.

I believe in some cases, not in all, that a very early operation, if you get the patient early enough, is the proper thing to do, but even then you should use your best judgment as to know just what is necessary to do, and do no more than is necessary.

I operated on a case last Friday morning for Dr. Mundy, a young man twenty-three or twenty-four years old. I think this was the third attack; he had an attack last summer or last fall and an attack prior to that time, some three or four months. The case had been going on for about five days, and when we went out to visit him last Friday morning the patient's symptoms were all better, the pain had subsided, temperature had gone down, and yet you could find over the region of the appendix a hardness that indicated that we had pus of considerable amount; but every other indication would lead you to believe that the patient would have gotten well if we had let him alone. There was something about the expression on the man's face and the character of the pulse that told us there was trouble brewing, and the proper thing to do was to make an incision and see how much pus was in the cavity, which we did. We removed from a pint to a pint and a half of very offensive pus, left open drainage, and the patient has been doing very well ever since that, without any bad symptoms, and is going to get well. If we had attempted to look for that appendix, or to investigate the matter more closely, after draining out the pus, the case would not have gone so well and we would have probably lost our patient.

I believe, in a great majority of cases, that the surgeon undertakes to do more, really, than he should do, and by so doing not only gets himself in trouble, but loses his patient. I think more cases get well if you drain out the pus and leave them alone; don't hunt for the appendix, don't try to do a lot of work that you don't know what you are doing, by probing around and letting the pus out in the abdominal cavity, resulting in peritonitis and death.

A PERSISTENT sinus after an operation for appendicitis in the majority of cases means that a portion of the appendix has been left behind. It may also mean that an exudate has broken down or that some foreign body has been left in the wound. One should give the sinus an opportunity to close by itself, but if it does not do so, a prolonged operation is necessary. The walls of the sinus must be carefully excised, all rents in the serosa of the intestine sewed over and drainage instituted, as there is often considerable oozing from raw surfaces. First and foremost, the primary cause of the sinus must be found and corrected.—*American Journal of Surgery.*

PROCTITIS DUE TO CONSTIPATION.—Empty the bowels, says Hughes, with an enema of warm water and soap, or an enema of four ounces of hot water, two ounces of epsom salts and one-half ounce of glycerine.—*Denver Med. Times.*

PYEMIA.—Tyson says: Remove primary focus if possible. Give the most nutritious and easily assimilable food and liberal doses of alcohol, quinine and strychnine.—*Denver Med. Times.*

𝔓𝔢𝔯𝔦𝔰𝔠𝔬𝔭𝔢.

The Significance of Pain in Pelvic Disease.

Novak, in his interesting paper (*American Journal of Obstetrics*, April, 1908), says:

1. That a careful physical examination is of first importance in the diagnosis of pelvic disease, but interesting information will also be derived from the character and distribution of the pelvic pain.

2. The exact nature of the disease should be determined in a given case, as nearly as possible, and not the advisability or inadvisability of an operation alone.

3. Pain in the pelvic viscera is governed by the same laws which apply to the causation of pain in the other abdominal viscera.

4. Neurasthenia may develop from neglected pelvic disease, with diffusion of pain and characteristic symptoms in other parts of the body.

5. Persistent neurasthenia following pelvic operations is frequently responsible for the continuance of unpleasant symptoms.

6. Hysteria with pelvic symptoms has the same characteristics as when associated with other diseases.

7. The removal of normal ovaries for pelvic pain is now regarded as unjustfiable.

8. Fibrocystic ovaries are often found in women who are in perfect health. Operation on such organs should be conservative.

9. Pain is the resultant of a lesion and a patient, and in order to understand its significance both these factors must be carefully studied.—*American Medicine.*

Echinacea as an Internal Antiseptic After Labor.

A new idea which I have been using in my practice of late may be of some use to others. *Echinacea angustifolia* has a reliable reputation for counteracting septic conditions of the fluids of the body. Knowing this to be so, I determined to use it for the purpose of heading off any slight septic post-partum condition from whatever cause. Very few labors occur without more or less laceration of the ostium vaginæ. A slight tear in this locality will result in some infection in spite of any local application which can be made. I believe that the slight fever which is so common about the third day, and which we were formerly told was due to the commencement of lactation, was due to nothing but septic infection. There is danger of septic invasion of the uterus from these slight tears, if left to natural trend. Again, often there remains in the location of placental implantation fragments of placenta, or shreds, or slight blood clots, which perchance become infected before being freed and washed away by the lochia. Again, there may be, and this is the rule rather than the exception, lacerations of the cervix, furnishing a door for the entrance of infection.

With some, if not all, these sources of systemic infection after labor it is not surprising that nearly every patient has "third-day fever." My idea is to give echinacea to ward off, counteract and prevent these feverish conditions by early use of its internal antiseptic action. Experience has demonstrated the correctness of this idea, and my patients do not have post-partum fever from "milk coming" or any other cause. I also find that lacerations of the perineum one-half to three-fourths of an inch deep do not require stitches when I use this valuable drug after labor. Another advantage in the use of echinacea is the tendency to prevent absorption of infection from cracked nipples and cause mammary abscess. Too much milk does not cause suppuration; there must be infection. Echinacea guards against this. Theory is all right, and the practical results are exceedingly gratifying.—A. D. HARD, *in Homeopathic Med. Recorder.*

Conjugal Diabetes.

In a recent address before the Berlin Medical Society H. Senator spoke of his experiences in this interesting phase of diabetes. Twenty-five years ago Betz first expressed the opinion that diabetes could be transmitted. and pointed out that it is relatively frequent in husband and wife in the same family. Further investigation, however, showed that among a large number of diabetics there was only about 1 per cent. of diabetic couples.

Senator, agreeing with Leo, emphasizes the fact that this statistical statement is not correct. It is not a question of the relative frequency of diabetic married couples as compared with the total number of diabetics. On the contrary, we must ask, How often does a husband or wife acquire diabetes after marrying a diabetic person? With this question in view, Senator gives a statistical record of cases of diabetes from his clinic and private practice. He found that there were 516 married couples in whom one of the two suffered from diabetes. He found that in 3.9 and 4.3 per cent. of his cases there was diabetes in both members of the family. He thought that these figures were still too small to show that diabetes is transmitted from one person to another, especially as hereditary diabetic tendency was often noted in one or both persons. Yet there are some clinical and experimental facts which point to the possibility of transmitting diabetes. Teissier reports the case of a laundress, aged sixty-two years, who acquired diabetes after having washed the laundry of a man suffering from a severe form of diabetes. Kulz reported that diabetes was present in five inhabitants of the same house, and found that a young woman who had acted as a companion to a diabetic lady had acquired the disease. In a similar case Naunyn and Senator reported that the second wife of a diabetic, whose first wife had died of diabetes, also acquired the disease.

Senator does not believe that the cases here quoted show definitely that diabetes can be transmitted. Thus, the disease may have existed before the patients had come in contact. Furthermore, the same causes which are connected with conditions of life, diet, etc., would act in a similar manner in persons living together. Still, it cannot be denied that there is a posibility of transmitting diabetes from one person to another, although we have as yet no definite proof of the occurrence of this transmission.—*La Tribune Medicale.*

The Family Physician and the Public.

There yet remains a means of educating the public which I believe will be the most potent of all. This rests in the hands of the family physician—the man who has the care of the household, who watches the growth of the children, who sees the father and mother bend under the strain of life, react and again assume their work, the counselor of the family—he it is who can carry into the homes of this country the judicious truth concerning disease. Well-educated people have recognized that the wave of specialism which threatened to obliterate the family practitioner was dangerous for the welfare of the whole. The trouble is that we all consider ourselves, when ill, as peculiar examples of some disease, when, as a matter of fact, all we need is the counsel and advice of a sound-minded family practitioner who has known us and our families for many years. This does not in the least deny the great advantage of having the benefit of special knowledge in reference to a special subject.

There is a distinct reaction, I believe, against the obliteration of the family practitioner. The well-educated family practitioner now has a new duty. He it is who should be the instructor of the family. This is particularly true in relation to the subjects which in medicine cannot with propriety be taught the public in masses; these subjects may be taught most appropriately to the parents, and, if need be, the children, by the general counselor of the family.

A great duty rests on the practitioner of medicine to-day. He must not shirk it; he must rise to his new burden, accept it and bear it. The reward to the medical profession for taking this new burden of judicious publicity in medicine will be a broader life for the practitioner, a greater consideration for his fellow man, better citizenship and the recognition by the world that the medical profession is a great public benefactor.— BURRELL, *American Medicine*.

Some Remedies for Headaches.

Ammonium Iodide.—Where your patient complains of a dull ache attended with dizziness and trouble in controlling the voluntary muscles, two grains of this salt, in water, given every three hours, will afford relief.

Specific Belladonna.—If the headache complained of is of a dull heavy character with drowsiness, add ten drops of the specific belladonna to four ounces of water and give teaspoonful doses every hour until relieved.

Specific Bryonia.—Headaches that are confined to the right side of the head and extend from front to back , with soreness of the head and severe pain, the right cheek being flushed, call for the use of specific bryonia. Add five to fifteen drops to four ounces of water and give in teaspoonful doses every hour.

Caffeine.—Occasionally you will see a headache that evidently is being caused by cerebral hyperemia, as indicated by the flushed face. Two grains of caffeine given every two hours will soon produce a marked change.

Specific Gelsemium.—Frequently your patient will tell you that the pain covers the entire head, there is perceptible throbbing of the temporal arteries, with bright eyes, flushed face, and the general picture of intense nervous irritation. Add five to fifteen drops of the specific gelsemium to four ounces of water and give a teaspoonful every fifteen minutes to every hour according to the severity of the case.

Specific Rhus.—If the pain is situated in the frontal region, particularly over the left orbit, and is described as sharp in its nature, especially if there is a redness of the papillæ on the tip of the tongue. small doses of this remedy will prove very effectual. Add five drops to four ounces of water and give in teaspoonful doses each hour.

Specific Nux Vomica.—Sick headaches, or those which are caused by any wrong of any part of the digestive apparatus, which is due to an atonic condition as indicated by pallor of the mucous membranes and a yellowish-white coating on the tongue, will be quickly removed by the use of the specific nux vomica. Put five to ten drops in four ounces of water and give in teaspoonful doses every fifteen minutes to every hour. If any stimulation is needed add also two to five drops of tincture of capsicum to this mixture and give in the same manner as before.

Specific Passiflora.—Headaches that are purely nervous in their causation are frequently relieved by the use of specific passiflora. This drug may be given in doses of from one to twenty drops every hour.— *Journal of Therapeutics and Dietetics.*

Physician vs. Surgeon.

It is said that every medical student cherishes a deep-seated hope to become, some day, a great surgeon, and shapes his work during the latter part of his college career with this end in view. If that be so, it is the duty of the medical faculty to correct this tendency by placing the chairs of practice of medicine and therapeutics foremost. Our graduates must be, above all, physicians. They should, of course, possess a fair understanding of surgical technique, but let not their knowledge along this important branch of practice be obtained at the expense of their thorough mastery of the principles of medicine and therapeutics.

Surgery has its legitimate field and, in many instances, surpasses any other means at our command for saving life, but it is unnecessarily fed and its sphere enlarged out of proportion by ignorance in matters of drug and physical therapy. Our young physicians ought to know about drugs and their indications in disease as much as they are eager to learn about appendectomy and herniotomy before they should consider themselves fit to practice their profession. Eagerness to attend surgical lectures and clinics should be encouraged only where the student attends his medical clinics and lectures on therapeutics with a similar degree of interest.—*Chicago Medical Times.*

Treatment of Scoliosis by Creeping.

Kuh (*Prager medizinische Wochenschrift*, Jahrg. 32, Nr. 52) observes that four-footed animals in walking bend the spine to one side at a certain phase of the progression, and to the other side at a subsequent phase. Following the example of Klapp, he has applied this knowledge to the treatment of scoliosis in the human being. In small children creeping is done without difficulty, as they simply follow their atavistic tendency. In older children whose spinal column is already stiffened the creeping motion must be modified. Klapp prescribes three modifications. In the first modification the child goes rapidly forward, and at the same time carries out rapid lateral movements with the entire spine relaxed, by this means producing considerable bending, which is increased by turning the head from side to side. The head is bent toward the side where the hand stands near the knee, and at the same time the child is instructed to look behind him.

In the second modification, the child creeps quite slowly while the bending is forcibly done. The leg which is set back is placed toward the concave side, the head and shoulder-girdle are forced over toward the concave side, and by this means the curve of the spine is accentuated; the next moment the opposite position is taken.

The third modification consists in a forced curving of the spine without locomotion. There occurs not only a marked mobilization of the spine but also a repression of the ribs. Finally in certain forms of scoliosis the child is required to creep in a circle. The knees and hands are protected by sandals. At first the exercises are for a quarter of an hour forenoon and afternoon, and later prolonged to two hours daily. The method is contraindicated in weak and anemic children. The author does not consider it of much practical value.—*The Therapeutic Gazette.*

Growing Old Gracefully.

In some measure longevity depends upon our heredity and the life insurance people are disposed to assume that we will live about as long as our parents. But the last few decades longevity is increasing, and one stands a pretty good chance of far outliving his progenitors. For all that we are going at a very rapid pace these days we are—some of us, at any rate—living longer than formerly. As proof of this assertion look at the octogenarians in the United States Senate. The immortal Shakespeare and many other notables of his time died at about the age of fifty. There are no valid reasons why we should not nearly all of us reach the century milestone. Any animal, including the genus homo, should live about five times as long as it requires such animal to fully mature and develop. There are many rules for making centenarians. One that we suggest is to learn to grow old gracefully. Studiously cultivate mental and physical relaxation. Cut out worry. The way to do this is to do new things and keep in touch with current events. A distinction should be made between worry and brain activity; they are wholly dissimilar. Active cerebration and good thinking tends to longevity and healthy old age. It seems that no special line of dietetics is especially conducive to healthy and extreme age, but most all observers are inclined to look with favor upon a system that approaches that advised by the vegetarians. The main thing about eating is not to overindulge. Long-lived people are usually sparing eaters and are rather abstemious in their dietary. It seems that it matters little what sort of nourishment is taken, provided it be not taken in too great quantities. The system appropriates what it needs. We repeat that to attain a healthy old age we should learn to grow old gracefully.—*Medical Summary.*

Staphisagria.

In an instructive article on this well-known Eclectic drug, Dr. Finley Ellingwood says in part:

"In chronic gleet I have been enabled to do more in the complete cure of the cases with this remedy than with any other single remedy, having succeeded nicely even in very protracted cases. It is not ordinarily advised in the acute stages of inflammation of the prostate, but in cases of subacute or chronic enlargement with chronic irritation it is useful, especially if combined with saw-palmetto. I have certainly found these two remedies to work very nicely together.

"In urinary irritation, common to old men with prostatic enlargement, with frequent desire to urinate, it overcomes the desire and the subsequent tenesmus, producing a sensation of restored tone. This result will occur if there is any inflammation of the bladder, provided it is combined with thuja or with chimaphila.

"There is a class of these stubborn conditions that will yield to a combination of these three remedies, with perhaps the addition of gelsemium or cimicifuga if the nerves are involved, and will induce results most highly satisfactory.

"In the treatment of certain forms of impotency I give this remedy with saw-palmetto and avena. It increases sexual power when imperfect and arrests excessive prostatic discharges. It is a remedy for nervous excitement and nervous irritability which depends upon sexual irritation or upon any disease of the genito-urinary organs. It should be given for certain forms of mental depression which occur in conjunction with hysteria or hypochondriasis, especially if accompanied with violent outbursts of passion.

Drugs Simulating Sugar in the Urine.

Coleman states that the following drugs, when ingested, may cause the urine to reduce Fehling's solution, and respond to some other tests for sugar: Acetanilid; arsenous, salicylic and dilute hydrocyanic and sulphuric acids; alcohol, amyl nitrite, chloral. chloroform, copaiba, glycerine, mercury, morphine, strychnine, turpentine.—*Medical Council.*

MAGGOTS IN THE NOSE.—The signs and symptoms include itching, crawling, gnawing sensations, intense pain and a bloody, purulent discharge. Inspection readily reveals the cause of the trouble. Bishop recommends the inhalation of chloroform, or inhalation followed by injection of the same.—*Denver Med. Times.*

THE ECLECTIC MEDICAL JOURNAL

A Monthly Journal of Eclectic Medicine and Surgery.

TWO DOLLARS PER ANNUM.

Official Journal Ohio State Eclectic Medical Association

JOHN K. SCUDDER, M.D., MANAGING EDITOR.

EDITORS.

W. E. BLOYER.	H. W. FELTER.	L. E. RUSSELL.	R. L. THOMAS.
W. B. CHURCH.	J. U. LLOYD.	H. E. SLOAN.	L. WATKINS.
JOHN FEARN.	W. N. MUNDY.	A. F. STEPHENS.	H. T. WEBSTER.

Published by THE SCUDDER BROTHERS COMPANY, 1009 Plum Street, Cincinnati, to whom all communications and remittances should be sent.

Articles on any medical subject are solicited, which will usually be published the month following their receipt. One hundred reprints of articles of four or more pages, or one dozen copies of the Journal, will be forwarded free if the request is made when the article is submitted. The editor disclaims any responsibility for the views of contributors.

Discontinuances and Renewals.—The publishers must be notified by mail and all arrearages paid when you want your Journal stopped. If you want it stopped at the expiration of any fixed period, kindly notify us in advance.

DEGREES.

As we are principally of European descent, it is not strange that we should be tinctured with European customs and tainted with its foibles. Some of these we may be proud of, while others may not be so universally admirable. High-sounding titles have always been held in great esteem across the water, and some Americans love to bask in the sunshine of their own greatness, reflected by high-sounding titles.

The time is not long distant, even if it has entirely flown, when those who were unable to afford degrees in England sent over to various shady institutions in this country and purchased them at moderate prices. Though rather questionable among the truly elect when thus obtained, the professors could congratulate themselves that they were at least "some pumpkins," even though not quite so good as those who had earned their degrees and obtained them at home.

The titles that some English doctors flourish at the end of their names are so lengthy as to be tiresome and unprofitable, for it requires valuable time and considerable trouble to read them. Few probably ever take the pains to even determine their significance; life is too short. If the title, "Doctor of Medicine," did not cover the whole field, there might be some reason for adding more than M.D. to their signatures; but so long as this includes everything a practitioner of medicine and surgery ought to require, why cumber the time and patience of people with more?

Dr. Osler furnishes us with an admirable example of modesty in this respect. Though highly honored by the entire medical profession, regarded as authority in many departments of medicine, and sought for abroad as well as at home, he was content to see his name on the title-page of his "Practice of Medicine" with only the addition of an M.D. Probably he possessed other titles and might have assumed them, but apparently he considered the title of Doctor of, Medicine paramount to all others in that connection, and others superfluous, because overshadowed.

Our own Professors Scudder and Howe were remarkably modest in this respect. Though the possessors of more titles than M.D., these were seldom paraded before the public. Because they had graduated at other institutions of learning than medical colleges, they did not seem to regard it in good taste to remind the world of it every time they appeared in print. It was a fair inference that if they possessed more than the average amount of knowledge the public would be apprised of the fact through their demonstrated attainments, and it was not necessary to append a string of doctor's degrees in order to remind people that they were on earth.

As a rule, Eclectics are commendably modest in this direction. Many years ago a tendency prevailed among some of the contributors to our medical journals and society transactions to string all the titles obtainable in the land to their names. They were Doctors of Pharmacy, Doctors of Laws, Doctors of Medicine, Masters of Arts, etc., through the entire category. A.M., M.D., Ph.D., LL.D., and all kinds of D's flourished—all in strings—until some Eclectics became almost as pompous a lot as a flock of London professors.

The practice at length became so nauseous to Professor Howe that he pricked the glittering bubble with his trenchant pen, and administered a well-merited rebuke. After this episode, the highly titled members of our persuasion gradually dwindled out of sight, as though their titles were the most that made them prominent. If a physician append M.D. to his name, he has assumed enough for all practical purposes, and possibly he has assumed more than he can make good. He may be a mighty poor doctor of medicine, even though he add titles galore. WEBSTER.

THE DANGER SIGNAL.

Every case of gastro-intestinal irritation in children, especially during the summer months, hangs out a danger signal in great big letters, which means STOP. Stop what? Why, feeding, of course. But you can't make the average man and woman pay any heed to the red flag. The great majority of the human family are so infernally afraid of starving that they insist on stuffing a cart-load of provender into their stomachs, even if said stomachs are bellowing loudly for just a little rest. But the baby is what we want to talk about more particularly, as this is the season of the year when children are having trouble and lots of it.

The danger signal I speak of is the frequent discharge from the bowels of a slimy, frothy, green, mucous stool, and perhaps occasional vomiting. This is the indication to stop feeding for a day or two in order that the alimentary canal may have a complete rest and recover its power to digest. It is seldom heeded, however, and the feeding goes on, the baby grows rapidly exhausted, and often dies as a result, or, having the vital power to resist the disease as well as the ingestion of food, worries along for days or weeks and finally recovers in spite of it all.

Children who are old enough to signify their wants and inclinations refuse to eat. Infants often make an attempt to do so, but the nipple, either natural or artificial, is thrust into their mouths, and they drink to their death.

Whenever a condition such as has been described arises, all food should be withheld for a time, varying in length according to the amount of irritation developed. Water is to take the place of milk during the time, and when, by means of fasting and appropriate medicinal treatment, the conditions change, food is to be given sparingly, first giving a *little* milk mixed with water, and gradually increasing the milk until a normal diet is reached.

The baby will not starve, but, instead, will show a rapid improvement, and the disease will pass without much reduction in flesh or strength.

I seldom have any difficulty in relieving those cases wherein the mother will follow my advice. It is those only where she will insist on feeding that the disease gets beyond control.

STEPHENS.

THE THERAPEUTICS OF SULPHUR.

Sulphur is one of the oldest of medicines. Though largely recognized and somewhat used as an external application, its value as an internal remedy has, we believe, been largely neglected.

There are some conditions for which we possess no better agent than sulphur in appreciable doses. These are largely disorders of the alimentary tract requiring the exhibition of remedies to act as a laxative without marked irritation or the excessive production of intestinal secretion. No remedy surpasses it for its laxative effect in cases of hemorrhoids, the stool produced being of a pap-like character and easily but plentifully voided. Again, when dry, hard, scybalóus feces are an annoying feature, the use of sulphur will produce the best of results. In such troubles as stricture of the rectum it is absolutely necessary to modify the stool so that it may readily pass through the contracted outlet. Here, again, sulphur is invaluable. By strict adherence to regularity in going to the toilet, with gentle urging, and the persistent use of small doses of sulphur, many cases of habitual constipation may be cured. The compound licorice powder, so valuable as a laxative during pregnancy, depends in part upon sulphur for its value.

While what we have written refers to the use of liberal doses of either sublimed or washed sulphur, there is another phase of the sulphur question which appeals strongly to us. It is a blood maker and a corrector of wrongs of that fluid. Its beneficial action in the form of sulphides is often fulfilled by the use of foods containing it in natural combination. Among these the best and most wholesome are eggs and onions. To these we would add the condiment mustard. They all tend to the more perfect elaboration of protein tissues. Most tuberculous patients require sulphur, and among the best foods for such subjects are the sulphur-bearing eggs. It is especially a remedy for anemia associated with tuberculosis. The classic condition for sulphur in minute doses we have fairly outlined before in the following:

"The cases requiring sulphur have a blanched appearance of the skin, the iris and the hair fade in color, and in the middle-aged there is an early tendency to gray hairs; the feces and urine are pale, and the latter contains cystine. If the mucous surfaces are bathed in a mucous flow, and there are itching and burning, the indications are stronger. If the secretions are fetid or cadaverous, and there is evident tendency to decomposition of the fluids and tissues, sulphur is indicated, and in small doses will greatly change the character of the disease of which these symptoms are a part. Again, if the bile be imperfectly elaborated, so that it fails to exert its antiseptic effects upon the gastro-intestinal contents, sulphur will greatly assist in rectifying the trouble."

Keeping before us the foregoing guides, we will find sulphur very valuable in headache due to cerebral fullness associated with dizziness and ringing noises in the ears; in tendency to cracking or fissure behind the ears, at the angles of the mouth and wings of the nose, so noticeable in ill-nourished and in some tuberculous children; and in amenorrhea and other female disorders with imperfectly elaborated menses, the flow being semi-leucorrheal. It is of value in dyspepsia, with heavy feeling after meals, and associated either with obstinate constipation or tenesmic diarrhea, with pale and offensive stools.

Many years ago sulphur was a very popular remedy for cough. It was then given in heroic doses. In our own experience we have found that its use in large doses does not begin to compare with minute doses of the trituration (1 in 100). This we have found a splendid agent in cough with heavy and copious secretion but lack of power to expectorate. It has thus rendered excellent service in the cough of pulmonary consumption.

Finally, though of value in many other conditions, it should not be overlooked as a remedy for pain, localized in character, as the darting and tearing pains of rheumatism and neuralgia, and in pain simulating the prick of a pin.

Of the external use of sulphur little may be said more than to refer to its value in scabies, acne and various forms of pharyngitis. In the latter instance the powder is used by insufflation; for skin affections chiefly as an ointment. For acne it may be given internally as well as used externally, and seems most potent in those cases associated with female disorders and with sexual disturbances in the male.

Though the classic specific for scabies, sulphur will disappoint if the proper preparation for its use be neglected. Wherever it can come in contact with the sarcoptes it will destroy it promptly. This is easy with the male, which travels on the surface of the skin. The female, however, burrows beneath the skin to lay her eggs, and is in a measure protected from the action of the ointment. Hence the necessity of softening the epidermis over the burrows by means of a prolonged and thorough soap bath and friction with a coarse towel to denude the surface where the pest is ensconced. Then the use of sulphur ointment applied every night for four or five nights, with proper attention to bedding and clothing, will be promptly effective.

Study sulphur for its many good qualities in chronic diseases, and you will be pleasantly surprised at the good it will accomplish for you.

FELTER.

CONCERNING INDIAN MEDICATION.

To one who has an opportunity of visiting the Indian country under the personal guidance of Dr. J. A. Munk, of Los Angeles, comes an instructive and most delightful treat. So many points connected with the comparatively unknown parts of New Mexico and Arizona are familiar to Dr. Munk as to make the journey, unconsciously to himself, one of continual education to his companions. It was our pleasure and good fortune, during the last six weeks, to be blessed with such an exceptional opportunity. In the multitude of problems connected with it all but a fragment can be satisfactorily presented at one time and in even those points under consideration connected issues dovetail so intricately as to render it impossible to satisfactorily draw the line between what should be said and what must be left unsaid.

Concerning Indian medication, or rather, sometimes, non-medication, one needs but to connect the past with the present to see that the Indian of to-day is moving in lines parallel with those followed by the Indian in the days of Tecumseh, of the Iroquois Nation, and of the time when Kentucky was the "Middle Ground," or the "Bloody Ground," for all the surrounding tribes. Then it was that superstition, incantation, charms, connected with the use of simples, prevailed. This is to-day true of the Indians in the Navajo and Moqui Reservations. Peter Smith, "The Indian Herb Doctor," a hundred years ago recorded much more than could be recorded to-day in the far West, because, for one reason, the multitude of plants in the rich middle West, with their great differences in nature, and the numbers of different tribes working independently, gave opportunities in the use of simples not to be found in the desert and in the rocky and sandy mountains of the present reservations. But there are yet possibilities, as may be illustrated by an incident.

The Indian guide who was taking me through the mountain stopped, dug up a plant, peeled a root, and handed it to me, having first chewed a portion of it himself, to indicate that it was not harmful. It tasted somewhat like ginseng, aromatically pleasant. With the secrecy of his people, however, he had not shown me the top, nor could I afterwards find a similar root. When finally we came to camp, the interpreter questioned him concerning the use of the drug. Said he, "Much good for the chest," tapping himself on the breast, "for cough, for lung trouble." Then he remained silent, nor could he be persuaded to give the Indian name of the drug or show a specimen of the plant. In the days of Peter Smith this drug would have been identified, given some common name, and its reputed qualities recorded.

As we passed through Canyon de Chelly, one hundred miles from the nearest settlement of whites, a weird sound came from under a cliff at our right. Approaching the spot, we discovered a cavern, in front of which hung an Indian blanket to block out the light. The weird sounds within were made by an old Indian medicine man, whose incantations had attracted us. Raising the blanket, we found a girl, over whom the old man was pow-wowing, but as we entered neither of them paid any attention to us. The pow-wow concluded, the old man left the cavern and rested in the sunshine against the cliff.

There, through our interpreter, he answered our questions, to the effect that a bad spirit dominated the girl, that she had been much worse the day before, but that by his art the spirit was being expelled, and that probably within a couple of days she would be much better. He informed us that he would sing again within an hour, and would keep up the incantation ceremony until relief followed. Drs. Munk and Welbourn examined the girl. They found a bruise on the foot, possibly complicated with a cactus thorn infection. The foot and ankle were much swollen, pus had formed beneath the infected part; a lancet was needed, and a lancet only, to give relief. It would probably break within another day, was the decision of Dr. Welbourn, after which the girl would recover. The old medicine man would probably then claim that his incantation drew the spirit out at the point whence came the relief. "Why not lance the foot?" occurred to us, but then came the thought, "We are in the Indian country, the prejudices of these people possess them. It would be a reflection on the medicine man, in whom they had confidence." What he might do by way of retaliation was a problem. What the girl's friends might do should relief not follow the incision, was another problem. Better let the girl suffer a day longer than intrude in a case like that. However, on our return. the girl was still being treated after the methods of the Navajo medicine man.

These are instances in the passing along, but I take it are sufficient to indicate the nature of the medication practiced by the wild men to-day, and also to indicate that the good offices of the United States surgeon and the physician who understandingly and sacrificingly attempts to educationally benefit such people as these, are deserving of the highest commendation.

However, on such testimony as this "cure" for chest troubles the most valuable remedies known to the materia medica have been discovered. Who can say that the plant of the Indian guide might not be invaluable could it have been located botanically. Nor can anyone find in the confidence the girl had in the medicine man's incantations a primitive belief in cure by faith.   LLOYD.

LOYALTY.

A condition which has always struck me as strange is the utter indifference among Eclectics for the welfare of their alma mater. It is usual for the alumni of an institution to refer with gratitude and pride and pleasure to that institution which has given them the position which they occupy and which has fitted them for the activities of life. Why is this not true of the alumni of our colleges? They have protected us, they have taught that which has made us successful in life. Why, then, are we not loyal to that institution which has done so much for us?

What we need to-day among us is loyalty and a strong fealty to that which has made us successful as a school. Rally to the support of our societies and to our colleges. Don't grumble, but encourage. Don't kick, but push. If you do not help to push, if you have never helped to push, you certainly have no right to kick. It is an easy matter to stand back on your dignity and tell what ought to be done. It is another matter to do it. If you know what ought to be done, why not add your mite and assist those who are willing and have been bearing the burden for these many years? Had our societies and colleges the united support of their alumni, as they ought to have, many changes could be brought about. We need to-day that support, undivided and unstinted.

The world admires a loyal and true man, no matter what may be his belief. It has no use for a traitor. You may be used, but after you have been thus used you will be discarded as was Benedict Arnold. We ask you as Eclectics to be true to your colors and cause. We have a system of therapeutics which possesses merit and certainty, and which has brought you success. You can learn it only in an Eclectic college. 'It can be taught only by those who have studied it, know it, and appreciate its merits by reason of experience.

We ask you to encourage those who have carried and are attempting to carry these burdens, and which you refuse to do, either for lack of time or disposition. This is no time for sluggards, shirkers or kickers. The need of the hour is for men, brave, true, loyal and unselfish, who are willing to make a slight sacrifice for the good of the cause

> "O brothers, blest by partial Fate
> With power to match the will and deed,
> To him your summons comes too late,
> Who sinks beneath his armor's weight,
> And has no answer but God-speed."

MUNDY.

EPIDEMIC REMEDIES.

We are firmly convinced that specific remedies for specific conditions is the only true or rational way of prescribing; that pathological conditions differ very greatly in different individuals suffering from the same disease, and in the same individual at different times; hence what will prove curative in one patient who is suffering from pneumonia will not benefit another, even though he have the same affection; nor probably the same remedy that benefited a patient this year would not prove efficacious a year hence, should he suffer a subsequent attack of the same lesion.

Ordinarily, toxins manifest themselves differently in individual cases and in the same disease. In one it will be represented by the dirty moist, pasty coating on the tongue, while in another the dry, red tongue will be seen, and still another will show a broad, dusky, moist tongue and full tissues, and there will be an offensive breath. In one the nerve centers are blunted and our patient is dull, inclined to sleep, the pupils are dilated, and he is impressed with difficulty, while another patient is restless, with flushed face, bright eyes and contracted pupils.

Again, the heart bears the brunt of the affection, and the full, strong, bounding pulse tells of excessive heart action, while in another the small, feeble pulse represents debility and feebleness. When a variety of symptoms are thus presented, each case needs special study though each patient be affected with the same disease.

Septic conditions do not always call for the same antiseptic remedy, and just in proportion to our skill in analyzing the different pathological conditions present, will success attend our prescribing. While this is true, there are some seasons when nearly or quite all our patients suffering from the same disease will show similar or identical symptoms, and the remedy that meets them in one meets them in all.

Thus, in some epidemics of dysentery white liquid physic is curative, is the epidemic remedy, while another year the same remedy might be used with but little benefit. Thus during the severe epidemic of dysentery that prevailed in Southern Ohio in the year 1868 the characteristic symptoms were a yellow, pasty coating on the tongue, a yellowish tinge to the skin, with full veins and tissues—symptoms calling for podophyllin, and the second trituration of this old and valuable remedy proved a specific. This year glyconda, a modification of that splendid old Eclectic remedy, neutralizing cordial, appears to be the epidemic remedy for summer diarrhea. Some will need the addition of a few drops of nux vomica, others a little bismuth, but in most cases it is the remedy without the addition of a single ingredient. THOMAS. .

TOXEMIA FROM BURNS.

Death occurring in a few hours from extensive superficial burns must be attributed to shock, but when it occurs from six hours to several days after the injury, an intoxication seems to be the cause. The clinical picture and pathological findings are much the same as in toxemia of bacterial origin. Delirium, albuminuria, hemoglobinuria, vomiting, bloody diarrhea, meningitis, pleuritis, pneumonia, neph-ritis, gastritis, and enteritis may be present, and at post-mortem degeneration of the kidneys and liver, swelling and softening of the spleen, thrombosis of small blood-vessels, and duodenal or gastric ulcers are sometimes found.

Many explanations have been offered to account for these conditions. Ten years ago this inflammatory stage, as it was called, was said to result from the marked congestion of the internal organs present during the stage of shock. Later, the destruction of the red blood corpuscles by the heat, the formation of thrombi in the small vessels by the partially disintegrated corpuscles, and the paralysis of the heart and vaso-motor centers by the overheated blood, have been advanced as explanatory of certain phenomena.

While the poison has not been positively identified, the weight of evidence points to a change in the albumin of the skin whereby a poisonous substance is formed, which, when absorbed and carried throughout the body, produces marked degenerative changes in the cells of the internal organs, especially in the kidneys and intestines, through which it is chiefly eliminated. That heat produces chemical changes in albumin, and that a slight change may convert it into an active poison, are well known. These facts, but more especially the clinical and post-mortem evidence, have caused this theory to be widely accepted. How much of the intoxication is due to the functional disturbance of a large area of skin and the retention of toxic substances usually eliminated by that route, cannot be accurately estimated, but it undoubtedly plays some part.

In the treatment of this condition emphasis naturally falls upon measures to secure the dilution and rapid elimination of the poison. The use of normal salt solution by infusion, hypodermoclysis, or, better, by continuous rectal instillation, will meet the indications and when used early combat shock. By the latter method eighteen to twenty-four pints can be introduced into the body in twenty-four hours, and a thorough flushing result. Hot applications should be made to the patient and the temperature of the room kept at 90° or above, thus stimulating the normal skin to activity. Early catharsis is contraindicated because of the great loss of blood serum from the exuding surfaces, but should be secured after this deficiency is supplied. These measures are suggested by the toxemia, but each case will have its own indications.   SLOAN.

CHRONIC MORNING DIARRHEA.—Blafield recommends castor oil in doses of five to ten drops.—*Denver Med. Times.*

THE ECLECTIC MEDICAL JOURNAL

ESTABLISHED 1836.

VOL. LXVIII.   CINCINNATI, OCTOBER, 1908.   No. 10.

Original Communications.

MEDICAL DISPENSING.

JOSEPH S. NIEDERKORN, M.D., VERSAILLES, O.

"Medical dispensing by physicians must stop." That's the proposition now being pushed the rounds by a source which claims the distinction of being "forceful and influential," and which is solicitous about the people's health and evinces the forethought of self-preservation.

The doctor should have no legal right to dispense any medicine. What do you think of that? How many of us have not often wished we need not carry with us our medicine-case on every sick-call! Simply too delightful, not to be permitted to carry it again; need have no apprehensions about stock running down or "bottle empty" when its contents are most needed. Decidedly clever promoter, don't you know—not only to make the doctor's work easier, but also (with special and vigorous emphasis on the also) to fill the drug-seller's pocket with shiny shekels.

Let me say to this, Mr. Scheme Promoter, that I and thousands of other physicians all over this great country of ours will ever be grateful to you if you will bring about a condition which will not permit us to dispense medicines for our convenience sake, for the protection of the health and life of our patients, and for the benefit of your own pocket-book. Do you not see what a good thing you will be doing?

But you can't do it. Why? Because your proposition is neither practical nor practicable; it lacks the substantial element of sincerity; it is devoid of the consideration which gives a fair deal to every one. The very method you are adopting in your endeavor to further your intentions, even with the help of physicians, invites criticism, could not resist and avert public search-light and public resentment, because the people themselves would not stand for it, and, again, because they would be the losers. Your proposition is so ridiculous and its purpose is so self-evident on the face of it that really you deserve at least some admiration for your exhibition of "nerve." Don't talk about quality of drug—it's too foolish even in thought. The national pure food and drug laws are to be obeyed by the manufacturers, the pharmacist, the druggist *and* the doctor, of course. If cheap and impure drugs can't be made or sold, by the strongest stretch of my imagination I can't conceive how the doctor can get hold of them to use them. He *must* use identically the same article the druggist has for sale. So, where's the kick? Many doctors have never prescribed or dispensed anything else but the product of the best pharmaceutical and chemical skill, and these they purchase either from the druggist or direct from the manufacturer.

Where do you get the "verdict of the best element in the medical profession" that "medical dispensing is a dead loss to medical efficiency?" Show me your "best element" and I'll show you a bunch of Osler disciples; a small bundle of men you call authority, but who never even thought of medicine as the present up-to-date therapeutist knows it to be by actual bedside, clinical demonstration, remdies administered with his own hands and dispensed from his necessary medicine-case. Do you think for a minute that any physician who has learned therapeutic facts *to know them* is going to stand idly by and allow a cluster of skeptical, medical nihilists dictate to him how he must conduct his business? You concede to him the right to know disease and how and what to use to alleviate or cure that disease, but you want to deny him the right to give; that, in other words, the doctor should have a legal right to know disease and how to treat it, but he should be denied the privilege of personally giving what he thinks his patient should have, because you say it is manifestly your special and exclusive right to dispense. That's the most prejudiced, asinine expression a supposedly mature and balanced mind ever conceived, and it is a proposition so foolish on the face of it that we feel inclined to take a whack at it; and since you accuse physicians of being ignorant of the "science" of medical dispensing, of ignorance, of carelessness, of criminality, and give utterance to these accusations with an evident impetuosity, you intentionally or not invite defensive remarks, and we propose to here say what we think of the situation.

The situation in medical dispensing will, with probably a little variation, always remain as it is. The people themselves will never be made to see things in medicine as you think you see it. Nine-tenths of the doctors will correctly insist upon a share of your exclusive right to dispense, because they know that that is the only correct way of supplying their patients with what they think their patients need. No legislature will ever enact any measure which has for its sole purpose a druggist pocket-feed paragraph, or which will deny the physician the legal right to dispense his own medicines.

Physicians do not dispense their own medicines for the sake of a financial profit on the *sale* of the remedies, but they do it because their patients ask it, are driven to it either by force of circumstances or by unfair business conduct on the part of druggists, or both. Doctors are paid for their services and time and not for the medicines they give. Many times an hour or more is consumed to thoroughly examine a case and careful discrimination is necessary to arrive at any positive conclusion. Then an ounce of some special medicine is given the patient, with directions, and a fee is charged and paid, *not* for the ounce of medicine, but for his time and services and knowledge of discovering the real pathological conditions of his case and for knowing what will cure the case. Why does he not direct his patient to purchase the ounce of medicine at the drugstore? Often he does, especially if he knows the druggist has what he wants and will give what is ordered; often patients object to pay what they think is "two fees for one service;" many times the doctor furnishes the ounce for the patient's convenience because a drugstore is ten or fifteen miles away (and which is very often the case), or for his own and the patient's protection, and this because he has learned that there are druggists who do *not* supply what is ordered.

To our shame it must be said that there are unscrupulous physicians; no attempt is made to deny this. But it is to be added that there are scalawags among druggists; men who rather than lose a sale will endeavor by hook or crook to convince the customer who is ignorant of drugs that one preparation of a medicine is of equal therapeutic value as any other; or he will insist that the prescription is filled as ordered, when, in fact, he substituted. To obtain desirable results the physician must know physiology and pathology, and, too, he must know drug action. He should know what and where the trouble is and what remedy will correct it. His familiarity with a particular class of remedies places him in the position of pretty accurately foretelling what results will follow. If he directs that this particular "make" of remedies be taken and the druggist substitutes another because he thinks "they're all the same," the probabilities are strong that results will be unsatisfactory, the doctor chagrined at his failure, the patient doubts the doctor's ability—but the druggist made a sale; *he* is satisfied. Where's the justice!

The doctor should not dispense; the druggist has a manifest exclusive right to dispense. The doctor should *send* the patient to the druggist to get what medicine the doctor orders. Let's see. There are sick people who frequently *first* go to the drug-store and there ask the druggist something like this: "I've got a pain in my stomach and a diarrhea; can you fix me up some medicine for it?" I'll venture that there is not a doctor who lives in a town where there are drug-stores but what has heard the druggist say something like this: "Yes, sir, I can; or if you would rather have something else put up, recommended and guaranteed for just such complaints as yours, I have it," and then see this same druggist stand there for minutes and extol the virtues.of some already-put-up or patent medicine and dwell upon its guarantee to cure or money refunded, and sell a twenty-five cent bottle of it. Does he *send the* sick man to the doctor? "Heads I win, tails you lose."

If I want my patient to have Lloyd's or Abbott's make of remedies and so order, if the druggist does not carry these or neglects to keep himself supplied with them, where does he get his "rights" to criticise me to the patient, and why should I be denied the right to furnish them myself? The doctor who does medical practice in localities away from drug-stores, by force of circumstances must, even against his own wishes, dispense what his patient needs; he has not the least desire to destroy the drug business.

I have always maintained that the doctor who "stocks up" on "all-ready preparations," no matter where he buys them, or employs stereotyped, shot-gun prescriptions and pharmaceutical jumbles, does not know his business; he has no right to expect results and is not to be trusted. Therapeutic exactness and results cannot be obtained in that way—utterly and positively wrong. But with the single remedy or remedies in simple combination definite results can and will be realized. It does not require a specially qualified pharmacist to add twenty drops of specific medicine gelsemium to four ounces of water; or to place twenty granules of Abbott's hyoscyamine 1-250 gr. in an envelope; or place any other remedy in a preferable or suitable vehicle. The physician in active practice needs fear no criticism from any source if he prescribes and dispenses his remedies in such simple manner. He purchases his remedies from or through his druggist or from where he pleases, gets what he wants, has always what he needs, knows his patients receive what they should have, results are satisfactory and everybody is happy, even the druggist.

Physicians make mistakes—who'd be so foolish as to deny it! But that does not relieve the druggist from identical possibilities.

"He who is without sin should throw the first stone." If the doctor diagnosticates his case, prescribes and dispenses, and the case dies from whatever cause, he is accused of ignorance, carelessness and criminality. If the doctor diagnosticates his case, able counsel confirms the opinion and approves treatment as prescribed and the druggist dispenses, but not precisely as the doctor ordered, and the case dies because the druggist tampered with the doctor's orders—some one else please give such conduct and results an appellation!

Medical dispensing by doctors is not a menace to the people. An assertion that it is, is a first-class insult to an intelligent body of men, and is no credit to him who utters it—and doctors are not usurpers of the rights of pharmacy; but the *best* doctors are antagonistic to dishonest medicine and allies to honest dispensers. The true doctor (not the medical nihilist) is a friend and supporter of the drug business. Such a thing as the annihilation of the druggist by dispensing physicians in any locality where the druggist did a legitimate business and proved that he appreciated the doctor's confidence has never been heard of. The druggist who is conscientious and conducts his business legitimately need not solicit the doctor's prescriptions with a proposition of a "rake-off" percentage, and it is fortunate that we have honest and conscientious druggists, just as we have honest and conscientious doctors.

My druggist is also a qualified pharmacist and is a business man from A to Z. He exercises good business judgment, has a well-selected stock of drugs, fills many doctor's prescriptions, cannot be induced to substitute, and treats the doctor with all business courtesy. Every doctor in this city and vicinity dispenses, at his office and at the bedside; they purchase some of their supplies from or through the druggist or through other sources, yet he has never said that we are the destroyers of his drug business.

It strikes me that a wail of this kind emanates practically altogether from a bunch of so-called druggists whose sole object in business has been to sell goods irrespective of quality and therapeutic merit, compelling the doctor, in defense of his own reputation and in defense and support of uniformity of drug quality, scientific preparations and direct medication, to purchase himself that which he actually needs, therapeutic effectiveness of the remedy necessarily to be of first importance. The doctor who prescribes and dispenses worthless, cheap stuff, some of which is too frequently supplied by druggists, and buys it just because it is cheap and without any consideration for his patient, deserves to have thrown about him all legal restrictions and penalties. But there isn't a single just reason why the doctor who prescribes for definite disease conditions medicines of the highest standard and best quality should be prohibited from dispensing that which his judgment dictates.

"The druggist or pharmacist, because of his proven qualifications, has the manifest exclusive right to dispense." Let's see, recalling a few instances. I order an original package of alkalithia and the druggist to whom the prescription was taken sells a can of antikamnia; an ingredient of another prescription is cannabis indica, the druggist uses Canadian hemp and mulishly insists that the prescription is filled as ordered. Instead of hydrarg. chlor. mite he dispenses hydrarg. chlor. corrosive. Instead of informing his customer that he has not the preparation of cod-liver oil the physician prescribed in stock, he lauds the special virtue of a preparation of his own make, insists to the purchaser that the already prepared mustard plaster has the identical therapeutic value as comp. tar plaster the doctor ordered, yet has never seen the action of either one demonstrated. Who will come out openly and accuse such a druggist of being specially qualified, or of ignorance, carelessness or criminality, or insist upon a coroner's inquest in case of "accidental death?" Where in all this wide world is there an unbiased mind which would even think of censuring a doctor for dispensing what he wishes to use under such unpleasant circumstances as related?

In reality, just such incidents are prominent considerations for the doctor; his patients and patrons demand of him the best his judgment dictates, and expect from his own hands to receive the medicine to cure their illness. That has been my experience.

Emergency cases too often require quick action and the employment of powerful and dangerous drugs. The right to dispense in emergency is conceded him, yet in the next breath the doctor is accused of being unfit to serve the people in this capacity—dispensing—because "physicians as a rule have no knowledge of that science;" they are ignorant. Emergency cases, it has been my experience, have no room for rattleheads and therapeutic ignorance, just as has not the everyday's work of the qualified practitioner. Inconsistency, thou art *not* a jewel.

Medical dispensing *is* a part of the practice of medicine; it adds efficiency from a source and in such a manner not to be attained by any other method. For physicians to be deprived of the right to dispense medicine would impose a serious handicap upon them—about as much so as an engineer would be without steam in his engine, or a civil engineer would be without theodolite. Medicines are a part of the doctor's paraphernalia, and he should understand how and when to use them; and when we come to consider his capability in these days of medical literature, medical training and education, it does seem hardly fair to accuse him of being ignorant and unqualified; to even intimate such would be adding abuse to insult. His college training is fully as thorough as is that of the druggist, and his every-day relation with drug effect simply adds to his efficiency. To become efficient in the application of therapeutic measures necessitates their employment in a single and simple manner in order to secure any definite and direct effect; compound prescriptions are a rarity with specific and direct medicationists, and are readily and easily prepared and dispensed from our medicine-case. And when we in this simple manner dispense to our patients who demand it, we dispense with the unnecessary services of the middle-man—the druggist.

It is quite possible that the proposition upon which we have briefly dilated emanates from some of the "higher luminaries" of those who are in the majority; that it is a fight among the "big 'uns" who look upon as fice and not to be considered. Let them devour themselves if they so elect; we can at least look on and see the show; and in the meanwhile continue to demonstrate the efficiency of direct medication, its efficiency enhanced by dispensing ourselves that which we think the condition of our patients demand. But it does seem that we are neglecting to protect our own rights as physicians if we refuse to take cognizance of the shrewd maneuvres of political apothecaries, for if all signs point right their purpose is more for personal financial gain than the protection of the health of the people, their statements to the contrary notwithsanding.

HIGH FREQUENCY CURRENT.*

O. A. PALMER, M.D., CLEVELAND, O.

Next to galvanism, the high frequency currents are the most interesting and promising agents that we have to consider in the whole subject of electricity. In the outset we must understand that high frequency affects the organism much different than galvanism, faradism or the static current.

In the use of high frequency we are on the borderland where electrical modalities appear to merge into force manifestations of visible and invisible light rays. The currents of high frequency are so remarkable in their conduct that it is not an easy matter to fully understand all their manifestations. They are closely related to currents of high voltage such as static machine currents, which makes it

* Read before the Northeastern Ohio Eclectic Medical Association.

almost illogical to separate them from the various modalities so closely related to them.

This high current undoubtedly is a link between electricity and light, and sôme day will occupy a therapeutic place which neither light nor electricity can attain. Ever since D'Arsonval and Tesla elaborated the principles of this current much has been done by other men to perfect it in a physiological way.

It must be remembered that the term high frequency is a relative one, and calls attention to the exceedingly high speed of alternations of the current which are oscillatory or alternating in character. It must not be forgotten that all oscillatory movements produce force manifestations. The alternations of this current produce a complex process of ethereal movement, consisting of at least two oscillations of each molecule given to each wave or undulation, which produces a distinct progressive movement. On this account the ether is traversed by impulses of varied intensities, direction and frequency. Many lines of force directions and vibrations are established which shows it has special force manifestations.

As has been suggested, the high frequency current is neither all light nor electricity, but contains the potentialities of many varieties of visible and invisible light. The therapeutic value of high frequency is contained in the close relationship exlsting between currents of high frequency and the rays emanating from the ultra-violet field of spectrum.

An organism treated with high frequency receives at least a current of 100,000 volts. The alternations, which are first positive then negative, run, according to some authors, to one billion or higher per second. The dose ranges from 150 to 3,000 milliamperes, and such a dose is not at all dangerous if judiciously applied and lured to 100 alternations, the usual rate. Where we have such enormous voltage air ceases to be an insulator.

Much has been said upon the physiological effects of currents of high frequency. One author considers the distinction between high and less frequency of great importance. He also states that the sensory nerves cannot be stimulated except within certain extremes of relative frequency. The same author says that cellular life is stimulated by high frequency currents in the same sense in which an increase of the positive potential of the organism will stimulate vegetative function, and it is through cellular elements metabolism is increased.

I have found that the functions of the stomach and intestines become more active. The excretory organs are stimulated to a great extent, so that the cleansing process is well done. It has been demonstrated beyond all doubt that patients treated with high frequency are better able to stand exertion. They digest better and sleep more soundly. All functional disturbances are improved.

In producing muscular contractions a current from twenty to thirty excitations per second is necessary. As the number of alternations increases the muscles become tetanized up to the rate of 2,500 to 5,000 alternations per second. From this point tetany becomes less marked until no appreciable sensation is experienced. Some claim that the enormous frequency of this current prevents it penetrating the integument, and places it side by side of the static current, which does not permeate but flows over the conductor.

It is possible that the sensory and motor nerves are so organized as not to respond only to vibrations of certain frequency, as does the optic nerve, which responds only to undulations between four hundred and ninety-seven billions to seven hundred and twenty-nine billions per second, according to the color.

The true order of things may not be readily determined, but it remains a fact that the effects of the current are felt in the body and have a powerful influence over nutrition. Blood pressure is increased and elimination is stimulated. The respiratory movements are augmented and there is a greatly increased absorption of oxygen and elimination of carbonic acid gas, varying from 15 to 30 per cent. This current has great bacteriological power on account of the large quantities of ozone generated.

The therapeutical effects of high frequency are both electric and radiologic. A current of comparatively low frequency, one-half million or more oscillations per second, produces nearly the same effect as the static current. The effect is to cause an over-stimulation which results in hyperemia and a subsequent over-nutrition of the surface treated. If the treatment is continued the hyperemia becomes more violent, often resulting in dermatitis.

We also find these currents of value in severe pains, and they generally give relief after a few applications, making them of great value in rheumatism and neuralgia. These currents have been used in the healing of ulcers and fissures as well as hemorrhoidal troubles, making one of the best remedies that we have for these conditions. It allays irritation, restores the tone to relaxed fibers of all structures, and imparts power and strength to all the muscles, which causes a better nutrition and a general restoration of the parts. All inflammatory conditions are much improved by them and marked relief is frequently obtained where least expected.

It must not be forgotten that this current is of special value in all cases of errors of nutrition, such as diabetes, nephritis, Bright's disease, obesity and gout. It has also been used in diseases of the liver, giving great satisfaction in many severe conditions. In fact, it has been used in the treatment of almost every organ in the body as well as in a general way.

In the treatment of skin diseases this current is a valuable agent, and is indicated in all cases of malnutrition of the skin, especially the dry form of eczema—in fact, in all disorders where the cuticle requires stimulation of the circulation and of the functional activity of the skin, in many cases of lupus, psoriasis, tenia, acne, and erythematosus. There is no better agent for general diseases where the quality and quantity of the blood is below par.

A distinguished professor of physiology in one of the universities of Paris used these currents extensively in the treatment of consumption with marked benefit. These patients usually begin to breathe more freely after local application over the chest of a shower from a vacuum tube about one-half inch long, and generally receive treatment lasting from thirty to sixty minutes daily for a long time. These currents are applied first by auto-conduction—that is, where the patient is enclosed in a solenoid of copper wire, the ends of which are connected with the terminals of a high frequency coil. By this means the electric currents are induced into the body. No sensation will be experienced, not even the slightest muscular contraction, but the surface blood-vessels will become dilated, which will in a short time become contracted with increased energy. The skin soon becomes reddened and covered with perspiration, but there is no increase of body temperature and the excess of heat is lost by vibration and radiation.

This current may be applied by general electrification, which is done by means of an electric couch which is known as a couch for auto-condensation. The patient may be brought in direct local contact with the electrodes, which are generally properly shaped vacuum glass tubes which can be used on the body externally or on any of the cavities of the body. The efficacy of the current may be increased by connecting the patient to the other terminal through the agency of the foot-plate, and the feet should be bare. Where the bodily electrodes are used the current from the tube of the resonator will produce the most marked effects.

Since it has been discovered that electricity favors the rapid growth of plants it has been used to a great extent, and beneficially, too, to stimulate animal metabolism, so that the changes that go on are more beneficial. When animals such as rabbits are placed in an electrical solenoid they will grow 20 per cent. faster and be more robust.

It has been used in the treatment of children suffering with marasmus as well as where they are suffering with backward growth, both physically and mentally.

The time has come when we have enough knowledge of this current to stimulate us to do better work, hoping for more light to guide our footsteps through its hidden pathways, hoping that what these currents promise will be worked out and our fondest hopes will be realized.

TYPHOID FEVER.

W. C. MILLER, BELMORE, O.

Owing to the fact that the time of the year is at hand for the typhoid bacillus to make his appearance, it behooves every practitioner to be on the lookout and be ready for an even start in the race.

It is not with the definition, etiology, pathology, symptoms, or anything else that I wish to deal in this paper, save the treatment as I have found it in my own experience.

Having been through but six seasons of fever, yet my experience has been very varied, and the success with which I have met has alone prompted me to pen these lines.

Every school of medicine differs in the treatment of typhoid fever, as also do graduates of the same school, for what sometimes proves a success to some may not be so successful to others. Yet on the whole we (Eclectics and some Allopaths) are on a common ground. Yet specific treatment according to symptoms never changes, for one might have a case of smallpox on the same treatment as a case of typhoid fever just as well as having two cases of typhoid on the same remedies, providing the symptoms were the same—in other words, treating the symptoms and not the name.

After being satisfied that we have a case of typhoid, the first thing we do is to stop short all solid foods and thoroughly empty the bowels of every vestige of their contents as near as possible. This is done with epsom salts given with a little aromatic cascara or lemon juice, as either tends to make the salts more palatable and not so hard to get patients to take it, knowing if we explain matters fully to the patient, and he wants to get well, he will not object to any medicine.

Next we select our antiseptic, which invariably is echinacea or baptisia, or both, according to the severity of the case.

As to sedatives, I use very little, if at all; aconite scarcely ever, veratrum only in cases where the heart-beat is strong and bounding, and the pulse runs from 130 to 150 per minute and the temperature runs above 105° F., and then used in from gtt. x to xxx to half glass water, teaspoonful every two hours, and then only continued long enough to bring the pulse down to say 100 per minute, even though the temperature does not fall very much, for temperature reduced under such conditions will not remain, but will soon rise again.

The object in using such remedies at such given times is not to reduce fever, but to save the heart and hold it in check, for somewhere down the road we are coming to a hill, and it is here that we will need all the force and strength at our command, and if the heart is not carefully guarded and saved from the start, and is worn out and weak when we gain the foot of the hill, no amount of whipping (stimulating) will make it climb to the top and reach the level ground on the other side. Such remedies—aconite, veratrum, gelsemium, the bromides, etc., are especially classified as sedatives, yet *any remedy,* when indicated, is a sedative. Never be afraid of a temperature even of 105°, so long as you have a good heart.

Gelsemium often finds a very important place in typhoid treatment, for the bright eyes, flushed cheek and restlessness, but do not suppose when given that these symptoms will at once disappear and your patient will lie down and sleep like a child; for if you do you will be sorely disappointed; but by the continued use, if your patient gradually yields and holds his own, and gets from four to six hours sleep in every twenty-four, you are doing well.

Hyoscyamus for the pale, trembling patient, when the limbs quiver like a flag in the breeze.

Belladonna for the pallid, cold skin, inclined to moisture, dilated pupils, tendency to coma, etc.

Sulphite of soda, when indicated, given in capsules of gr. j to ij, if the patient is rational and can swallow well, if not, give in solution.

Hydrochloric acid when the tongue is dry, brown, parched and fissured, enough in half glass water to make it pleasantly sour.

Many other remedies, as ipecac, rhus tox., bryonia, phytolacca, xanthoxylon, asafetida, sulphurous acid, sulphocarbolates, the bromides, and many others which the keen observer will know when indicated and so use them. I have only mentioned those most commonly indicated, as it takes too much space to name all.

We recognize typhoid as a septic fever or condition affecting the mucosa of the small intestines and Peyer's patches.

I spoke in the beginning about clearing the bowels. Now I will explain more fully what I mean: Not to move the bowels once, twice or three times a day, but copious, watery movements from three to six times in each twenty-four hours.

The bacilli with their products are highly poisonous, and the longer such material lies in contact with the mucous membrane of the bowel the greater will be the absorption of poison, the higher the temperature, the greater the danger of ulceration, perforation and hemorrhage.

Every one has noticed the fall of temperature after a thorough watery evacuation of the bowels, and if they fail to move for twenty-four hours how the fever will rise one or two degrees. So I use salts, and that freely, too, to cause several watery movements every twenty-four hours, and just in proportoin as we keep the bowels clean and sweet, just in that proportion will be the duration and severity of the disease.

I do not know that I would use salts so freely in a case where it had not been practiced from the onset, especially during the latter part of the second and the third week, when the ulceration is greatest, as it might cause perforation, or a rupture, or a fatal hemorrhage, but if used from the first there will be no danger.

Baths are to be recommended and used two or three times a day when fever is high and patient is restless, as it is refreshing and tends to lower temperature and quiets nervous irritation—using tepid water with soda or acids as indicated.

Echinacea, two to four drachms to half glass water, and baptisia in another glass half full of water, using one to two drachms, forms the basic treatment, to be used from the beginning to the end, and is a solid foundation upon which to place other indicated remedies, using teaspoonful alternately every hour.

Salts first, last, and all the time.

Let your patient sleep all he possibly can. I never disturb a patient after midnight till five o'clock in the morning unless he is restless and awake. If a patient will not get well by giving medicine eighteen or twenty hours in a day, he will not get well by giving it twenty-four.

Last of all, but not least, feed your patients well. If a well man requires food to live, a sick man requires it just that much more.

Milk, from one to three quarts a day, broths of every variety and description; boil a pot full of beans, meat, potatoes, cabbage, and feed all they will eat; tapioca, corn-starch, buttermilk, pieces of oranges, lemonade (though I am careful not to give it soon after taking sweet milk, as it is apt to form a curd and make patient sick and vomit), raw eggs, break and beat a raw egg thoroughly in a glass of sweet milk, sweeten, flavor with a little vanilla and give three or four times a day, or as often as a patient will take it. Make everything as pleasant and palatable as possible; they enjoy it.

I should have spoken of complications, but will say only this, that they are many—bronchial, gastric, complications of liver, kidneys, brain, lungs. In fact, every organ or structure may become affected, and should be treated as though they existed alone.

I have followed the above treatment, and I have never lost a single case, neither have I had a drop of hemorrhage, nor never had a heart to stimulate climbing the hill.

Surely, treatment that has given me such good results in the past will be safe to follow on, and will give success in the future.

Some one may say that I have never had very severe cases, but I have had my share, from the mildest to the most severe, when they were unconscious for a period of ten days, with all discharges involuntary, necessitating the change of the bedding from three to five times a day; cases of mild delirium, where it required two or three men to keep them in bed; cases of almost complete coma, constant picking at the bedding; cases of nervous tremor, where for days the bed would shake from the constant quiver of the musclar structure of extremities; cases where consulting physicians said no possible hope, will not live twenty-four hours; cases where the fever went to 107° F., some stood at 105° for fourteen days without even a morning remission—and they have all gotten well.

I do not mean to say that I will never lose a patient with typhoid fever, for people are prone to die, and some are going to die with this disease, but I do mean to say that all curable cases can be saved by careful treatment.

APPENDICITIS.*

A. S. McKitrick, M.D., Kenton, O.

There still is much to learn regarding appendicitis. While the diagnosis in a classical acute case is relatively easy, there are many times that a diagnosis is not easy, and may be impossible. A few years ago I saw a case brought into the polyclinic at Chicago with a diagnosis of acute fulminating appendicitis by a capable Chicago surgeon, and after making the usual incision found a perfectly healthy appendix, but found a little free bile in the peritoneal cavity. He then decided that it was a ruptured gall-bladder and proceeded to make an incision in that region, only to be disappointed and find an ulcer of the stomach with perforation, which he closed and made an unfavorable prognosis, but the patient recovered. Recently I saw a

------

* Read before the Northwestern Ohio Eclectic Medical Association, July 9, 1908.

case operated by a world-renowned surgeon, with a diagnosis of appendicitis, and upon operation found a case of ectopic pregnancy.

Given, a case with pain in right iliac fossa, with tenderness over the appendix, vomiting and fever coming in that order, the diagnosis is easy. Dr. J. B. Murphy says when the symptoms do not occur in that order he doubts the diagnosis. But a great many cases are not so easy. Many times the pain in the beginning is referred to the stomach and to the left side, but if you palpate carefully you are likely to find the greatest *tenderness* over the appendix. Sometimes the pain is referred to as the pleurisy, and often is around the navel. Morris has discovered a point of tenderness at the right and below the navel that he considers pathognomonic. Rigidity of muscles over the appendix is an important symptom. I read recently of a case diagnosed as appendicitis that operation revealed a tumor of an undescended testicle which was twisted upon itself.

In chronic appendicitis with occasional pains and symptoms of indigestion, or *so-called* indigestion, and about three-fourths of the so-called indigestion and disease of the stomach, if carefully diagnosed, proves to be chronic appendicitis or disease of the gall-bladder.

The treatment is to put patient to bed, wash out stomach if vomiting, and move bowels with an enema. Put absolutely nothing in stomach unless it be a little hot water. Nourish per rectum and wait for localized abscess or recovery, and you will nearly always get one or the other if this plan is observed. If you must use aconite and echafolta, etc., take them out and pour them in a rat-hole where they at least will do no harm.

If an accurate diagnosis is made and you can get the patient to a hospital, it is better to operate in the first twenty-four hours, not that you cannot tide the patient through, but that any person who has one attack of appendicitis is very likely to have another, and the danger of operation in the first twenty-four hours or in the interval is a very safe one, but shun operations at the third, fourth and fifth days as you *should* shun the devil, provided you carry out the above don't-meddle-treatment; but if you insist on feeding and keeping up action of the bowels, operation might be necessary, but the grim reaper will reap an abundant harvest, with or without operation, if you persist in feeding and purging the patient. If you keep your patient quiet and get a localized abscess, open as you would any other abscess, and see how little disturbance you can make, and not break the adhesions that nature has put up to save the patient's life.

The operation is done perhaps in various ways with equal success. The peritoneal opening should be as small as is consistent with good

work. An inch or inch and a half is often sufficient. But if you need
a large incision enlarge it sufficiently to allow good work. Morris, of
New York, ties mesentery, ligates appendix, cuts it off, touches stump
with carbolic acid, and closes abdomen. He has splendid success.
Edebohls inverts the whole appendix.

I rather prefer the Ochsner method, which consists of a purse-
string suture around the base, ligation of mesentery, ligation of appendix, removal of all but one-half or three-fourths of an inch, which
is inverted, purse-string tightened stump covered with omentum,
wound closed, peritoneum first with catgut, then muscle sheaths to
each other, and finally skin, being careful, as in all surgery, not to
draw sutures too tightly and strangulate tissues.

If no complications occur, patients sit up at six days and leave
hospital at twelve. I sent one case home at seventh day, but that is
too soon.

There are many more things to say regarding appendicitis, but
I think with as long a program as you have you do not want me to
say more at this time.

BABY'S FOOD.

John Fearn, M.D., Oakland, Cal.

There are some physicians, who, if they would give less attention
to medicine and more attention to baby's food, would have more success in caring for children in sickness. Not that I would decry medicine, not for one moment. But the child does not need much medicine, but it does not need much nourishment. But the food must be
right.

This thought arises out of some quite recent experiences with
children. I shall illustrate.

Called to see a child about eight months old. Soon as I entered
the house I heard the wail of the child, and even before I saw it
I said to myself, that is the wail of a hungry child. Examination
showed a very puny infant, wasted and thin, vitality almost spent;
there was soon given me the history. For weeks the child had
always been hungry, and though it took large quantities of food, just
such food as other babes thrived upon, it cried night and day, and
was seldom quiet except when taking food. I shocked them by saying
the child was starving. Then they told me of the food it took. I at
once had other food prepared, and when given the child took it and
was soon asleep. The change worked well for the time, but it was too
far gone; it passed away. That child needed not medicine, but food.

The second case was a child about four months old, a healthy child when born, but nutrition had been interfered with. What a picture it presented—its limbs, face and body so wasted and wrinkled, but abdomen large, regular .pot-bellied; always hungry, would have to be fed frequently night and day, cried much, the little thumbs turned tightly into the palms of the hands, impending convulsive trouble. It needed circumcising, but it was so very feeble I advised delay. They told me the child had been dosed with strong medicine. Bowel discharges green and very unhealthy; vomiting much of its food. The food of the child was changed. Calc. phos. 3 x trituration and chamomilla 2 x trituration were given in small doses. A few drops of olive oil was given three times a day, and the child was treated to inunctions of olive oil every day. They were very anxious, but I told them I could not give them any hope. A few days after I saw the child again. There was less bloating of the abdomen, and the child did not need food so often; it cried less and the bowel discharges were more healthy. The same food was given, but more at a time and less frequent, and a few small doses of calomel well triturated. This child has been under my care a little over a month. It sleeps well, takes food about six times in twenty-four hours. It has improved in every way but one. Though it looks better nourished, yet it has gained scarcely any in weight. I am now giving calc. carb. 3 x trituration. That is all the medicine except as I will note hereinafter. I am not without hopes of this child; it may recover even yet.

The third case is something like last case. A bottle-fed child, principally fed on cow's milk. Bowels constipated, stools not healthy, feeding too often, crying much at night, not well nourished. Changed the food, gave small doses of olive oil internally, inunctions of olive oil. Gave larger amounts of food, but not so often. Gave chamomilla 3 x trituration. The child had not been out of doors, though some twelve weeks old. Had it taken out and in the daytime sleep out of doors. Gave sodium phos. in small doses. There was soon a great change for the better. He is putting on flesh and enjoying life in sunny California.

Now for the food. In these last two cases I have had them take rolled oats, one of our breakfast cereals. Cook it well making it into a thin gruel. Then strain, add it to good milk from a suitable cow. Sometimes I give more of gruel and less of milk, at other times most of milk. The gruel is made fresh every day, and to each dose of food add one-half teaspoonful of Parke-Davis fluid Taka-Diastase. This addition I have used for some time, and I like it much. The child will get more good out of a given quantity of food while using the Taka Diastase; it is pleasant and it is a good thing for bottle-fed babies. I shall not mention the proprietary foods that were given to two of these children, as they are good, and I would not even appear to cast a slur upon them. But they simply were not the food for these two children.

Moral—do not give the babies much medicine, though they should have the indicated remedy. But study closely the food question. I remember a case where the food was just the thing, but the child did not do well on it. A little seasoning of salt was all that was needed. And let me say it is often the case that nat. muriaticum, either straight or in trituration, makes all the difference between a sick child and a well one.

THUJA—ITS VALUE DEPENDS ON ITS RELIABILITY.

THOMAS M. STEWART, M.D., CINCINNATI, O.

A recent experience in which thuja (a drug-store preparation) failed to do that which thuja (Lloyd's) had done a year or so previously, and which thuja (Lloyd's) "again did do" as soon as it was given in place of the inert preparation, proves that *reliability* is a primary requisite to curative effects from internal medication.

The case was one of papilloma of the larynx in an elderly patient, to whom the advice had been given to submit to operation, in face of the prognosis that an operation would endanger his life. Between the alternative of choking to death or dying on the operating table, the patient's friends advised a consultation with the writer.

We recognized the alternative referred to, and suggested that it might be wise to take some medicine internally, which medicine had cured papilloma.

Lloyd's tincture of thuja was given in three-drop doses, diluted with a teaspoonful of water, six times daily. Improvement resulted in one month; the use of the voice was regained in a few months, and the patient resumed his business.

For about two years no trouble was noticed. The laryngoscope showed only a flattened base to the growth. But a vocal strain, due to "trying a case," started the trouble again.

Thuja (a drug-store preparation) was prescribed with no results. The patient was discouraged, of course, but with the use of Lloyd's thuja, a second time, the relief was soon apparent.

With this remedy this patient has received and will continue to receive an amount of physical and mental relief that can only be appreciated by the patient and his friends.

Ohio State Eclectic Medical Association.

Proceedings of the Forty-fourth Annual Session.

W. N. MUNDY, M.D., EDITOR.

SECTION III.

MISCELLANEOUS.

J. K. SCUDDER, M.D., Chairman..........................Cincinnati.
IVADELL ROGERS, M.D., Vice-Chairman.....................Delaware.
JAMES HAYS, M.D., Secretary..............................Dayton.

THE MEDICAL PROFESSION AND PURITY.

JEROME D. DODGE, M.D., COLLINWOOD.

We use the word purity in a special sense, having reference to the sex life.

In so far as the enlightenment of the general public is concerned, this subject has been strangely neglected, through a shameful prudery, until evils of gigantic proportions have resulted. There was formed in Chicago in 1905 an organization called "The National Purity Federation." Its object is to "unite all reform forces in one great society, and arouse the conscience of the world to the awful facts relative to individual, social and organized vice, and the deeds of their promoters, and assure to all a high standard of morality and a right knowledge of the pure life."

There has been formed within the ranks of the medical profession itself "The American Society of Sanitary and Moral Prophylaxis." A similar organization has been formed in Europe. Under the auspices of the Chicago Medical Society, "The Chicago Society of Social Hygiene" is doing much effectual work in enlightening the people.

The New York Society for the Suppression of Vice, which has been thirty-six years in the field, has destroyed over forty-one tons of immoral book and sheet stock, more than 3,000,000 obscene pictures, and large quantities of utensils for making the same, and over 3,000,000 circulars, catalogues, songs, poems, booklets, etc., which were unfit for use. That sort of immoral poison is sent among the youth of the land, even into the schools and colleges, by human vampires, to do its deadly work.

The times are ripe for purity organizations. The psychological period has come when they can do a great and necessary work in reforming our local and national life.

It is quite in order for medical societies to take up this subject and promote an educational scheme which will uplift the social world and make our work pleasanter than it now is.

We think we are, as a nation, building the highest civilization, but we are leaving 'out of our educational structure an important cornerstone which ought to be placed in its proper position.

Among other things, the people must know that children, even those of tender years, of high and low degree, in families of all grades, unless early and wisely instructed and safeguarded, are in great danger of nervous and bodily exhaustion, from an evil habit, which will greatly impair their physical, moral, intellectual and spiritual development. Children as young as three years are known to indulge in the secret vice, and girls are said to be as unfortunate as boys in this respect.

Young people approaching the age of manhood and womanhood must be taught, by those qualified, in regard to the nature of the phenomena which will appear in their lives at that time.

The youth of the land must be taught the dignity and true meaning of the powers of the sex life with which they then become endowed. They must understand its purpose, its proper care and its dangers. They must be taught not only the "Thou shalt not," but the why not. They must be taught to keep the thoughts as well as the actions pure, for thoughts are living things, and as a man thinketh, so is he.

No young couple should be permitted to assume the sacred compact of marriage until they have been taught what constitutes proper matrimonial life according to the best judgment of our time, and be able to present a satisfactory certificate of health.

It is the duty of physicians to teach their married patients, when fair opportunity presents, that the purpose of sexual union is reproduction, not pleasure; that "the exercise of the sexual function is accompanied by the most exhausting expenditure of nervous and vital energy of which the body is capable;" that "excess in a normal way tends to make men hate their partners in excess; the unhappiest marriages are those in which there is the greatest indulgence; irritability, aversion, positive hatred and disgust toward the object of former love follow protracted sexual debauch;"* and that continence is compatible with health and should be observed during the period of utero-gestation. In short, marriage should not be made a sort of legalized prostitution with one woman, and married people should be made to understand it.

---

* Beard and Rockwell, "Sexual Neurasthenia."

Children six to eight years of age should be given a correct, be it ever so brief, knowledge of the mystery of life. If they are not, they will be given an incorrect knowledge, by impure companions, which will be a lasting injury to them.

A considerable use could be made of physicians in teaching this subject in the schools, and the expense need not be great. Lady physicians could be obtained, if necessary, to teach those of their own sex.

After a generation has been properly trained, lay teachers may develop who can do the work as well or better.

Pupils thus taught who later marry and bring children into the world will teach them the laws of life, and safeguard them, from their earliest years.

The instruction in the home should begin early. Luther Burbank, the marvelous producer of new forms of plant life, and many others, have wisely said that a mother must not neglect her child before it is born. Prenatal culture is of inestimable value to the child. Heredity plays an enormous rôle in the life of man.

Emerson has reminded us that we often hold intelligent communion with people even when no audible words are spoken. In much the same way a mother influences her offspring and teaches it from the day of its conception. Such teaching, supplemented by that of spoken language in due time, should not end with its birth, but go on up through each year of childhood, youth, manhood and womanhood.

I believe that the aid of the medical profession is necessary to accomplish the greatest possible results in this work. Physicians have a more intimate knowledge of human life than any other class of people. We have a far better understanding of the evils resulting from impure living, because we see more of those evils, study them more and comprehend them better. All that we need to make us the best purity workers extant, other things being equal, is, first, the divine love for humanity in our hearts; and second, the best possible opportunity for the work. Certainly many physicians have that love, and, if this plan is developed more of that class will develop with it; and I believe that the best possible opportunity can be made by creating a department of health in every school in the land, to be presided over by a physician who shall teach the pupils in regard to the care of the general health, not omitting a knowledge of the care and functions of the reproductive organs, together with a wholesome knowledge of vices and venereal diseases. It is mockery to teach physiology and never mention this important part of the physical being. A shameful prudery permits destroying evils to flourish.

We must break the traditional policy of ignorance, and place in its stead a rational, national policy of general public education in these matters which are of such vital importance to humanity. And this on the principle that prevention is better than cure; recognizing the fact that parents do not do their duty in teaching these matters to their children, and that they, as a rule, are not thoroughly informed themselves.

In harmony with a suggestion of Dr. Morrow, of New York, State boards of health could request their State medical societies to formulate plans of instruction and submit them to the boards which would perfect and promulgate them. Such a plan of instruction, coming from such a source, would command the respect and confidence of all. The plans thus prepared by different States can be compared and improved as experience shall dictate.

Medical colleges all teach this subject to their students, well knowing that there will be many victims of sexual diseases coming to the doctors for relief.

Physicians already instruct a surprisingly large number of people, but usually not until they come to them as victims of disease. How much better it would be, if, instead of acting this rôle, which is somewhat analogous to that of the spider and the fly, we could act the more rational, humane and noble rôle of instructing the youth of the land before they fall. It is a uniquely delicate task, but physicians are already trained for it, and could, generally speaking, do it best until others are better trained.

Until it is made the definite duty of some one to do such teaching systematically it will never be done. When teachers are justified by their superiors and backed by public opinion they will do a divinely important work in this line. As a people we are not given to avoiding work simply because it is hard.

The microscope and the combined experience of the medical world . have been revealing some valuable secrets. They tell us that from 60 to 80 per cent. of young men in the larger towns and cities acquire gonorrhea; that 60 to 80 per cent. of pelvic suppurations requiring hysterectomy or oöphorectomy are due to the same disease, and that no class of society is spared by the terrible scourge. They say that that disease is the cause of a large per cent. of the cases of impotence and sterility among men and women; that 80 per cent. of the world's blindnes is caused by it, and that from 60 to 80 per cent. of that blindness is inflicted upon innocent babes by infection at birth. They tell us that there are more married women in the cities innocently affected with this disease than there are abandoned women in the same cities, although it is said that there are upwards of 25,000 of the latter in Chicago and 50,000 in New York. They say that absolutely no other disease has such a destructive effect upon the health and procreative power of woman.

We really never know when we have gonorrhea cured, and Dr. C. B. Parker, one of the leading physicians and surgeons of Cleveland, said recently in a lecture to men that no doctor in the world can cure it.

Young men illicitly contract the disease, and supposing themselves cured, when they are not, marry; and the aggregate results in diseased wives is becoming frightfully large. One medical writer relates the case of a man who killed three wives in succession by this disease, and he thought himself cured before marrying each time. It often causes inflammation of the prostate gland, bladder and kidneys. It causes the so-called gonorrheal rheumatism. It invades the brain and spinal cord, the eyes, heart, pleura, peritoneum and other tissues. No part of the body is exempt from its attacks. Gonorrhea until comparatively recent times was thought to be of minor importance, but it is now known to be more destructive to human life than syphilis, which is far more dreaded.

Then there is this other disease prevalent which the sensual libertine is likely to acquire, syphilis, which is said to cause from 50 to 90 per cent. of the cases of locomotor ataxia; 50 per cent. of the cases of hemiplegia which occur under fifty years of age; and a death-rate of 60 to 85 per cent. among children whose parents have it, to say nothing of the impaired development in those who survive such conditions. They tell us that syphilis causes 40 per cent. of all cases of abortion and miscarriage; that most syphilitic women abort, and that it would be a blessing if all did.

Syphilis attacks with destructive energy the blood, bones, brain and nervous system. Every tissue of the body is subject to its ravages, and no man knows its end. Diseases which bear other names, may, so far as we know, be its ultimate termination, even in succeeding generations. After slumbering twenty-five or thirty years it may break out and end the life of its victim.

I can never forget the case of a woman who was said to have been beautiful in her youth, who innocently married a syphilitic man. She was infected with the disease and it ran a destructive course. Her nose was entirely destroyed, her eyelids distorted, her face blanched and splotched, and offensive odors from the decaying bones filled her rooms. She was a woman of good character, but she suffered a living death for years because of this terrible affection. In another case of a young woman, the frontal bone dissolved, and the disease went on until it destroyed her life. In the case of a young man, loathsome abscesses formed on his face and a few years later the disease reappeared in his larynx and dragged him down to the grave. A tale could easily be made up from hospital and private reports which would "freeze the blood" and shock the world out of its position of indifference.

"A considerable percentage of the idiotic, imbecile and insane in our charitable institutions are a curse to themselves and a burden to the community through the venereal taint implanted before their birth."*

It has been said that no other disease makes such fearful ravages in the human constitution, nor subjects its victims to such terrible sufferings and disfigurements as syphilis.

Keyes, in his work on syphilis, quoting from the Surgeon-General of the Army's report for 1904, says: "There are more soldiers rendered permanently unfit to follow their profession by syphilis than by any other disease; 27.83 per thousand among officers are syphilitic. The ratio of syphilis to gonorrhea among the men is 1 to 4, among officers 1 to 1. . . . By far the most important diseases affecting the efficiency of the army during the year have been the venereal . . . causing 16 per cent. of all admissions, 28 per cent. of all non-effectiveness, and 18 per cent. of all discharges for disease. . . .But if we measure the importance of a disease by the damage it does, syphilis immediately jumps into far greater prominence. Taking as a criterion the number of days sick, we find syphilis, 70,398 days, second only to gonorrhea, 146,609, and well ahead of dysentery, 49,518, and tuberculosis, 49,195. . . . Syphilis stands first as a destroyer of careers, causing 166 discharges, whereas tuberculosis caused only 101. . . . In general, there is one-eighth to one-fifteenth as much syphilis as gonorrhea."

Dr. F. C. Valentine, of New York, said in a lecture before the Ohio State and local Boards of Health, January 16, 1906, that "it is most conservatively estimated that of the million people walking the streets of New York, at least 200,000 are infected with venereal diseases." This was based on a report of the New York Medical Society. He says that "there is no purpose in denying Bulkley's calculation that the New Yorkers infected are increased by 50,000 annually, and that there is reason to believe that these figures under- rather than over-state the facts." He further states that "although the figures given must under-state the truth, yet if we accept them we must also accept that to-day there are walking the streets of the United States some 16,000,000 people infected with venereal diseases. The same conservative estimate would give these polluted ranks an increase of

---

* Chicago Society of Social Hygiene.

three and one-half millions annually. The power of this immense army for evil to each unfortunate and to others, is beyond discussion. The cost to the nation produced by venereal diseases is beyond computation. The disasters directly and indirectly wrought to the innocent cannot be even estimated. Venereal diseases are more widespread and more dangerous to the individual, the family and the State than all other diseases combined."

In view of all this, justice demands an equal standard of purity for men and women. A licentious or venereally infected man is quite as obnoxious and dangerous as a woman similarly affected. We must think of and treat them as fallen men on a par with fallen women.

When we reflect that a great army of regular and clandestine prostitutes, laden with disease, is scattered throughout the towns and cities of our country, and that the children, young men and women of the nation are practically ignorant of the seriousness of venereal diseases and sexual vices, it requires very little thought to see that honesty and fairness and the law of self-preservation demand a general diffusion of sex knowledge among the young.

They are now telling us that in the city of Chicago alone from 38,000 to 50,000 criminal operations occur annually; and when we reflect that this is probably but a fair sample of the condition of our other American cities, we can readily see that in this wrong life we have a potent force working for the degeneration, the depopulation and the suicide of our race. Yes, in the wrong sex life lies the secret of a vast amount of wasted life, disease, poverty, insanity, drunkenness, suicide, domestic discord and divorce. The sensual libertine cannot go far in sowing wild oats without causing and reaping a terrible harvest. The hospitals are full of the crop.

Venereal diseases, because of their insidious, destructive nature are worse than leprosy; they are as a cancer gnawing at the vitals of the nation. The house of prostitution and its fostering evil, the saloon, can never be tolerated by a right-minded people. There is no more use trying to regulate them than there is in trying to regulate hell. If they could be regulated they would still be—hell.

It is now known that there is an international traffic in girls which has become as strongly intrenched and as compactly organized as was ever the traffic in negro slaves. It has its agencies in many lands, its bureaus of exchange in many cities. It has its means of transfer, its system of distribution, its supply and demand, and all the features of a protected and legitimate commerce. Five and one-half years is said to be the average duration of the life of these victims of man's barbaric lust.

It easily becomes apparent that children, youths and young men and women are not taught enough in the schools unless they are taught the fundamental principles of correct personal and social sex life; for those are what concern them most. It is those principles upon which the foundations of a strong body and a strong life are built.

We may take it as an axiom that personal and social purity mean personal and social life, while personal and social impurity mean ultimate personal, social and national death.

This is really everybody's work. Everyone should do everything possible to become well informed, to teach those under their care or influence, and assist in the formation of a public opinion which will not only permit, but insist upon, this needful educational reform.

I believe that the medical profession will rise to the occasion, put its shoulder to the wheel and become a mighty dynamic power in uplifting the morals of the people.

We well know that many nations of the distant past have risen to power and worldly glory only to sink into oblivion through preventable vice largely of this nature; and that if we do not pursue a more rational course than they, we, too, will walk the same downward course.

If we were ascending a mountain with a company of people, and having arrived safely at the top should look back and behold any who were unable to surmount the last obstacle, we surely would put down our hands and help them to the summit. Our duty is equally clear in this situation.

We who believe, and have faith in the ultimate consummation of these lofty ideals, should endeavor, according to our ability, to leaven the world's thought, and thus aid in the establishment of a splendid civilization—a civilization having the permanent power within it to advance onward and upward forever.

DISCUSSION.

DR. J. H. HUNTLEY: The medical profession is not used to discussing that kind of a paper. If that man had been a minister he would not have gotten a chance at this body. It was a good paper, but is hardly susceptible of discussion.

DR. E. FLORENCE STIR SMITH: It seems to me that physicians should take advantage of every opportunity to explain to people these things which he has spoken of. There would be less evil if the physicians would make themselves a moral standard, as well as the minister attempts to do; but when people know that the physician does these things why need he hesitate?

DR. W. B. CHURCH: That was a very excellent paper. We were all doubly interested, but it occurs to me that there would be a difference of opinion as to the propriety of instructing young girls and young boys in regard to the sex knowledge spoken of. I think there will be in most minds still a mooted question as to the propriety of it, and especially until we know just what those instructions cover, the extent of it and the effect of it, whether the effect will be to draw their minds too much to that part of their nature. Now I have known myself of a number of women who told me that up to the time of their marriage they were absolutely innocent of any knowledge whatever of sexual life. They had no thought of it, no anxiety in regard to it, and no care about it. I think most men would prefer such a woman for a wife to one who had from very early years, from infancy, been drilled as to the nature of all her organs, and the uses to which they might be put at some future time. This is the only point that I care to make, and I confess that in my own mind the question is not settled. I don't understand yet what would be the effect of such knowledge. I confess to a preference for allowing young people to develop in the natural way, without forcing any premature knowledge upon them.

Dr. T. E. Griffiths: It is a vital question, and one that confronts every physician. In the town that I live in, about six thousand people, it is a terrible question. It comes up before us on every side, and unless physicians and men that have self-respect and will stand for right and virtue will come to the rescue, we are going to lose all our young people; and I believe it is pretty much the same all over the country. It is terrible. I surely cannot help but admire the essayist for bringing that up, and I think the physicians ought to take hold of this question, because they are supposed to know more than other men, and I think we ought to do our duty along this line if we are going to save our young people.

Dr. J. D. Dodge: The argument which our brother advanced in regard to leaving people ignorant, that has been the one that the world has been using and that is the position that I desire to jar the world out of. It is because of that ignorance that the young people fall into these errors. I am positive of that. It would be foolish for us to suppose that if the majority of young people knew all of these facts in time, that the majority would choose the wrong life. The majority of people want to get health and strength and happiness in this world, and when they find that there is a road which leads in the opposite direction I believe and I know that the majority of the young will prefer the right life. Hence, I think that the instruction should be imparted, and I believe the medical world should forward the movement.

DEATH—PHYSIOLOGICAL AND PATHOLOGICAL.

A. F. Green, M.D., Cleveland.

The Psalmist says: "We spend our years as a tale that is told. The days of our years are three-score and ten; and if by reason of strength they be four-score years, yet is their strength labor and sorrow; for it is soon cut off, and we fly away."

The evident meaning of this passage is that the average limit of a complete and full life is seventy years, and but few, "by reason of strength," exceed it. David's measure of life, expressed three thousand years ago, answers well to human longevity at the present time. But as we read of the age of the patriarchs before the flood, running six hundred, seven hundred, eight hundred, and, as in the case of Methuselah, nine hundred and sixty-nine years, we wonder why men cannot live as long to-day. This thought often arises in the mind: Why should not he, barring accidents, who comes from a good ancestry, is well born and raised and faithfully observes the rules of hygiene, live on indefinitely. Let us see what the facts are and then try to answer the question. Approximately, out of every 100,000 persons born into the world, one-fourth, or 25,000, die before they reach the age of five years; one-half, or 50,000, are dead before the fiftieth year; about 99 per cent. have passed away before the ninetieth year; while only two of the original 100,000 live to see the one hundred and fifth year of life. Thus tradition and statistics are agreed that few attain three-score and ten, and beyond that age they die off so rapidly that seventy years may be practically regarded as the extreme limit of a long life.

Therefore, as we observe that the human body, even under the most favorable environments, has an end as well as a beginning, we must admit that death from old age is the result of a physiological development, and is uniformly linked with structural change. We are so much accustomed to associate development with growth merely that it seems a somewhat startling thought to connect it also with decay, and therefore but few are in the habit of regarding the development of the body as naturally ending only with its death. Nature unobstructed works during a definite period in building up the physical structure, and during another period in taking it down. But in some cases this process is more rapid than usual, giving us a precocious development or a premature decay. The development of man is a physiological process dependent upon tissue change, and not on years; and it may attain its natural completion before, or after, the allotted threescore and ten.

In early life the body grows rapidly because of the abundance of nourishment with which every part is nourished. In infancy the arteries, as compared with the length of the body and size of the heart, are very large, and the heart is located, as it were, in the center of a circle. Hence there is low blood-pressure and a rapid pulse-rate. The large amount of fluid in the tissues, the abundant supply of nutriment, and the low blood-pressure, together with the shorter time in which the whole circuit of the vascular system is traversed, all favor the diffusion of blood-plasma and the rapid growth of the body. These conditions prevail during early life, but are most marked during the first year. During early life the whole body grows in every part, but the growth of the arteries in calibre does not keep pace either with the growth of the body in length or with the growth of the heart in capacity and strength. The natural result from this condition is a gradual rise in the blood-pressure and an equally gradual slowing of the pulse-rate, as growth and age increase, until in early manhood growth is completed and the blood-pressure reaches its highest point. At this period the body is full of life and vigor, and is at the best for the performance of bodily and mental exertion. We have now reached the summit of life's hill; but as development progresses, the arterial coats, after many million stretchings from the action of the heart on the blood, slowly lose their elasticity and become gradually converted into more or less rigid tubes. The effect of this loss of resilience in the arterial coats is that, while these coats yield as formerly to the advancing blood invasion, they yield more slowly and they do not spring back to their original size, so that the arteries undergo gradual dilatation. The heart, suffering from the same arterial changes within its own structure, tends to fail, and senile atrophy begins. We now find ourselves descending the other side of the mountain, but we are faithfully walking in the physiological pathway.

Because of the dilatation of the arteries there is a tendency to the lowering of the blood-pressure, and to this failure of blood-pressure is probably due the drying up of some of the capillaries, which is the cause of the dry and wrinkled skin, the gray hair, and cessation of the sexual functions.

In youth the relatively large calibre of the arteries has no ill-effect on the circulation, because, though the blood-pressure is not great, it is perfectly sufficient to keep up a steady and continuous flow into the capillaries. In age, however, the case is different; the loss of arterial elasticity, while it throws a greater strain upon the heart itself, makes the outflow into the capillaries approximately intermittent, and thus lowers the blood-pressure in the capillary area, though it still remains high within the arteries themselves.

From our earliest days the growth of our frame is accompanied by a gradual condensation of tissue, till the gelatinous pulp of the primitive embryo is converted into the withered old man. Every tissue partakes of this change. The skin becomes dry, flaccid and wrinkled. The bones are denser and more brittle. The muscular fibers are more rigid, diminished in bulk and impaired in contractility, so that they are less readily and less powerfully excited by stimuli. Hence, the shrunken limbs, the tottering gait, and withered aspect of the aged man. Worn with his weary tramp through life; no longer able even to totter about, he at last lays himself down to his final rest. Partly from the loss of the stimulating effect of the exercises he was able to take, and partly from a similar cause to that which has occasioned the wasting of his muscles, his powers of assimilation give way, his blood becomes diminished in quantity and defective in quality, the brain centers for intellectual processes and for organic life get poorly nourished, the production of nerve force becomes more and more imperfect, and death from weakness closes the scene. Death comes from weakness which is due to the failure of oxidation, and this failure of oxidation follows the failure of assimilation, which was primarily induced by changes in the circulatory system which reduced the blood supply to the various cells of the body. We cannot trace the changes in the capillaries and arteries beyond the vessels themselves, but it is an advantage to know that the arterial system, which leads the van in the development of the body, is also that upon which the finger of decay is earliest laid. Decay and death are thus the necessary and final stage of physiological development.

Physiological death, or death from normal old age, commences at the periphery and terminates at the heart, *i.e.*, death begins at the circumference and ends at the center.

Pathological death, or death from injury or disease, begins at the heart and spreads to the skin, or begins at the center of vitality and gradually extends to its outmost bounds.

THE ADVANCEMENT IN MEDICAL PRACTICE AND MEDICINE.

J. L. HENSLEY, M.D., MARION.

Who would dare say that the past three-quarters of a century has not been fraught with wonderful advancement in the practice of medicine?—each year witnessing great strides in this direction.

Memory reverts back to the days of my youth, and calls up the time and the fright of the entire family when we saw our father fall from his chair in a faint due to the loss of blood from the use of the lancet in the hands of the grave old family physician. I have stood by and watched him as he dished out the huge doses of calomel and jalap, gamboge and castor oil and other nasty potions. I well remember the annoyance I experienced when holding the basin to receive the saliva that poured from their mouths, due to the salivation produced, and as they picked their teeth one by one from their mouths, all due to the continuous use of the same drug without regard to indications or reasons for its use. In case of fevers or other grave diseases, all food must be withheld in order to starve out the fever, but, unfortunately, the patient was usually starved out much sooner than the fever. The only nourishment allowable was a little badly made beef-tea. Milk was considered a deadly poison in fevers, but is now considered the best obtainable food. Water was strictly forbidden, no matter how much the patient might suffer from thirst. If any should be allowed, the friends or nurse were required to get from the wood fire coals, which were to be dropped into the water until it was warm and had the taste of lye, and was to be given in teaspoonful amounts at long intervals. I have seen patients under this form of treatment suffer the torments of the damned.

This cruel form of treatment awakened the people to such an extent that they demanded something better, and gave rise to the crude system of Samuel Thomson, consisting of emetics, cathartics, sudorifics and steam baths, sometimes almost to scalding, with its massive doses of decoctions. Yet the people hailed it with delight, notwithstanding the flood of persecution which was poured out against Thomson, causing his arrest and confinement in jail for months. His system would not down, however, at the bidding of his persecutors.

Later, Wooster Beach, anxious for a better system of practice, established the Eclectic system, a great improvement over the others, though far inferior to the Eclectic system of to-day. His contemporary, Thomas V. Morrow, came to his assistance, and these two, with others, established an Eclectic college at Worthington, Ohio, where they did much good, notwithstanding a relentless persecution was waged against the enterprise. They recognized the importance not only of a radical reform in the practice of medicine, but the need of a thorough education as a prerequisite qualification for the study of the profession. This small beginning led to the founding of the Eclectic Medical Institute of Cincinnati, Ohio. Her graduates are scattered from Maine to California and are thoroughly equipped physicians and surgeons. Long will live the names of John M. Scudder, John King, Robert S. Newton, A. J. Howe, I. G. Jones, L. E. Jones, E. Freeman, Z. Freeman, F. J. Locke and Jeancon, all of whom have gone to their reward. Their places are filled by others who are doing much good work. A number of other most excellent Eclectic colleges have been located in different parts of the country, all of them teaching Eclectic practice and doing good work.

The large doses of medicine given by the early Eclectics were objectionable to many patients; hence Prof. John King relieved the situation somewhat by the introduction of alkaloids, making a concentrated tincture, then evaporating it by means of a sand bath, so as to reduce it to a powder. For a time this method met with favor from both physician and patient. The matchless and fertile mind of the late Professor Scudder was in the meantime busy with the work of bringing about specific medicines. Not that he believed, or ever taught, that a medicine could be made that would be a specific in any disease, without regard to the conditions or symptoms, but that each medicine must be preceded by specific diagnosis. That the thorough study of each medicine would reveal to the student or physician its effects on certain conditions of the human system, and that it would meet these conditions, no matter what might be the name of the disease.

The appearance of the tongue must be thoroughly understood as to the coatings, as they call for different remedies. The pulse in its various actions, the skin, the eye, the expression of the countenance, etc., each has its combinations which should be thoroughly understood. The physician who is thoroughly posted in specific diagnosis and medication and practices it is a sure winner.

Some doctors say they never could get any good results from specific medicines, but on inquiry you will find that they use it indiscriminately, without reference to the indications, simply loading up the professional blunderbuss and firing at the name of the disease. I have confined myself to the advancement in medical practice and medicine as I have been able to see it in the past sixty or more years. I can well remember when it was considered sure death to open the abdomen. The advancements of surgery have been simply marvelous, and have been sufficient to convince the most skeptical. I shall not dwell upon its advancement.

—————

Eating by Chemical Rules.

It is nice to know just what per cent. of proteid, carbohydrate and fat our food contains and how many calories a given quantity of food will yield. But in the case of normal men with normal appetites, who work at least a part of the time in the open air—as all men should—the chemistry of food is an unnecessary nuisance. We believe that the normal appetite is a safer guide than the theoretical dicta of such an infantile and capricious science as physiological chemistry. By the way, do you remember that in the days of Liebig proteid was the real stuff, carbohydrate being anathema; now proteid is the cause of all our troubles. Isn't moderation in all things the best and safest rule?—*Critic and Guide.*

Eye, Ear, Nose and Throat.

CONDUCTED BY CHARLES S. AMIDON, M.D.

Care and Knowledge in Operating.

This was suggested by a recent case that came ihto the clinic. When the mother brought the child in she said: "This boy has been butchered once, but we think there is something wrong with him yet."

The case in question was a boy seven years of age, who one year previous had been operated on for adenoids and tonsils. The examination showed a condition that coincided with the mother's remark that "the boy had been butchered once." Inspection showed the tonsils greatly hypertrophied, but in the operation a small piece had been taken off of each tonsil on lower anterior part; this, of course, could be easily remedied by a properly performed tonsillotomy, but the soft palate was where the butchering had taken place. The uvula had been almost completely torn away, and the soft structures had been lacerated on either side to such an extent that in healing the parts had been drawn together, forming a mass of scar tissue that greatly constricted the opening.

I do not know the method of previous operative procedure, but if performed with the forceps, probably in the excitement of operating, the uvula and soft palate had been grasped and torn away; if with the curette, the instrument, instead of being guided in such a manner as to carry it back of the soft palate, was forced through, producing the condition as described above. It is needless to say that the boy still retained the adenoid mass.

The points emphasized by this case are: Know your anatomy before beginning an operation; be familiar with the technique, and the complications that may arise, because without this knowledge you are sure to meet defeat.

Treatment of Exophthalmic Goitre.

The paper of J. M. Jackson and L. G. Mead is an analysis of eighty-five cases personally treated. Of this number eighty were women and five men. Nothing unusual is presented under the headings of diagnosis, but the authors claim that many cases are not recognized until they have become advanced. Their favorite remedy has been the more or less continuous use of the neutral hydrobromide of quinine, first proposed by Forchheimer. The acid salt does not act as well. The neutral salt is given in five-grain capsules three times a day and this is as much as can ordinarily be borne, although the authors have found patients who could take four capsules a day for a long time without the unpleasant symptoms of tinnitus. On the other hand, they occasionally find a patient who cannot take more than one or two capsules a day. At the beginning of treatment patients are told that no marked effects may be seen short of a month and they must be prepared to continue it for, at least, two years. Great stress is laid upon this because patients become very easily discouraged if no immediate results are obtained. Usually after a week or two of treatment the pulse rate will be slowed, the thyroid diminished, and the sweating and tremor lessened. It should be continued until all the symptoms have disappeared, which may be in four months or as long as three years. The order of disappearance of the symptoms seems to be: first, the tachycardia subsides, then the sweating, then the thyroid gland diminishes, and finally the exophthalmos and tremor, the last two after only a prolonged course of treatment. In a few instances the goitre and exophthalmos persisted more or less marked after all other signs had disappeared and the patient was practically well and at work. They have never seen any bad permanent effects follow from the administration of the quinine, and the only unpleasant effect is occasional tinnitus, especially if large dose be given. It is advisable to continue the drug in small doses, one capsule three times a week during the second year, and the patients are cautioned to return immediately to former doses at the first indication of any reappearance of their old symptoms.—*Homeopathic Eye, Ear and Throat Journal.*

Infection of the Middle Ear Following Treatment of the Nose and Throat.

Dr. Ferdinand Alk (*Wiener klin. Rund.*, April 19, 1908) says Stoerk has long since drawn attention to the need of gentleness in cleansing the nasal chambers. Any vigorous efforts to douche the nose are likely to result in direct damage to the ears, and inflammation readily follows unwise efforts to use the syringe in cleansing the nares. The writer believes that infective matter is even more likely to be carried to the ears during nasal washing if the patient happens to swallow while the nose is being syringed. The act of swallowing opens the Eustachian tube, and if acute rhinitis, ozena, accessory sinus disease, or even hypertrophic rhinitis be present, infection of the middle ear is thus easily brought about.

The author thinks the glass or rubber "boats" so widely advertised as the ideal nasal douche for "patients' own use," are especially likely to cause damage to the ears. The common habit of cleansing the nose by sniffing saline solution from the palm he also condemns, particularly if the solution is used cold. He has seen a number of cases where middle ear inflammation could be traced directly to this habit. He thinks the numerous cases of middle ear disease seen in ozena patients are to be explained in one of these ways.

The repeated and forcible sneezing of patients suffering from influenza is undoubtedly the cause of much of the middle ear infection found in these epidemics. The importance of never blowing the nose by compressing the two sides is also insisted upon. Patients and school children should be taught to cleanse the nose by blowing one side at a time, holding the other to give the necessary expulsion force. When both sides are compressed a valsation inflation of the ears occurs and infected secretion is easily carried into the tubes.

Even in the most careful hands an occasional case of otitis media will follow operative treatment of the nose or naso-pharynx. The writer believes that palpation of the naso-pharynx for example, after an adenoid operation is responsible for such infection of this part and of the middle ear in some cases.

Posterior plugging of the nares is very likely to cause infection of the ears, especially if the plug is left *in situ* more than twenty-four hours. The posterior tamponade is for this reason to be avoided whenever possible.—*Post-Graduate.*

Periscope.

Why I Write for Independent Journals.

While attending one of the sections of the A. M. A. at the recent Chicago meeting, I was asked by a certain ethically (?) hyperesthetic medico-literary snob, who industrially seeks for motes in his confrères eye regardless of the beam in his own, why I wrote articles for "that fellow X's journal." My answer was that it pleased me so to do. Although I am heartily in sympathy with the moral of a certain Rabelaisian story, which, in effect, is "to h—l with the other reasons," I'm going to expatiate, enlarge, amplify, elucidate and—"conflagrate" the theme a bit, earnestly hoping that the multitudinous ultra-ethical self-labeled medico-literary perfecto will eventually be told what I have to say. Indeed, I'm sure he will, and, moreover, that he will stop browsing among the thistles of discontent just long enough to gather new notes for his raucous, discordant bray—that bray of narrow-minded, illogical protest wherewith alone he attracts the attention of the professional rank and file to himself and, incidentally, of course, to his literary holy of holies, choked to the brim with intellectual sweepings from other men's garrets.

Obviously I am not bidding for popularity with certain self-styled journalistic "leaders."

The feature of the better class of independent journals that appeals most strongly to me is the mere fact of their independence in wearing no brand or collar. As matters medico-literary are now trending, the day is not far distant when the average practitioner of medicine will have no medium of expression, no literary representation and no literary pabulum of practical value within the comprehension of the average medical mind. Medicine is fast becoming so scientific, so turgid with "things that ain't so," or which are at least "under suspicion," that the main purpose of medicine, the healing of the sick, bids fair to be lost in the maze of laboratory experimentation and illogical deductions from mentally indigestible "facts"—scientific bricks without straw—from which none but a wizard could build an enduring fabric. What boots it to the practitioner of the cross-roads that there be opsonins and opsonic indices? He has neither the technical training, the appliances nor the time to practically apply them in his daily work. Besides, who knows how soon the opsonins will be gathered to the snows of yester-year?

I fancy I hear the ultrascientific ones cry: "Let the practitioner of the cross-roads and the hamlet hie him to the post-graduate school and cultivate—at so much a cultivate—'the optic sharp I ween that sees things which are not to be seen.' Let, also, the student of medicine be more thoroughly prepared in things scientific." ·

As to the post-graduate school, it often makes confusion worse confounded. Abdominal and other special surgeons "made while you wait," men who entered the mouth of the hungry P. G. school, passed immediately through its short, angleworm-like *prima viae* and promptly tumbled down the back steps with a special-course certificate in their hands, have not seldom out-heroded Herod—which means that where the haughty professor of the special P. G. course has slain his dozens, some of his half-baked special students have slain their scores, aye, hundreds. . . .

Our medical schools are responding with alacrity to the demand for ultrascientific training. The *ultima thule* of medical teaching in some quarters apparently is the manufacture of half-educated scientists, not trained physicians. Here is an illustration of some of the brilliant results. I recently had occasion to inquire into the knowledge of materia medica and therapeutics possessed by a recent graduate of a well-known school, who, by the way, was one of the ten "Honor Men" in his class:

Question—"What is the botanic name of the plant from which opium is derived?"

Answer—"Poppy, I think."

Q.—What is papaver somniferum?"

A.—"Poke root."

Q.—"What are the alkaloids of opium?"

A.—"Morphine and atropine."

Q.—"What preparations of aconite would you ordinarily prescribe internally?"

A.—"Why, aconite."

I suggested that the tincture was an eligible preparation, and informed him that there were two tinctures.

Q.—"Which tincture would you give to a child?"

A.—"The tincture of the root, because it's the milder."

Q.—"What dose of the tincture of the root would you give to a child six months old?"

A.—"Oh, about one-half a dram every hour."

Q.—"Given the same child and a stimulating expectorant being indicated, what would you give?"

A.—"Carbonate of ammonia."

Q.—"In what dose?"

A.—"Oh, twenty grains every three hours."

Be it remarked that materia medica and therapeutics are taught in the sophomore year in the school from which this gentleman graduated. The treatment of disease is taught before the *raison d'etre* of treatment has dawned on the student's mind. But, this newly fledged graduate knows a lot about the embryology of the chick—he has watched it for weeks—the nervous anatomy of the frog, neurons, opsonins and things—which knowledge is not likely to save from massacre the first hapless infant he treats.

The independent medical journal meets the demand of the every-day practitioner who wants to know "what to do." The self-styled high-class medical journal—and there is really only one "high-class" journal, you know, which is climbing so high that its head looks from below very like that of a pin—often gives him a stone when he asks for bread. He seeks for light on the treatment of disease, and on looking over the menu card presented by the "most high," he finds such things as "My Last Thousand Cases of Excision of the Calamus Scriptorius," "My New Postural Method of Catheterizing the *Iter a Tertio ad Quartum Ventriculum*," "The Opsonic Index in the Care of the Second Bicuspid," etc.; and editorials in which the mantle of dignity conceals vast intellectual abysses. In despair he turns to that cemetery in which so many fond therapeutic hopes lie blasted and buried under tons and tons of therapeutic nihilism, Osler's "Practice" —and still he finds no balm in Gilead. And then he turns to the independent journal and is consoled—which is a blessing, e'en though he be sometimes cajoled into belief in things unsubstantial. And the proof of the pudding is that thousands upon thousands of doctors buy and read the very journals upon which the "lily whites" of medical journalism frown so blackly.

The practitioner knows full well that his patient wants something more than a diagnosis. . . . The ultrascientific one who does not overmuch believe in treatment and recognizes naught but the scalpel and hemostatic forceps sometimes marvels that anyone could condescend to read, much less contribute to, our independent journalistic media of medical expression. "Nothing in drugs," he wails; "send 'em to me and I'll cut 'em." He forgets that modern science has not yet conquered the lay aversion to the knife, nor the honest practitioner's belief that, after all, the knife is often a confession of our limitations and weakness. And there is much in the training of the experienced practitioner which inspires him with the therapeutic hope in a vast number of the ills of the flesh. By drugs he can produce anesthesia, local or general, relieve pain, produce sleep, stimulate or depress the circulation, allay nervous irritability, aid digestion, relieve constipation and hepatic torpor, produce emesis, diaphoresis and diuresis, antidote malaria, and cure syphilis. What wonder that he has confidence in drugs *per se* while rather skeptical of our knowledge of them? "There must be a remedy. If I only knew" is a brow-contracting reflection familiar to the conscientious practician. And so long as there are sick ones to heal so long will he search for remedies—and so long will he read and believe in the literature that offers therapeutic hope. —G. FRANK LYDSTON, M.D., in *Daniel's Texas Medical Journal*.

Molecules, Atoms, Corpuscles, Ions.

We have been taught in school for years, in the study of physics and chemistry, that the molecule is the smallest particle of matter that can exist in a free state as matter, partaking of all the properties of the mass, and that a molecule consists of two or more atoms. We are also taught that the atom was the smallest divisible particle of matter, and that it was supposed to be about one twenty-millionth of an inch in diameter. More recently we have been working on a later theory that even the atom was a complex body, containing one thousand other smaller particles, which are called corpuscles. Now we go a step further toward infinitessimalism, and believe that even the corpuscle is a community, consisting of ions, which are one five-thousandth of the diameter of a corpuscle. Now, going down through the division of the scale, through the successive stages of imaginative conception, through the different theories, viz.: molecular, atomic, corpuscular to the ionic, with our pencil we can figure out the supposed size of the ions. Thus we find that one hundred quadrillions (100,000,000,000,000,000), or one hundred thousand thousand millions of ions can be placed on the flat point of a needle which is small enough to go inside the central canal of the finest hair you ever saw. Can imagination go any further? Whether this is correct or not—and it remains yet to be proved or disproved—we only offer it, not as a practical fact, but to further carry out our statement previously made, that each ultimate particle of human tissue is independent and free to move, and is possessed of its own individual polar affinity, and follows the laws of electrification, that likes repel and unlikes attract. Therefore, if we conceive of such a condition, it will help us to understand how electrification can exert its catalytic effect upon the vasomotor mechanism, controlling circulation, and also the endosmotic and exosmotic processes, by which nutrition is affected.—*Allbright's Office Practitioner.*

How to Use Old Dry Batteries.

M. K. Orton says: "Cut out the bottom of the dry battery and clean thoroughly. Punch three or four holes with a nail or pointed instrument near the top of the cell. These holes will allow the air to escape when the battery is set in the solution. Make a five-ounce solution of sal. ammoniac and place it in a jar which should be a trifle larger than the dry battery. Set the battery prepared as above in this solution and you will have a good battery."—*Popular Mechanics.*

How to Mend Plaster Casts.

Contributed by G. Robbins, M.D., Salem, Mass.: "In mending plaster casts I have tried everything, shellac included, with very poor results, until one day I tried oxyphosphate of zinc, a cement used by dentists for filling, and have never had a failure in any case. The cement should be made thin and then the edges of the broken parts brought firmly together and held in place for a few minutes."—*Popular Mechanics.*

CATARRHAL DIARRHEA OF LARGE INTESTINES.—Richter advises an early morning injection, followed by astringents, subnitrate of bismuth, etc., postponing breakfast for a few hours.—*Denver Med. Times.*

THE ECLECTIC MEDICAL JOURNAL

A Monthly Journal of Eclectic Medicine and Surgery.

TWO DOLLARS PER ANNUM.

Official Journal Ohio State Eclectic Medical Association

JOHN K. SCUDDER, M.D., MANAGING EDITOR.

EDITORS.

W. E. BLOYER.	H. W. FELTER.	L. E. RUSSELL.	R. L. THOMAS.
W. B. CHURCH.	J. U. LLOYD.	H. E. SLOAN.	L. WATKINS.
JOHN FEARN.	W. N. MUNDY.	A. F. STEPHENS.	H. T. WEBSTER.

Published by THE SCUDDER BROTHERS COMPANY, 1009 Plum Street, Cincinnati, to whom all communications and remittances should be sent.

Articles on any medical subject are solicited, which will usually be published the month following their receipt. One hundred reprints of articles of four or more pages, or one dozen copies of the Journal, will be forwarded free if the request is made when the article is submitted. The editor disclaims any responsibility for the views of contributors.

Discontinuances and Renewals.—The publishers must be notified by mail and all arrearages paid when you want your Journal stopped. If you want it stopped at the expiration of any fixed period, kindly notify us in advance.

THE COLLEGE OPENING.

For the sixty-fourth year in her prosperous history have the doors of the old Institute swung widely open to those who would learn Eclectic medicine. The Eclectic Medical Institute was the fountainhead of Eclecticism, and after all these long years is unabating in her zeal and work for the dissemination of the principles and practice of that cause. If one does not want Eclectic medicine the Institute is not the school to select. If one does want Eclecticism he will get it here in all its fullness.

If one would take pride in Eclecticism; if one would be a loyal Eclectic; if one desires Eclecticism perpetuated, an Eclectic college is the only institution to rely upon. While often convenient and possibly involving less pecuniary outlay to enter some neighboring medical college other than Eclectic to begin the medical course, in the long run it is poor policy to thus begin and then attempt to finish in an Eclectic college. Let us urge, then, if you would be a good and well-prepared Eclectic physician, do not fail to grasp the opportunity to begin aright and learn Eclectic medicine from foundation to finish in a reputable and well-equipped Eclectic college.

The Eclectic Medical Institute offers every possible advantage in the way of a thorough college clinic and hospital education. Good men are invited; idlers and triflers asked to stay away. It means work to pursue a course of study in this college. It means hard study, diligence and close application, for nothing less will fit the student to meet the requirements she demands. But as hard labor has its reward in rest, so he who studies faithfully and diligently can enjoy the mental satisfaction of having done his part and done it well. It is this insistence upon good student service that has given the old Institute her good name and marks her diploma with a value coveted by every Eclectic and honored everywhere in the world. The student who would fritter away valuable time, dissipate and carouse, and "live the pace," had better seek elsewhere for medical instruction. But if a man means business, loyalty, honest work, a clean life, and a career which will do honor both to himself and his alma mater, he will find in the Eclectic Medical Institute an hospitable welcome, and his every desire for good work will be fostered, encouraged and aided.

Stability and progress are everywhere the marks of success. During the vicissitudes of the years of the last half century the old Institute has remained unshaken. Though she lost by death valued and valuable teachers, yet have their places been filled promptly by those who have brought the knowledge acquired of their predecessors and the added progressive ideas of the times. By this process of previous training has the school kept up with current medical thought, and never has she been found wanting in the essentials of progression that should mark the live teaching institution. To those who know the Institute it is not necessary to write this, but naturally we feel a pride in referring to the successes of the past and the present outlook of the school—an outlook far more hopeful than could have been dreamed of by her fondest admirers.

As with all progressive schools, the college has undergone some changes during the past year. The faculty has been strengthened by new teachers of exceptional qualifications—men who have been for some years in special preparation for the chairs they now occupy. In addition, special lecturers have been secured who will deliver brief courses upon important topics. This is one of the most important accessions to the curriculum. Interwoven with all the work done is the great and strong thread of specific medication—the very woof and warp of modern Eclecticism. Since its inception this feature has never been allowed to flag, until now it has grown to be the distinguishing feature of modern Eclecticism. Day in and day out the student meets this feature in every study in which a possible therapeutic thought can be injected. Specific medication had its beginning here; here it has been zealously studied, verified and extended. He who would have Eclectic medicine must necessarily have specific medication, and here it is taught fully, simply and eternally.

The aim in teaching in the Institute is simplicity and practicability.

The fad finds here no place and the faddists no comfort. Men are taught to be practical bedside physicians, and the highest interests of the patient are inculcated. The Eclectic physician trained in the Eclectic Medical Institute has no cause to regret his choice; neither may he be ashamed of his preparation.

To be an Eclectice physician is to be a successful physician. Few Eclectics leave the ranks to enter other pursuits. To be a good Eclectic one must have good Eclectic training. The mission of the Eclectic Medical Institute is to give such training. Moreover, a diploma from the Eclectic Medical Institute is a passport readily recognized everywhere. It pre-supposes good preparation. It makes the possessor of it secure by the laws that gave the school the right to issue it and the doctor the opportunity to earn it. The graduate of the E. M. I. should foster his school, that these laws and these opportunities be maintained. He should see to it that his student should be sent where his medical education may be as complete as this school gives. He cannot send too many good students, for the demand was never greater for Eclectic doctors than now.

The sixty-fourth year of the Institute opened September 14. Already the teaching is in active operation. Students have until October 12 to enter, and still have the benefits of the session. After that date credit for a full term cannot be given, but lost time will have to be made up by the delinquent. Those contemplating taking the course this year should begin at once, thus getting the full benefits to be derived from the instruction given. Let each alumnus send a student, and send him now.   FELTER.

ON THE USE OF CATHARTICS IN PNEUMONIA.

I do not believe that cathartics are always contra-indicated in the treatment of pneumonia. I do not believe that a pneumonia patient to whom a cathartic has been administered during the course of this sickness will necessarily have to die because of that cathartic; neither do I believe that cathartics should not be given to patients ill with pneumonia; nor that an unfavorable prognosis should be wholly based on an admission to the fact that a cathartic had been administered.

All of this is at variance with an opinion expressed by Dr. Church in an able article in the August number of the *Chicago Medical Times*. It is not my intention to be understood that cathartics should be given to *every* pneumonia patient, but I do wish to say that frequently we have patients ill with pneumonia whose condition is materially benefited by the proper use of remedies which produce thorough bowel evacuation, and I believe that every observing physician in active practice will bear me out in this.

This brings us to the proposition: Which of our pneumonia patients should have cathartics and who should not? And the answer is as easy as any proposition in therapeutics or in medical practice can be.

I have no patience with all this "bug" talk one is compelled to hear, any more than I have with a man who must cause active elimination from the bowels in every case he is called to treat. Cathartics are medicines used to produce evacuations of the bowels, and the selection of any particular cathartic agent depends upon its individual action and what it is expected to do. Given any case, pneumonia or what not, where we have marked manifestation of morbid accumulation of bowel contents and further evidenced by a dirty, foul-coated tongue, foul breath, disgust for food, and a history of unsatisfactory bowel evacuation, a cathartic is indicated.

Of what good is a cathartic in such a case? The properly selected cathartic will not only cleanse the stomach and the entire alimentary tract, but it will also stimulate secretions and prepare the way for a better absorption of other agents which may be indicated or which have a direct effect upon the pneumonitis. It has been my experience that a dirty, heavily coated tongue is among other manifestations indicative of a condition of the stomach which will prohibit the immediate digestion and absorption of whatever is introduced into it, and the sooner that stomach is cleansed the sooner you will be in a position to be of material benefit to your patient. And this is especially true when treatment is instituted in the incipient stage of the disease.

If the stomach alone would be in a condition unfavorable to a ready absorption of its contents, an emetic would in all probability be the correct thing to give; but usually the intestines also are implicated in like manner, and a properly selected cathartic will not only cleanse them and overcome torpidity, but it will also stimulate intestinal secretions, as well as animate the functions of other organs which have in any manner anything to do with secretions, assimilation and elimination. The entire chylo-poietic system will be beneficially influenced. If veratrum is selected to be the specific remedy for the pneumonia condition, that remedy will act quicker and better where the stomach and *prima viae* are clean and in working condition, if I may use that expression. Who will want to say how much of the elevation of temperature is the result of the absorption of toxins and how much to the actual inflammatory process?

Every case of pneumonia does not necessarily need a cathartic; neither are cathartics always contra-indicated in the treatment of pneumonia; but when they are indicated they should be given, but not to the extent of producing debilitating effects. Jalap and senna, small doses of podophyllin, or podophyllin and calomel followed by a saline, castor oil, leptandra, among other remedies in proper doses and in selective cases, will prove of undoubted worth and enhance the value and action of any other indicated remedy. Treat the patient, and let the actual condition of this patient govern you in the selection of your remedies. I am not afraid of the diplococcus if my patient's condition permits of the ready absorption of my medicine, and I know that a clean stomach and bowel is preferable to one loaded with impurities and inactive, and that is what we generally have when the conditions which I have mentioned present.   NIEDERKORN.

ILEUS.

The number of conditions in which surgical treatment is paramount has greatly increased in the last decade. In their enthusiasm some surgeons have no doubt gone too far and merited the criticism of medical men, who have offered a stubborn resistance to encroachment in fields which have been so long allotter to medicine. On the other hand, the tardy employment of surgical measures in many conditions has brought upon the followers of medicine the just rebuke of the surgeons.

Too much emphasis cannot be laid upon the early recognition and surgical treatment of acute intestinal obstruction, a condition in which the mortality following operation is in direct proportion to the delay in its employment. The responsibility for death cannot be placed at .the door of the surgeon when his services have only been sought after the lapse of days.

Morphia and cathartics, so frequently used, have practically no place in its treatment. Morphia serves to disguise the real condition, and gives physician and patient ungrounded confidence. So long as his pain is relieved just so long will the patient turn a deaf ear to suggestions of more radical treatment, hence morphia should be used only after an operation has been decided upon.

Cathartics increase pain and vomiting and rarely aid in relieving the obstruction, while in most cases they do positive harm. If they are not vomited they increase the amount of fluid, with more rapid dilatation of the intestine above the obstruction, and aid in the strangulation of the gut.

The careful and repeated use of fluid or gas in distending the colon may relieve in the small percentage of cases where the obstruction is due to volvulus, intussusception or impaction of the large bowel.

Such measures should not be employed after the first twenty-four hours, and have no effect upon obstruction above the colon.

Thus in the large percentage of cases an operation is indicated from the beginning, and is the truly conservative treatment. The less accessible to surgeons and hospitals the shorter should be the delay. The recovery of the patient largely depends upon the promptness with which the physician acts.   SLOAN.

INTESTINAL INTOXICATION.

In these days of bacteriologic exploitation it is not strange that this subject should occupy a prominent place in the mind of the dominant school. Nor would it be strange if a few Eclectics were captured by it. In former times, before so many microbes were lassoed, the common location for most diseases not so well defined that he who ran might read, was the liver. The liver was the seat of almost all ills; and calomel, to wake the offending organ up, and cathartics to carry the objectionable dose off, was the stereotyped plan of medication in both acute and chronic troubles.

"Gut-scraping," as Professor Scudder was wont to facetiously term such practice, was the practice of the dominant school, as a rule, and Eclectics were for years a good second, except as regards calomel, which was substituted by various vegetable cholagogues. Will Eclectics of to-day repeat the history of the past and be led into another unprofitable field? Must the much-abused alimentary canal still bear the brunt of professional stupidity, and be raked by cathartics in all seasons, on account of germs of putrefaction?

Let us not deny that intestinal putrefaction may occasionally be a source of auto-infection. We will not deny that hepatic disease not only now, but formerly, might occasionally call for treatment; but this does not argue that such conditions are so common that nearly every case should be medicated for them, on the routine plan. There is a way of determining if intestinal putrefaction exists—at least, a way of determining its absence—which is very simple.

Intestinal putrefaction is always indicated by the presence of an abnormal amount of indican in the urine. Why then not look for this before subjecting the patient to the disagreeable effect of treatment for a condition which may not exist. The test is soon made, and though indican in abnormal amount may indicate empyema, gangrene, putrid bronchiectasis, breaking down carcinoma in various organs— in fact, putrid decomposition of body albumen and its entrance into the blood steream from any cause—intestinal putrefaction will not go on long before the kidneys begin to separate an abnormally large amount of indican. Excluding other causes of indicanuria, and this ought not to be difficult, we will not find it hard to determine with tolerable accuracy whether we are justified in subjecting our patient to treatment for an intestinal intoxication or not.

Fill an ordinary test-tube two-thirds or three-fourths full of equal parts of the suspected urine and strong hydrochloric acid, and to this mixture add an eighth or tenth part of chloroform by bulk. Now add, drop by drop, shaking well at the addition of each drop, several drops of a 10 per cent. solution of sodium hypochlorite. As soon as the agitation ceases the chloroform will settle to the bottom, carrying with it the indican, which will then present an indigo-blue color. Normal urine contains a trace of indican, but when the urine is not in an abnormal condition in this respect the bluish tint will only be slight.

Would it not be fairer to the patient and more scientific on the part of the physician to investigate every suspected case from a positive standpoint before subjecting him to a treatment that can hardly promise beneficial results unless actually demanded? A patient who is free from intestinal intoxication can hardly be benefited by treatment for it, especially if he is to be treated upon the cathartic plan. If he needs scouring out then scour him out—if there is no better way.

But there *is* a better way. Raking the alimentary canal with cathartics will hardly sweep out putrefactive agencies, though it may possibly temporarily alleviate the condition. However, digestion and assimilation may be impaired and other important functions disturbed, but the microbes of putrefaction will remain, to multiply, if well fed; and such is liable to be the case upon an average diet. People consume too much sugar and butter as a rule, and they are good food for germs of putrefaction in the alimentary canal, when digestion is not going on properly. Milk is another objectionable element of food in such cases. Meats incline to coprostasis, and this encourages the condition. Swill is famous feeding ground for putrefactive germs, and this is what the intestinal contents are liable to become, if all kinds of fluids are poured down without reason or restriction.

Let the patient adopt a new mode of living until a change for the better occurs, which will soon be if the new regimen is faithfully adhered to. In fact, it would be best if he adopted it permanently. Let him live on two-day bread, or that which is at least two days from the oven; though greater age will not impair its virtue. Home-made bread is better than that from the baker's shop, for it is less likely to contain alum or ammonia. It should be eaten without butter or other dressing; dry and plain. This, with dry boiled rice, taken without other condiment than salt, and without sugar or milk, should constitute the principal diet. It may not taste good at first, especially where the appetite has been pampered, but it will taste better when he patient has become hungry enough to eat. Let him be taught that he is eating to live, not living to eat. A little fruit may be allowed, but it should be served without sugar. Plain baked apples; plain stewed, baked or raw tomatoes; stewed prunes. All should be served without dressing. A little chicken or mutton once or twice a week may possibly be allowed, after a time. No eating between meals.

Fluids should be taken sparingly and without sweetening. Tea and coffee are never good, even for well people. Water is pretty good, if not overdone. The amount ought not to exceed one pint per diem, and twelve ounces would be better. Fluids encourage intestinal putrefaction and fermentation. The meals should be eaten without drink, and fluids postponed to two hours after eating. When taken they should be sipped slowly and incorporated with saliva. The best way to take fluids is with a teaspoon, to insure against gulping excessive quantities down at a time. If water is not good enough all the time, a small amount of cocoa without sweetening may be taken once a day. The fluid taken, even if plain water, would be best taken hot.

Medicamentous treatment is not of much importance compared with such measures. Sodium sulphite temporarily arrests fermentation and putrefaction, if it reaches the spot. How far toward the seat of trouble it would get in intestinal intoxication might be a question. The sulphocarbolate of zinc is highly thought of in some quarters. Medicine, however, can only palliate, unless radical measures as to diet are adopted.

Coprostasis is to be averted when depending upon removable causes. It is not likely to persist long upon an appropriate diet. Rectal troubles, when present, should be attended to. In obstinate cases of constipation an opening dose of epsom salts might be administered for temporary purposes, but let there soon be an end to it. Of course, intestinal stenosis would render a case more than ordinarily trying, but even here an appropriate diet will be the best means of cure.

WEBSTER.

RHEUMATISM.

We have had reason to recently re-study this subject as it appears in childhood, by reason of being called upon to treat two cases of rheumatic pericarditis. This experience has emphasized anew the necessity of establishing a routine habit of carefully watching and examining the heart in rheumatic children, no matter how mild the attack of rheumatism.

It should be remembered that rheumatism in children does not pursue the typical or routine sequence that it does in the adult. The typical symptoms, such as the swollen joints, fever and profuse acid sweats, are rare in children under eight or ten years of age. In fact, the swelling and tenderness in the joints may be entirely wanting or extremely moderate. The number of joints affected may be small, or the arthritis may be confined to one joint. The child may complain of only a stiffness of the joints or muscles sufficient only to render it disinclined to exercise, preferring to sit quietly in a chair, or to lie down occasionally. The pains may be such as are usually called growing pains, or it may be styled "malaria," until an endocarditis or pericarditis awakens us to a realization of its true nature.

It is claimed that cardiac symptoms may follow, precede, or even be present when arthritic symptoms are absent. In other words, there it no regular order or sequence of rheumatic symptoms in the child as there is in the adult. Endocarditis is the cardiac difficulty usually found, and it is said to attain its maximum as a rheumatic affection in childhood, arthritis its minimum. We have at present two cases of pericarditis under observation in young girls. Each has been for some time complaining of vague, wandering pains in the joints and muscles, and at times of only a slight stiffness and disinclination to move about. They were allowed to go about as they desired or felt able to. Examination in each case revealed a heart tumultuous in action, beating from 120 to 130 per minute, and even more rapid on the slightest exertion, such as standing on the feet. Under treatment the action has become more quiet, but still increasing in rapidity upon the slightest exertion. No valvular lesions are discernible at present, neither is the apex beat displaced.

The prophlyactic treatment for these cardiac conditions of rheumatism can be summed up in the simple word—rest. Rest prevents these complications, just as it does complications in other infectious diseases. It is difficult at times to maintain quiet in these young patients, when they are able to be about, yet it is necessary for the prevention of serious complications. We have learned this lesson by some bitter experiences, and we have also seen dire results follow a neglect of this caution in the practice of others. Therefore, the first consideration in the treatment of rheumatism in children is rest, absolute rest in bed, should there be any elevation of temperature. The other indications are met by anti-rheumatics as they arise.   MUNDY.

JOHN K. SCUDDER, M.D.,   NEWARK, N. J., Sept. 18, 1908.
    1009 Plum Street, Cincinnati, O.
    Professor Wilder peacefully passed away to-night at ten thirty of pneumonia.   DR. G. E. POTTER.

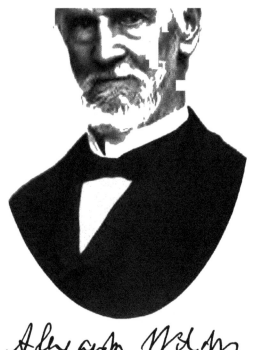

The Eclectic Medical Journal

ESTABLISHED 1836.

VOL. LXVIII.   CINCINNATI, NOVEMBER, 1908.   No. 11.

Original Communications.

ALEXANDER WILDER, M.D. (1823-1908).*

HARVEY WICKES FELTER, M.D., CINCINNATI.

Dr. Wilder died of pneumonia at his home in Newark, N. J., September 18, 1908. There then passed from the arena of this world's life one of the most remarkable of men.

Alexander Wilder, M.D., erudite philosopher, philologist and historian, whose monumental accomplishments the Eclectic profession is ever ready to honor, and whose portrait is herewith presented, bore well these titles to distinction. His very ideals of mental freedom made his life necessarily a part of the structure and history of Eclecticism.

Alexander Wilder came of Massachusetts parentage, his father being Abel Wilder and his mother Asenath (Smith) Wilder. A distinguished line of ancestors backs these parents. Of English, Scotch, and Irish stock, he was born at Verona, N. Y., May 14, 1823, being the eighth of a family of ten. The district school furnished his early education. At the age of fourteen he left school, and at the precocious age of fifteen began teaching. Always a student, he read everything that came in his way, and at this early age had mastered the branches ordinarily taught, and made a good beginning with such academic subjects as botany, chemistry, rhetoric, algebra, Latin and Greek. He never had a college education, but acquired his great knowledge by diligent study, aided by a remarkably retentive memory. Spending several seasons in Massachusetts, he began reading medicine with his cousin, Dr. George H. Lee, a Regular physician, and Dr. J. A. Gridley, a Bo-

---

* A portion of this biography of Dr. Wilder appeared in the May, 1905, issue of the *Gleaner*. This fuller sketch is here put upon record, and will take the place of the usual biographical sketch of another, to have appeared in this issue.

tanic physician. Many of his brothers and sisters dying upon reaching adolescence and adult age, and not being robust himself, Dr. Wilder began to question prevailing medical methods, and thus was led to examine into the new notions of the day, such as mesmerism, the water cure, etc. This began his independent career, in which, however, he had at that date no purpose of becoming a practicing physician. At the age of eighteen, desiring to be an editor, he learned to set type. Here he laid the foundation his ambition sought, and subsequently, in many conspicuous journalistic positions, displayed his remarkable intellectual powers and capacity for learning. In this connection it may be said that for thirteen years he was connected with the editorial staff of the *Evening Post*, of New York.

As early as 1848, while still working on the New York home farm, he organized a county botanic medical society, which a year or two later took the name Eclectic. He was now fairly heretical in medicine, but he regarded Beach's practice as safer and more complete than Thomson's. Though disliking illiteracy, he never ceased to admire the energy and courage of Thomson. In 1850, upon request, he attended the session of the New York Eclectic Medical Society. He was made secretary to the society, and subsequently lectured in the Syracuse Medical College. Here began his long and conspicuous service in Eclectic medicine, which is too well known to JOURNAL readers to require special notice. During the interval between 1853 and 1864, however, he took little interest in the proceedings of medical bodies. From 1876 to 1895 he served as Secretary of the National Eclectic Medical Association, editing during that period nineteen volumes of its Transactions. Four times has the honorary degree of M.D. been conferred upon Dr. Wilder, but, while appreciating such and other collegiate distinctions, he made no selfish use of the honor. Dr. Wilder's influence procured for Dr. R. S. Newton the charter for the New York Eclectic Medical Society. The bulk of his medical and public career is in the domain of the future historian's pen, and, much to our regret, owing to lack of space, cannot now be even touched upon.

In person Dr. Wilder was of striking appearance, tall, sparely built, with a massive head and remarkably piercing eye. He was a ready, fluent and pleasing speaker, kept his temper in debate, and by reason of his great wealth of knowledge seldom found his match in discussion. Born with a liberal sprinkling of stubbornness, he has enjoyed mental freedom in all his acts, more than once making great personal sacrifices in behalf of friends. We believe this will be recognized when, in a time to come, his biography is written in detail. Though temptation to do so had often arisen, Dr. Wilder carried no malice, possibly not treasuring sufficiently Carlyle's wise injunction, "It is well to think well of mankind, but ill to trust them too much." While his service to Eclecticism has been long and exacting, his erudition and philosophical trend will ever stand conspicuous in the historian's record of deeds.

From early manhood, as has been said, Dr. Wilder never failed to hold the most intense passion for knowledge, and this was particularly apparent in the fields of philosophy, archeology, philology, common law, and whatever may tend to improve human life and conditions.

In religious belief Dr. Wilder was as free to exercise his freedom of mind as he was liberty-loving in all his acts.

All his writings are marked by the touch of a master in the subjects discussed. The one that most concerns us is, naturally, his "History of Medicine," which, as a model of conciseness, displays a keen insight into the field of ancient and medieval medicine, while that part relating to the rise and progress of "irregular" American medicine, and particularly of that period in which, as a protesting reformer, he was an active participant, furnishes the only reliable collected data that has yet been published in book form concerning comprehensive American medicine.

Loyal to the medical friends of his earlier days, he frequently contributed reminiscent and biographical sketches of them to various Eclectic medical journals.

Dr. Wilder resided in Newark, N. J., and in recent years was hard at work upon a series of papers on Platonic philosophy, appearing in *The Word,* a philosophic magazine. A man's worth and character may sometimes be best shown by the testimony of those closest to him. Of Dr. Wilder, Prof. Henry B. Lord, of Cornell University, wrote: "Dr. Wilder is a man to be remembered." A. Oakey Hall, ex-mayor of New York and celebrated in New York politics, characterized him as "an encyclopedia of political knowledge." Major-General Ethan Allen Hitchcock wrote: "I would that Wilder's mantle fell on me." A. Sammis said: "His style is superior to that of Emerson," while Edgar Saltus wrote: "His erudition is marvelous, his style agreeable without being pedantic, and his views are broad and powerful."

This journal loses one of its strongest contributors and our school of medicine a most eminent man.

FOR SCURVY.—Tyson recommends good ventilation and outdoor life; plenty of fresh vegetables, fruits (especially lemon juice), and fresh meats; iron, quinine and strychnine.—*Denver Med. Times.*

DIAGNOSIS FROM SEVERAL VIEWPOINTS.

M. F. BETTENCOURT, M.D., GLADEWATER, TEXAS.

Diagnosis has been sneeringly defined, "the science of guesswork." That it involves an element of guessing is undeniable; but that the "guessing element" is directly proportionate to the lack of knowledge in the guesser, is indisputable.

The value placed upon this so-called guess-work may be estimated when one becomes aware that "all schools" of medicine look upon it as the essential crowning piece of the art. By all it is recognized as the compass which indicates to the pilot of human life the selection of the means that must be utilized in the attempt to steer safely the human craft through the many maelstroms which threaten its earthly existence.

In itself, the art of diagnosis is of no greater, if even of as great, importance as many other things in medicine. Though the compass be essential to navigation, it will not of itself control the ship, feed the starving crew, or repair the torn sail; but it is, however, the thing by which the whole must be guided.

To have it tell us that the bark is drifting reefward and will finally be shattered upon the shoals, would of itself be of no material value; but if in these moments of danger it suggests to the pilot, or causes him to decide what must be done, how and when to do it, then it is indeed most valuable.

Surgically, diagnosis is of use in so far as it reveals to the diagnostician the organs involved, how and to what extent diseased, and suggests to the surgeon the proper method of procedure in the effort at bringing about a cure.

Therapeutically, it is essential to the physician in his selection of remedies to assist nature in her endeavor to restore health.

To him of the one school, if he be not a medical nihilist, it is of value because, primarily, it names a disease, and, secondarily, it suggests the use of a certain agent or combination for its relief. This he uses because it has been reported good in that special *disease* or is theoretically adapted to it, or because some "authority" recommends it in that ill, or possibly because of the prescriber's knowledge of the action of the agent as regards the law of "antipathy." This is all good, but was better in the past than it is in the present.

To him of another school a certain remedy is suggested because by the law of "similia" that agent is, above all others, the one called for in the case, independent of what name may be given the ill which affects the one diseased.

And to him of a third school a certain remedy or remedies are suggested because there are present certain definite or "specific" or pathological conditions or symptoms which experience, through the experimentation of thousands of careful observers, has repeatedly proved to be successfully met by that agent or agents, independent of the nosological appellation of the ailment. He is not held in fetters by any "law," but is a firm believer in that universal law, that under like conditions like causes produce like effects, because daily results prove its truth in medicine as in other things.

He sees his remedies successfully meet certain definite symptoms to-day, sees them meet those same symptoms to-morrow and the next day, has seen them do so for years, and consequently reasonably believes they will do so next week, next year, and in all time to come. He cares not whether the drug acts by the "law" of "similia" or "antipathy." What he wants is results, and he usually gets them. He believes disease a departure from health, tending to weaken the body and rob it of the vital forces; and, realizing the need of nature's aid in accomplishing his end, he keeps ever uppermost in his mind the one thought: "Vires vitales sustinete."

Thus we see that to the one school, diagnosis, in so far as it relates to medicine proper, is seemingly a synthetic procedure, a building up or putting together of the prominent symptoms present in order to arrive at a nosological whole—that being the main point in view, seemingly the goal to be reached. It looks upon disease as an entity, such as is a building after its completion. It seemingly forgets or willingly overlooks the fact that in the make-up of that building there are varied apartments, stairways, hinges, floors, locks, roofs, doors, etc., any of which may need special attention; and that if it is desired to repair the structure by simply slamming one or several bucketfuls of paint up against it, one can hardly conscientiously call the job done. It groups the prominent symptoms to name the disease; the disease-name suggests the medication. This will be a certain conglomeration if a certain "authority" says so; or quite likely it will be another because, theoretically, antiseptics and germicides must accomplish the work.

The second school is primarily comparative and secondarily synthetic in its diagnostic procedures. Comparative, inasmuch as it compares the symptoms present in the one ailing to the known physiological action of drugs, then administers in potentized form the one or two drugs capable of producing in the healthy individual, in physiological dosage, a state closely resembling that present in the sick. It is secondarily a synthetic procedure, since it groups together the prominent symptoms to realize the existing pathology and thereby give the disease a name. That there is much truth in its teachings, no thinker will deny.

The third system spoken of is primarily analytic and secondarily synthetic. Like the other schools, it groups the major symptoms to arrive at a name. This it does for the purpose of a more correct prognosis, for the protection of the public, and for the information of the patient and his friends. To this school the analytic procedure is of prime importance. It analyzes, dissects, each major symptom to learn, as it were, its very molecular make-up, by means of which close pathological study it picks out the causal symptoms, thereby obtaining the indications which are direct calls for definite remedies. Thus it is seen that the remedial measures used depend entirely on the existing conditions and not at all on the disease-name. Because a dozen patients are being treated for a "cold" is no reason why any two of them may be receiving in all respects the same treatment. In one case it has possibly caused a rhinitis, in another a tonsillitis, in a third a pharyngitis, etc. In one case the patient is dull, drowsy, inactive; in the other there is a cerebral hyperactivity; in the one the cough is dry, harsh; in another the secretion is abundant, etc., etc. No one can deny that they have all contracted a "cold," but certainly no one drug or combination can be expected to be the appropriate treatment for all cases.

This minute differentiation between cases and a corresponding variation in the medication must certainly be admitted as reasonable, and at least savoring of science, even though much of the knowledge may have been obtained through empiricism.

The drug study and drug application of the third class is, then, based upon the proven relation between the remedial action of drugs and minute pathology, not physiology; tried and tested on the sick man, not the well one; studied with reference to human beings, not on the laboratory guinea-pig or the poor outcast dog.

NOTES FROM INDIA.

G. E. Miller, M.D.,* Mangeli, Central Province, India.

Some time ago I had an experience here which my fellow-practitioners at home never will have unless a menagerie should break loose.

The other missionary worker of this place and myself went over to one of the native States on a business trip. This place contains some of the wildest jungles in India. While there we went out on a

---

* E. M. I., 1905.

hunting expedition in the midst of a chain of hills and spent the night in a cleared space near a small village. We slept out of doors, spreading our bedding upon some cut twigs and green leaves.

About 4 A.M. a tiger came by and grabbed our host by the foot, and began to drag him out of bed. He gave a series of wild Indian war whoops and threw his sheet toward the beast and thus succeeded in frightening it away.

Examination showed that the upper and lower canine teeth of one side had met. There was a neat hole through the foot. I had foolishly left antiseptics, bandages, etc., behind. I had with me a small pocket case in which was a vial of baptisia. I applied this to the wound and bound it with a clean handkerchief, and covered the foot with a bath towel wrung out of cold water.

We then started to our host's house, a journey of about five hours. The pain, shock and fever that resulted from such a small wound was surprising to me. I was afterward told that a tiger bite or scratch is usually fatal.

On reaching the man's house I syringed the wound with carbolic solution and bandaged it. I repeated the operation the next day and left. A week has now elapsed and the man writes that the wound is healing. I am of the opinion that the early application of baptisia had something to do with the successful issue. I shall try it on other wounds.

* * * *

I am just getting into hospital work here. Language study has occupied most of my time until quite recently. I have not had time for continued medication and observations yet, but a few facts concerning hospital work here may interest Eclectics at home.

The amount of disease here due to sin is astonishing. We have about thirty patients daily. Of these about two-thirds have specific disease. A patient comes up to the desk.

"Well, what is the matter with you?"

"Syphilis, Sahibjee."

"All right, go out there and get some medicine."

Then follows a woman with gonorrhea, another man with syphilis, a woman with syphilis, a poor child with the hereditary taint. And so it goes through the morning.

I see the most sickening sights daily—ulcers, rotten buboes, decayed noses and palates, fistulæ, abscesses, tumors—all because of syphilis.

I circumcised a chancroid case yesterday. There was so much thickened tissue that I was at sea for a while, and was glad when I discovered land in the form of the glans penis. There are many such cases here. Even now one of them waits while I write this. Iodoform heals them. The odor does not matter. Nothing gets ahead of the odors of India.

I have performed one cataract operation. It seems that every fourth person in this country has cataract. There is also much ophthalmia and trachoma. There has been one case of trichiasis.

I met with a tumor here which I never saw at home, and of which I do not remember ever having heard. It seems to be a cystic tumor under the tongue, filled with a viscid, gelatinous secretion. One such case came yesterday. The sac was emptied and full strength thuja injected.

One hydrocele case of three years' standing came recently. The scrotum was nearly the size of a half-gallon tin. There is much hydrocele, due to the hot climate.

There are also many cases of general edema, especially amongst the poor and illy nourished people.

We discovered a new test to-day for sugar in the urine. We noticed some large black ants around the urine of a new ward patient. We suspected sugar, and a chemical test corroborated the tale of the ants.

* * * *

And so day after day interesting cases come and go—a splendid opportunity for trying Eclecticism. A fellow-Eclectic who is here on the field with me wrote the other day and said: "Don't forget that specific medication takes the cake."

I have some difficulty in administering drugs, as the people want powders and pills. They bring all sorts of little pots and crazy-shaped bottles, and it taxes one's ingenuity in arranging doses for them. Sometimes they take three days' medicine in one day. I look for someone to take a ten-drop mixture of aconite in one dose.

I am planning to get all the drugs in the powdered form that I can, and use triturates. The trouble with this method is, I am sure to get hold of inferior or spurious articles. Our Eclectics at home ought to be glad that they have men who devote their lives to drug preparation, and that they have patients who know how to drink out of a bottle.

The specific drugs I have found most use for are: Phytolacca, echinacea and thuja. I use quite a bit of cactus also. The infants are getting coryza these days, and I have opened my bottle of euphrasia.

* * * *

As time passes and I obtain greater experience here, I hope to be able to send a few useful notes home now and then for JOURNAL readers. I am not forgetting the Eclectic cause, though so far removed from the strife. May every Eclectic be true to his colors, first, last, and always.

But I would have my readers bear in mind that I am first of all things a missionary, engaged in the Master's work. Medicine opens up people's hearts to the saving gospel. May our many Christian Eclectics not forget the work in which I am engaged, and above all, may they not forget their own obligations and opportunities as Christians.

VERATRUM VIRIDE.*

P. F. PRICE, M.D., MILO, IA.

I am going to talk for a short time about veratrum, called American hellebore and swamp hellebore.

This is one of the most important remedies in the materia medica. The physician who studies the therapeutical value, and uses it, and knows how and when to use it, can testify to what I shall have to say. This is true of many of our remedies, that the more we study them the more we discover of their valuable properties and actions.

A short historical sketch of this remedy may be of value.

The earliest reference to this plant is by Josselyn, in 1672, who considered it the European veratrum album. This plant was introduced into Europe in 1763 by Collenson. The name is due to William Solander. Frederick V. Coville informs us that sheep fatten on the leaves and stems, and that stockmen call it wild Indian corn, and owing to its emetic qualities the drug is seldom fatal to man.

With Prof. A. J. Howe veratrum was a great favorite, and it has occupied an important position in every modern Eclectic work on materia medica and practice.

Of its toxicological action Prof. Felter says: "In toxic doses veratrum produces an exceedingly weak heart action, reduced temperature, cold, clammy sweat, extreme retching, and incessant vomiting, dizziness, faintness, failure of sight, dilatation of pupils, complete muscular prostration, slow, shallow breathing, coma and unconsciousness, with stertorous breathing, and the prompt emesis induced undoubtedly prevents lethal effects. I have never heard of a death from the effects of this remedy."

As early as 1820 the United States Pharmacopeia recognized tincture of veratrum viride. Excepting the British Pharmacopeia and the Homeopathic works, Europe ignores it altogether. The tinctures and

---

* Read before the State Eclectic Medical Association, at Muscatine, Iowa, May 27 and 28, 1908.

the fluid extracts and the alkaloids are not always pure nor satis-factory. Only the Eclectic preparations can be called standard. Lloyd's specific medicine veratrum, Merrell's normal tincture and Merrell's special veratrum are worthy of use.

The veratrum prepared by Lloyd and Merrell is clean, energetic, stable, and a standard preparation. It will mix with water, alcohol, syrup and glycerine, and is used by thousands of physicians, and thou-sands more should use it.

Veratrum is a remedy of great value and power. It is the remedy *par excellence* when indicated, but when not indicated even small doses cannot be tolerated. It is contra-indicated when the tongue becomes long and pointed and reddened at tips and edges, and nausea and other unpleasant gastric phenomena are present.

Veratrum increases secretion from lungs, kidneys and liver. It is an admirable remedy in all sthenic conditions with full, bounding pulse.

Prof. Tully called attention to the value of veratrum in gout and rheumatism, declaring it equal, if not superior, to colchicum. Dr. Osgood in 1835 affirmed it to be an excellent remedy in all diseases in which it is required to diminish the activity of the· heart, and this observation has been confirmed by many others.

The popularity of veratrum as a specific agent in specific condi-tions is due to the writings of Prof. J. M. Scudder, M.D. He de-clares it to be the remedy in sthenic diseases, high grades of fever, pulmonary and other active inflammations, when there is a full and hard pulse, a full and bounding pulse or a corded and wiry pulse, when there is a frequent but free action of the heart and serous in-flammation, in determination of blood to the brain and in delirium, and to increase the action of the excretory organs.

It lessens the frequency of the pulse in small doses and improves innervation through the sympathetics, removes obstructions to the free circulation of blood, also the irritability of the circulatory system, the power of which it increases, and promotes a uniform and equal cir-culation. In small doses veratrum is a stimulant to all the vegetative processes, acting through the sympathetic or ganglionic system of nerves. It removes obstruction to the capillary circulation, gives tone to the vascular system and strength to the heart. As the obstacles to a free circulation are removed, and the vessels through which the blood is distributed and returned regain their normal condition, there is less necessity for increased action upon the heart; and as the power of the heart is increased there is less necessity for frequent contrac-tion. By this process all nervous irritation is allayed, temperature re-duced and inflammation subdued. The hard and full and bounding pulse is the guide.

Prof. Webster, in his very able work, "Dynamical Therapeutics," gives veratrum a weighty value. He says it is specially indicated in the early stages of inflammation of the areas of distribution of the bronchial blood-vessels and in inflamed throat. All sthenic inflammations of the throat are controlled by it. It is the one remedy in acute tonsillitis, when indicated. Veratrum, when indicated by the full bounding pulse, the hard, full pulse, the corded pulse, is an excellent sedative and remedy in acute pneumonia, in sthenic cases. The dose should be small and frequently repeated until the temperature and circulation respond, when the pain will be lessened, nervous excitation allayed, secretion established and cough controlled. With bryonia it is valuable in pleuritis, and in bronchitis when specifically used.

Prof. Howe regarded this remedy as one of the best alteratives that could be used in chronic lung diseases, being especially valuable in pulmonary consumption, and for the control of the inflammatory conditions.

Prof. Webster writes that this remedy is useful to control irritation in the nervous centres resulting in neuralgia, headache and convulsions. In puerperal convulsions it is one of our best remedies. He has been much pleased with the action of the remedy in such cases, and would make it his first choice.

This is a popular remedy with a large number of the profession in the treatment of pneumonia. In this disease, when not contra-indicated, it is pre-eminent, and possesses an affinity for the area of distribution of the bronchial arteries. It acts remarkably well in the treatment of rheumatism. He has seen it clear up a badly treated case of inflammatory rheumatism after the patient was partially convalescent with a badly swollen knee, in a few days, lowering temperature, promoting secretions and relieving vascular tension.

Felter says when convulsive disorders depend upon an excited circulation it proves a powerful remedy. Few remedies have been more praised than veratrum in puerperal eclampsia. There is marked cerebral engorgement, and the indications for veratrum must be present as in other disorders, for one to get good results. The dose must be quite large and be regulated to produce sedation. "We have given as high as forty drops every hour for three days to control puerperal eclampsia, for which it is the very best remedy."

Locke says it is of much value in many forms of convulsions, especially in undue excitement of the spinal nervous system, cerebral meningitis and acute mania with excited circulation. "It will restore quiet and allow sleep in delirium tremens, when the pulse is full and bounding, and eyes red and bloodshot, with evidence of inflammation. In cardiac hypertrophy and palpitation, where there is a full, strong and bounding pulse, the carotids pulsate forcibly, the eyes are bloodshot, and there is cough, headache, and weight in the epigastrium, while the heart may beat so violently as to shake the bed, and sleep is entirely prevented, this remedy relieves the excitement, the heart action becomes normal, the cough improves and the patient is every way better."

Prof. Foltz always employed veratrum after cataract operations, and used it locally for mastoid disease.

Dr. Frost claims that as a stimulant, given in a fraction of a drop, veratrum was effective in the collapse of Asiatic cholera, while Prof. Paul. W. Allen states that in a case of diphtheria, in a pulseless state, in which veratrum was given, recovery followed. He believed it antidotal to the blood poisons of diphtheria, erysipelas and zymotic diseases.

Prof. Ellingwood in his up-to-date work says that the characteristic indications for veratrum are found in pneumonia in strong men previously healthy.

The use of veratrum as an antispasmodic is very common with our practitioners. It may be given in convulsions with active cerebral hyperemia. It is especially reliable as an emergency remedy in persistent cases of convulsions of childhood, while the cause is being removed.

In puerperal convulsions the mass of evidence in favor of veratrum is overwhelming. One old physician reported in the *Medical Record*, of 1888, that he had treated an average of eight cases per year for twenty-eight years, without the loss of a single patient, with veratrum alone. Another reported twenty-three cases treated with veratrum, with recovery in all.

Dr. A. L. Clark, writing on the subject in 1889, said: "As an alterative, especially as an antisyphilitic remedy, there is no better agent in the vegetable kingdom. Indeed, there is room for doubt whether the animal, vegetable, or mineral kingdoms furnish a better remedy in purely syphilitic cases."

Prof. J. M. Scudder, the first teacher of specific medication, who is second to none, writes that in small doses veratrum is a stimulant to all the vegetative processes, that it is the remedy for sthenia. A full and bounding pulse, a full and hard pulse, and a corded wiry pulse, if associated with inflammation of serous tissue, call for this remedy. He has treated inflammation of the lungs with veratrum alone, with a success he never saw obtained from the use of nauseants and counterirritation. Scores of our students who have learned this practice give testimony to its success. We employ veratrum in treating chronic diseases for its stimulant influence upon the vegetative processes, by increasing waste and excretion, and finally to stimulate digestion and nutrition.

Now, I have given the testimony of others who have used veratrum, and in conclusion will add mine, and will guarantee that if you know how to use veratrum, and use Lloyd's and Merrell's, and in accordance with the specific indications, it will do just what those witnesses say. In these two standard preparations we know just what we have. Not so with the fluid extracts, officinal tinctures and alkaloids; the amount and strength are uncertain.

We use Lloyd's specific medicine veratrum and Merrell's normal tincture of veratrum, from a fraction of a drop to one or two drops, and if larger doses are continued will induce emesis. But Merrell's special veratrum can be given to adults three to six drops every hour, for children one to three drops, without any nausea. This preparation is void of emetic properties, can be used hypodermically in two-drachm doses, and will not cause abscess. I have used Lloyd's veratrum hypodermically in drachm doses with no local inflammation following.

I use the special veratrum of Merrell's, because I can give it to children or adults if there is vomiting or nausea. It allays irritation and the vomiting ceases. I have been called to see pneumonia patients where they were vomiting, and began the use of this veratrum and a few doses would calm the tumultuous action of the stomach.

It makes no difference what disease or pathological condition I find in the patient. I look for indications, and the symptoms for remedies to give treatment. If I find a patient with pneumonia I will look for indication for treatment. If I find a high temperature (and we always do), a full hard pulse, a full and bounding pulse, a full and wiry pulse, there will be flushed cheeks, a full broad tongue, delirium, dry skin, these conditions call for veratrum. Use the remedy freely, with a cleansing out of the intestinal canal and rest. Use it in any disease when these conditions are present, diphtheria, tonsillitis, bronchitis, measles, pleuritis, whooping-cough, typhoid fever, etc.

In nearly all cases of croupous or lobar pneumonia these conditions exist and veratrum is the one remedy we must use. In children when the pulse is small and wiry, the indication is for aconite. I give a few drops of veratrum with it to establish secretions and excretions from the skin, kidneys and mucous membranes. I have treated many patients when the whole right lung was consolidated or hepatized. In this condition there is great danger. There is congestion or stasis of blood in the lobes, red hepatization. The heart is pumping away, throwing great volumes of blood coursing through the left lung, which gives the patient two-fifths of area for oxygenation for his life. The brain is on the whirl, carotids bounding, pulse bounding, breathing from forty to fifty times per minute, and a groan every breath, temperature 104° to 106°. In this condition, if there is one remedy that can settle this state of affairs, veratrum can do it, and has done it many times for me. I treated fifteen cases of pneumonia during the past winter without the loss of any, and all got veratrum in good gospel doses. In this condition, in pneumonia, when things are desperate so many make the grave mistake and treat the heart with digitalis and strychnia and lose so many patients. There is no worse fallacy than to give those heart stimulants, as they are called, in the treatment of pneumonia; no wonder they lose their patients and say but few can be cured. More work or harder work is thrown on the heart by stimulating the nerve centers with such treatment. Giving digitalis, strychnia and opium in pneumonia is destructive. What should be done is to relieve the congestion of the lobe or lobes, by using the indicated remedy to open up the capillaries and let the blood flow to the surface, away from the lung. This can be done by giving sufficient doses of veratrum, which will make the patient sweat profusely. Keep the room warm so the temperature will stand at 76°, but have fresh air. It must not be below 75° if you want your patient to recover. The cool air must be kept from the patient's body. It is a crime to put cold applications to the chest of a pneumonia patient. Keep them from the cold air. Cover the chest with libradol, warm, or the compound powder of lobelia and capsicum, warm. Keep his feet hot, give plenty of cold water to drink. I have given in extreme cases of pneumonia Merrell's special veratrum in ten-drop doses from forty-eight to seventy-two hours until I made the patient sweat until his clothes would be wet. The pulse would soften up, the capillaries would dilate and let the blood course to the surface, and the blood in the lung would find room to move out and expectoration be established, pain will be relieved and improvement will begin.

Unless this condition is brought about with the indicated remedies by the seventh to the ninth day the patient will die about the twelfth day with a few exceptions. The blood can be aerated and carry oxygen with one lung about seven to nine days, and some will die in a few days or do die, and then the amount of carbon and effete material and the ptomaines will render the blood so impure that no more oxygen can be carried. The nerve centers fail for want of oxygen and pure blood, the nervous system fails to respond, and of course the heart stops and the patient dies, and then they say he died of heart failure and all the time treating the heart, run it to death. Let the heart alone and look after condition that calls for specific medication, or you will give the undertakers a job every time.

I have made pneumonia a study for fifteen years and I have the first dose of digitalis or strychnia to give. I gave one small dose of opium about eighteen years ago to a pneumonia patient and came near killing him, and that is the last.

Some one is ready to ask, why not sweat the patients with jaborandi. Because that remedy is too depressant and is not indicated in pneumonia.

Well, some one will ask, does veratrum depress the patient? I have never seen any such effects nor will there be any if given in doses to agree with the condition of the patient. In regular medicinal doses it has rather a stimulating effect. Give it when the tissues are full, even if livid and purple, if lips are blue or livid mucous membranes, face and nails. With a full pulse, hard and wiry, give veratrum and see this condition fade away. It shows that it has with its sedative power a vital force to start along the blood vessels the venous blood filled with broken down tissue and blood cells to the dumping ground by the stimulating forces. In this one process it is allied closely to belladonna.

Another will ask, do you give any other remedy with veratrum? Yes, if there is much pain in the pleura I give asclepias; if there is much soreness in the chest and a dry cough, give bryonia. You ask if there is an irregular and weak pulse in pneumonia, would you give veratrum? No, for it is not indicated. With such conditions the patient will probably die, but this calls for small doses of aconite and belladonna, with cactus. If there is a valvular lesion in the aged who have pneumonia they probably will die, and if the pulse is full and hard, of course give veratrum. I stated that during the past winter I treated fifteen cases of pneumonia without the loss of any; the winter before treated fourteen with no death. In October, 1907, lost an old lady, eighty-nine years old, with pneumonia. The previous winter to this treated twenty-seven, lost two, one old lady, eighty-seven years of age, one child, after convalescence began; the mother sat it down on the floor, it took relapse and died.

During the month of April last treated an old lady of eighty-five. She was seized with a violent chill, high temperature, 104°, pulse full and hard, 120, râles all through every portion of the right lung, cough dry and constant, great excitability, a case of bronchitis. Gave veratrum in five-drop doses every hour, and varied this, of course, as she improved. The sweat poured off and the abundant muco-pus was expectorated profusely. In one week fever subsided, cough lessened, and she made a good recovery. The other patient, eighty-two, at the same time was seized with a chill, high temperature, 104°, was seized with pleuritic pains, râles in the middle lobe of right lung, harsh dry cough, full hard pulse and delirium. I gave this patient five-drop doses of veratrum, with asclepias, every hour, saw her twice and she made a good recovery.

This was a case of pneumonia aborted, and this is only one of many which I have aborted and shortened the time and lessened the severity with veratrum.

I have given hypodermically, in puerperal convulsions, my syringeful of Merrell's veratrum at once. There were no more convulsions and recovery resulted.

I have given five-drop doses every hour for a severe headache across the top of the head with a full hard pulse and no temperature and brought relief.

I have given to many patients five-drop doses to establish suppressed lochia without a failure.

I have given three-drop doses of Lloyd's specific medicine veratrum every half hour for six hours and reduced the temperature from 106° to 100° in that time and saved the patient from convulsions and puerperal septicemia.

I gave to a man of forty years five-drop doses of Merrell's special veratrum every half hour for two hours, and relieved renal colic caused by calculus passing along the ureters into the bladder.

In the treatment of puerperal septicemia I want no other remedies but veratrum and echinacea for the temperature and sepsis.

When the pulse is full and hard in tonsillitis I give veratrum with phytolacca. Veratrum will level up the uneven road in pathological conditions caused by the mad rush of blood to and fro as if to find an exit from its great channels, made so by an eruption at the fountain head by a disturbing element in the nerve centers.

The greatest battlefield, and where it does the most and surest executive business and becomes victor of all surroundings, is when there is a general storm in the system from morbific influence, and everything is on the mad rush, and the brain is on the whirl, and everything in the human economy is crashing and smashing and lashing and splashing and all in a tumult. I say give good and frequent doses of veratrum.

You can find this general's headquarters in the highest rank in the therapeutic office of the Eclectic materia medica.

MALARIAL NEURALGIA.—Papine in one or two teaspoonful doses every three hours.

OPTIMISM.

H. L. HENDERSON, M.D., ASTORIA, ORE.

"This world is exactly what each one chooses to make it," was truthfully said by some wise philosopher. It is a truth that should be deeply impressed upon every man or woman who essays to practice medicine, and should be the guiding star of their every professional act. All wish for success in their profession, and this is one of the principal energies or forces that will contribute to that end. With success come fame and financial independence and all the train of pleasures and luxuries that necessarily follow in the natural course of such events.

"Thoughts are things," is another fact that may be rather too abstract a problem for many to thoroughly appreciate and digest. Yet it may be true, notwithstanding the incredulity of many skeptical scoffers. If thoughts are things, then it naturally follows that "birds of a feather flock together," and so the aggregation of a large flock of dark or even black things may serve as a cloud and obscure the most brilliant sunlight or the clearest sky.

We are told in the Sacred Writings, that as man sows, so shall he reap, which may have been said in the sense in which we are now speaking, and would apply to physicians as well as to the humble layman. I feel very certain that a large part of the success of the most successful physicians rests, not in the amount of technical knowledge which they possess in comparison with that of their less successful neighbor, but it does rest in the mental attitude of the successful one, which at all times points toward recovery of his patient, and self-satisfaction, not egotism, and self-confidence in his own ability. This will give him an air toward his suffering patient that at once inspires confidence, instills hope in to the suffering mind; effort is brought forth and recovery follows. Think of the brilliant successes of the old-fashioned country doctor, how he often snatched his patient from the very jaws of death, and then scrutinize and weigh the extent of his real scientific knowledge, and we are forced to find some other explanation than that of professional ability to account for his successes in battling with the "Grim Destroyer." Let each one look about and note the varying degrees of success of his professional neighbors. Nine times in ten the man who is scientifically best equipped for the practice of medicine is barely eking out an existence, while the one who is his direct opponent, certainly far less instructed in the science of medicine, is reaping a rich harvest in both the confidence of the people and in the emoluments that necessarily follow. This must not be understood as decrying learning, far from it, but it is to show that there is something else necessary to bring about success than that of technical knowledge.

One of the things necessary to bring that success for which we are all striving is that peculiar state of mind known in metaphysics under the name of optimism. If that is necessary, it certainly is not amiss to inquire about what it is and how it may be attained? Lexicographers tell us that optimism is "the opinion or doctrine that everything in nature, being the work of God, is ordered for the best, or that the ordering of things in the universe is such as to produce the highest good; a disposition to take the most hopeful view." An optimist: "One who holds the opinion that all events are ordered for the best." This is directly opposite to what is called pessimism, and we are all ready to admit that of all the unhappy and detestable creatures with whom we come in contact, the confirmed pessimist is the one that we seek the most to avoid. If we seek to avoid the avowed pessimist in a general way, how can one blame the people when they avoid the physician who is the least particle tainted with pessimistic views, especially if these views touch upon the profession of which he is a member. To the contrary, how we all love the optimist! His sunny disposition, his smiling face, his cheering words and hearty laugh are always welcome, and we soon in his company acquire the same feeling of jollity.

In the literary world, the most popular author is the one who caters to our sense of mirth. I believe that I am right when I assert that the popularity of our own "Mark Twain" lies not in his great degree of literary ability, but in the fact that the whole trend of his writings is in the direction of optimism and mirth. The same may be said of Riley and a host of others. As a literary genius Ella Wheeler Wilcox stands high in the list of fame, and her writings literally bubble over with optimism! If these things are true in the literary field—and who will dispute that it is so—they will apply as well and as forcibly in the practice of medicine.

But, you say, what has this optimism to do with the successful practice of medicine? Let the optimistic doctor enter a sick-room and note the result. He may be an absolute stranger to the patient. The patient may even be a small child, but even then a bright smile loaded with hope at once illuminates the fact of the sufferer, and in many cases the turning-point of the case has been reached, the patient enters upon convalescence; that family is ready to sing the praises of the "new doctor" and recommend him to their friends. Now in such a case what happened? That "new doctor" perhaps recommended that the same treatment that you had been using all along in the case be continued, offered no new medicines or appliances, but his thoughts, his actions, his tone of voice and his very air diffused hope and confidence and called out the latent energies of the patient which had lain dormant under the ministrations of the pessimistic attending physician.

People demand that which pleases them, and they repel that which savors of asceticism. The doctor who does not act up to this standard of life will find his patrons drifting to the doctor who adjusts himself to these demands of the people. I have often thought that to the average medical student, it is just as important that he should learn normal psychology as it is that he should learn normal anatomy, or any other of the subjects that go to make up the college curriculum. I am almost persuaded that the time is not very far distant when such a chair will be found in the faculty of every up-to-date medical school. These things have to be learned by the average medical man after he has left college, and the learning of them is often at the cost of many heart-burnings and financial losses, even sometimes at the sacrifice of a whole professional career. To be able to know what people want, and to adjust one's self to the flow of the tide, instead of vainly battling against it, is an art that often requires years to master. To me, the practice of medicine was a distinct labor, ofttimes irksome, until I learned by sad experience to adjust myself to existing conditions. Then, what a revelation! I began to get ahead in the world, my patrons began to look to me for counsel and cheer, not alone on matters medical, but along other lines as well. The practice of medicine became an absolute pleasure, and success was in proportion.

I have in mind a certain physician who is not to be credited with any superior amount or degree of medical learning, at least not above that of the average, who has been doing a thriving practice for a period of twenty-six years, and who during all that time has had a death loss amounting to ninety-six. This includes all cases, such as consumption, cancer and all causes. Many physicians as well posted in the science of medicine as is the one mentioned, living in the same locality, working under the same conditions, have lost as much as five times this number of patients. What makes the difference? The successful one goes into the sick-room with an expression of face that says far plainer than words, "Don't fear, I will save you," and his language and acts carry out the conviction; while his opponent goes into a similar sick-room, expresses doubt, looks doubt, says he has no faith in the action of medicine, tells the family and friends that it is to be hoped that the patient will get well, but is very doubtful, and the result soon follows—death of the patient and a funeral, loss of confidence and patronage of the people—and the real fault was in the pessimistic mood of the doctor himself.

If "thoughts are things," as expressed before, then the physician who in his own heart even thinks that his patient will die is contributing toward the death of that patient, and indirectly toward his own failure as a physician. Many are not inclined to subscribe to the abstract philosophy of metaphysics and psychology, but willing to admit that there is something that makes a difference in men in the way of success and popularity. They are sometimes inclined to believe that it is "blarney." Be it what it may, the one who has not a full supply of it is unfortunate.

The demonstration of that mysterious power possessed by every one to a greater or less degree, called telepathy, opens a field of investigation that is especially rich to every practicing physician. That every mind has more or less influence over other minds, even without spoken language, and possibly at great distances, has been demonstrated beyond the possibility of a doubt. If this be true, then the state of mind prevailing in the attending physician may tend strongly toward the recovery of his patient, or it may cause the balance to swing in the opposite direction. If the last prevails, then the physician really becomes an accessory to the death of his patient when he permits his mental balance to bend toward pessimism. To some this may seem like a rather far-fetched theory, but to the one who has kept abreast of the times in the development of the science of psychology and occultism, it is not a theory without possible demonstration. On my own part I lay no claim to extensive knowledge along these lines, but I am very certain that there are some things of this nature that affect the welfare of the suffering patient that may be employed by the attending physician. It is all very well to ridicule Christian science, but no well-informed man can succesfully claim that they as a cult do not and have not performed some veritable cures on which perhaps some ultra-scientific physician has made an ignominious failure. The whole secret of the successes of these faddists lies in the state of mind of the operator. Who ever heard of a pessimistic Christian scientist? Such a monstrosity would be as rare as a white crow! So with other cults. The osteopath does some good with his persistent massage, but his optimism plays no unimportant part in bringing about his cures. The faith-curist also does his work by arousing the dormant hope and building up an expectation of cure in the mind of his ecstatic patient, all produced by the optimistic mind of the curist. These things are and these things will be. The progressive and successful doctor will take advantage of them, but the confirmed mossback will ridicule that which his mind is too infinitesimal to comprehend, and will add one to the ranks of the chronic kickers and croakers!

Some are so egotistic that they think they could improve on the divine works of creation, and every effort of their puny little lives is directed toward that end, to the discomfort and often disgust of those who are so unfortunate as to be brought in contact with them. If the doctor happens to be so constituted, he carries that same sentiment into the sickroom. He is dissatisfied with the action of his medicines; he is dissatisfied with the work of the nurse; he is dissatisfied with the weather; he is dissatisfied with the cut of his coat, the temper of his wife and the color of his child's hair! This kind of people are sometimes enough to make a well man sick, much more so if their unhappy victim is so unfortunate as to be sick to begin with. Why not look on the bright side of life, and view everything through the roseate light of hope and satisfaction with everything as it is, except possibly the one single effort to make one's self and others better and happier? These people who are constantly endeavoring to diffuse the seeds of dissatisfaction with this world and all things therein, had best be careful and enjoy this world to its full extent, for possibly it may be more enjoyable than the next one they are permitted to visit!

Practice and preach optimism in all its myriad applications. It is a state of mind that any one may attain and hold for an indefinite period. Some one may say, "My temper is so high that I cannot control it." The man who says that simply admits that he is a poor weakling, not capable of doing the same thing that others do. The man who makes such a claim as that should be ashamed to look an honest man in the face, or else he should be committed to an asylum for the care of the feeble-minded!

Doctor, you who are not succeeding in the world as well as you should, and you that are not so successful in your efforts to cure the sick as you think you should be, try this everlasting and never-ending optimism. Carry it into the sickroom with you. Approach the operating-table on which lies the mutilated and suffering mortal pleading for your best efforts with this state of mind predominating. Give him the encouragement that can only come from a man who is satisfied with the world and all things therein. Buoy him up with the elixir of hope and a smiling face, and you will be astounded with the degree of success that you attain in your chosen calling. Never allow your mind to dwell for a moment on the possible failure, and failure will not approach you.

BILIOUS DYSENTERY.—Butler recommends powdered ipecac, twenty grains every four hours.—*Denver Med. Times.*

PAIN IN THE EYE.

THOMAS M. STEWART, M.D., CINCINNATI.

A patient is certain to direct the physician's attention to the presence and general location of pain, if it be a symptom in its affliction. The patient's manifestation of suffering furnishes a very imperfect guide as to the severity of the pain. One patient will complain little, and yet the pain may be so severe as to rob him of sleep. Another patient will grunt and groan over pain of moderate severity. Again, the same disease, running apparently the same course, will cause severe pain in one patient and in another very little.

Pain cannot, therefore, be taken as an indication of the severity of the disease of which it is a symptom. Pain may vary considerably without that fact having much to do with the progress of the case; generally, marked relief from pain accompanies an improvement.

Now eye patients complain of several kinds of pain, such as smarting and burning; a feeling as of sand or grit in the eye; stinging, aching; neuralgic; a full feeling in the eye, pressing it out or drawing backwards of the eye; aching back of the eyeball; headache. In this connection we might mention the fact that often there is an absence of pain in diseases usually accompanied by it; and lastly, a loss of sensibility of the eyeball to touch, even though great subjective pain is complained of.

The smarting and burning pains are usually due to conjunctivitis. At times these symptoms are exceedingly annoying, and, simple as the case may seem, they often tax the physician's patience and exhaust his skill. These pains are made worse by the use of the eyes, and by wind, dust, heat and light.

To cure the case a careful examination of the refraction may be necessary, as a small error may be the cause. Glasses prescribed for distant use, for reading, or for constant use have many cures to their credit. Often these cases show decided inflammatory symptoms.

Muscular weakness is a frequent cause of eye pain, and one that is not only overlooked in the examination, but sadly neglected when it comes to treatment. A special equipment is needed for the treatment of such cases.

If due to acute conjunctivitis, attention to the general habits and diet of the patient is often a necessary step in the treatment. The eye symptoms and the general symptoms will point to one of several remedies, and internal medication should be given a chance to cure. A chronic conjunctivitis may be the cause; in some cases a pale conjunctiva is often noted.

In addition to the internal remedy, diet is an important element in the removal of the cause, as, indeed, it is often the secret spring to unlock many a stubborn case, and the one thing needful to start it along the right road wherein the remedy can do its work and do it well.

The sand and grit feeling may be due to a foreign body. An inspection of the cornea by the aid of a good light, particularly the so-called oblique illumination, and an examination of the everted lids will disclose the presence or absence of the foreign body. Its removal, if present, generally completes the cure. Often such an examination shows little white granules in the mucous membrane. These are most often lime deposits. The cure is made by snipping them out. At other times the mucous membrane is seen to be rough, a sand-paper appearance, at the corners near the canthi, often accompanied by the same condition along the lower edge of the everted lid. To aid in the cure, if remedies fail, a thorough massage or curettement of these places is necessary. Stinging pains often accompany faulty action or cramp of the ciliary muscles. At such times the vision is suddenly blurred; the effort to again see or focus the eye is also painful.

Aching pain is found in the inflammation of the deeper tunics of the eye. It denotes a decided degree of tension of the parts, and it is most often found in iritis, irido-cyclitis, and glaucoma. An iritis will show a discolored iris, sluggish-acting pupil, the latter usually contracted; in such a combination the diagnosis is cleared by using a mydriatic, viz., atropia in 1, 4 or even 8 per cent. solution if pupil does not respond to weaker solution. The characteristic irregular dilatation of the pupil makes the diagnosis sure and the treatment clearly outlined. Atropia should be used to secure a still greater dilatation of the pupil, and to preserve as much as possible of the pupillary margin of the iris from being bound down to the lens capsule. Paracentesis of the cornea is an aid, often needed, to the action of the mydriatic.

Irido-cyclitis is iritis plus cyclitis. Cyclitis is diagnosed by palpation of the ciliary body, a zone one-eighth inch wide from the margin of cornea. Extreme tenderness of one or more points is diagnostic. The treatment is much the same as iritis.

Glaucoma is diagnosed by pressing with the forefinger of each hand, through the closed lid, as the patient looks down. If the eyeball does not dimple to the touch, or does not dimple as much as the fellow-eye or your own normal eye, *look out. Don't use atropine.* Blindness is not far away in any deep eye inflammation, and it lurks dangerously near when the eyeball is harder than the normal. Use ½ per cent. solution of eserine. If in doubt as to whether the case is an iritis or a glaucoma, use a 5 or 10 per cent. solution of dionin. Dionin sometimes causes pronounced redness, and if it increases the swelling and the congestion, cold applications will relieve it. Cold is not well borne in iritis. Iritis and glaucoma are two dangerous eye diseases; the general practitioner, when in doubt as to the diagnosis in other disorders that threaten life or are liable to impair the function of certain parts, calls in a fellow-physician to help solve the problem and assume part of the responsibility. Eye diseases that threaten blindness are on a par with fatal disease. It is, therefore, necessary to act with the same good judgment in regard to them as one does with regard to general disorders. In glaucoma the attacks are preceded by a prolonged, and often an unrecognized, tardy tissue elimination. Operations are made to save the eye from ravages of such faulty elimination. Sclerotomy, when well done, offers as much relief as an iridectomy.

Neuralgic eye pains usually accompany lesions of the fifth nerve. The pains are severe and persistent. Discriminating care is necessary to differentiate the pain of a neuralgia from the pain due to an eye inflammation.

Headaches, with fullness and discomfort in the eyes, are very often due to eyestrain. Headaches accompany fevers, organic disease of the brain and its membranes, or may be a reflex from disease of ovaries, etc., and headaches often are toxemic in origin. Excluding these as causes, eye-strain is a cause of a large percentage of headache. There is no special character to the pain. The refractive and muscular errors of the eye have caused headaches located in various parts of the head, with pain of a constant or intermittent type, felt on use of eyes or coming on at variable times after their use, recurring at regular and irregular intervals. Again, these headaches may be aggravated by hunger, exposure to heat or cold, indigestion, etc., or they may be independent of these. In a great many cases eye-strain and muscular weakness may be but one factor in the chain of causes; but until this source of nerve waste is checked a cure cannot be obtained. When the eye is one of the causes it is an important one, because it can be reached in a direct manner, perhaps paving the way to a cure by additional means. A prolific cause of headache and eye-strain is enlargement of the anterior end of the middle turbinated bone, removal of which is a positive cure.

Loss of sensibility of the eye, especially the cornea, to touch, may be found in herpes and glaucoma, and yet intense pain may accompany it.

Absence of eye pain has been noted in optic neuritis, retinitis and plastic choroiditis. Sometimes a quiet iritis may be encountered. Cataract is quite a painless affection. All of which proves that the presence or absence of pain demands a careful examination when eye or head symptoms are present.

Ohio State Eclectic Medical Association.

Proceedings of the Forty-fourth Annual Session.

W. N. MUNDY, M.D., EDITOR.

SECTION IV.

PEDIATRICS.

R. R. BARRETT, M.D., Chairman..........................Mansfield.
C. P. KROHN, M.D., Vice-Chairman....................Pleasant Plain.
J. V. ATHEY, M.D., Secretary................................Belpre.

SCOLIOSIS.

W. B. CHURCH, M.D., CINCINNATI.

A degree of lateral or rotary-lateral deviation from the normal axis of the spine is quite common. Angular antero-posterior deviations are due to tubercular spondylitis. Two other varieties of this form are lordosis and a total kyphosis of the whole column. A combination of these two varieties constitute the hollow round back observed in strumous, weakly children. The various obliquities so frequently seen in the spinal column suggest that the human body was not originally intended to meet the requirement of an upright posture. No other structure required such extensive modification to adapt itself to such a radical departure as the spine. Nature for a very long period rested content with invertebrates, the spine itself being the result of ages of evolutionary progress.

In addressing a body of educated physicians, one may take for granted that organic life, as we behold it, is the result of continuous adaptation of organism to environment. Man has made such wonderful progress by the working out of the principles of evolution that he is himself able to co-operate in the work of creation. Indeed, this is the special office of the physician. No time is likely to arise for suspension of the great work which nature has in hand for developing life on this planet. For intelligent co-operation nothing is more important than appreciation of the natural methods of evolution. It is our good fortune to come upon the stage after the work is so far along that the climax seems to be nearly reached. It is difficult to conceive of further progress along the same line. The advantages of an upright posture are so manifest that notwithstanding the serious consequences traceable to it, no one will now be found to advise a return to the primal position on all fours. It is evident, however, that nature has not fully conformed to the altered attitude.

When tired or ill, a return to the horizontal position is very agreeable. Many important functions are performed more easily and more perfectly while reclining. The muscles which support and maintain equilibrium in the upright posture have not yet become entirely involuntary. They do not act effectively during sleep. Soldiers on a march often become sorely fatigued; if the march is prolonged into the night, they will sleep fitfully in their tracks; but as the sleep grows deeper, they weave back and forth until threatened loss of equilibrium rouses them to consciousness. Even in a sitting posture we are all familiar with the nid-nid-nodding which ends with a jerk as the limit of motion is reached. We find it advisable to have our patients resort promptly to bed when attacked with a grave form of sickness, and warn them against the danger of too early getting up after the disease has spent its force. The limit of endurance is implied in saying, "I have been on my feet all day." The strongest and most enduring find it expedient to spend a considerable part of each twenty-four hours in a recumbent posture. Such are some of the proofs of incomplete adaptation.

More serious still is the increased labor imposed on the heart by the acquired erect position, causing a long list of pathological conditions and weaknesses. To even mention these would take too much of your time. The provision for sustaining the weight of the body in the erect posture, and at the same time yielding and flexible enough to prevent shocks, or jars to the brain and cord, is the spinal column. At birth two backward curves exist, one dorsal, the other sacral, to accommodate internal viscera. Efforts to sit or to stand erect develop later a forward cervical curve, and a forward lumbar curve, which are compensatory, and adjusted to bring the chords of each curve in the same vertical line, corresponding to the gravity line of the head. Marvelous as its adaptation for this great purpose, and completely as it serves in the great majority of cases, from youth to old age, failures are common enough to give genuine importance to the causes and conditions which impair its efficiency. The majority of cases of serious deformity are based on some obliquity of the vertebral column. A young girl's life is frequently blighted by the discovery of an unsuspected curvature when the dressmaker is called upon for the first careful fitting of gowns. The elevation of the shoulder, projection of a scapular wing, and prominence of one hip, has caused such asymmetry that an attempt must be made to conceal it by resort to pads of various shapes and sizes. The outcome even so was far from being satisfactory. Her mother had doubtless for years upbraided her for supposed carelessness, for holding one shoulder higher than the other, and for her habit of standing on one foot in a lolling position. She had been distressed to think her daughter was not going to have a good figure, was growing all out of shape. It often happens that the real cause of the deformity is not suspected until the curvature becomes so extreme that nature makes the best of a bad situation by producing ankylosis of the vertebræ. Weak muscles, maintaining too long positions exaggerating the normal curves, infantile paralysis, congenital inequality of length of · legs, are some of the causes of rotary lateral curvature. Whatever tends to keep the spine in an abnormal position for long periods of each day will change at length the bones, intervertebral cartilages, and ligaments in a way to confirm the deviation. This is the most common form of spinal curvature, and the one had in mind in preparing this paper. Until recent times, treatment of scoliosis was barren of good results. It must be conceded that prevention here is far better than cure. Slight deviations, before permanent. changes have occurred in the bone and before fixed by ankylosis, are quite amenable to treatment. After such changes, complete restoration is not always possible. The problem has been attacked by surgeons in many ways. Conclusions reached and promulgated one year have been retracted the next. The efforts of orthopedists have been directed mainly to various mechanical braces and appliances with very indifferent results. Sayres' suspension and plaster jacket treatment was accepted for a time as a solution of the problem; but expectations have not been realized. The scheme of every attempt has been to forcibly correct the curvature, and by some form of jacket or corset maintain the corrected outline. This is not so simple as it seems. The curvature, for unknown reasons, is usually to the right in the thoracic region, with a compensatory curve in the lumbar. Bulging outward of the thoracic spine is accompanied with rotation outward and backward of the vertebræ of this region, dragging the attached ribs in the same direction. The costal angles become acute and there is marked prominence of the right chest midway between the lateral and dorsal borders. It is plain that direct pressure toward the center of the body over this prominence increases the acuteness of the costal angle, and must also aggravate the rotation of the vertebræ. The combined action of two forces is needed, one inward, the other forward, to straighten and untwist the vertebral column. To accomplish this, a variety of apparatus has been devised, the design of each being the application of forces in different directions to straighten out the curves, and then maintain the corrected position by plaster-of-paris jackets. In some cases of my own a much simpler device has proven very satisfactory. Two strips of adhesive plaster, two inches wide and long enough to paritally encircle the body diagonally, are applied over the prominence in such direction that the upper strip, when brought around the body, will just cover the crest of the ilium. The lower strip, applied in an opposite diagonal course, terminates on the left scapula. Both strips are reinforced by a vertical strip applied over the initial extremity to prevent slipping. Then, with an assistant making pressure over the apices of the costal angles forward, the two strips are forcibly drawn into place. After the adhesion of the plasters is made perfect, the patient is prepared in the usual manner for a plaster jacket by donning a woven undershirt with suitable pads to protect bony projections. He is then suspended by Sayres' apparatus, and the plaster jacket is applied as usual. Soon as it hardens it is cut through in the median line in front. The cast is then removed. About one-fourth of an inch of each edge is cut away, and then the edges are bound with stout drilling; the top and bottom of the cast are trimmed and bound with soft leather. A strip of stout leather provided with hooks such as are used for lacing men's shoes is then sewed to the cast, so that the hooks are even with the vertical edges. If the cast has been well made with fine dental plaster, this jacket will be very serviceable.

It will be a great mistake to consider the work now complete, even though the curves have been corrected, and the correction can be maintained by the jacket. In fact, you are just ready to begin the treatment upon which a permanent cure depends. Restoration to the normal is only possible by restoring flexibility to the spine, and so increasing general muscular tone that no support is needed. The erector spinæ muscles in the vertebral groove are the chief dependence; but the co-ordinate action of so many other muscles is essential that prolonged and systematic general massage and special gymnastic exercises are required. The jacket can hardly be regarded as curative, and should be laid aside as soon as possible. The patient is sure to attach great importance to the jacket, and there is constant danger that he will come to depend upon it to the neglect of the real curative treatment. If constantly enclosed in this rigid jacket, all efforts to restore flexibility will be defeated; and, besides, the muscles grow weaker from lack of use. It will soon be noticed that when the jacket is taken off the patient immediately feels helpless, and cannot easily be satisfied until it is replaced. It should only be worn at first for a short time while standing or walking. Reliance for cure must be based wholly on such roborant measures as I have mentioned, supplemented by liberal diet, tonics and reconstructives. The massage and exercises are too important to be delegated to professional nurses and masseurs. The surgeon should officiate himself if he is ambitious to secure the best results. He can emulate to good advan-

tage the zeal and manual dexterity of our osteopathic confrères. In- ·
deed, it will not be surprising if these energetic and enterprising if
not always scientific fellows monopolize this field, and score many
successes that should have fallen to us. Their opportunity is plain.

The object of this paper will be missed if insufficient emphasis
has been placed on prophylaxis, and early management of those cases
that are liable to develop spinal curvature. Careful examination
should be made of all patients that raise a suspicion of deviation. If
stripped and made to bend forward, an unsuspected curve may often
be demonstrated. In such incipient stages the disease is readily
cured.

THE SICK BABY.

J. L. HENSLEY, M.D., MARION, O.

The late Professor Howe used to say to the class: "To the average
student or young physician, a subject that is not baptized in blood is
considered a very tame affair, and not worthy of consideration." Yet
it is a well-known fact to every medical man that in his early experience a case of capital surgery, such as an amputation or laparotomy,
was as rare as a hundred-dollar bill in a young doctor's pocket. But
it is also well known by every physician that among his first calls he
receives is to see the sick baby. Possibly the results attained decided
his success in the practice of medicine.

No physician should spurn a call to see a baby, whether it be in a
palace or in a hovel. He should recognize the fact that it is just as
much the idol of the humble home, though occupied by a washer-
woman, as it is in the home of the millionaire.

Occasionally the physician's attention is called to an early cyanosis,
occurring at birth. This arises from a congenital malformation, the
fetal circulation persisting in a measure; the blood is not properly
oxygenated. In common parlance, this is known as "blue skin disease."
Little can be accomplished by medication in this condition. The baby
is placed on its right side in a warm bath. Endeavor to keep it on its
right side, thus assisting as much as possible the circulation.

Sometimes a malformation, such as a hare-lip, imperforate anus,
congenital talipes, umbilical or scrotal hernia, are met. These call
for surgical interference.

With proper care as to clothing, feeding and the use of mother's
milk as a diet, it is not often that a baby needs the services of a physician. The culpable habit of feeding the babies catnip tea, molasses
and whisky, or many other disgusting mixtures, frequently mixed

with ignorance, meddling with the laws of nature, are calculated to make sick babies and fill many tiny graves.

Red gum disease, or baby rash, is a disease which makes its appearance within from four to seven days after birth, and is caused by the action of the atmosphere on the skin. It needs but little treatment, but for the satisfaction of an over-anxious mother should receive careful attention, so as to reassure her of its harmless character.

Jaundice sometimes makes its appearance early in infant life. It is readily recognized by the yellowish color of the skin, conjunctiva, nails and highly colored urine, staining the napkins a saffron color. Though alarming to the parents, it is not of a dangerous character. The symptoms call for nux, often combined with rhus tox. or ipecac.

These simple conditions frequently cause anxiety to the parents, and should receive the careful attention of the physician. They may assume grave symptoms if allowed to go untreated and be a cause of reproach for the indifference shown earlier.

Diseases of the Brain.—A delayed visit by the physician may cause him to be confronted by a high fever, patient restless, rolling its head from side to side on the pillow, uttering that familiar cry to the experienced physician. The face may be flushed, eyes bright, or he may find the patient dull, pupils dilated, and the little patient inclined to coma. In either event he may rest assured he has a serious condition to contend with. The indications in the first-named condition are for gelsemium or rhus tox., combined with veratrum viride if indicated. The second condition calls for belladonna, usually with aconite. Wet cloths are applied to the head—cold if there is much heat, hot if the vitality is low. Quinine inunctions may also be used.

Sore Throat.—The new-born babe is seldom attacked with a sore throat of a serious nature. Later in life we may be informed by the mother or nurse that the baby seems to have an earache. On examination, we find high fever, swollen glands, and on examining the throat we may find the tonsils swollen and covered with the characteristic ashen-colored exudate of diphtheria, or we may find the dark red throat and strawberry tongue of scarlatina. Examining the body we find the rash and verify the diagnosis. In the first-named condition the indications call for veratrum, phytolacca, and acids. In the second, aconite, rhus tox. and acids, with inunctions of quinine and lard.

Pneumonia.—The little patient may have a high fever, quick, short respiration, dilated nostrils, and a short, hacking cough attended with pain. By auscultation and percussion we recognize symptoms of pneumonia or of a congestion of the lungs. These conditions demand prompt treatment. The full pulse calls for veratrum, the small, quick pulse for aconite. The sudden starting in the sleep, attended with the shrill cry, plainly says rhus tox. and bryonia. The oppressed breathing calls for the compound powder of lobelia and capsicum on the cotton cloth spread with lard. If the temperature is very high, frequent sponging with tepid water will afford some relief.

Croup.—This is one of the most alarming diseases of the nursery. There are two or three forms of the disease, all of which are distressing and dangerous. The most common form is spasmodic or catarrhal croup. Another form is the pseudo-membranous, which is a much more dangerous malady, and requires vigorous and prompt treatment. The disease usually develops suddenly in the night. The child wakes up suddenly with a hoarse or metallic sound to its cough, and great distress of breathing. The remedies indicated are aconite and belladonna, three drops of each to a half-glass of water, teaspoonful every hour. Bathe the throat with the compound stillingia liniment and give one drop on sugar, internally, every hour. The more severe form partakes of the nature of diphtheria, and in addition to the remedies above named, acids should be resorted to at an early stage and the treatment recommended for diphtheria used. Such surgical relief as may be determined upon should also be employed.

Diseases of the Alimentary Canal.—Among these we will mention cholera infantum, summer complaint, the usual diarrhea arising from improper feeding, with the attendant indigestion. A marked difference will be found to exist between cholera infantum and summer complaint. The former comes on suddenly, is attended with severe vomiting and watery discharges from the bowels resembling that of Asiatic cholera and attended with great prostration. If relief is not promptly rendered the result is collapse and death. Summer complaint comes on more gradually, often continues through the entire heated term, and if neglected continues until frost. Indeed, it used to be considered that nothing could relieve it until cool weather brought relief. Emaciation is marked, the child being reduced to a skeleton. The old-time treatment consisted of hydrargyrum cum creta, kino, opium and acetate of lead. This has given way to a more rational treatment, such as aconite, 'rhus, gelsemium, and other remedies as indicated, with the emulsion of bismuth in mucilage of acacia, to which may be added a few drops of tincture of peppermint and syrup q. s. to make it pleasant to the taste. If the abdomen is swollen and tympanitic, apply the liniment previously described every three hours.

Take care of the baby; it may prove to be a king, president, statesman, minister or doctor in embryo.

Seton Hospital Reports.

L. E. RUSSELL, M.D., SURGEON.

Case 500.—Man, sixty years of age, admitted to the clinic with a history of severe peritonitis of long duration, with a complication in the nature of partial obstruction of the bowels.

On examination of this case we find a severe tympanitic condition of the bowels, with here and there across the abdomen the outlines of the intestines, which is a marked indication of obstruction or partial obstruction of the lumen of the intestines.

I have advised the patient to submit to a laparotomy for the purpose of giving relief to the obstructed intestines.

We find, on making the median incision from just below the umbilicus to near the pubes, that the whole anterior abdominal wall is attached to coils of the intestines, so that on making the intrusion into the abdominal cavity the intestines must be wiped away from the abdominal parietal wall.

We are now within the abdominal cavity and the intestines are adhered, coil by coil, by lateral attachments, and the involving parts are bound down for two or three inches where the coils angle and curve. It will therefore be necessary in the completion of this operation to carefully dissect and break up all the adhesions from the duodenum to the head of the colon. And it is here, at the head of the colon, that we find the cause for this aggravated intra-abdominal condition, namely, appendicitis with sloughing of the appendix, followed by a very severe appendicitis, which has at this time become chronic.

There is not a single inch of the intestinal tract of the jejunum or ileum that has not been burned over very thoroughly by this high grade of inflammation.

We shall, and do now, take out of the abdominal cavity all of the ileum and jejunum into hot towels, and into the abdominal cavity we pour many gallons of normal salt solution to wash out the débris caused by this inflammatory attack.

The intestines are now carefully wiped with gauze, moistened with the normal salt solution, and replaced in the abdominal cavity, which is now filled with two or three gallons of normal salt solution.

The peritoneum is closed with continuous catgut sutures without drainage, for it is the intent and purpose of the normal salt solution to cause the intestines to float in this fluid until nature completely absorbs the same. The normal salt solution has another purpose, namely, the extreme stimulation to the abdominal viscera, and this is made manifest by the increase and strength of the pulse, the flushed face and the entire absence of shock.

The hospital report now, two weeks following the operation, shows a complete and uninterrupted recovery; the abdomen is flattened normally, and the action of the bowels free and regular.

We make the report of this case thus carefully to show that oftentimes cases *in extremis* may be rescued by surgical relief after the above method.

Eye, Ear, Nose and Throat.

CONDUCTED BY CHARLES S. AMIDON, M.D.

Injuries of the Conjunctiva.

Foreign bodies, like particles of dust, cinders, ashes or particles of coal, which so often get into the eye, fall first upon the surface of the eyeball. The movement of the upper lid brushes them away from the spot, and the substance usually sticks to the inner surface of the lid just back from the free border. The pain, which is often quite severe, does not originate in the conjunctiva itself, which has very little sensation, but is caused by the foreign body scratching over the cornea. By everting the lid the offending substance is brought into view and can be easily removed.

Sharp-pointed substances, like pieces of steel, emery powder, etc., striking the eye with force, often penetrate the conjunctiva, and may remain there a long time without giving rise to irritation. However, when located, it is best to remove them, and this is done by picking up the tissues with forceps, incising, and bringing away the offending body in this way.

If a foreign body lodge on the cornea, the removal should not be attempted without the use of cocaine, 2 per cent. solution. A blunt eye-spud is probably the best instrument, but if this is not accessible and the foreign body is not embedded deeply, the end of a match or toothpick, sharpened and smoothed, will answer.

Burns of the conjunctiva are frequent, and are the result of hot ashes (from cigars), hot water or steam, molten metals, exploding powder, alkalies and acids. Those that arise from lime are the most frequent. It is of the greatest importance when we get an eye under treatment that has been injured by caustics, to thoroughly remove all of the corrosive substance that may be present. The solid particles may be removed with a pledget of cotton or forceps; then we should wash the conjunctiva with a gentle stream of water.

The inflammation following injuries of the eye should be treated according to indications—boric acid dr. ij to water O. j, used several times a day as a cleaning solution; atropine if there is any iritic complication, cold compresses, etc. Following severe injury there is usually a tendency to the formation of adhesions; this should be opposed as far as possible by often drawing the lids away from the eyeball, and by laying a strip of gauze soaked in oil between the opposing denuded surfaces. Adhesions once formed can be removed only by an operation.

As a rule traumatic conjunctivitis will get well in a few days, in spite of the violent symptoms presented in the beginning.

— — —

Hygiene of the Eye in School Children.

W. M. Carhart (*American Journal of Obstetrics*) July, 1908) draws the following conclusions:

1. The increase of late years in the number of children wearing glasses is not due to an increase in the number of weak or diseased eyes so much as it is due to the greater strain upon the function of vision necessitated by our more extended use of the eyes for close work in the complex civilization of the present day.

2. The normal child is born hypermetropic and without astigmatism. The myopic child is either defective from birth or has acquired myopia from the stress of eye-strain, usually through the "turnstile of astigmatism." Astigmatism is not congenital, but is practically always acquired in the normal child during the early years of life by excessive strain upon the muscles of accommodation.

3. Kindergarten and primary work should be arranged so as to avoid the strain upon the muscles of accommodation of the eye in the plastic years of childhood. Hence sewing and all weaving exercises should be limited in amount, if not absolutely eliminated.

4. Systematic study should be only begun when the delicate and soft tissues of the child's eyes have attained sufficient formation to resist distortion on moderate use of the accommodation. This means, in my estimation, that prolonged, close work should not be allowed until the age of ten or over. A child beginning systematic study at that age will, with suitable care, be able at sixteen or eighteen to acquire all the knowledge possible to its more precocious companion, and will have the inestimable advantages of normal eyes and healthy physique.

5. No young child should be encouraged to compete with its companions for prizes. Mental and ocular over-strain are the inevitable results of such educational monstrosities. In the primary schools, especially, there should be no grading of the children.

6. A child incapable of the prolonged use of the eyes at the proper age should not be classed as culpably lazy. In the majority of cases there will be found uncorrected refractive error.

7. Inability to concentrate the mental attention and deficient powers of observation are often caused by bad visual memory resulting from eye-strain.

8. The symptoms and physical signs of eye-strain in children can be easily recognized, and there is no more brilliant success in medicine than follows the correction in children of refractive error. Ocular hygiene is all-important in preventing educational over-strain.

Periscope.

The International Tuberculosis Congress.

The sixth triennial meeting of the International Tuberculosis Congress, held in Washington during the past three weeks, was, no doubt, the most important medical meeting ever held in this country. Its importance is due not only to the fact that it was called to devise and consider methods for the eradication and cure of the greatest enemy of mankind, tuberculosis, but because it brought into close and sympathetic co-operation representatives from almost every civilized country on the globe. In the language of one of the delegates, it was "the greatest peace congress ever held." What can bring nations closer together than a united effort against a common foe? Every quarter of the world brought its offering and secured what it needed from the common store.

Not only was it valuable from the standpoint of international progress and comity, but it also served to bring us into closer relations with the people at large, who attended the meetings in large numbers with untiring interest and enthusiasm. The appreciation and enthusiasm of the medical men were unbounded, and when they parted it was with the determination to return home and resume their work with renewed inspirattion and ardor.

Delegates from no less than thirty-five countries were present. It is not possible to state accurately the number of those from across the ocean, but three hundred will no doubt be a conservative figure. Among them were many whose names are familiar to the medical world—Koch, Calmette, Pirquet, Detre, Arloing, Landouzy, Denys, Bang, Febinger, Jee, Newsholme, Stafford, Latham, Raw, Williams, Paterson, Philip and Liceage. The thousands from our own country were headed by Trudeau, Theobald Smith, Flick, Ravenal, Fisher, Biggs and Phipps. Through the efficient efforts of the Executive Secretary, Dr. Livingston Farrand, everything was ready and the various sections proceeded at once with their work.

Section I was devoted to pathology and bacteriology, and was presided over by Dr. Wm. H. Welch, of Johns Hopkins.

Section II—Clinical Study and Therapy of Tuberculosis—Sanatoria, Hospitals and Dispensaries. President, Dr. Vincent Y. Bowditch.

Section III—Surgery and Orthopedics. President, Dr. Charles H. Mayo.

Section IV—Tuberculosis in Children—Etiology, Prevention and Treatment. President, Dr. Abraham Jacobi.

Section V—Hygienic, Social, Industrial and Economic Aspects of Tuberculosis. President, Mr. Edward T. Devine.

Section VI—State and Municipal Control of Tuberculosis. President, Surgeon-General Walter Wyman.

Section VII—Tuberculosis in Animals and its Relation to Man. President, Dr. Leonard Pearson.

In subsequent issues of the *Lancet-Clinic* I shall take up in detail the work of the various sections, and also show, where it is practicable, conditions in Cincinnati that are related to the subject.

The exhibit alone would have justified a long journey. Photographs, models, charts, radiographs, stereopticons, stereoscopes, phonographs, pamphlets, pathologic and normal specimens, animal and human, mounted and fresh, illustrated and explained every phase of the tuberculosis problem. Many of the most valuable of' these came from across the water. The model dairy was quite a feature, all modern methods being employed. The milk was examined daily at the government laboratory, and during three days the count was respectively 900, 1,200 and 600 bacteria c.c. The exhibit also has a negative virtue in that nothing that savored of commercialism was evident. The drug vendor, the condensed food purveyor, the instrument exhibitor and the book seller could not seduce with their wares those who are wont to dally outside the precincts where the intellectual pabulum is served.

The opening session of the Congress was presided over by Secretary Cortelyou, who called upon representatives from every country.

The Congress went wild with enthusiasm when Professor Koch was introduced and walked to the front of the stage. The delegates rose to their feet, cheering for the famous scientist.

"The tuberculosis situation in Germany has been distinctly favorable during the last three decades," he said. "The rate of mortality due to tuberculosis in Prussia has been reduced one-half. This is equivalent to a gain of 30,000 lives per annum.

"We are active in trying not only to maintain but to increase this diminution. For this purpose many sanatoria have been established, in which 40,000 patients are cared for every year. You may be sure that Germany watches the work of the Congress with the keenest interest.

"The task which medical men face in their crusade on tuberculosis is admittedly a gigantic one. In many parts of the world great progress is being made in checking the disease, while in others, chiefly because hygienic principles are not understood, the course of the disease appears to be gaining. It will require a great campaign of education to check consumptoin, and this seems to be the chief duty of medical men. We are all bending our efforts to rid the country of this disease, and it may be said that we are doing well."

The press had considerable to say during the Congress about the disagreement of the younger investigators and Koch concerning the transmissibility of human and bovine tuberculosis. The majority of those at the Congress knew nothing about the matter except what was seen in the papers. The reason given why Dr. Koch takes the stand that bovine tuberculosis is not so dangerous to the human family is that the German government stands behind Dr. Koch, and that Kaiser Wilhelm is much perturbed lest the pure food inspection of America and the strict meat laws will cause American beef to become so popular in Deutschland that a German slaughter-house will be a rarity. If the world accepts the Koch theory, then it is evident that the meat need not be inspected for tuberculosis, or, at least, not so strictly examined. If the world throws Dr. Koch down, then not only will meat be inspected as in the past, but the influence of this Congress will cause more stringent measures to be taken everywhere, and a concerted action will some day be taken up by every nation.

If the Koch theory is accepted, all the pasteurizing plants for the purification of milk will be counted as useless. As New York is vitally interested in the milk problem, Dr. Abraham Jacobi was a participant in the discussion. He is reported to have said, when Dr. Koch demanded that no resolutions be passed against him: "The lives of thousands of babies are of far more importance than the reputation of one scientist."

Those present at the secret session were: Professor Koch, Professor Arloing, Dr. N. P. Tendeloo, Professor of Pathology at the University of Leyden; Dr. Bernard Bang, Professor of Veterinary Pathology of the Royal Veterinary School, University of Copenhagen; Dr. Febinger, Professor of Pathological Anatomy at the University of Copenhagen; Dr. Sims Woodhead, Professor of Pathology at the University of Cambridge, England; Dr. Eastwood, also of Cambridge University; Dr. Adami, of Montreal; Dr. Theobald Smith, of Boston; Dr. Mazyk P. Ravenel, of Madison, Wis., and Dr. Leonard Pearson, of Philadelphia.

At the closing session of the Congress Dr. Livingston Farrand, of New York, read the resolutions prepared by the Committee on Resolutions, which were adopted without a negative vote. They were:

"*Resolved,* That the attention of the States and central governments be called to the importance of proper laws for the obligatory notification by medical attendants, to proper health authorities, of all cases of tuberculosis coming to their notice, and for the registration of such cases in order to enable the authorities to put in operation measures for prevention.

"2· That the utmost efforts should be continued in the struggle against tuberculosis, to prevent the conveyance from man to man as the most important source of the disease.

"3· That preventive measures be continued against bovine tuberculosis, and that the possibility of the propagation of this from man to man be recognized.

"*Resolved,* That we urge upon the public and upon all governments the establishment of hospitals for the treatment of advanced cases of tuberculosis.

"2. The establishment of sanatoria for curable cases of tuberculosis.

"3· The establishment of dispensaries and night and day camps for ambulant cases of tuberculosis, which cannot enter hospitals and sanatoria.

"*Resolved,* That this Congress indorses such well-considered legislation for the regulation of factories and workshops, the abolition of premature and injurious labor of women and children, and the securing of sanitary dwellings as will increase the resisting power of the community to tuberculosis and other diseases.

"That instruction in personal and school hygiene should be intrusted to properly qualified medical instructors.

"That colleges and universities should be urged to establish courses in hygiene and sanitation, and also to include these subjects among their entrance requirements in order to stimulate useful elementary instruction in the lower schools.

"That the Congress indorses and recommends the establishment of playgrounds as an important means of preventing tuberculosis through their influence upon health and resistance to disease."--B. F. Lyle, M.D., in *The Lancet-Clinic.*

A Malaria Theory of History.

A new theory as to the cause of the decay of ancient Rome and Greece was recently advanced by W. H. S. Jones, of Cambridge. Practically the first occurrence of the Greek word for malaria is in "The Wasps" of Aristophanes, in 422 B. C. Three years before that date the Athenians had been engaged in military operations on the island of Sphacteria, now one of the most malarial spots in the Mediterranean. The Peloponnesian war soon afterward led to great tracts of land going out of cultivation, which would give the malaria-bearing mosquito ample breeding grounds. When the word for malaria became common the word for melancholia (black bile) began to appear. The melancholia of the ancient Greek writers resembles the mental effects of malarial fever; Hippocrates found it to occur especially in autumn (the malarial season), and Galen considered that it caused enlarged spleens (a feature of malaria). Malaria seems thus to have become prevalent in Greece in the fourth century B. C.; and the change which gradually came over the Greek character from 400 B. C. onward was one which would certainly have been aided, and was in all probability at least partially caused by the same disease. The Greeks commenced then to lose much of their intellectual vigor and manly strength. Home life took precedence of city life. Patriotism decayed and lofty aspirations almost ceased to stir the hearts of men. Dissatisfaction and querulousness are marked characteristics of that age.— *The Medical Times.*

Pure Drug Law and Eclectic Medicine.

"Prof. John Uri Lloyd, in the *Eclectic Medical Gleaner,* says that while the materia medica and practice of the dominant or "regular" school of medicine "has been practically brushed twice from the map" during the past century, there is not a single Eclectic drug of the early "fathers" that "does not stand the test of present-day experience." He also declares that not one Eclectic drug is mentioned in the pure food and drug act and regulations, although "the harmful remedies, the harmful compounds, the deleterious drugs, substances that need to be guarded by the strong arm of the national law, insidious nerve-racking narcotics, the criminal synthetics," comprise a "mighty list."—*The Druggists' Circular,* June, 1907.

Combinations.

In renewing a JOURNAL subscription or subscribing new we are frequently asked to make a combination offer with a *late* book. Consequently we offer until January first the following:

THE JOURNAL (new or renewal) and Thomas' Practice, Cloth, $7.50.

THE JOURNAL and Ellingwood's Treatment, $7.50.

THE JOURNAL and Mundy's Children, $4.50.

THE JOURNAL and Stephens' Gynecology, $4.50.

THE JOURNAL and Foltz on the Nose, Throat and Ear, $5.00.

Cash with the order in every case.

The Eclectic Medical Journal

A Monthly Journal of Eclectic Medicine and Surgery.

TWO DOLLARS PER ANNUM.

Official Journal Ohio State Eclectic Medical Association

JOHN K. SCUDDER, M.D., MANAGING EDITOR.

EDITORS.

W. E. BLOYER.	H. W. FELTER.	L. E. RUSSELL.	R. L. THOMAS.
W. B. CHURCH.	J. U. LLOYD.	H. E. SLOAN.	L. WATKINS.
JOHN FEARN.	W. N. MUNDY.	A. F. STEPHENS.	H. T. WEBSTER.

Published by THE SCUDDER BROTHERS COMPANY, 1009 Plum Street, Cincinnati, to whom all communications and remittances should be sent.

Articles on any medical subject are solicited, which will usually be published the month following their receipt. One hundred reprints of articles of four or more pages, or one dozen copies of the Journal, will be forwarded free if the request is made when the article is submitted. The editor disclaims any responsibility for the views of contributors.

Discontinuances and Renewals.—The publishers must be notified by mail and all arrearages paid when you want your Journal stopped. If you want it stopped at the expiration of any fixed period, kindly notify us in advance.

CELLULAR VITALITY AND OPSONINS.

While the discussion of opsonins seems to be fashionable at the present time, we should not forget that they occupy but a minor position on the stage of pathology and therapeutics. In infectious, diseases they may be interesting as a matter of curiosity, though we learn little new of value in their inspection.

Thanks to the inductive philosophy of Professor Scudder, we had provided for them with our specific antiseptics and antizymotics long before the revelations of pseudo-science in this respect were on the ground. Does present knowledge of opsonins afford any practical advance upon what was then taught? Doubtful.

The basis of life is the cell, and therefore opsonins must depend upon cellular activity for their existence. In acute cases we might hope to correct faulty conditions of the circulating medium with direct means; but in the majority of cases in practice, especially in chronic affections, our proper aim would be to provide means for improving cellular vitality and activity. Here is where the secret of success must lie in the treatment of chronic diseases; and so far as the practitioner is capable of arriving at correct conclusions as to the seat of trouble and the remedy applicable to lack of structural integrity, will his success lie in chronic practice.

Experience has taught us that various remedies selectively influence various parts and functions. In other words, remedies possess

their affinities—possibly better put that cells possess their affinities—
and knowledge of these affinities is important for the proper education
of the successful therapeutist. A knowledge of them, with all their
subtle individualities, should be the lifelong study of the physician;
for he can never memorize them sufficiently to continually qualify
for the many phases of disease he is liable to encounter.

These remarks apply more particularly to chronic lesions. There
comes a time in the lives of many old physicians when acute practice becomes irksome and repellant. It becomes so much a matter of
routine, and its demands are usually so simple, that its repetitions
become humdrum. To such there is an irresistible desire to dig
deeper into the mysteries of therapy in chronic disease, even though
they never get to the bottom.

We may limit our remedies in acute disease to a small number of
agents; but not so in chronic disease. Tissue selection is not the only
object to be considered. Quality and character of action are important
elements in the adoption of remedies. Another important element is
permanence. Many remedies which act well are evanescent in their
effect. They must be continually renewed in order that the effect
may be kept up. They may even then wear out, and need to be
changed for something else in order to keep up desired improvement.
Many of our remedies are acute-disease remedies. They do not afford
us permanent results in chronic affections. They do not reach deep
enough into vital reinforcement. They may stimulate normal processes temporarily, but the disease returns as soon as they are withdrawn, if their effects do not cease entirely with steady use. They
are inadequate to bring about permanent restoration of normal structure and function. They are superficial in effect, and do not restore
normal energy and integrity of the cellular basis of life.

We can never hope to cope successfully with such diseases as
tuberculosis, benignant and malignant new growths, chronic nephritis,
and other stubborn affections, therapeutically, until we possess more
knowledge in this direction. We must learn of remedies which penetrate deeper into the vital activities of cells, in order to reach affections depending upon serious alteration of structural integrity.

We know a great deal about superficial remedies. We are well
qualified with them to treat acute affections, but we are not well
enough posted upon remedies which bring about restorative processes
in chronic structural affections which seriously threaten vital organs
and operations. There is yet a great field open before us.

Some of us know that certain remedies are capable of curing structural changes. We know from observation that silica will cure en-
chondroma in young subjects. We know that thuja and magnesium

sulphate will effect the removal of warts from the skin of young subjects through their constitutional effects. We know that saw palmetto will sometimes bring about a revolution in the nutrition and development of the mammary gland. We know that conium and hydrastis will remove hardened new growths from these organs when not malignant. These are a few of the facts of therapeutics which should stimulate us to further investigation along such lines.

Let us learn to make better distinction between acute and chronic remedies. In other words, let us study materia medica and therapeutics by separating remedies into two classes; a new classification, if you please, or an old classification revived, for the idea is not at all new. Two classes at least, until we have progressed a little further: remedies for acute diseases, and remedies for chronic structural lesions.

However, we must not expect to draw the line too closely, for a few remedies will occupy both sides of the field. Yet such a differentiation would be useful for purposes of emphasis, and to stimulate investigation along well directed lines of study. It is the searching—slow, perhaps—but deeply acting agents we are after in the treatment of chronic affections; agents which have to do with cell nutrition and cell vitality; agents which permanently normalize the structure and functions of cells upon which the life of the diseased part or parts depends.

Surely we may search profitably for these in all three kingdoms—vegetable, mineral and animal—though it seems as though we may get the best results from the last of these. Criticize as we may, animal products are affording surprising results in the treatment of chronic disease in more than one instance. We can afford to allow them a fair share of our attention. Where else can we expect to find remedies capable of curing spastic paralysis, locomotor ataxia, exophthalmic goitre, paralysis agitans, etc.? It is claimed by many good observers that this can be done with certain animal products. The proof of the pudding is in the eating. Many apparently hopeless cases of such kind come to us with hope and depart in sorrow. Have we reached our limitations? WEBSTER.

PREVENTATIVE MEDICINE.

It must be admitted that some of the greatest achievements of medicine in the past twenty-five years have been along the lines indicated by the above caption. If the study of bacteriology has achieved or resulted in the finding of specific bacilli, or if doubts have been cast upon some which we have accepted as pathogenic in the past, there is no doubt its study has resulted in immeasurable benefit to mankind, by reason of the improvements in sanitation, purer foods and better habitations. It has taught mankind the advantages to be derived from cleanliness. Surgery has been brought to its present high standard by reason of its study. Though the spray of Lister has developed into strict cleanliness of the operator and person operated upon, yet the former was evolved through the study of bacteriology, or the desire to rid the field of operation of the pathogenic bacteria, and has been the means of enlarging the field of surgery as well as lessening its mortality.

Municipalities, States and nations have taken hold of the subject, and by reason of the enforcement of pure food laws, better drainage and care of sewage, improvement of water supply and of habitations, they have succeeded in lowering the mortality records to a notable degree, and have prevented the spread of contagious diseases. Possibly one of the most notable achievements of recent date along this line of work has been the practical elimination of yellow fever from the canal zone and Cuba. It might be claimed these belong to the domain of sanitary engineering. Granted. Yet the physician paved the way for the work of the engineer. Physicians have been bending their best energies along the line of the prevention of disease, taking a humanitarian view of the matter rather than a sordid one.

The activity along the line of pediatrics has resulted in an intense study of the subject of infant feeding. This study has not inured to the benefit of the physician only, but to the laity as well. The result has been that we do not see so many of the severe cases of enteric and ileo-colitis of twenty· or more years ago. Why? Because the laity as well as the physician have learned how to feed and care for the food of the babe. The physician's attention has been called to the necessity of a better care for the welfare of those who will become the men and women of to-morrow. The making and developing of a robust youth means the making of a robust, well-developed mankind, physically and mentally, and this inures to the benefit of the State and nation. This is not a theoretical dream, for if we turn to the introduction of the American edition of Pfaundler and Schlossman's "Diseases of Children," we find some statistics that are rather startling. Holt reduces the mortality records of New York, Rochester and Yonkers to a uniform scale for the sake of comparison, and we find that in New York City (Boroughs of Manhattan and Bronx) the mortality of children under five years of age, per 100,000 of population, has fallen in eighteen years from 1,160 to 620, or nearly 47 per cent. During the same period in Rochester, an inland city of 180,000, it has fallen from 584 to 340, or 42 per cent. In Yonkers, a suburban city of 60,000, from 880 to 660, 25 per cent. A calculation, based upon the present population of children under five years, shows an annual saving of the lives of 12,000 children of this age in New York alone.

Surely the care devoted by municipalities to the water and food supply; the care of the disposal of sewage; the providing of parks and breathing spaces for the unfortunates, and the better housing, has brought a large reward upon the investment. Who can foretell what the same energy, displayed in the next quarter century as in the past one, will bring forth? Possibly a curtailing of the ravages of tuberculosis. We rejoice in the achievements of the past; let us labor and hope for greater achievements in the future.   MUNDY.

THE PSYCHICAL AND THE PHYSICAL.

The influence of the mind upon the body should be well understood by physicians, and he who disregards the relations which a patient's mentality exerts in medication will not be as successful in practice as otherwise. But there is also an influence of the body upon the mind which must be taken into consideration in therapeutics. Man is not all mind, but also possesses a body which makes itself evident, which has needs and tendencies that must be considered. The body is not always the servant of the mind, but often the master. The calls of the body for food and raiment, and for the necessities of life, urge the mind to greater activity, and while we may speculate learnedly upon the superiority of the mind, and call man the "higher animal" because of his mental faculties, yet starvation, exposure or pain will reduce the intelligent and learned to the level of the beast, even to cannabalism, so much does the body dominate the mind. On the other hand, mental illusions, delusions and hallucinations may bring the body to a deplorable state. It must be admitted that man is both a mental and physical being, and these attributes should work in harmony for the best interest of the body. To assume that all is mental, and that every physical ailment can be removed by faith, is an extreme; yet, on the other hand, we cannot wholly disregard the psychical in our treatment of disease. A judicious middle course is best. However, extremists do good, inasmuch as they cause discussion, which in time establishes the standing of important facts. As science has no emotion, but deals alone with demonstrable truths, many things occur which are outside her realms. For instance, certain symptoms of disease exist without pathological basis; still we cannot say there is no cause, notwithstanding science can find none. In mental disturbances slight causes may be evanescent and transient, but are still causes, and if our methods of diagnosis were delicate enough we would find a physical basis for the trouble. The body must be reckoned with in therapeutics; to refuse or neglect this as a tangible entity is a mistake equal to that of those who ignore the mind as a factor in disease. Scientists are prone to consider the body as a machine, as material, and this body is liable to wear and accident like other machines, and to assert that it requires attention to keep it in order and repair. Even the mental is regarded as the result of the material, and when the material is destroyed the mental ceases. It was a part or product of the machine and died with it. A disposition upon the part of the profession to look lightly upon "mere mental phenomena" has given rise to faith healing, absent treatment, Dowieism, and many forms of charlatanry which, after all, have a modicum of good in them. WATKINS.

PNEUMONIA.

The time of year again approaches when diseases of the lungs become prevalent, and a warning against too vigorous treatment to overcome pronounced symptoms should be sounded.

I know that some physicians; who ought to know better, resort to depressants to lower the extremely high temperature which prevails in pneumonia, and to narcotics to allay the *necessary* cough, which is decidedly wrong. I know that gentleness in the treatment of pneumonia means' recovery, and that sledge-hammer treatment means death and a funeral forty times in one hundred.

Let us not forget that an exhausted heart is the cause of death in nearly all cases, and remembering, let us give nothing to the patient which tends toward weakening that organ.

The temperature range is high, but fever will not kill; cough is troublesome, but cough will not kill; pain is wearing and hard to bear, but pain alone will not kill. *The wrong kind of treatment will kill.*

If I did not know anything about specific treatment of disease, and was compelled to confine myself to few remedies in the treatment of pneumonia, I would count them on my fingers, so: Veratrum, gelsemium, ipecac, bryonia, iron. Veratrum for the full, strong, bounding pulse; gelsemium for excitation, with flushed face, bright eyes, etc.; ipecac for irritation of the mucous membrane; bryonia for sharp pain and cough; iron for inflammation of the lung tissue. These may be combined by those who do not know specific medication as follows: R. Spec. med. veratrum, gtt. x-xx; spec. med. ipecac, gtt. x-xx; aquæ dest. q. s. ad oz. iv. M. Sig. Take a teaspoonful every two hours. Then R. Spec. med. bryonia, gtt. v; spec. med. gelsemium, gtt. x-xxx; fer. et ammon. cit., grs. v; aquæ dest. q. s. ad oz. iv. M. Sig. Take a spoonful in alternation with the first prescription every hour.

Feed not at all until fever abates and a desire for food returns, although fruit juices will do no harm at any time and will often be relished by the patient. Give all the cold water the patient desires. Keep the bowels moderately free, but do not physic. Bathe the patient as often as may be agreeable, but not otherwise. Let the patient have plenty of air and sunshine by keeping windows open and shades up. Keep everything clean about his bed and in the room.

If an application to the chest must be had, use the compound powder lobelia and capsicum on a larded cloth.

In seven to fourteen days 95 per cent. of your cases of pneumonia will be convalescent.

If you know specific medication, use your judgment as to changes of treatment. If you are ignorant of this method of treatment, stick persistently to the above remedies, and by the providence of God, the benefit derived from your treatment, and the avoidance of remedies that kill, you will be successful far above the man who adheres to a bastard scientific treatment. STEPHENS.

THE SELECTIVE FUNCTION OF THE CELLS AND THE ACTION OF DRUGS.

The doctrine of the selective action of the cells, by which they are enabled to choose out from the blood those elements which they have need of, and appropriate them to the supply of their wants, while they reject all other elements, and send them along to be used by such other cells as may have need of them, is one which offers an easy solution of many things in physiology and medicine which are otherwise hard to understand.

Stated a little more at length, the theory may be illustrated as follows: In the general blood-stream as it comes pouring out of the left side of the heart, and goes pulsing through the arteries to every part of the system, there is to be found every kind of matter which goes to make up the different tissues and structures of the body. There is oxygen to purify the blood and revivify the tissues, phosphorus for the brain cells, lime and gelatin for the bones, albumin for the muscles, and the proper materials for all the different kinds of cells, mucous serous, glandular—in short, the things which are needed for evry part of the body.

Nor can the material which is needed for the nutrition of one part be made use of by any other part. Each cell claims for its own and takes unto itself that kind of material, and only that, which can be elaborated in its own factory and made up into the substances which it needs and uses in its daily life and work. Unto each part its own, and every part unto its own place, is the law of life. So through all the parts of the body this one fluid goes coursing on its way, while at every station there is thrown off by the blood and taken up by the cells those particles of matter which are needed there, and only those. There is a selective affinity of each part for its own material. The hair cells pick out with unfailing accuracy those substances which go to the making up of hair. The liver chooses only those materials which can be changed into sugar and bile and the other liver materials and liver products.

Again, the quantity which is normally appropriated by any cell is the amount which is needed to restore and preserve the physiological equilibrium, or proper balance of the functions. As the processes of waste are always going on, so the repair of tissue must go on apace, and these two are normally equal, no more being taken up by the cells than is needed to carry on the natural functions of the part or than can be carried off by the organs of excretion.

To be sure, just as in nature everywhere we find a normal action and an abnormal one, so here there is such a thing as loading down the circulation with matter which is not needed by any of the tissues, yet which cannot be gotten rid of except by the regular physiological processes of nutrition, and hence it has to be taken up by the cells. And there is such a thing as overburdening the system with the best of materials, so that the cells will take up more than they need or than they can properly dispose of. In either case the result is that the functions dependent on these cells are rendered abnormal in their action, or are depressed in their character, or unduly stimulated. We then see the symptoms of innutrition, or overnutritrion, or of poisoning. This is only in line with what is done by reasoning creatures every day, for there is none of us who live up to our light and knowledge all the time and under all circumstances. We all of us eat too much at times, and improper food at that. If we did not, there would be few cases of colic or typhoid fever or gall-stones or rheumatism for us to treat. Nature carries on her operations automatically to a certain extent, it is true, but she makes false steps at times, and needs an intelligent mind to direct her in her work.

To carry the theory a little further, the same principle holds good with medicinal and drug substances as with food and dietetic materials. When active remedies are given in small amounts and repeated at the proper intervals only, we find that there is produced a definite effect—

and if the drug was properly indicated, a remedial effect—on some definite organ, tissue, or structure, while the other organs, tissues and structures are apparently uninfluenced thereby. Hydrastis has an especial action on the mucous membranes; bryonia influences especially the serous tissues; jaborandi acts primarily on the sweat glands of the skin, and in a less degree on the other excretory glands. Strychnine is the great nerve tonic, while iron builds up the blood. But if too much strychnine or any other active substance is administered, it is not in the power of nature to properly dispose of the additional quantity, and harm results to the individual. The same is true of all remedial substances, in greater or less degree in proportion to their activity and their power to accomplish good or ill.

The proper application of these principles gives us *definite medication, for specific indications, and in therapeutic dosage only.*

There may be objections to this theory, and it is quite possible that the statement here given can be improved upon. But as a whole, it is certainly a most convenient peg upon which to hang a large number of known facts; and without it or its equivalent in some form, we have very little foundation for any advanced science of therapeutics.

FRENCH.

COAL OIL.

"Oil workers are never bald. Visit oil regions, such as those of Russia, examine the workmen's hair; it is soft and thick and glossy. For petroleum cures incipient baldness, and if your hair is thinning, rub some in. Never mind the smell. It will do you good."—*Pharmaceutical Era,* October 17, 1907.

In connection with the above clipping from the *Pharmaceutical Era,* we will remark that about forty years ago, when petroleum was a matter of some scientific inquiry, and its qualities practically unknown to the people, a marvelous remedy for the provocation of the growth of the hair, and as a remedy for baldness, was introduced under flaming advertisements in a proprietary manner. This marvelous remedy proved to be nothing more nor less than kerosene, the price, $1.00 for an eight-ounce bottle, making probably the record mark.

LLOYD.

Installment Plan.

We will send any number of late Eclectic books only, on the installment plan, with suitable references, on the following terms: *Five* dollars down and *three* dollars per month till paid for. Send for price-list.

ERRATA.—On p. 475, "coal oil" should read "cod-liver oil."

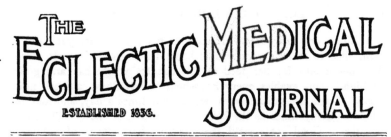

THE ECLECTIC MEDICAL JOURNAL

ESTABLISHED 1836.

VOL. LXVIII.   CINCINNATI, DECEMBER, 1908.   No. 12.

Original Communications.

SOMETHING ABOUT GOAT'S MILK, WITH REFLECTIONS.

A. GARFIELD SCHNABEL, M.D., TUCSON, ARIZONA.

When one stops to reflect upon the many articles that are suggested and put upon the market as infant food, if he be conscientious in his work he will hesitate and be sure of his ground before he will offer to the critical medical profession anything new. I doubt not but that every physician who shall honor this paper by his reading, has some one baby food that he "ties to," and if you tell him you have something better, he'll tell you, "I'm from Missouri." However, it is a self-evident fact that no very satisfactory food has as yet been found, else our shop shelves would not be filled with a score or more of baby foods, and our records be filled with infant mortalities. What I have to offer is not new, but an old article dug up and polished a little with two years of experiment and experience, for I believe goat's milk has been used as an article of food since the time of Babylonia, and those of you who have sojourned in Europe know it is a common article of food there even to-day.

My attention was first attracted to goat's milk as an infant food about ten years ago. While reading a story in German, I was particularly impressed by the fact that the baby hero of the story regained his health by the old doctor prescribing goat's milk for him to drink. That impression was a lasting one, so when it became necessary for my boy to be weaned at four months I naturally looked for a goat. She was obtained and the youngster has thrived on it ever since. So satisfactory was the use of the milk, that I resolved to try it with other babies and invalids. I purchased eight nannies and have furnished milk to twenty-five babies and ten consumptives, and from these experiments and information taken from Bulletin No. 68, Bureau of Animal Industry, I have the following to submit in favor of the goat.

1. *Goats are easily kept.* It requires but a small dry yard and a warm shed to make a comfortable home for a goat. It costs about $1.50 per month for her feed in this country where hay and grain are high. This enables every household to have first, a fresh milk supply. Goats are milked from two to four times a day, and may be milked as many times as the baby is fed, provided she is milked dry each time. Good goats yield from two to four quarts of milk per day, some species as much as seven quarts. Second, a pure milk supply. The bacterial count of goat's milk obtained under good circumstances is less than 1,000 c.c., and usually below 500 (cow's milk obtained under the very best circumstances is rarely less than 10,000 per c.c.).

2. *Goats are by nature very clean animals.* Their excrements are of such a nature that a few minutes' contact with air and sunshine makes them dry and compact and not easily pasted and smeared upon the animal's hair and udder. Goats do not lie down in filth, but seek dry places. (Compare this with cattle.)

3. *They are practically immune from infectious diseases and especially tuberculosis,* the percentage being about .001. It is stated in Paris that out of thousands of animals slaughtered not one was found to be affected with tuberculosis (cattle have a percentage of from 35 to 51 per cent.). And not only this, but it has been proven that one tubercular cow in a herd will render the milk from the whole herd tuberculous; that is, it will contain tubercle bacilli from the fact that her excrements contain millions of tubercle bacilli. The excrements coming in contact with the food will make the excrements of other healthy animals contain bacilli. It is practically impossible to obtain milk which is not contaminated with the feces. (Bulletin No. 99, pages 12 to 20.)

4. *A goat is the only natural foster mother we have.* She will adopt and care for almost any animal. When a doe is shown the baby that receives her milk as food, she will come to her place to be milked at the baby's cry. It is no uncommon thing among the less refined Spanish people of this country to turn baby and doe in the yard together, and the doe comes at the baby's cry and places herself in such a position that the baby can suckle her.

5. *Goat's milk is the nearest to the human.* It is alkaline in reaction, sweet and practically inodorous. Casein and paracasein are formed slowly when treated with acids or rennet. The precipitate formed is loose and flocculent (not tough and compact like cow's milk under similar treatment). The quantity of proteins is nearly the same and proportion of casein to albumen is about 4 to 2.5 (human 4 to 3, cow 6 to 1). Like human milk it contains small amounts of

lecithin and nuclein. The fat globules are small and the capsule easily dissolved. It is rich in lactose.

COMPARATIVE ANALYSIS.

	Goat.	Human.	Cow.
Water	85.6	87.3	87.5
Dry substance	0.7	0.3	0.7
Casein	3.5	2.0	3.5
Albumen	1.3	1.6	0.5
Fat	3.2	2.8	3.5
Lactose	5.7	6.0	4.3

These analyses will vary from time to time in different species and according to period of lactation, food, etc.

Experience has shown that babies do better on milk taken from does that are confined to a clean, dry yard and fed upon dry, well-cured hay, such as clover, alfalfa and natural grasses, together with one 'pint of oats or barley as grain twice a day. No green food of any kind, especially carrots, turnips, beets, etc., should be allowed.

For very young babies it is well to select a doe about two weeks fresh, the milk for the first month being diluted with two parts of pure warm boiled water (not distilled). After the first month the strength should be gradually increased so at the fourth month it is given pure. Some infants will require stronger milk than others, but it is easy to watch the stools and regulate the dilution by their appearance. If the stools are curdy, add more water. If white and pasty, allow milk to stand eight hours and skim off the cream. If acid, add lime water or sodium citrate. If any intestinal trouble occurs, allow the goat no alfalfa or clover hay, but only hay made from grasses with her usual grain. Another thing, keep a lump of rock salt within easy reach of the goat so she can get what she needs each day and not salt at intervals, for colic and diarrhea are sure to follow these salting days.

Just a word in closing this paper regarding milk and tuberculosis. In Bulletin No. 93, Bureau of Animal Industry, is to be found a very elaborate and worthy discussion on "The Relation of Tubercular Lesions to the Mode of Infection." This bulletin will prove to the fair mind the unreasonableness of the respiratory theory of tuberculosis, and the reasonableness of the theory of direct infection, from abrasions in either skin or mucous membrane by fresh tuberculous material. It is to be believed that the vast majority of cases of tubercular infection are due to the use of the food products of the tubercular cow. This statement is made in view of the following facts:

1. Cattle seem predisposed to tuberculosis, the percentage being from 35 to 51 per cent.

2. That milk from tuberculous cattle is used more extensively than

any other article of food, almost every person at some time in his life subsisting upon it.

3. Milk from a herd of cows in which one tubercular cow is kept will contain tubercle bacilli.

4. Milk is almost entirely relied upon by physicians as a food for patients suffering from acute infectious diseases and fevers, especially when the temperature ranges the highest.

5. This continued, elevated and gradually declining temperature fills the space which makes it possible for the bovine bacillus to become acclimated to human soil.

How often have we heard the story, "Doctor, I had typhoid fever and tuberculosis set in; or, I had la grippe, or pneumonia, and my lungs did not clear up." We have all heard it many times, yet I doubt if most of us have given a possible thought that the food might be the possible reason that the case didn't clear up. Suppose a case of typhoid fever, milk used as a food, the third week, ulcerated Peyer's patches, the digestive functions not properly performed. Now the milk containing tubercle bacilli comes in contact with abrasions in the mucous membrane, is absorbed and carried through the lymphatics and thoracic duct and empties into left subclavian vein. It then goes to the right heart and thence to the lungs where it meets with the first set of capillaries. It is common in typhoid fever to have the capillaries engorged with blood, or plugged with clotted blood. Some of the infectious material is thus carried into what might be termed a dead end, with no immediate way of getting out. Phagocytes, ever active to remove foreign material, pounce upon it, and by virtue of the ameboid movement take it in. The poison of the bacilli kills the leucocyte and the bacilli are thus practically encapsulated and free from invasion of other leucocytes. The proper conditions for their acclimation are present, such as a temperature around 102° F., proper culture media, etc. In the course of a few days they begin to multiply and thus we have a deposit in the lung. The temperature now falls gradually, completing the conditions for the acclimation.

Bacteriologists will tell you that human and bovine bacilli are not the same, their cultural peculiarities are different, etc., but ask any of them from a pathological standpoint if there are any differences between a tubercular lesion in the human, bovine or any other animal tissues. They cannot answer in any other way but in the negative, for under the microscope a section of tubercular tissue has the same characteristics no matter what animal it is taken from.

I do not wish to be understood as claiming that no case of tuberculosis is due to respiratory infection by germ-laden dust, for a small percentage of cases are contracted in this manner, but I do believe that sufficient data can be obtained to warrant the assertion that the vast majority of cases are caused from the use of food products from tubercular cattle. Already the movement against the use of cow's milk is gaining ground in the United States. Large herds of goats are being imported into California, Arizona, New Mexico and Texas. The Department of Agriculture has taken it up, and when the movement is started, backed by facts and a horrible fear of a dreadful disease, it is reasonable to predict that in the near future cow's milk will be shunned as a filthy food, and replaced by the milk of the most misunderstood, abused, cleanest and healthiest of animals, and the only natural foster mother of the human race.

BY RIGHT OF AUTHORITY.

JOHN URI LLOYD, PH.D., CINCINNATI.

In a recent editorial we called attention to the fact that scientific authority too often labors under difficulties that are unreachable from the stand of the party making the investigation, regardless of his talents in other directions. This fact, for it is a fact, explains why the marked advances in that which concerns life and civilization, are instituted largely from sources outside precise professional science. Take medicines for example. In America alone, over one hundred thousand physicians who make no pretense to other than that of a practicing professional life, are concerned in observing the action of medicines in disease expression.

These men are often likely to meet conditions that the scientific experimenter in his laboratory, or the too busy internes in the hospital who follow their leader, are but seldom called upon to observingly combat. Then, too, such men have illimitable opportunities of acquiring knowledge concerning unknown materials, used by empiricists in disease expressions, and of observing what comes to them from empirical sources about them. This gives to these men an opportunity both of observingly balancing the actions of old remedies in disease, and of studying the possibilities of unknown substances, by which term, "unknown substances," is meant materials that mere chance alone, and very scant chance at that, would ever bring before the wall-encased scientist in his laboratory, wheresoever that laboratory might be.

Hence it is that if no one will take the established vegetable remedies, it will be found that they are to be first credited to persons engaged in outside affairs, to be next utilized by the profession at large, and, after being thus established, at last, to drift into the hands of the men involved in pure science, who experiment thereon, and record what comes to them in their restricted directions. In this manner, such drugs as jalap and ipecac and belladonna and ergot and cascara and lobelia and opium, and nearly every other item that could be mentioned in the direction of the invaluable and established vegetable remedies, have become known. And on such empirical authority as this (not on the researches of the professional scientist) were they established.

Nor are these substances accepted, in some directions, without the most violent opposition from the men most needing their services. As a rule, they travel the same road, first into empirical home use as household remedies, then into the practice of local physicians, then into a brief mention in some book on medicine or pharmacy, or a contribution to some medical journal, blossoming at last into conspicuity as established therapeutical agents. Too often, in the end, they meet with a hostile reception by the man of pure science in his laboratory experimentation, who from his observed results decides that the opinions of the thousands of practicing physicians are illusions.

Even such a world-renowned remedy as cinchona ran the gauntlet of all the opposition that "authority" could give to its employment, for that despised "Jesuit's bark" was reviled and abused most inhumanly, and berated viciously by the very men who most needed its help. Books appeared from professional authorities calling it a quack remedy, and telling of the terrible effects of cinchona. Thus good men (much prejudiced) attempted to beat the life out of "Jesuit's bark," the greatest remedy ever discovered.

The record of most of our American drugs is largely a repetition of that of cinchona. Seldom did they get a cordial reception from so-called "authority." Even after they have been established in the practice of thousands of physicians, are they too often slurred by inexperienced persons occupying authoritative scientific positions. Very ignorant, too, these talented men may be of the substances which their positions give them authority to berate. Gelsemium, an exceptionally useful drug, met with an indifferent reception in "professionally regular" America until Dr. Richardson, of England, became enthusiastic over its merits as voiced by him in the London *Lancet*.

Such also is the record of other drugs that might be mentioned. America has too often awaited the opinion of Europe concerning what belonged to America by right and by priority.

A side thought in this connection is illustrated in the fact that qualified authority (men who speak by the right of experience) is often resisted by inexperienced men, who apprehend that they themselves, being authorities sufficient unto themselves, must be considered so by others. For example:

About forty-five years ago, Pond's distilled hamamelis was quietly introduced into the Homeopathic school of medicine. With almost irresistible force it came gradually into the practice of Eclectic physicians, creeping then into that of the Allopathic physician. The chemist found little in that distillate other than traces of essential oil. He united with the laboratory scientist in assering that the value of distilled hamamelis must, therefore, depend on the water and the alcohol it contained. But thousands of practitioners of medicine thought otherwise, and acted for themselves.

Distilled hamamelis became an important article of commerce, being finally employed in immense amounts by the profession of medicine. It next crept into home use, the laity becoming acquainted with its name and its asserted qualities. To-day, after practically four decades have passed, distilled hamamelis stands firmly intrenched as one of the most largely used remedies in America, and that, too, in the face of such authority as Drs. John Marshall and H. C. Wood, of Philadelphia, who, in 1886, gave hamamelis a strenuous scientific *laboratory* investigation, and decided that there was nothing in the distillate, ending their article as follows:

"The much used and still more lauded witch-hazel, or the so-called distillates of witch-hazel, must depend for their virtues upon the alcohol which they contain and the faith which they inspire."

But for fear that some who do not know better may infer that we are opposed to legitimate scientific investigation, let us assert that we are opposed only to so-called scientific attempts to accomplish what is outside the legitimate field the scientist irrationally invades. In his proper sphere the scientist deserves, and receives, our highest encomiums, and in medicine he is accomplishing much that lies within the true domain of science.

For example: In that same year, 1886, a substance was introduced in England, and had a start as a remedy under the name "Hopeine." It was asserted to be an alkaloidal substance obtained from the "wild hops of America." The botanist knew of no alkaloidal hop vine, and the chemist took hold of this so-called "hopeine." He assayed it, and determined it was a fraudulent mixture, principally of morphine and cocaine, with some atropine. The result of this scientific investigation was published, and in a short time the office of the great "Hopeine Company," in London, was closed.

A similar record is that of "Husa," the wonderful "Everglade

Remedy" for the opium habit, which in our laboratory was on scientific assay shown to be composed of morphine only.

Give to the scientist the credit due to legitimate science, but do not discredit over a hundred thousand physicians and sixty thousand pharmacists of America who intelligently comprehend what lies within their own sphere.

OBSTETRICS FROM A PRACTICAL STANDPOINT.

A. J. KEMPER, M.D., WEST MILFORD, W. VA.

It is not our intention or expectation to produce anything new from a scientific standpoint, but to sum up in a short article the various facts and factors of a successful obstetrician.

When the student of medicine receives his diploma he has had a thorough course in all the technicalities of this line of work, and he imagines that no case can present itself that can exhaust his skill. But when he comes face to face with a variety of cases, as well as a variety of dispositions, he frequently concludes that theory is one thing and practice is another. This paper is directed more especially to the young practician than to those who from years of experience have learned the needs and peculiarities of mankind.

I once heard of a physician whose first obstetrical work ran like this: Upon his return from a case of labor he was asked "how he got along." His answer was: "Very well; I lost the mother and the child, but I saved the old man all right."

I've never yet met with just the same experience as the above case, but have seen the time when I had more trouble with the husband than the wife. And so it runs—sometimes it is the wife, sometimes a midwife, or some woman who has given birth to six or eight children and imagines she knows more than the most skillful physician; and sometimes a big two-fisted husband who imagines the doctor can so aid the woman as to bring about childbirth at his pleasure, and if you don't some very unkind words are spoken, as well as severe threats.

Under these circumstances the physician must be self-possessed and not listen to the discouraging expressions of the patient, nor the ignorant and old-time suggestions of a midwife, nor the threats of a man. We should, of course, deal kindly and respect any kind suggestions of a bystander, but in an uninsulting way convince them that you are master of the occasion. Yet if the case should be of such a nature as to necessitate the assistance of another physician, don't hesitate to say so.

It sometimes occurs that we are inclined to see clouds through the brightest sunshine, and, again, we fail to recognize a cloud when it presents itself. Which is the more detrimental, to be an optimist or a pessimist? We are inclined to think the former to be the more acceptable to the laity. Yet if proper judgment is used, it sometimes pays to be pessimistic, but would not recommend it in every-day life.

No one is thrown on his own responsibility more than the country obstetrician. I have seen the time when the presence of a second doctor would have brought sensations of joy to a troubled mind, beyond the description of man. But the condition of the patient and the vast distance between another physician and me compelled me to rally all my energy to do such things as version and high forceps delivery. Too often we go to a case unequipped to do whatever might present itself. This, to my mind, is a sad mistake. Go prepared as if you knew you were to encounter the most grave condition that can befall the lying-in woman (except it be a craniotomy or Cæsarean section), for many times a short delay or unclean methods means death to the mother, child or both, as well as an injury to your reputation.

Then the question naturally arises, what should our obstetric bag contain? To some extent this is a matter of individual choice. But there are certain things that should be in every obstetrical bag. I will give what seems to me to be the practical, common-sense contents of a ready-packed grip. Among the therapeutic agents are:

Lloyd's tincture, ergot, tincture macrotys, tincture veratrum, Dover's powder and quinine.

As antiseptics: Bichloride tablets, green soap or ethereal antiseptic soap.

Instruments: Placental forceps, obstetric forceps, curette, volsellum, hemostats, needles, needle-holder and uterine douche.

Among other things that cannot be classed under any special head are: Scrub brush, aseptic umbilical ligatures, aseptic perineal pads, sterile plain gauze, baby scales, bottle white vaseline, tube of sterile vaseline, rubber catheter, fountain syringe, Kelley pad, and a tube of No. 2 or 3 catgut.

Some object to the use of chloroform except where profound anesthesia is needed. I do not use it in every case, but don't hesitate to use it in *any* case where the woman is nervous and easily discouraged, labor tedious and parts rigid. Some explanation of its use and effects should be made to the patient and bystanders so as to establish confidence in its value. I've had some object to its use until they had once used it, but have never had a woman to say she would never use it again. But it should not be used till the second stage of labor is well advanced.

If an oxytocic is necessary, I depend on specific tincture macrotys in fifteen-drop doses every twenty or thirty minutes till a drachm has been given. Sometimes quinine sulphate in four-grain doses every twenty or thirty minutes till three or four doses have been given has a better effect.

Aseptic precautions are many times dealt with .too carelessly. The hands of a physician should be thoroughly asepticized before making an examination per .vag;nam. Not by carelessly washing them with unsterile water and soap and drying them on an unsterile towel, as you will in most cases be asked to do, but by a thorough scrubbing in sterile water with green soap or ethereal antiseptic soap and followed with a bichloride solution. And not only is it necessary to be sterile for the first examination, but for all examinations, for the further labor advances the more likelihood there is of infection. A bowl of bichloride solution should, therefore, be kept by the bedside for this purpose.

Too frequent examinations should not be' made; it is not only a vexation to the woman, but increases the chances of infection. In brief, we say, whatever you do, do it *clean*.

A Kelley pad is not generally used in this section, but in our estimation it is doubly worth the trouble you are to in carrying it. It is not only a benefit to the doctor, but is highly appreciated by the patient and all bystanders.

We so frequently hear physicians speak of having so many cases of retained placenta. I do not say there is no such thing as an adhered placenta, but I do say that many of the so-called cases are imaginary. My routine procedure for the last three years has been as follows, and I have not had any trouble of any note since adopting the method:

As soon as the child is born I seize the uterus with both hands and grasp firmly for five or ten minutes; then tie and sever the cord, hand child to nurse and order it to be washed. While the little fellow is being washed I again resume my grip on the uterus and hold till the child is washed and cord ready to dress. After dressing the cord I again return to the bed and usually find her complaining of uterine contractions; then by slight traction on the cord with my right hand and firm pressure of uterus with left hand, the placenta is readily expelled.

Great care should be taken in washing the patient and dressing her and her bed. Never leave a woman in her soiled condition nor the bed undressed unless her condition demands it. It shows untidyness and a lack of interest. Look after laceration of perineum and repair it at once if there is such a condition. If it has been a tedious case of labor and some distance from your office, it is advisable to catheterize before leaving. It many times saves considerable worry and a subsequent visit. I frequently leave four or five five-grain doses of Dover's powder, with directions to take one every four or five hours if after-pains are severe, but not to take them if she can rest without them. If everything is looked after carefully, a subsequent visit will not be needed in one case out of ten.

Post-partum douches as a routine is, in the writer's opinion, more of danger than a benefit. The natural inclination of drainage is downward, and by the force from a fountain syringe septic material may be driven upward into the uterine cavity and there taken up by the open-mouthed vessels. In some cases the douche may prove beneficial, but only under the most strict aseptic procedure by the physician or a competent nurse, and never as a routine treatment administered by Tom, Dick and Harry.

The day was when the laity looked for the doctor who would attend a case of confinement for the least money, regardless of how it was done. But not so to-day. The people have learned to appreciate the advances in the medical.profession, and are hunting for the physician who does his work in accordance with modern methods and does it well.

APHASIA AND SOME IMPEDIMENTS OF SPEECH.

THEODORE DAVIS ADLERMAN, M.D., BROOKLYN, N. Y.

The question of the pathology of aphasia, as well as the general subject of aphasia, is one of more than ordinary interest, and the declaration of some authors that there is no evidence that there is such a thing as sensory and motor aphasia, that aphasia is a unit, and is merely a variety of intellectual deficit deserves careful consideration and study.

Aphasia, as we are used to understand it now, is a condition in which the function of expressing ideas by articulate sounds is perverted or destroyed, and for the general subject we can divide aphasia in two great varieties: (1) one in which the memory of words is lost; and (2) the other in which the function of articulation is lost or destroyed.

The general problems concerning speech defects are especially complicated because of the existence of four different kinds of word memory, each having its seat of registration in a definite part of the cerebral cortex. In cases where the memory of words is lost, or destroyed, when you contrast the utterance of your patient with that of a normal person, the great departure from normal articulation is prominently apparent, and the earliest indications will consist in a loss of substantives and names, other parts of speech being properly applied. Sometimes a loss of a language, with which the patient had been thoroughly conversant, may take place; terms are persistently misapplied, and a general periphrasis employed, and here we must also mention a peculiarity of this particular variety: you will notice a peculiar weakness of the right angle of the mouth and a deviation of the tongue to the right.

In the second variety the function of articulation is completely lost, the patient is only able to indicate by signs that he is conscious of the idea conveyable by the term; in some cases only a very slight memory seems to exist about different words—thus "do" will stand for dollar, "wa" for watch, and so on. In these cases the intellectual deficit is very prominent; some even are unable to comprehend a single word.

In establishing a diagnosis we first determine whether a defect of language, function or aphasia is present. We must exclude simulation, hysteria, mental disease and defect of the organs of speech.

The tests necessary here are voluntary speech, repeating lines, repeating spoken words, indicating the number of syllables in a word to show that the patient knows that it is a word, humming tunes, naming things seen, smelled, tasted, or touched; gesturing, reading letters and numerals, general intelligence, naming abstract things and qualities. In going over all these tests we get the various special symptoms by which to qualify aphasia. The principal symptoms, therefore, are: (1) Aphonia, or inability to speak; (2) agraphia, or inability to write; (3) amusia, or inability to sing; (4) anomia, or inability to name objects; (5) word deafness, or inability to understand words or sentences; (6) alexia, or inability to read words; (7) mind blindness or inability to recognize things seen, and the general difficulties in repeating and understanding gestures.

I do not think it is necessary here to dwell much on the prognosis and treatment; it can be summarized in a few words. Find the cause, if possible, and train your patient in the use of words until the lost power of expression is gradually acquired. Much more difficult and tiresome is the treatment of stuttering, which can be regarded as a functional nervous disorder without any structural changes, leading to erroneous action of the muscles concerned in speech. There seems to be an intermittent inability to omit certain sounds, and the very peculiar thing here is that the disability in a great many cases is noticed only when the patient speaks in a conversational voice, and this disability seems to be very rarely present when he sings or hums. You will also find that the stuttering is very much worse when the patient is nervous or excited and when he is in bad health.

The prognosis in most of the cases can be said to be good, as there seems to be a tendency to a cure. As I said before, the treatment is very tiresome, and each individual case has to be studied carefully and distinctly, and the common feature of all is steady, regular and long-continued practice. The patient must be instructed to speak slowly with a full resonant voice, and when he comes to a word on which he stutters he must be made to direct his energies not to articulation, but to vocalization. Singing exercises are very useful; the progress made by the patients is very slow the first few months, and the supervising medical attendant must encourage the patient and persist on further exercises.

Another interesting impediment of speech is lisping, which is often asquired by affected adults, and sometimes taken up by youths as a fad. As a purely normal condition lisping is seen in children and in infants who are learning to speak, and in these cases the difficulty is soon overcome; in others, while it may take a little longer, the ultimate results are very satisfactory.

SCUTELLARIA IN HYDROPHOBIA.

Thos. F. Collins, M.D., New Castle, Pa.

During the past summer, I received Lloyd's Drug Treatise on Scutellaria advocating the use of that remedy for the preventive treatment of hydrophobia. Almost simultaneously Dr. I. A. Thayer, Health Officer of this city, an ardent Eclectic but now retired from active practice, directed to me two cases for treatment as outlined in the above-named treatise.

Case I.—E. T., aged fourteen years. On July 5, while passing along the street was attacked and bitten on the right knee by a supposedly rabid dog. The dog was killed, no pathological examination being made. Began treatment July 11 and continued four weeks. Sp. med. scutellaria was given on alternate days every two hours. A mild, non-stimulating, easily digestible diet was prescribed, active exercise was forbidden, as well as exposure to the extremely hot weather and to exciting scenes and circumstances. No symptoms of clinical importance appeared except the pulse-rate, which ranged around 100 to 120 per minute during the last three weeks of treatment. This was probably due to the alcohol in the scutellaria, or was it a reaction to the hydrophobic virus?

Case II.—W. McC., aged eleven years. Bitten on the forearm July 17. Pathological examination made in the laboratories of the University of Pennsylvania revealed the fact that the dog had rabies. The wound was not cauterized. Began treatment July 21, continued five weeks, same treatment as in previous case. Rapid pulse was the only symptom manifested, though at one time the temperature was 101°, which I attributed to a trip to the office in the excessive heat then prevailing.

At the present time both patients are enjoying their usual health.

My chief object in reporting the cases is to encourage the more extended trial of this treatment in remote sections where a Pasteur institute cannot be reached on account of distance, and more often on account of an anemic condition of the purse.

In this city there are sixty physicians; more than fifty are of Regular persuasion. Naturally, they were up in arms as soon as they learned the city had employed me to treat these cases. Their county society began a vigorous fight on me, through the papers and otherwise. One article I herewith quote to show their attitude:

"WHEN DOCTORS DISAGREE ON VITAL QUESTIONS.

"It is no credit to the city to use other than the Pasteur treatment in the care of those unforunates who have been bitten by dogs suffering from hydrophobia; furthermore, it is subjecting those treated to the dangers of death in a terrible form to offer them to a treatment not generally recognized by the medical profession as being an efficient one.

"These were the sentiments voiced by the Lawrence County Medical Association before council last night, when several members addressed those bodies in the interests of the citizens and children who had been bitten recently by mad dogs. It is stated this morning by those who do not agree entirely with the views of the Lawrence County Medical Association members that an incentive to the interest of the doctors is that Dr. Collins, who holds the health committee's contract for the care of patients who have suffered dog bites, is not a member of the school of medicine recognized by the association members. The matter will be taken up at a meeting of the health committee that meets this evening."

The law of Pennsylvania provides that the Department of Charities shall furnish proper treatment to all persons applying for aid who have been bitten by rabid animals, which treatment may include that known as the Pasteur method. As it is a serum treatment, the Allopathic crowd had to stand up and defend their honor against this, to them unheard of treatment not born in Germany, the kindergarten of most of their beloved fads. However, these cases are now on record for their sober contemplation, and subject to their closest scrutiny.

Many physicians are so located that they can test this method thoroughly without arousing this rabid antagonism, and it is for such that this article is written.

In a letter from Prof. J. U. Lloyd, he instructs that the remedies be used as follows: "Four ounces sp. med. scutellaria should be mixed with a quart of water and boiled until the alcohol has disappeared, this reducing the volume to about one and one-half pints. Of this one-half glass should be administered six times a day every other day, and on the omitted days a teaspoonful of flowers of sulphur in molasses should be given in the morning, fasting; at bedtime the same amount in a little new milk. I should also apply a compress to the bite, keeping it saturated with a mixture of sp. med. scutellaria one part and water three parts."

This is about the treatment of Thatcher, and can be applied at any season of the year, as well as when the scutellaria is in blossom. The treatment, according to Thatcher, should be continued three weeks. For cattle or horses four times the amount should be given. The object of the treatment is the thorough saturation of the patient with the remedies' before the virus can exert an influence, on the same principle that echinacea is antagonistic to rattlesnake virus, or typhoid toxins in the systems, as has been demonstrated hundreds of times.

Physicians should write and get the treatise on scutellaria, and those trying the method should always take pains to determine definitely whether the animal had rabies, either by confining the animal a sufficient length of time or killing it and submitting the brain to a disinterested pathologist for examination and proof. Then let us have some definite and accurate reports as to results obtained. In this way a year will definitely establish or disprove the efficacy of the treatment.

In closing, I will state that in any case any specific indications of prominence should be met by the indicated remedies in addition to the above treatment, and here, doubtless, is where our Regular brother will stumble when he tries this method.

CONVALLAMARIN.

W. C. Abbott, M.D., Chicago, Ill.

Convallaria, the lily-of-the-valley, has won considerable repute as a very useful and important cardiac medicament, and many physicians who know digitalis only through the galenic forms, prefer convallaria. The plant contains two active principles—convallamarin, a cardiant glucoside, and convallarin, which Marme pronounced a purgative. The former has the power of increasing cardiac energy, correcting arhythmia, moderating excess of the heart's pulsations, augmenting arterial pressure and promoting diuresis.

The therapeutic applications of convallamarin are those of digitalis. It may be preferred to the latter when through idiosyncrasy it is not well borne, or when the menace of collapse defies digitalis. Here strychnine, caffeine and even atropine in small doses have an urgent and legitimate indication. Digitalis and its official preparations should then be prescribed, or employed only with the greatest prudence and incessant vigilance, since they may produce, besides gastric and cerebral troubles, collapse and even an arrest of the heart, prolonged and perilous.

Convallamarin is indicated in organic cardiopathies with arhythmia and failing compensation, especially in lesions of the orifices and the valvules. It is especially indicated in regurgitation of the tricuspid and insufficiency of the mitral. By rectifying the heart action and consequently the flow of blood in the greater and the lesser circulation, it ameliorates with rapidity the respiratory, cerebral and renal functions. In general this remedy may be described as a succedaneum of digitalin, in some cases usefully replacing it. That is all that Laura will say to its credit; but the Italians as well as the French have for many years adhered to their digitalin as the one perfect representative of digitalis, and feel that they have no occasion to look further.

The dose of convallamarin, according to Laura, is for an adult one-twelfth to one-sixth grain, rarely more, large doses causing toxic phenomena. Convallamarin itself does not act on the bowels, but convallaria does; this advantage, however, if it be one, is overbalanced by the exceeding variability in strength of the extracts found in the market. Moreover, as this drug is costly and rarely employed, the chance of obtaining a fresh extract that has not decomposed is very small. If one desires to employ this agent, the granules made with milk sugar as the excipient preserve the contained glucoside without change for many years. The writer has in his cabinet granules of convallamarin made by a pharmacal company that ceased active work fifteen years ago, and these granules recently displayed full and unimpaired activity.

Bound Journals.

This issue of THE JOURNAL completes the sixty-eighth year. Many of our subscribers bind their journal—seventy-five cents each for half sheep style; sixty cents for plain green cloth, plus carriage each way.

To *new* subscribers we can furnish 1906-1907 or 1908 in green cloth at two dollars each.

Ohio State Eclectic Medical Association.

Proceedings of the Forty-fourth Annual Session.

W. N. MUNDY, M.D., EDITOR.

SECTION V.

SURGERY.

J. F. WUIST, M.D., Chairman..................................Dayton.
J. D. SOUTHWARD, M.D., Vice-Chairman......................Carey.
B. K. JONES, M.D., Secretary...............................Kenton.

CONCERNING ABDOMINAL ADHESIONS.

A. RHU, M.D., MARION.

In the year Anno Domini 1886, also the year after my graduation in medicine and surgery, by courtesy of my preceptor, the late Dr. R. L. Sweney, I was present to see the operative work of Ohio's greatest abdominal surgeon, as he was then known and pronounced to be by the profession, Dr. Dunlap, of Springfield, O. The operation was for the removal of an ovarian cystoma, at the home of the patient.

It is well to remember that this was before the day of careful preparatory treatment for such cases, hence the doctor ordered a dose of castor oil the evening before the operative work, had the housekeeper boil a few tubs of water, strain through cloths and put into some large crocks for use.

In the early morning we proceeded to the home of the patient, a lady of some fifty-seven years of age, the abdomen was carefully scrubbed and washed with ordinary soap and water, and a long median incision was made. The doctor found a few bread and butter adhesions along the anterior abdominal wall, which he dexterously separated, brought the tumor into view, tapped the same, and then began the work of ligation which caused him no little trouble. The doctor was somewhat nervous and possessed with a mercurial temperament and an abundance of ego; nevertheless, he perspired enough to permit numbers of droplets to be uncomplainingly received into the peritoneal cavity. This wonderful surgeon completed the work in an hour, made a fairly good toilet of the abdomen, left the patient in his son's care for a few days, and departed happily on his way rejoicing, with a $300 fee and expenses. On the second day the junior doctor left also for home.

On the morning of the third day we were hastily called and informed that the patient had vomited incessantly, which would not yield to hypodermatic medication of morphia. The dressing was moist and ill smelling, hence it was deemed best to inspect the same before the doctor arrived, who had been telegraphed for during the night, and found that the entire wound had burst asunder, spread wide open, the omentum curled up above, the coils of the intestine covered with a plastic, septic, exudative inflammatory mass of adhesions. Enormously distended abdomen; anxious facies; pulse 160, temperature 105°; respiration 30. of costal variety. Surely you will agree this was worse than the tragic stage. In a few hours the scene was shifted by sleep that knoweth no awakening. Am also sure the everlasting impression is indelibly engraven on the tablets of my memory; the post-mortem examination showed adhesions too numerous ever to be effaced from my mind during my life.

In a general way, much is known about abdominal adhesions and the frequency of their occurrence by surgeons who have a working experience in abdominal work. So much has been written concerning the pelvic inflammatory diseases that we seem to fully understand and comprehend much concerning the causes producing them. The knowledge came to us through the pelvic surgeon who finally evolved the splendid record of American achievement in this interesting department, and made it possible to enter the abdominal zone above the pelvis, and for all time settle the question of gastric, pancreatic, splenic and hepatic surgery, with its numerous complications. For be it remembered all pelvic, as well as those of the upper zone, inflammatory adhesions, are caused by trauma of some sort or other. Localized pain is the constant expression of injury within the abdominal cavity where inflammatory adhesions are likely to happen; hence, any localized pain either in the pelvic or abdominal zone or perchance in the subphrenic region, are the truest clinical evidence of beginning adhesive formation.

The inflammation occurring in the pelvic zone, according to Joseph Price, who, by the way, is one of America's greatest pelvic surgeons, whose common-sense ideas have helped to place American surgery on the highest plane in scientific circles the world over, and whose surgical teaching has never been equaled in our country although he holds no professorship in a medical college, yet he. with the great John B. Deaver, made it possible for Philadelphia to be known again as a medical center, for since the days of the elder Gross surgery was at a low ebb. To go to Philadelphia and not visit the clinics of Price and Deaver would in the coming years fill any heart with regret, provided you have the true medical and surgical instinct within yourself. And, if endowed with an artistic feeling in your heart for "Ars Medica," you will make the effort of your life to listen to these past masters in surgery. Go where you will in the old country and you will not likely find God has made many such.

Pardon for this digression, for I was just about to call your attention to the fact that the pelvic inflammation and its adhesions are by all odds the most dangerous ones to life. On the right side of the abdomen, however, the appendix vermiformis lies adjacent to the pelvic organs; hence, a large number of cases are directly affected from the appendix; or, in the female, also from the ovarian and tubal ends. Adhesions are usually firmly attached to the inflammatory masses by its extremities or its lateral walls; by adhesive inflammation due no doubt to infection. In a majority of cases the etiologic factor is a Neisser complication; hence, the consensus of opinion among abdominal surgeons is to remove infected tubes and involved appendices as a rule. It is my experience in all secondary abdominal work to find adhesions as the result of imperfect surgical technique. Those commonly met with are the adhesions to the pelvic walls, pelvic floor, the omentum, appendicial regions, liver, bladder, stomach, pancreas, etc., varying in character from the very brittle bread and butter adhesions to the very dense and unyielding ones. Uterine adhesions are found in most pelvic cases, involving all pelvic and adjacent tissues, bowels, etc.

. A few weeks ago I operated on a strangulated inguinal hernia for Dr. J. E. Baker, of Caledonia, O., in a child seven years of age. Found a mass of half necrotic tissues, omental and intestinal, with an ulcerated caput coli; appendix tied off by adhesive inflammatory action; end of bowel ulcerated, with a perforation large enough to admit my thumb. The appendicular artery was beautifully tied off by omental adhesions; an enterolith was also found. All this in the hernial sac, yet this patient's life was saved and convalescence established with no event of note. Besides the recovery, a complete cure was effected so far as the hernia was concerned. Gentlemen, the surgeon's knife in obscure cases is a safer procedure than to temporize with therapy. No harm can come to any case by a mere exploratory incision. It is imperative at times to do so in order to save life.

One of the functions of the omentum is to remove foreign materials from the abdominal cavity, or to encapsulate them. If the mass is small it may envelope it completely. Where the whole pelvis is choked, it often walls off the inflammatory area and acts as a secondary diaphragm to separate the abdominal cavity by forming adhesions to the brim, or to the uterus and bladder. As a rule, all pelvic inflammations are directly followed by adhesion formation in at least 50 per cent. of all cases.

Adhesions may be light velamentous or dense indurated; some covering and encapsulating areas of purulent exudates, etc. Abdominal wall adhesions are the rule after pelvic and other abdominal opera-' tions.

Now a word concerning sigmoid and rectal adhesions, which are, the most troublesome because they are situated deep down in the pelvis, and because the bowel is more rigidly fixed, and, as a rule, the adhesions are more dense, with frequent and very strong bands of diverticulate formation in the sigmoid region, needing a wide surgical contact experience in order to deal with such wisely, and which are the ones overlooked most frequently.

Intestinal adhesions are usually of a mild velamentous variety. They are readily stripped off without injury to the bowel.

Intestinal adhesions are of a low organization and poor vascularization; hence, if handled in good surgical form are easily dealt with. Not so, however, the dense, e.g., flat Meckel's diverticulæ, etc. The variety where the plastic lymph has undergone organization and the peritoneal surfaces are bound intimately together by newly formed connective tissue richly supplied by blood vessels, are handled with great difficulty. This class of adhesions are mostly found with pelvic abscesses, and, as said before, all pelvic inflammations are dangerous, more than the zone above.

Adhesions to benign tumors and cysts are dealt with in a more facile manner than any others.

Quite a large number of pelvic inflammatory diseases and tumors of this region are found with adhesions to the appendix vermiformis, usually firmly attached to the mass by its extremity or its lateral wall. An inflamed right tube and ovary is frequently involved by adhesive inflammation due to infection, either originating from the appendix or from a tubal inflammation as ordinarily found in Neisser infections. Such tubo-appendix involvement with firm adhesions are best removed.

Sigmoid adhesions are found to occur in the shape of diverticulæ in any part of its course, a few of which might be regarded as congenital. Most of them, however, are acquired by trauma and their resultant adhesive inflammatory action. Meckel's diverticulæ are the probably congenital variety, and are more frequently found in the lower part of the descending colon and the sigmoid flexure. There we also find them usually multiple, of fairly constant anatomical features, and prone to undergo secondary pathologic changes; with a symptomatology of its own, producing a train of clinical phenomena chiefly by localized obscure pain in the sigmoid region, no pathologic evidence recognizable with the proctoscope. In the sigmoid flexure these adhesive bands are usually found multiple, closing over the gut close to the mesenteric attachment. These adhesions are rarely found in the young, and occur with some frequency in the middle aged and advancing old age, chiefly in persons complaining with a history of persistent constipation.

The secondary process to which sigmoid diverticulæ are liable are summed up as follows by Telling (London, *Lancet*, March, 1908):

1. Infection of general peritoneal cavity from thinning of sac walls without perforation.

2. Acute or gangrenous inflammation—diverticulitis.

3. Chronic proliferative inflammation, with thickening of the gut wall and stenosis of the bowel.

4. The formation of adhesions, especially adhesions to the small intestine and to the bladder.

5. Perforation of the diverticulæ, giving rise to general peritonitis, general abscesses, submucous fistulæ of the gut wall, and fistulous communication with the viscera, especially the bladder.

6. The lodgment of foreign bodies.

7. Chronic mesenteritis of the sigmoid loop.

8. Local chronic peritonitis.

9. Metastatic suppuration.

10. The development of carcinoma.

11. Perforation into the hernial sac, etc.

Now a few words concerning adhesions occurring in the upper abdominal zone. The pathologist has not shown us much help until modern surgery revealed to us living pathology, studied in situ. The past decade has revolutionized the trend of medical thought, and we have acquired valuable knowledge. Chronic dyspepsias, gastralgia, etc., we now know are but the clinical syndromes presented by numerous diverse lesions. As a result of the surgeon's observations we now are enabled to make correct diagnoses founded upon exact chemical and pathological basis. I shall refrain, however, to engage in the discussion of diagnoses, between gastric, duodenal and intestinal ulcers from the ordinary gastric diseases and even malignancy.

However, it is probably true beyond the venture of a doubt that all pathological processes with probable adhesive tendencies are clinically manifested first by pain and abdominal distress and nausea.

The consensus of opinion in surgery is that 50 per cent. of such cases result in adhesions in this zone, principally to the pancreas, liver, and stomach. These adhesive formations cause constant and periodic pain and distress. Pain, in fact, assumes and is the clinical picture of importance; nausea is also a clinical phenomena, depending upon obstruction and stenosis. Ordinarily one must not forget the likelihood, when associated with pain, to take into consideration abdominal adhesions. In the diagnosis of probable intra-abdominal pathology, a correct interpretation of these symptoms, *i.e.*, pain, distress and nausea, will lead us directly to a rational diagnosis, and bring to our realization the fact how frequently we overlook adhesive formation within the peritoneal cavity; how we should be on our guard and study the constant and never to be downed pain and distress so persistently found in such cases.

Much of value could be presented concerning duodenal ulcers, the pain of acute cholelithiasis, the pain and plastic adhesive formation in ectopic pregnancy, etc., for which we have not time this day, and reserve the privilege for a further communication. This subject goes to confirm the present trend that we, as internists and surgeons, must draw nigh unto each other more than ever, co-operate and study anew how best to treat and relieve a suffering humanity.

DISCUSSION.

CHAIRMAN: The discussion will be opened by Dr. B. K. Jones.

DR. B. K. JONES: I believe I am assigned the privilege of opening the discussion, which is now open. Dr. Huntley will please speak.

DR. J. H. HUNTLEY: I expected to hear something from Dr. Jones as he was to open the discussion of this paper, but I feel that the paper is too important a one not to have a discussion, not to do something to bring out its merits, because I fail to see any demerits in it. There is one thing that speaks well for the man who wrote this paper, and that is this, that literature, surgical literature, tells very little on the subject he is trying to handle, and surely gives him very little light by which to be guided and guarded; and the most of the knowledge that he has given in his paper I feel has been brought to him by work of his own. It is most valuable knowledge, and more so than if compiled from surgical literature, for we have very little on the subject. The pathology, the treatment, the etiology of adhesions following abdominal operations, pelvic inflammations, abdominal inflammations, is lightly treated.

The doctor's paper is not only well put and well worded, but it is surely very *apropos*. It is new material to the most of people who do surgery.

I believe the greatest cause of adhesions, either pelvic or abdominal, is infection. You may operate on a clean case, in which you are liable to have no infection, to operate on which you are very liable to have no adhesions follow.

The time was once when it was thought unwise to tap the abdomen in an ovarian cyst, if it was a case in which an operation was afterwards contemplated. That is not necessary to consider now, because I don't believe tapping makes your operation any more hazardous.

I once had a case of a large ovarian cyst, before I did any surgery, and Dr. Russell was doing my surgery. I couldn't get the consent of the lady to have an operation. In fact, there was a little division of opinion between myself and some other physicians as to it being a case for operation. In the meantime I had tapped the lady eleven times, drew off the water, and it was suggested then by some pretty good men that it would be a very difficult operation on account of the many adhesions. Finally we got the consent of the lady to have an operation. At the time she was about ready to pass to the glory land. The evening before the operation I was sent for. She was in a state of collapse, and I telegraphed Dr. Russell not to come. The patient died the next day. I got the privilege of a post-mortem. We made the post-mortem and found no adhesions at all, with pedicle as thick as your finger. And so, if an ovarian cyst in a patient without fever needs to be tapped, to give breathing space, do it; it doesn't hinder successful operation in the future. I have found that nearly all of our adhesions are in cases that have had high degrees of infection.

Where I operate on an abdominal or a pelvic case, and I feel that I have a clean one, in which I can close up the abdomen, a case in which I don't fear infection, I will have that patient to turn over, literally on one side and then on the other, then lie on the back, and turn every few hours, in order to avoid adhesions. But, if I have a case of infection, and I cannot do a thoroughly clean operation. I must put that patient to rest and take the chances of adhesions.

PATHOLOGY AND TREATMENT OF CHRONIC JOINT DISEASES.

J. H. HUNTLEY, M.D., LIMA.

In the endeavor to write a comprehensive paper on the above subject, I wish it fully understood in the outset that an exhaustive rehearsal on the subject would mean more time than is allowable in a medical meeting where many are to be heard from.

The day has arrived when there need not be a very great amount of speculation on local diseases of the joints.

Research work by orthopedic surgeons, the experience of doctors who constantly care for joint disturbances, pathologists whose conclusions have been and are based on microscopic findings, make the subject I am dealing with, a fixed factor when compared with what we knew of these ailments twenty-five years ago.

Many a limb was sacrificed in the far past in order to save a life that to-day can be handled with a degree of certainty, showing that facts are born of experience and investigation. I believe the surgeons of a half century ago were conscientious in their endeavors to save life and limb. Their shortcomings only foretold the age in which they lived. The doctor who in that day would absolutely immobilize a joint for six months was thought cruel and ignorant. The liniment, the poultice and the passive motion have long since died, and in its wake we have local germicides, immobilization and complete rest.

Classification, pathologically speaking, may be grouped under four distinct heads in their primary manifestations: (1) Those affecting the synovial membrane; (2) those affecting cartilages; (3) those affecting the ends of the bone; (4) those affecting primarily adjacent structures to the joint.

Usually one of the distinct classes mentioned is prominent in the primary onset of the disease, but soon becomes mingled with one or more of the other classes, making it a confirmed affection. The synovial membrane may become chronically affected by a continuation of an acute attack, or it may be primarily sub-acute.

After persisting for a time the synovial membrane becomes thickened, with increased secretion and a retrograde metamorphosis of connecting tissue. This retrograde condition may serve to set up unhealthy granulations and may attack the bone or cartilage in its germicidal travel; or as in rheumatic arthritis it may continue to confine itself to the synovial membrane. We have a serous synovitis that is chronic, as in hydrops articuli, non-purulent. A certain amount of fluid is always present, and some cases show no pathological change except this fluid. Such cases were at one time held to be non-inflammatory like hydrocele, but such views to-day are not well taken. The laboratory has shown that the fluid contains more mucus and albumin than the ordinary dropsical fluid.

The synovial dropsies are now taken as inflammatory processes of low order with slight tissue change. The simple dropsies of the joints should not mislead us, as frequently they go on to positive tissue change. We may have hypertrophy of the synovial fringe, and thickening of all the adjacent membranes. We also have gradual degeneration, which will often lead to purulence and destructive invasion. If effusion is extreme, we will have stretching of the posterior and lateral ligaments, with loose and lax joint conditions. Sometimes thickening of the cartilage will be found to such a degree that bony plates will be found in the joints. The synovial membrane will become thickened and encroach on the cartilage, the same as pannus does on the cornea. This is simply an extended condition of what we have described above. These conditions do not always become purulent, but sometimes do. The ending of such a case of synovitis may be by resolution, or, in an obstinate condition, of persistent disability with over amount of lateral motion. It is always possible that this condition is tubercular, but the condition described may and does more often exist; that is, non-tubercular. Where foreign and hard bodies are found in the pent-up fluid, such as rice or melon-seed bodies, this increases the liability of tuberculous suspicion. In these days of laboratory diagnosis, where the microscopic findings are accessible, with our clinical experience of to-day, much is expected of us. Conditions as above mentioned, coming on very slow, are often unexplainable in their causes.

Gonorrheal rheumatism should not be overlooked as a possible cause for these joint affections in the male. Gonococci are to be found in the effusion; and the history of gonorrhea may serve as a cause for microscopical examination. Chronic purulent synovitis is only a continuation of the serous form speaking of it as a primary disease. We can have chronic purulent synovitis as secondary to ostitis or traumatic infections.

DISEASE OF THE CARTILAGE.

Primary disease of the cartilage is rare and infrequent. Many causes are apparent for this, the most prominent of which is the anatomic or rather the histological make-up. Cartilage is a structure of low grade, non-impressible and non-vascular.

It is slow in its reaction, late to be impressed by inflammatory deposits, and slow to take on fatty degeneration.

As it is non-vascular, it is slow to take on secondary infections, and almost proof against primary invasions.

It is a bluish-white, opalescent structure, void of nerves and almost of blood supply. It is surrounded on one side by the synovial membrane of the joint, and on the other by bone. It receives all its nourishment from these two structures and will live sometimes after its source of supply is necrosed before it degenerates. Hypertrophy of cartilage is sometimes found, but is secondary to rheumatoid arthritis. Atrophy of the cartilage is sometimes found in old people as a primary condition. We may have primary degeneration, with fatty deposits of the cartilage in some forms of gout. We may have deposits of ivory-like bodies, which are almost identical with true cartilage, histologically speaking, which find their way to different parts of the joint and sometimes entirely spoil the easy motion, giving rise to great distress and disuse. Such bodies are known as floating cartilages, and may be present without any other diseased condition.

Primary inflammation of the cartilage is denied by some authors and conceded by others. The etiology of secondary inflammation is sought for by the primary disease which preceded it, and is often found in gouty troubles.

The interesting features found in this class of joint disease are the loose bodies found in the joints. These bodies are mostly fibrous and of the same structure as the cartilage but not always. They are sometimes lipomatous. These are of a softer nature, and while they encroach on the cartilage, they are not so apt to cripple its workings as the harder fibrous variety. Neither have they as much movable latitude.

CHRONIC JOINT DISEASES BEGINNING IN THE BONE.

This part of the classification I have used in describing joint diseases is of great importance. This might be divided into degenerative changes and formative obstructions. The latter can hardly be called a type of disease, and yet the exostoses which occur in joint vicinities must be looked upon as pathological, inasmuch as they hinder free joint movement and are surgical in their treatment.

I will not dwell on the formative obstructions of joint motion as they all come under the head of articular exostoses, but will dwell more on the degenerative changes.

We may have as a primary disease a true ostitis, or a periostitis, or an osteomyelitis. We may have a malignant disease of the shaft of the bone, near the joint, as an osteosarcoma. All these can become chronic before the patient is aware that his trouble is of a serious character. We first have a hyperemia of the bone circulation. We next have a fatty degeneration of bone cells. These in themselves form mechanical reasons for any amount of degenerative changes. This feature of disease forms itself near the spongy ends of the long bones, often at the junction of the epiphysis, sometimes under the periosteum near the joint. There are various names given to these many formations. However obscure may be the starting-point, it is necessary that we learn to differentiate malignant conditions from those of tubercular type. The microscope is the safe guide, and should be used in all suspected cases.

The first you will notice is a hyperemic condition on the shaft of the bone near the joint not involving the synovial sac. The surrounding tissue will look boggy, with no indication of pus in the soft parts.

The patient will sometimes complain of pain in the onset, but not unless the periosteum is involved.

Where we have very little pain we may presume we have a true ostitis or an osteomyelitis. Could the bone be seen at this time we would find a cheesy degeneration. Later we would find nodules filled with soft degenerated tissue in which would be found spiculæ of bone. Occasionally at this point where a patient has great resisting power, resolution will take place, reorganization will occur and a small abscess will burst through the soft parts and the disease stop without great destruction. This fortunate occurrence is so seldom, however, that dependence upon it is bad judgment. At other times the first diseased focus may be absorbed and a cure occur. More often, however, the invasion goes on, breaks through the epiphysis and invades the true joint.

Infection of the joint almost always takes place even though the focus of disease is sometimes quite distant. In non-strumous persons there is often a very great effort in nature to supply the degenerated bone tissue, and a new formation will start up and entirely surround the necrosed bone. The seat of disease is often very close to the epiphyseal line, and the joint will not suffer for some time, but sooner or later the inflammation will extend beyond the epiphysis and joint destruction will begin at once. When once the pus has broken through the cartilage, destruction of the joint goes on at a rapid rate. It matters little at this stage whether the trouble began in the bone or in the synovial sac, the clinical aspect of destruction is the same. Any amount of destruction is now within the bounds of expectation.

I might speak here of arthritis deformans, as coming under the obstructive class. The reason I did not make this more prominent is because it is a mooted question, whether there is true bone deformity, or whether it should be classed under hypertrophy of the cartilages. It is believed by most authors that arthritis deformans is not a bone deformity, but is a cartilaginous development.

The fact, however, is established that it is rheumatic or gouty in its origin. Whether this is bony or cartilaginous in its mechanical obstruction to the joint matters very little when treatment is taken into consideration.

While I feel that I have dwelt very briefly on the osseous classification of joint diseases, yet I also feel that a longer dissertation of the pathological changes would be of little value to the doctor who has a case under advisement.

I will now dwell very briefly on the last of my classifications.

DISEASES OF JOINTS,

Depending on pathological changes of the soft parts that are periarticular, are not very common, yet are sometimes met. Joint ailment may be the local manifestation of a constitutional disorder, gout, rheumatism, tuberculosis, or many troubles coming on from low resisting force.

Rickets I have failed to mention, and yet it often involves the joint, but more often the shaft of the bone.

Strumous joint troubles often begin in some of the ligaments, and is carried to the joint by continuity of structure.

Accidental sprains in which muscles, blood-vessels and nerves are involved, often result in joint troubles following highly inflammatory processes.

This part of my classification is not as important as the others, yet traumatisms outside of the articular structures often lead to joint invasions.

Tertiary syphilis, as in tabes dorsalis, often brings articular disturbance that is a serious hindrance to good joint action. With this amount of descriptive pathology I will now briefly review the present-day treatment.

There are a few points in diagnosis that must actually be learned before intelligent treatment can be carried on.

We must be able to differentiate bone diseases from affections of the synovial membrane. We must know malignancies from simple disorders. We should be able to tell a tubercular ostitis, or synovitis, or osteomyelitis from one of simple form. Each clinical manifestation will ask for different treatment.

Treatment of chronic joint diseases may be properly divided into two general classes, local and constitutional.

Constitutional treatment is provided for in many ways aside from internal medication. Climate, water, environment, exercise or rest, has much to do with patients who have struma. Good food and plenty of it, is also one of the essentials. The salicylates, the iodides, in the form of syrup hydriodic acid, iron and arsenic, and remedies along this line. Syrup hydriodic acid is always a favorite remedy in cases where the iodides are thought necessary.

Constitutional remedies can do very little in cases where the body is suffering as a secondary manifestation of a local infection. Yet it is very important that the general condition be looked after, and as there is no specific for such local trouble, your internal medicines must be prescribed after very careful investigation of each case. Local treatment is the important feature in the case, and should be guided by very great judgment, and you should know whether you have a case of synovitis, arthritis, periostitis, or otitis. You should know whether it is rheumatoid, syphilitic, gonorrheal, tubercular or simple inflammation, or possibly traumatic in origin.

All these things have a great bearing on the treatment.

It is impossible for me to lay down any set of rules to govern the treatment of chronic joint diseases. Every case is a law unto itself, and calls for very great discrimination in its treatment.

Most cases, without regard to their origin, can be treated under three heads: Rest, good drainage, and aseptic or antiseptic dressings.

When I speak of rest to a joint, I do not mean that the patient shall stop his exercise or moving around, or that he shall be put to bed or on crutches. I mean by rest that the joint shall be put to absolute immobility. This is the only way a joint can be put to rest, and unless this is accomplished and the inflamed joint surfaces stopped from grinding on each other, muscular spasm with pain will continue. This can be done with splints or plaster of paris cast. If you have a synovitis or arthritis of any of the joints of the long bones of the arm or the leg, and you have reason to believe it is tubercular and not a bone lesion, you would at once put the limb up in a plaster dressing. Should there be a synovial dropsy and your joint is not affected, you may aspirate the dropsical sac and inject it with pure tincture of iodine; and after a few treatments of this kind, if no relief follows and the sac refills, you should incise the sac freely, and keep packed with gauze until the space is closed.

Sometimes these synovial sacs have to be dissected out entirely, then the wound packed until healed. In simple synovitis, where the sac is opened the joint need not be immobilized, but the patient kept at rest. Where there is any arthritis, the joint should be fixed. Should you have a purulent synovitis or arthritis, the joint should be opened at once under the most aseptic precaution, and washed out with a 5 per cent. carbolic solution, or 1 to 2,000 bichloride, or a 10 per cent. iodide solution, then packed with iodoform gauze. If there is much pain, a fixation splint should be applied. Daily cleansings are necessary. Should you have an ostitis from any cause, or an osteomyelitis, this should be opened at once, and any necrosed bone removed and curetted thoroughly.

For me to give the necessary steps, covering all cases of joint disease, is impossible. All cases, however, come under the general conditions of free drainage, aseptic dressings, complete rest. Many limbs can be saved that were once sacrificed. Most of the knee-joint cases which formerly went on to amputation to save life under old management, can now be generally saved if seen early. Hydrarthrosis, or white swelling, was once thought to be fatal to a limb, but it is not so under the recent mode of management.

I have said very little about the treatment of floating cartilages, but will say here that it is strictly surgical and should be done under the strictest aseptic precautions. There are so many things I should like to say of the different types that come under the head of my paper. Hip-joint disease should have a paper to itself. The description of the various mechanical methods of treating morbus coxarius would take a whole evening alone. Yet what I have said will apply to all joints.

Don't treat a purulent joint without first evacuating the pus.

Don't immobilize a joint until it is free from necrosed substances, if such is suspected.

Don't put off operating on a joint after you know you have dead tissue either in bone or in soft part.

Don't make a small opening where a large one is needed.

Don't wash out a cavity through a small sinus, thinking you can heal it.

Don't operate on a joint case unless you do it thoroughly and under clean surroundings.

Don't use peroxide of hydrogen in any joint case.

Don't compromise with any patient and allow him to dictate to you what should be done in a joint case, unless he knows more than you do.

DISCUSSION.

CHAIRMAN: The discussion will be opened by Dr. McHenry.

DR. O. P. McHENRY: I think it can be agreed upon by all present that the paper has been a most excellent one. I think all will agree with me that what Dr. Huntley knows, he knows; and I agree with the doctor, particularly as to making a free opening, making an incision large enough to get free drainage.

DR. W. B. CHURCH: I understood the writer to say that a case of arthritis was of rheumatic or gouty origin. That information is new to me. If it is true, it is somewhat singular that rheumatic treatment for arthritis is without any good result. I have been interested in the subject of arthritis for some time, have treated a number of cases successfully, and written some articles upon the subject that some of you may have seen. I have regarded the disease as of nervous origin. I find it most likely to present itself in debilitated nervous condtions, and the great difficulty in regard to these cases, which are generally considered very little amenable to treatment. is that they are regarded as rheumatic. The bone is not as stiff as in rheumatism. It differs from rheumatism in all respects. It is mainly a disease of the cartilages of the joints, although these sometimes undergo ossification.

The habit of regarding and calling these cases rheumatism is an unhappy one, because many patients are subjected to treatment for years, to one form or another, extending from macrotys and rhus tox to the mud bath, without any benefit, and are generally more or less debilitated and injured by the treatment. The subject is of itself wide enough to occupy a whole paper.

DR. C. W. RUSSELL: I only came in as the paper was being read, and I don't know very much that was said. What I did hear I considered excellent, with very little to be discussed, other than what has been already said. He covered the field very thoroughly. The main thing of any diseased joint, whatever it may be, as the author has said, is to open it thoroughly and drain out. Wash out with bichloride or carbolized wash or iodoform. If there is any suppuration, and the joint seems to be in an inflamed condition, use local applications, iodine treatment of the joint, and. if possible, hot applications.

DR. J. H. HUNTLEY: In the treatment of joint diseases there are several things that are prominent now among American surgeons, that I did not have time to speak of or recognize. Concerning the etiology of the subject, spoken of by Dr. Church, I still feel that my position is backed by some of the best men we have, that it is believed to be rheumatic in origin, or gouty in origin, and the fact that the rheumatic remedies have no effect on it is not speaking at all for or against it, because, how many cases of true rheumatism do we have going on day after day and year after year, that are drenched and saturated with salicylates, iodides, and everything, and yet they go on with the pain and rheumatic drawings and articular deformities, gouty cartilages, and so on. On the other hand, neurotomy done on these cases never has stopped the disease from going on, nor have the salicylates done so. Now, I don't say positively that this is a disease of gouty origin or rheumatic origin, but I say I believe it is.

I don't know of any other class of diseases to which a surgeon should give his every-day attention and his good judgment, to see that no mistakes are made and thorough cleanliness is maintained, and everything done that is necessary—I don't know of any other class of diseases in which he can make as many mistakes if he does the wrong thing, or as much good if he does the right thing.

LATE SURGICAL IDEAS.

L. E. RUSSELL, M.D., CINCINNATI.

I present my paper by title, and I want to say, in presenting it, that there is not as much attention paid to the care of surgical cases in the use of the thermometer as there should be. Too often the patient's temperature is reported either by axilla or under the tongue, when the fight has been going on in the pelvis. If you wish to take the temperature in the right place, you must take it where the fight is going on, and it will be correct and enable you to pass upon your case and know whether it is doing well or not doing well. Temperature reported under the tongue of 101° sometimes means pelvis of 103° or 104°. It may mean an abscess formed in the line of the incision in the abdomen; it may mean pus formation in some part of the body, which, having had correct warning by the proper taking of the temperature, you can relieve the patient by opening up and by drainage.

Oftentimes we have in the use of the catgut some defect in which we have pus forming in the line of the incision in the abdomen. If your temperature shows above a hundred you must commence to look for the cause, and on stripping your wound you press carefully along the line of the incision on either side, and if you come to a hardened point, you can depend upon it that you have pus, and that your thermometer has given you warning at the proper time.

Recently I received a letter from one of our prominent physicians, who had a case operated upon, a laparotomy, in one of his best families. He never attends our State conventions; he never attends any of the State meetings; he fights out there by himself. Every two or three days he reported the patient doing well, everything doing well, and on the ninth day sent a report of temperature of 101° by the mouth. "What does it mean?" I replied as soon as I could, "You have pus somewhere; drain." And before he had time to get the letter his patient had passed to the great beyond. He was taking the temperature with the thermometer by the mouth, whereas he should have taken it where the fight was going on.

I instruct all our nurses to take the temperature at the nearest place that they can to the seat of the operation.

In all cases where the thermometer gives warning it is your duty to look after the condition of the field of operation at once.

Sometimes you will have cases of auto-infection, in which your patient has not been properly prepared by the removal of the contents of the bowels, and this produces temperature.

You may have cases in which your patient has taken a little cold, or a little pneumonic condition has taken place, and you want to get down to the truth as speedily as possible.

Again, another thing I want to call your attention to, and that is the position of your patient. In all of your cases where you have pus in the pelvis, where your operation has been of a pelvic nature, it is better to have your patient in a semi-reclining position. Much is to be obtained in the position of your patient following the operation. Don't place them down flat. Don't raise the foot of the bed, if you have your trouble in the pelvis or the abdomen. Don't place them down if you have your trouble, your adhesions, in the region of the liver or gall-bladder. Set them up. Let an aged patient sit in a rocking chair, and let the rocking chair be tipped back. You will do better if, instead of putting an old person to bed, you encourage them to sit up. They will do better to sit up.

Where you have pelvic lesions, oftentimes you will remove the pus tube, where you have done a hysterectomy, either vaginal or abdominal; where you have a pus appendix, turn your patient right over on their side, right on their face. Insist on their lying that way, so as to make drainage available, so as to get rid of every drop of pus that nature puts in there, and get rid of it at the very earliest possible time.

Salt water solutions are valuable. Normal salt water solutions are valuable in resuscitating your patient, given both by enema and by the use of the needle anywhere in the flank or breast.

I think that the greatest dangers that we have to encounter are in the first twelve or twenty-four hours following any serious operation or condition. The nursing and the care and the position that your patient is placed in are important. I emphasize this, because if you can get your patient twelve or twenty-four hours away from their surgical operation, you will nearly always see that they will get along all right after that. The bowels, of course, are important, and you must look out for peritonitis. Possibly you may have hemorrhage. These are conditions that all of you understand pretty well.

The importance of the position of your patient following an operation is of more value than any of us have heretofore thought in these cases.

DISCUSSION.

DR. J. S. HAGEN : I want to say one thing in regard to the position of the patient following operation. In doing a prostatectomy—the removal of the prostate gland—within one or two days the patient can sit in a chair, a rocking chair with the bottom cut out, and it allows drainage. A position of that manner helps in recovery in half the time that a patient lying in bed would. In operation on the gall-bladder the inverted position comes in very well.

The selection of suture material is a question that I believe is troubling all surgeons to-day, and is something that has never been thoroughly settled. All surgeons should be careful in the selection of their sutures. I believe that a great deal of post-operative trouble, adhesions, etc., are caused by the character of the sutures.

DR. J. R. SPENCER: I would like to ask Dr. Hagen or Dr. Russell what is the best material, what is the best make, for sutures, and where we can obtain it, so that we may not have this trouble.

DR. J. S. HAGEN: I might say that various surgeons advise various kinds of sutures, and very often the material may have to be handled as carefully as possible. It must be absolutely sterile, and I am not prepared to say what should be used in each and every individual case, but I think experience will prove that we have been making mistakes in the material which we use for sutures.

DR. L. E. RUSSELL: Silkworm gut I think is the best material for suturing wounds of the face, scalp, in fact, any part of the body. Silkworm is about the only suture that I have much faith in. If you wish to suture deep wounds, you can do it with the figure eight and remove your silkworm gut. It will not digest; it will not dissolve. I have taken out silkworm sutures that have been in the tissue for two or three years and it remains just the same as the day it went in. It is not very expensive.

———•———

A MEDIASTINAL tumor may be present for some time without other symptoms than cough, expectoration, loss of flesh and slight fever—thus simulating pulmonary tuberculosis. A skiagraph will determine the condition; laryngoscopy is also helpful, for adductor paralysis is frequently an early sign.—*American Journal of Surgery*.

FOR LEAN PEOPLE.—Einhorn commends the free use of butter, a quarter of a pound daily. In addition to the regular meals, two or three smaller meals, consisting of milk and buttered bread, may often be given with advantage.—*Denver Med. Times*.

Seton Hospital Reports.

L. E. RUSSELL, M.D., SURGEON.

Case 501.—Girl, fourteen years of age, with lateral curvature of the spine. Presented to the clinic for the application of a plaster-of-Paris cast.

In this case it is the duty of the surgeon to super-correct the deformity before the application of the plaster cast, and in doing so the patient is placed underneath a hanging bar and the torso torsioned in the opposite direction of the curvature, super-correcting the distorted or crooked spine.

An assistant now holds the patient's arm and helps to carry the shoulder far above the opposite side and the plaster cast is applied, commencing over the pelvic bones and tightly encasing the same so that the thorax and upper part of the body has a fixed support, and we continue the winding of the plaster bandages, extending up well into the axilla on either side.

Just as we reach the epigastric region we place a folded towel over the stomach, allowing it to extend upward under the chin where later on it can be removed, leaving a cavity so that the stomach can expand when food is introduced.

Loose plaster of Paris, fairly well moistened, is now applied by one or two assistants, reinforcing the places most liable to give way in carrying the upper part of the body from its lower support. Absorbent cotton is provided in either axilla and across the bony part of the hips. The tightly fitting undershirt, as used in this case, is always advisable in the application of the plaster cast, as it prevents the irritating effects of the plaster when it comes in contact with the body.

This little girl will be allowed to wear this support for at least three months, holding the body in this super-corrected position, and relieving the softened condition of the bones that is accountable for this deformity.

We take a measurement of the child before the application of the plaster cast, and also before the re-application of a second cast, and we will find that the child, instead of remaining at the present height, will have gained two or three inches in the next three months.

I think the fixed position of the distorted torso, by the plaster-of-Paris method, of greater advantage in accomplishing a cure than the other methods of mechanical jackets as applied in orthopedic work.

Case 502.—Miss M., forty-five years old, unmarried. Has been complaining of severe vaginal discharge for ten months; no pain and no offensive smell to the débris.

On making a digital vaginal examination we find the whole vaginal tract impacted with a malignant disease; much of this impacted mass can be torn out with the fingers and as there is danger of tearing into the bowel, we shall carry the index finger of the left hand into the rectum and with the right finger into the vagina tear away and remove enough of the malignant tissue so that a speculum can be inserted. We find now that the whole uterine cervix has been destroyed. Let us use the uterine curette and we can now remove nearly all broken down tissue and treat the cavity with gauze moistened in pure alcohol. Much good than thus be accomplished.

Eye, Ear, Nose and Throat.

Conducted by Charles S. Amidon, M.D.

Ophthalmia Neonatorum.

A purulent conjunctivitis occurring in the newborn. It may be produced by various causes, but the majority of cases, and particularly the severe ones, owe their origin to the gonococcus.

As a rule, the infection occurs during the passage of the head through the parturient canal. The eyelids are covered with the secretion contained in the vagina as the head passes, and this is either forced through the palpebral fissure into the conjunctival sac, or the infection passes through as soon as the child opens its eyes.

The disease manifests itself, as a rule, on the second or third day after birth, but may be as late as the fifth day. Cases that develop later are surely due to infection from other sources than the parturient canal.

The disease is usually bilateral, but one eye only may be affected.

The time of onset, the redness of lids and conjunctiva, with the swelling and purulent secretion, make the diagnosis easy.

The integrity of the eye depends upon prompt and thorough treatment. Cleanliness is of the greatest importance and should be repeated often enough to keep the eye free from secretion. Pus should not be allowed to accumulate, so the eye should be cleansed often, possibly every fifteen or twenty minutes in some cases.

A saturated solution of boric acid may be used. First cleanse all secretion from the lids, then gently retract lids, allowing solution to wash over eyeball. If the swelling is so great that it is difficult to cleanse the eye, a canthotomy should be performed; this not only facilitates the cleansing, but relieves pressure.

A 2 per cent. solution of silver nitrate should be used once a day.

Lloyd's hydrastis .... dr. ss.
Morphine sul. .... gr. jss.
Sol. boric acid, q. s........................... oz. ss.
Sig.—One or two drops in afflicted eye every two hours.

Or the following is possibly more effective:

Argyrol sol. .... 6 per cent.
Sig.—Two drops in eye every two or three hours.

Atropine should be used if there is any corneal complication.

Cold compresses give relief from pain, and tend to allay the inflammation.

These should be applied to the eye directly from ice and should be changed every minute for a period of half an hour, and repeated every hour or two as the case demands. If corneal complications develop, hot compresses should be used in place of cold.

Internally aconite, belladonna, rhus, apis, and apocynum are the drugs usually thought of, and should be prescribed according to their indications. Lime in some form should be given in every case.

Prophylaxis.—The measures proposed by Créde should be used in every case where the physician suspects a gonorrheal infection in the mother, or where there is any irritating vaginal discharge. This consists in thoroughly cleansing the parturient canal with a 2 per cent. solution of carbolic acid, and instilling a drop of 2 per cent. solution silver nitrate in the child's eyes as soon after birth as possible.

The Eye as a Contributing Factor in Tuberculosis.

E. Park Lewis, in the *Journal American Medical Association,* believes the eye is a great contributing factor in tuberculosis. He bases his idea on the following propositions:

1. Errors of refraction, or marked muscle imbalance, may so disarrange the nervous functions that gastric or intestinal disturbances may result, and metabolism be retarded in consequence, with lowered resistance and increased susceptibility to infection.

2. The continued existence of such conditions, especially in the neurotic, may so lower the vitality as to retard recovery from tuberculous infections of the lungs.

3. Relief of the abnormal visual conditions is a necessary prerequisite to recovery from pulmonary disease.

4. In view of these facts the complete examination of a suspected tuberculous patient has not been made until the condition of the eyes, including the refraction and dynamics of the ocular muscles, has been investigated and carefully recorded.

Periscope.

Advantage of the Small College.

Americans are nothing if not extremists. We have acquired the habit of running in ruts and are a nation of faddists. Some men can only see one side of a question, although, naturally, every question has at least two sides. When a man gets such a one-sided idea he sees nothing else, and carries it to the limit regardless of what the result may be. Because any one thing contains something that is really good is no reason for adopting it to the exclusion of everything else. To make a right choice of everything it is first necessary to look at the subject from all sides.

This statement applies to education as well as to other mundane affairs. The time was, and not very long ago, when institutions of learning were small and few, and the times such that men who sought an education had to depend more upon themselves than on colleges and teachers. Notwithstanding the difficulties of such a course, some men struggled through, and are numbered among the greatest men that our country has produced. It did not take any kind of a college to make them. They acquired their knowledge in the liberal school of self-education. This is not said in disparagement of modern progress, nor of improvements in our educational system, but simply to show that more depends on the man than upon the method of schooling. The fallacy consists in supposing that it requires a college or university training to make the man. On such a basis of reasoning it is considered necesary to build up great institutions, as students are inclined to flock in the direction of the largest crowd. Such a course is apt to be far from wise, as is being discovered and commented on in these later days.

Success is the god that is usually sought, but merely going through and out of college does not qualify a man to succeed. Many a young man, after taking a full course in some university and with the best of teachers, ends his career in disappointment and failure because he depends on the college and teacher to put him through, and fails to get in and dig for himself. Instead of depending on merit, things are measured superficially, and their value estimated by dimensions and quantity rather than by true worth. Unless a man can count his dollars by the hundred millions he is no longer considered rich, and if he does not hold a parchment from some large college or university he is not educated. The tendency has been for some time in educational affairs to go to extremes in a combination of the large colleges against the small ones, by creating an educational trust to control knowledge. This state of affairs exists in a medical education even more noticeably than in a literary or scientific course, and the time has arrived to call a halt. Experienced educators have become alarmed at the situation and are now advising against the exclusive university course and in favor of the small college. In a small college the instruction is more individual and personal, and therefore is much more direct and effective. In the crowded classroom of a large institution the individuality is merged in the mass and lost, and teacher and pupil cannot get into close touch except by favoritism to the few.

A late writer has said that "The State universities almost everywhere are growing to such an extent that they threaten to undo the very purpose for which they exist—education. It becomes a hard matter to maintain discipline to any extent over thousands of young men and women who, full of ardent ambition and life, are flocking to the great educational centers. The advantages there sought, namely, contact with truly great teachers of reputation, is more than counterbalanced by the practical certainty that the size of the classes will forbid all personal touch with these great teachers and will compel the student to learn from a tutor. This hallucination of seeking great teachers is therefore usually dispelled early in the university experience of the student. The numbers are too vast, and the dangers of this multitudinous herding of men and women together is beginning to worry the heads of these institutions themeslves."

President Angell, of the University of Michigan, is quoted as saying:

"I am inclined to think that most of the State universities are suffering from excessive attendance. It is apparent to me that one of the greatest problems before the universities of the nation during the next twenty years will be how to administer these rapidly growing institutions properly."

The Chicago *Record-Herald* says:

"The day of the smaller college is coming again. Of course, the special inducements offered by the State universities as public institutions will always make them popular, but may there not be some relief because of the preference which many people now express for the small colleges? The country has scores of these colleges. and not a few of them enjoy an excellent reputation. They can give as fine discipline as any of the larger institutions, have the advantage of bringing faculty and students together, and are freer from distractions than the big rivals. A professor in one of these vast State institutions said some time ago that he would never intrust his son to it for training. In answer to a question as to the reason of this strange remark he expressed himself oracularly: 'The gains are too little, and the possible losses are too great. I prefer the small college.' "—J. A. MUNK, M.D., Los Angeles, Cal., in *California Eclectic Medical Journal*.

State Board Examinations: Chemistry.

A review of the statistics resulting from the examination of candidates by the various State boards shows that the average results were notably low in chemistry. This was especially the case with mature practicians, those who would naturally be considered the safest men to whom the lives of citizens could be entrusted.

During our college course we gave the requisite attention to medical chemistry and passed our examinations in it. We graduated and went to work. As problems arose in practice in which chemistry figured we drew on our memory and referred to our textbooks. Result—what chemistry we needed and could use we retained and developed. The rest we soon forgot.

New and pressing duties monopolized our attention and our energies. We had to win a livelihood among a crowded press of competitors. Suffering, dying human beings demanded our aid, and we soon found that every ounce of energy, every bit of knowledge, the utmost exercise of every mental power we possessed, was requisite to enable us to do our duty to our patients. Many a time we have wrung our hands, crying, "Oh, if we only had more brains."

Twenty, thirty years pass by and we are growing old. We have won the love and confidence of the community. Blessings follow our footsteps from many a grateful heart. But some one of our loved ones has grown pale, and ominous symptoms indicate that the limit of our skill has been reached, and the Destroyer is camping on her trail. Still there is a chance, and under the sunny skies of a favorable climate the vital powers may yet win the fight. Such a climate awaits us; but how are we to earn our needs there, if not by the exercise of that art to which we have given our lives and souls?

Facing the examiners we meet such queries as these: "Give the formula of nitric acid and tell how it is prepared."

Answer: "Formula, $HO\,NO_5$. I don't know how it is prepared. I never had occasion to make it, and cannot conceive of any set of conditions that would render it advisable for me to do so. If such were to occur I would get the latest texts and learn the most recent improved methods."

"Wrong—formula, HNO_3."

"Give the meaning of the words monad (univalent), diad, triad, valence, quantivalence, and state the valence of (CN), (OH), (NO_3), (CO_3), (HC)."

"How is a clinical thermometer made and graded?"

"Define empiric, molecular, rational and graphic formulas."

"Give the graphic formula of sulphuric acid, representing S as a diad, also as a hexad."

"By what means are anions and cations designated?"

"Complete the following equation and give the name of each resulting compound: $C_2H_5OH+C_2H_5—H_2HSO_3=$?"

"What is methane? Give its formula, chemic importance and method of manufacture."

"How would you proceed to detect arsenic in a case of suspected poisoning?"

To the last question the candidate replies: "When I graduated I could give Marsh's and other tests. But then and now, with a life depending on the result, I should not trust my memory, but should consider myself criminally negligent were I not to take the textbook and follow every direction, constantly referring to the text. Moreover, if there were a competent chemist within reach it would be my duty to put this work on him, lest through my inexperience a fatal error might be made. As to the other questions, they relate to matters that have never arisen in my practice and never will. They treat of a new chemistry developed since I studied, and in which I am too remotely interested to justify me in devoting my time and attention to them. When, as is always the case, I have patients hovering between life and death, I dare not take up my time studying the manufacture of sulphuric acid and the production of methane. The recent graduate should know these things; the old practician who does has violated his obligations as a physician and neglected his duty to his patients to waste time on matters that do not come within his sphere."

And so our friend gets a zero in chemistry, and is not allowed to practice legally in that State unless he turns quack, for the bars, strangely enough, seem to be down to all but real doctors.

Moral: If you wish to change your location, get a modern textbook on chemistry and a laboratory outfit, and take time to read yourself familiar with the new chemistry.

Haven't time or means?

Or agitate for a law limiting the examinations in chemistry to points on which a busy practician can legitimately be expected to be posted.—*American Journal of Clinical Medicine.*

A FEELING of discomfort in the mouth while eating may be the first signs of a calculus in one of the salivary ducts.—*American Journal of Surgery.*

THE ECLECTIC MEDICAL JOURNAL

A Monthly Journal of Eclectic Medicine and Surgery.

TWO DOLLARS PER ANNUM.

Official Journal Ohio State Eclectic Medical Association

JOHN K. SCUDDER, M.D., MANAGING EDITOR.

EDITORS.

W. E. BLOYER.	H. W. FELTER.	L. E. RUSSELL.	R. L. THOMAS.
W. B. CHURCH.	J. U. LLOYD.	H. E. SLOAN.	L. WATKINS.
JOHN FEARN.	W. N. MUNDY.	A. F. STEPHENS.	H. T. WEBSTER.

Published by THE SCUDDER BROTHERS COMPANY, 1009 Plum Street, Cincinnati, to whom all communications and remittances should be sent.

Articles on any medical subject are solicited, which will usually be published the month following their receipt. One hundred reprints of articles of four or more pages, or one dozen copies of the Journal, will be forwarded free if the request is made when the article is submitted. The editor disclaims any responsibility for the views of contributors.

Discontinuances and Renewals.—The publishers must be notified by mail and all arrearages paid when you want your Journal stopped. If you want it stopped at the expiration of any fixed period, kindly notify us in advance.

OUR FUTURE.*

Those who have kept posted in medicine are aware that marked changes have occurred during the last twenty-five years. The great commercial world has undergone almost a revolution in its methods of conducting business. Great manufactories have found that by pooling their interests and merging into one or more great plants much cheaper production can be secured. The big institutions are swallowing the smaller ones, the large banks absorbing the little ones, and we are face to face with new conditions.

What has taken place in the commercial world is rapidly taking place in the medical world. Through the American Medical Association plans are being formulated with the object of eventually merging all schools into one, and all colleges into universities. This Association has taken upon itself the power or authority to grade all medical colleges and say which are entitled to live. The minor schools of medicine are facing one of the greatest crises in their history. What of the future?

Shall Eclecticism, with her splendid history of good works accomplished, cease to exist as an independent school? No; a thousand times no. The fact that so many are present this evening and enrolled under her banners, is proof that you rejoice in her splendid past, glory in her present and believe in a crowning future.

* Read before the Chicago Eclectic Medical Society, November 11, 1908.

There are those who, having seen the harsh medication of the fathers give way to a humane system of medication, say that our mission is ended, and the only proper thing to do is to kindly give up the ghost, while admiring friends place flowers upon the remains.

We hear on every side that the schools are getting together, that after all there is not much difference between one doctor and another, and that the only rational and decent thing to do is to merge into one school. What of the future of Eclecticism? The whole question, as it appears to me, depends upon whether or not Eclecticism still has a work to perform in the medical world that cannot be accomplished by any other school. I firmly believe that there are problems to be solved that, unless worked out by our school, will never find solution; therefore I firmly believe her mission is not ended, and that a splendid future awaits her.

Many have mistaken the purpose of her birth and mission. There is a widespread impression that Eclecticism was founded to combat the harsh medication that was in vogue eighty-five years ago, and that had been practiced for centuries. I am here to emphatically refute any such claims or idea. Eclecticism was not born to combat any school or system of medicine. It was founded for only one purpose, and that was to combat disease. Her mission has *always* been to heal the sick. It is true that in this warfare against diseased conditions she has often come in serious combat with forms of medication, but the one great purpose of Eclecticism from the time of her birth to the present hour is *how best to treat the sick*. For more than eighty-five years she has studied the relation between diseased conditions and drug action, and to-day believes in the therapeutic action of her splendid materia medica.

What is the position of the *dominant* school to-day as to medication? If we are to take their most prominent disciples as authority, we can only come to one conclusion, and that is that they have lost all faith in the curative action of medicine. To-day Osler is regarded as a therapeutic nihilist, while Dr. Bevin proclaims to the world that pneumonia is incurable. If the dominant school, therefore, admits its inability to heal the sick, then there certainly is still need for a school that can, and I firmly believe that there never was a period when Eclecticism was more needed than it is to-day.

One of the most serious questions before us is not how to simply fill the ever-depleting ranks occasioned by death and retirement from age, but how to increase our numbers. We are getting letters from various parts of the country asking for Eclectic physicians, but the supply is not nearly equal to the demand. We could place five hundred graduates every year for the next ten in good locations, yet there are not that many students in all our colleges combined. In some manner our men have allowed themselves to become lukewarm or careless as to our general cause, or have become so engrossed in their own work as to neglect the school at large.

Last year there were 20,936 students in 123 Allopathic colleges, or 170 students per college. In 16 Homeopathic colleges there were 891 students, or 55 students per college; while in 8 Eclectic colleges there were 479 students, or 60 students per college. One out of every five Allopaths sent a student to an Allopathic college. One Homeopath out of every ten sent a student to a Homeopathic college, while one Eclectic out of every fifteen sent a student to an Eclectic college. You see, therefore, the Eclectic colleges are getting only about one-third as many students as we are proportionately entitled to. Unless we can bring about a radical change, we certainly cannot occupy *new* territory.

What is the solution of the problem? One important factor in its solution is a better organization of our men. So long as Eclectics fail to unite with their State and national associations, just so long will they remain apathetic as to the general welfare of our school. I believe that when our men become acquainted with the true conditions they will respond to the needs of the hour, and the best way to become acquainted with all matters pertaining to Eclecticism is to become members of our organized bodies. Here they come in touch with every need and every advance made in medical legislation, and they will learn that our schools are abreast of the times. The law is no respecter of persons; hence our colleges must be equipped to do the work required by the best colleges in the land. We *need* recruits, we *must have recruits,* and loyal Eclectics will see to it that we get them.

I believe that every State should have an organizer, whose business should be to marshal the Eclectics and round them into the State society and then into the National. If this can be done, the question will soon be solved. THOMAS.

HODGKIN'S DISEASE.

This affection, known also as pseudo-leukemia, adenia, general lymphadenoma, multiple malignant lymphoma, malignant lymphosarcoma, lymphatic anemia and lymphoadenosis, is a disease of rather rare occurrence, and especially so in a patient so young as in the one under consideration.

It is defined as an anemic disease, characterized by a progressive hyperplasia of lymph-glands, occasional secondary lymphoid growths of other organs, and the absence of the distinctive blood-changes of true leukemia.

It derives its name from Hodgkin, who first described the disease in 1832. Two varieties are at present recognized, one which presents simply an enlarged spleen, and the other in which the lymphatic glands are chiefly involved; yet it is claimed that the spleen is enlarged in four-fifths of the cases. No well-established predisposing condi-

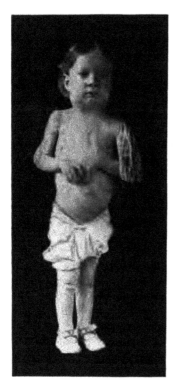

tion to which this trouble can be referred seems to be known. It affects males most frequently, in about 70 per cent. of the cases reported. Tuberculosis was thought to have a distinct influence, yet this is untenable, as it is not uncommon to find it developing in one who has previously been in good health. Its name, pseudo-leukemia, conveys at once the impression that it resembles leukemia in its course and the appearance of the patient. Some observers are of the opinion that the same irritation produces pseudo-leukemia and leukemia, according to whether it affects only the lymphatic glands and spleen or medulla also; whilst others place the affection in close relation to leukemia, owing to a relative lymphocytosis which was always found in pseudo-leukemia.

The symptoms vary somewhat, and it is often difficult to distinguish the disease from tuberculosis or chronic adenitis, both of which it resembles, and a microscope ought to be employed for a study of the blood.

There may at first be some impairment of the general health, or the glandular enlargement may appear first. This latter usually begins in the submaxillary and cervical glands, and later involves the axillary, inguinal and internal glands. The extent and rapidity of their growth vary considerably.

With the progress of the disease the impairment of the general health increases. The paleness increases with the progress of the disease, and symptoms of anemia appear. Languor, loss of physical strength, emaciation, gastro-intestinal disorder, headache and palpitation of the heart appear. Hemorrhages, epistaxis, hemic murmurs and an irregular and moderate fever also occur. It is claimed that this fever pursues an intermittent type, and the paroxysms may last for several days or weeks.

Symptoms due to the mechanical compression by reason of the enlarged glands are varied and numerous, depending upon their number, size and location. Unless pressure be made upon adjacent nerves, the disease is said to be painless.

As we have said in the beginning, it is more apt to be confused with tubercular adenitis than with any other disease; especially so at its onset. Tubercular adenitis is much slower in its progress and is more common in the young. It is more often unilateral, and attacks more often submaxillary rather than the entire cervical group. Periadenitis, adhesions and suppuration occur in tuberculosis, and tubercular foci are apt to be found in other organs also. An intermittent pyrexia is said to favor Hodgkin's disease. The case that called forth this study is as follows:

E. M., aged three years, had in February, 1908, what was diagnosed "scarlet rash," previous to which time he had always enjoyed good health. From this he made a poor recovery. The submaxillary glands were swollen and continued so, enlarging very slowly. The child was pale and complained only of being tired. Appetite poor and capricious. I saw him in July, just previous to his going to Oklahoma. The glands were swollen, child pale, pulse very rapid, but no lung affection could be discovered. During the stay in Oklahoma he was continually under the care of a physician for a gastro-intestinal disturbance. On his return I was again called, and found not only the sub-maxillaries enlarged, but both the anterior and posterior cervical chain, as far as I could trace them. The child was exceedingly anemic and emaciated, the abdomen distended, the veins standing out prominently in sharp contrast to the pallor of the skin. Examination of the abdomen revealed the liver enlarged, its border being felt on a level with the umbilicus and to the left of it, and nodules were distinctly felt upon its surface. On the left the spleen was so distinctly palpable as to be felt by the uninitiated. The pyrexia was of the remittent type, 100° F. in the morning and 102° to 103° in the evening, the latter being the highest temperature recorded. Repeated examinations failed to reveal any tubercular lesions elsewhere. The anemia and emaciation were progressive, as was also the enlargement of the glands. Gastro-intestinal trouble slight, though present, and finally we had some epistaxis, and twenty-four hours before death some slight hemorrhage from the bowels. Death was due to asthenia.

We are sorry that an accident prevented the securing of a microscopic examination of the blood, which, though not absolutely necessary for a diagnosis, would have proven corroborative.   MUNDY.

ANESTHETICS.

Which is the safer anesthetic, ether or chloroform? Is the cause of sudden death under chloroform, respiratory, cardiac or vaso-motor failure? Does the danger of pulmonary and renal disturb-ances following the administration of ether counterbalance its greater safety during the anesthesia? What part does the method of admin-istration play in lessening the danger, and what method is best adapted to each drug? To what extent should local anesthesia, nitrous oxide, ethyl chloride, scopalamine-morphine, spinal anesthesia, and rectal etherization be used?

Some of these questions physicians have been trying to answer for years. Commissions and individual investigators have reported their findings from time to time, but have not been able to settle the matter to the satisfaction of all. The controversy between the advo-cates of ether and chloroform still wages.

The preliminary report of the Anesthesia Commission of the American Medical Association has just been published, and in it we find answers to some of these questions. Its recommendations are as follows:

"1. That for the general practitioner and for all anesthetists not specially skilled, ether must be the anesthetic of choice—ether by the open or drop method.

"2· That the use of chloroform, particularly for the operations of minor surgery, be discouraged, unless it be given by an expert.

"3· That the training of skilled anesthetists be encouraged, and that undergraduate students be more generally instructed in the use of anesthetics."

This must not be interpreted as an unqualified endorsement of ether. It simply means that the more potent, rapidly-acting drug, chloroform, is more dangerous in the hands of an unskilled anes-thetist, and that since the death from chloroform usually occurs in the earlier stages of anesthesia, it is just as dangerous in the short operations of minor surgery as in the longer major operations. There-fore chloroform should be given by a trained anesthetist, and in minor surgical cases some less dangerous anesthetic should be used. The importance of trained anesthetists cannot be too strongly empha-sized. Given a case in which neither anesthetic is contra-indicated, the danger is greater from the anesthetist than from the anesthetic.

Until recently nitrous oxide has been turned over to the dentists, but now, by the use of sufficient air or oxygen to prevent asphyxia, operations requiring more than an hour are performed under its in-fluence. Since it is the safest general anesthetic it should have a wider field, and with perfected appliances for its administration its use will be greatly increased.

Local anesthesia is making rapid strides, and some surgeons are performing 50 per cent. of their operations under it. With a wider diffusion of knowledge concerning this method, the cases requiring general anesthesia will be greatly lessened.

Spinal anesthesia, after passing through severe criticism, bids fair to establish a place for itself in a limited field. Rectal etherization has its advocates, and is being carefully studied. Scopolamine-morphine anesthesia looks dangerous. In a series of ninety-two cases, three deaths are reported. Experience will probably show that it should be limited to small doses before ether or chloroform.

As our knowledge of anesthetics increases, fewer surgeons will give one anesthetic exclusively, and a greater number will select the anesthetic to meet the indications in each case.   SLOAN

SLANDERERS.

Dr. J. N. McCormack, organizer of the American Medical Association, told his colleagues of Cincinnati, in a public address, that out of 120,000 physicians of the United States, only 30,000 belonged to their organization, and that half of the physicians of his school of medicine lived in rented houses worse than the skilled mechanic or laborer. He furthermore says:

"As a rule, the doctor is a slanderer or a backbiter toward his competitors, and medical colleges are the hotbeds where strife and discord are engendered in the young medical student, and even before he leaves college he has been infected with this strife."

Think of it! I take this statement of the doctor as self-explanatory for the conduct of so many of the men of his school towards reputable physicians of other schools.

I would like to have *our* men read these burning words and then tell me what they have to gain by casting aside their college associates and joining this band of backbiters under the pretense of brotherly love. I am firmly of the opinion that when the old school of medicine gets through with using our men for political purposes only, then the bulk of our boys will drop back into our rank and be contented when they have been "sufficiently used" by our old-school competitors.   RUSSELL.

FETID FEET.

One of the annoying affections that are accentuated during the winter months is stinking feet, an affection most probably due to bromidrosis, a functional disturbance of the sweat-glands by which the sweat takes on an offensive odor. This sweating is sometimes so profuse as to keep the stockings constantly wet, and we have seen the shoes so saturated that the stain could be seen on the surface of the leather. When it has progressed to the latter stage, a change of shoes following treatment will best prevent its return. A form of this affection is so severe in some cases as to cause the epidermal layer of the sole to lift in great patches, or to become white, macerated and stinking. The treatment is simple, usually, unless there is marked debility of the patient requiring supportive treatment. The feet should be washed daily with Asepsin soap and warm water, carefully rinsed, and then soaked for ten minutes in a solution of salicylic acid (first dissolved in alcohol). At least a drachm should be used to two quarts of water. Or the feet may be painted with the alcoholic solution after bathing and rinsing. The shoes should be washed with the same and put away to dry, or, if they must be worn at once, should be sprinkled with a dusting powder composed of salicylic acid, boric acid, alum and talcum powder, using one part each of the first three to six parts of the latter. Other agents of value for bathing are potassium permanganate, beta-naphthol, and formaldehyde in solution, using the latter with caution. Stockings which have been soaked in solutions of either boric or salicylic acid should be worn, a fresh pair being put on every half-day or day.   FELTER.

Club Rates.

The various Eclectic publishers have decided to offer special club rates to March 1, 1909. If you are not familiar with any of these journals, a sample copy can be obtained on request.

JOURNALS.	PRICE.	CLUB RATES.
American Med. Journal, 5255 Page Ave., St. Louis......$1 00		$ 80
California Med. Journal, 818 Security Bldg., Los Angeles. 1 00		80
Chicago Med. Times, 412 Fulton St., Chicago.......... 1 50		1 20
Eclectic Med. Gleaner, 224 Court St., Cincinnati........ 1 25		1 00
Eclectic Med. Journal, 1009 Plum St., Cincinnati........ 2 00		2 00
Eclectic Review, 140 W. Seventy-first St., New York..... 1 00		80
Ellingwood's Therapeutist, 100 State St., Chicago........ 1 00		80
Medical Harbinger, 910 Lami St., St. Louis............. 50		40
Therapeutics, 703 Washington St., Dorchester District, Boston 1 00		80

You can subscribe for any or all of the above through this office, the only condition being that you include a "paid in advance" subscription to the ECLECTIC MEDICAL JOURNAL at Two Dollars.

The ECLECTIC NEWS

A MONTHLY NEWSPAPER

Vol. XIII.   JANUARY, 1908.   No. 1.

BOOK NOTICES.

Personal and Social Purity. By Jerome D. Dodge, M.D.   Price, fifty cents.   Published by the author at Collinwood, Ohio.

Had this little book reached the reviewer's desk two decades ago, he would probably have considered it in the light of something that violated the ethics of good society, something that should not be tolerated in the line of home instruction to either young or old.   Good men there are to-day in whom these views are yet engrafted, men who cover their faces to fact and sacrifice their loved ones to the false teaching that prevents the young from receiving authentic information concerning facts, a knowledge of which none can escape.   This false idea of wrong protects the licentious who prey upon the ignorant and the innocent by reason of this unwritten law which commands society to view as forbidden those things that because they are covered turn the innocent into paths that lead to destruction.

Could this book of Dr. Dodge's be studied by those charged with the instruction of the young, and the facts therein portrayed in it discreetly taught those who need such facts, a multitude would be benefited, and none would be harmed.   Could the precepts engrafted in this book in language that cannot be misconstrued, be taught to those who need to learn these facts, untold misery and suffering and shame would be avoided.   Let it not be misunderstood that Dr. Dodge in his book handles candidly, kindly and vividly, the wrongs that are committed by those who take advantage of the ignorance that comes through lack of needful information.   J. U. L.

Foods and Their Adulterations. By H. W. Wiley, M.D.. Ph.D.   Price, $4.00.   P. Blakiston Son & Co., Philadelphia, Publishers.

This book of 625 pages, illustrated, is from the pen of the foremost man in America concerned in the helping of the country to better foods and medicines.   It is a monument, carrying a fund of information to be found in no other publication. It treats of every form of food and of food sophistication, whether it be in its natural condition, or manipulated and preserved. The subjects of sophistications and adulterations, as well as of inferior qualities, are naturally given much attention. Dairy products and canned fruits are also naturally conspicuous. The diseases that afflict fish, flesh, fruits and vegetables, are so treated as to furnish a fund of authentic information from the foremost authority on the subject in the United States, if not in the world. The appendix is made up of decisions of the department in Washington, concerning the food and drug acts, flavoring extracts, fish and meat inspections, wines, sulphurous acid in wines, false labelings, preservatives in sausages and foods, mixed flours, blended whisky, coloring of butter and cheese, physicians' prescriptions, etc., etc. To sum up, this book will be as valued in the future as it is in the present, a book of information and of reference it is to-day, and will so remain.

J. U. L.

Handbook of Cutaneous Therapeutics. By W. H. Hardaway, M.D., and Joseph Grindon, M.D. Pp. 606. Lea Brothers & Co., Philadelphia. Price, $2.75; cloth.

Hardaway's *Manual of Skin Diseases* is the basis upon which this useful volume has been built, the therapeutic and descriptive sections of the former having been utilized, revised and extended. All that relates to the descriptions, general and medicinal treatment has been written by Dr. Hardaway, while Dr. Grindon has furnished special sections on the physical and mechanical treatment, including minor surgery of the skin, galvanism, faradism, high-frequency currents, and radio-therapy. The opsonic theory has received adequate notice. Rare and unimportant diseases receive but little attention, but great stress is laid upon the diseases most likely to be encountered by the general practitioner. Much attention is given to differential diagnosis and treatment is especially full. We regard it as one of the most useful of the books on dermatology.   H. W. F.

Physical Diagnosis. By H. S. Anders, M.D., with case examples of the inductive method. 456 pp. Cloth, $3.00. D. Appleton & Co., New York.

Each chapter on the different methods of physical diagnosis is very complete and is treated in a progressive manner. The work is especially strong from a practical point of view, in that the physical diagnosis of the diseases of the respiratory tract are *inductively* considered. This method is logically pursued, and it teaches the student to rely upon his own observations and to think and reason for himself points that are most needed by the student and practitioner in the study of its application in physical diagnosis.

The illustrations and plates are clear and clean, and are of great value, especially to the student. J. C. E.

Physical Examination of Infants and Young Children. By Prof. Kilmer. Price, 75 cents. F. A. Davis Company, Philadelphia, Pa., publishers.

This work treats of many points in the examination of infants generally overlooked in the larger text-books. Kilmer mentions the different types of children and the ways of handling each. The causes of a baby's cry are enumerated with the means of distinguishing them. The various steps in a physical examination—mensuration, palpation, examination of eyes and ears, etc.—are given, and each step is shown in illustrations. The book should be of value to every general practitioner, and especially to the recent graduate.

Surgical Diagnosis. By D. N. Eisendrath, M.D.; 482 ill.; cloth $6.50. Philadelphia: W. B. Saunders Co., publishers.

This work by Eisendrath is well worthy of the attention of the busy practitioner, as it very graphically illustrates many of the lesions that are encountered by the busy practitioner along the line of clinical work, as pursued by Prof. Eisendrath with the advantage of a very large clinic.

The work contemplates a grouping of injuries in a general manner so that the practitioner can easily differentiate in many of the lesions, and arrive at a very positive diagnosis in these troublesome cases.

Much attention has been given by the author in illustrating his method of making his examinations, and the book is well filled with illustrations that are of great value.

We shall commend the work as of much value, and a book that should adorn the library of the up-to-date physician. L. E. R.

Obstetrics. By J. Whitridge Williams, M.D. D. Appleton & Co., New York. Cloth, $6.00.

The author of this book has divided it into eight sections. The first section is devoted to a description of the anatomical structures of the bones of the pelvis and the female organs of generation; the other sections are utilized in discussing such subjects as the physiology and development of the ovum, the physiology of pregnancy and labor, obstetric surgery, the pathology of pregnancy and labor, and the pathology of the puerperium. The book is well illustrated by numerous well-designed illustrations. The writer is very clear in his statements, and has given to the medical profession a book thoroughly up-to-date in every respect. _____ J. R. S.

Wellcome's Photographic Exposure Record and Diary. By Burroughs Wellcome & Co., 45 Lafayette Street, New York City.

For any one doing photographic work out of doors, especially when traveling, this handy little book will be almost a necessity. Besides the pages for recording the subject, time of day, light, etc., and the usual memorandum found in any diary, there are many valuable hints and information for the photographer. It is a handy companion, as I can testify from personal use of the Record. K. O. F.

_____

Practical Observations Upon the Chemistry of Foods and Dietetics. By J. B. S. King, M.D.; 147 pages; second revised edition. $1.00 net. Boericke & Tafel, Philadelphia, Pa.

As stated in the title, this little book is a practical one, and gives the clearest and best idea of food and dietetics, in the simplest and most condensed form of any I have seen. Every student and practitioner should have a copy, and read it often. J. L. P.

_____

A Text-Book of Physiology. By H. Howell. Second edition, thoroughly revised; 939 pages. W. B. Saunders Co. Cloth, $4.00 net.

The second edition of Howell brings the work up to date. There has been some elimination and some addition, but the scope and size of the book remain about the same as heretofore. The treatise is interesting and complete. _____ L. W.

Text-Book of Physiology. By Isaac Ott, M.D. Second revised edition. Illustrated. Royal octavo, 815 pages. Cloth. Price $3.50 net. F. A. Davis Co., publishers, Philadelphia, Pa.

This is one of the best works on the subject of physiology that has been offered to the medical profession for many years. It is complete without being verbose; it is scientific without being absurdly technical, and instructive without being tiresome. It will be read and enjoyed by both student and practitioner. L. W.

_____

"**King's Medical Prescriptions**" is one of the most curious and interesting books that can be found in any physician's library. It is a selection of the famous prescriptions of prominent doctors, from Sydenham down to the present day. Good for reference and also makes an attractive and profitable present to physicians to whom you would like to tender a remembrance. Large type, 350 pages. Cloth,

$1.00. Paper covers, 50 cents, postpaid. Practical Science Co., 14 Dutch Street, New York.

"**The Physicians' Visiting List**" for 1908 has been issued by P. Blakiston's Son & Co. for the fifty-seventh year of its publication. The dose-table has been revised in accordance with the new U. S. Pharmacopeia. The contents, as usual, contains practical matter, such a table for calculating the period of utero-gestation, table of signs, treatment of poisoning, and other matter necessary to have always at hand. This little book is well known and popular with the profession. The price is only $1.00.

So great has been the demand the W. B. Saunders Company, the medical publishers of Philadelphia and London, have found it necessary to issue another revised edition of their illustrated catalogue of medical and surgical books. In looking through the copy we have received, we find that since the issuance of the last edition six months ago, the publishers have placed on the market some twenty-five new books and new editions—truly an indication of publishing activity. The colored insert plate from Keen's new Surgery, which enhanced the value of the former edition, has been replaced by a new one from the second volume of the same work, and this alone gives the catalogue a real value. A copy will be sent to any physician upon request.

COLLEGE AND SOCIETY NOTICES.

Sigma Theta Notes.

Fellows, your fraternity extends to you greeting, and wishes you *all* the prosperity which you so well merit.

Sigma Theta is in a flourishing condition, and possesses that same fraternal spirit which has ever characterized its existence.

With the dawning of the new year let it ever be uppermost in our minds to follow out that line of life laid down within our walls, for by carrying out the precepts here enjoined we will become useful members of the medical profession and ornaments to society at large.

During our leisure moments let us keep in touch with our fraternity, and by so doing we will keep in touch with one another.

Regarding the future, the sun is already upon the horizon, and the meridian not far distant.

As we all know, the bulwarks of our fraternalship were weakened at the close of the session of 1907. This temporary weakness must be overcome, and to do this we must have material. The forest has been earched far and wide, and with success, we have selected four trees; from these trees we hope to obtain the necessary Sigma Theta timber with which to make this repair.

As a parting word, we will remind the fellows that the characteristic Sigma Theta spirit, when once imbued, is ever after present; and last, but not least, let us always do unto our fellow-man as we would have him do unto us.   SCHANTZ.

Kentucky Notes.

I have the following to report:

Organization of State Auxiliary Medical Societies, which are to meet annually or oftener if necessity demands.

Officers of the Eastern Eclectic Medical Association, November 7, 1907, at Fullerton, Ky.: G. W. McGinnis, M.D., Hoods, President; M. W. Meadows, M.D., Fullerton, Secretary.

Officers of the Central Kentucky Eclectic Medical Association, November 18 and 19, 1907, at Salt Lick: L. F. Robbins, M.D., President; T. A. E. Evans, M.D., Farmers, Secretary.

I was present at both of the above two.

Officers of the Western Kentucky Eclectic Medical Association, Mayfield, November 14, 1907: G. T. Fuller, M.D., President; R. T. Rudd, M.D., Fulton, Secretary.

A fair attendance was had at each one, and everything was in good order. Some new members were obtained for the State Association.

Our State meeting in May, 1908, promises to be the best we have ever had. With the three above auxiliary to the State, it will afford opportunity for our men to attend their own, and will feel less like paying any attention to the opposition.

The object being the betterment of medical education, and antagonize none.   Yours respectfully,
            LEE STRAUSE.

PERSONALS.

Drs. Herbert & Florence Truax are conducting a new medical and surgical sanitarium at 497 Cherokee Avenue (Grant Hill), Atlanta, Ga., and are doing well.

As noted in a former issue of the JOURNAL, Dr. M. H. Hennel, formerly of Coshocton, O., and a prominent member of the Ohio Society, is now located at Asheville, N. C., where he expects to do a general business, making a specialty of pulmonary cases. Dr. Hennel is in a location with seventy-five other physicians, and, being the only Eclectic, the editor hopes that his many Ohio friends will send some of their pulmonary cases to Asheville rather than the West.

THE ECLECTIC NEWS

A MONTHLY NEWSPAPER

No. 3.   MARCH, 1908.   Vol. XIII.

BOOK NOTICES.

Essentials of Medical Gynecology. By A. F. Stephens, M.D., Professor of Medical Gynecology in the American Medical College, St. Louis, Mo. 12mo., 428 pp. Fully illustrated. Cloth, $3.00. Scudder Brothers Co., Publishers, Cincinnati, O.

Professor Stephens has given us a new book on medical gynecology, which is creating quite a flurry in medical circles. The idea that diseases of the reproductive organs of women can be cured without the use of the knife is so strange to many physicians that in instances they have developed strong symptoms of hysteria. It is the belief of Professor Stephens as well as myself, that more than one-half of the cases of gynecological surgery are done without any definite idea of what the conditions really are, and that such operations are wholly unnecessary. A very large per cent. of the ills of women come directly from a simple congestion, and the right medicinal agents administered under the direction of a trained intellect will remove its hidden cause, and she gets well. It is a blot on the high standard of medicine to see the physician start to whetting his knives when he spies a lady entering his office. Of course, there are many cases where the knife is the only hope, and here the writer says so, and does not mislead the reader by advising the use of medicines where he knows the remedies will do no good.

This subject has been woefully neglected, and this book should appeal to every physician in our broad domain. The unsexing of our women has gone too far, and should never be sanctioned by the physician unless it be as the last resort. I have known Professor Stephens for the last twenty-five years. He was a good student when we sat together at the old E. M. I. in the early eighties. He is still a good student, a close observer, a good thinker, a good writer, a good lecturer, and a good fellow. His hat is not too tight on his head, nor has he ever suffered an attack of intellectual constipation. If a man knows his subject he can tell it, and this is what Professor Stephens has done. There is no conglomeration of meaningless words, but each sentence tells something, and each page tells a whole lot.

E. R. WATERHOUSE, M.D., St. Louis, Mo.

Atlas and Text-Book of Human Anatomy. Volume III, completing the work. By Prof. J. Sobotta, of Wurzburg. Edited by J. P. Mc-Murrich, Ph. D. Quarto of 342 pages, containing 297 illustrations, mostly all in colors. Philadelphia: W. B. Saunders Co. Cloth, $6.00 net.

This volume, the third, completes this sumptuous collection of anatomical plates, with descriptions, suitable for the ͺuse of the student in anatomy. For accuracy, beauty, and usefulness, these plates stand unexcelled by any work in the English tongue. The student who uses this work will thank the publishers again and again for putting it within their reach, and the authors deserve the highest credit for the contribution they have made to our working manuals on this subject. This volume covers a portion of the circulatory system, the lymphatics, the central nervous system, and the organs of sense. The plates on the brain and nervous system are marvels of beauty and helpfulness, and alone are worth the price of the volume. To see this work is to purchase it.   ―――――――   H. W. F.

Progressive Medicine. Vol. IX, No. 4—Quarterly Digest. Edited by H. A. Hare, M.D., assisted by H. R. M. Landis, M.D. December 1, 1907. Lea Brothers & Co., Philadelphia. $6.00 per annum.

The fourth number of Progressive Medicine for 1907 covers the advances, discoveries and improvements in medical and surgical lines gathered from a vast field of book and journalistic literature. This number contains Diseases of the Digestive Tract and Allied Organs, the Liver and Pancreas, by J. Dutton Steele, M.D.; Diseases of the Kidneys, by John Rose Bradford, M.D.; Surgery of the Extremities, Fractures, Dislocations, Tumors, Surgery of Joints, Shock, Anesthesia, and Infections, by Joseph C. Bloodgood, M.D.; Genito-Urinary Diseases, by William T. Belfield, M.D., and Practical Therapeutic Referendum, by H. R. M. Landis, M.D. These volumes are of inestimable value for present use, and will be consulted for years to come as containing the cream of medical and surgical literature of the years of which they treat.   H. W. F.

Syphilis in its Medical, Medico-Legal and Sociological Aspects. By A. Ravogli, M.D., Professor of Dermatology and Syphilology in the Medical College of Ohio ; Dermatologist to City Hospital of Cincinnati ; member of the Ohio State Board Medical Registration and Examination ; 8vo. cloth, $5.00. The Grafton Press, New York.

The author of this most excellent work has an international reputation as a dermatologist, and his experience in the clinics of the Medical Colleges of Ohio gives Professor Ravogli the undisputed right to treat upon the subjects set forth in this admirable work in a masterly way, which is manifest throughout the volume of over 500 pages, forcefully backed by the best authorities on the subject in the new and old world. The book is well illustrated with photo-engravings, and gives marked evidence of high art of the publishers. We bespeak for Prof. Ravogli and the publishers great success for this up-to-date book. L. E. R.

A Text-Book of Practical Gynecology. For Practitioners and Students. By D. Tod Gilliam, M.D. Revised Edition. Illustrated ; 642 Royal Octavo pages. Cloth $4.50, net. Subscription. F. A. Davis Co., Publishers, Philadelphia.

This work on gynecology covers the subject most conclusively and practically. The text is complete, but not irksome as to details ; the illustrations really illustrate, and we consider them the most valuable part of the work. The chapters on examinations and differential diagnosis are especially valuable, and ought to be worth many times the cost of the volume. The author also dwells at some length on the preparation of the patient for operation, subsequent treatment and diet-making is especially useful to the man whose hospital experience has been limited. In short, we have only praise to offer for the work, and consider it invaluable not only to the student, but to the general practitioner and gynecologist as well. V. P. W.

Infectious and Parasitic Diseases, Including Their Cause and Manner of Transmission. By M. Langfield, M. B. Illustrated. Cloth, $1.25. Philadelphia : P. Blakiston's Son & Co.

This little book is an introduction to the study of bacteriology, and should be in the hands of that large class of practitioners who, though interested in this subject, have had no practical training in it. The author's style is clear and simple, and written in such a fascinating manner that one's attention is held to the subject to the end, and one feels sorry when he comes to the last page. This little work is a gem, and will undoubtedly stimulate the reader to further study in the field of bacteriology. THOMAS.

Pharmacology and Therapeutics. By R. W. Wilcox, M.D. Seventh Edition, Revised. With index of Symptoms and Diseases. This is a companion book to the author's " Materia Medica and Pharmacy." Price, $3.00. Philadelphia : P. Blakiston's Son & Co.

Full attention is given to pharmaceutical processes, to the various kinds of preparations, their dosage, and to the art of prescribing. It is believed that the substance first should be learned and then its uses. In the volume before us the classification is based upon the particular physiological systems upon which the various agents principally act ; there are elaborate accounts of their pharmacological action and their therapeutic, and in these descriptions the latest views of the highest authorities in these departments are presented in an effort to make the book practically usefnl. While as a whole the work is much better than the usual work on the subject, from an Eclectic standpoint the advice as to the giving of a medicament is too general. w. e. b.

The Compend of Surgery. For Students and Physicians. Including minor surgery and a complete section on bandaging. By Orville Horwitz, M.D. Cloth, $1.00. P. Blakiston's Son & Co., Philadelphia.

This new (sixth) edition, containing 334 pages with 195 illustrations, at $1.00 per volumes, enables every practitioner and medical student to make an investment worth one hundred cents, and then some, as the compend touches topics used by the various State boards in formulating their examination questions, and suggests the latest researches on medical and surgical subjects. The book is a handy reference for the surgeon who wishes to glance for a moment at surgical problems. ———————— L, E. R.

Surgical Applied Anatomy. By F. Treves, F.R.C.S. Revised by A. Keith, M.D. 12mo., 640 pp. Cloth, $2.25. Lea & Febiger, Philadelphia.

A most pleasing and practical little volume, in which the study of applied anatomy is presented in a manner as interesting and entertaining as a work of fiction. To the beginner of the study of anatomy it commends itself as a collateral text-book, to give him a selective ability as to the parts of the systemic treatise upon which he should spend especial effort, and especially to the advanced student who desires a review of anatomy in connection with his study of surgery, or when reviewing for examination ; and likewise to the busy practitioner, whose time may be limited, and who, perhaps, has allowed himself to forget, so that he is required to " brush up " a little, this book is a valuable asset.

B. V. H.

The Practitioner's Visiting List for 1908.

An invaluable pocket-sized book containing memoranda and data important for every physician, and ruled blanks for recording every detail of practice. The Weekly, Monthly and 30-Patient Perpetual contain 32 pages of data, and 160 pages of classified blanks. The 60-Patient Perpetual consists of 256 pages of blanks alone. Each in one wallet-shaped book, bound in flexible leather, with flap and pocket, pencil and rubber, and calendar for two years. Price by mail, postpaid to any address, $1.25. Thumb-letter index, 25 cents extra. Descriptive circular showing the several styles sent on request. Lea Brothers & Co., Publishers, Philadelphia and New York.

COLLEGE AND SOCIETY NOTES.

Calendar of Society Meetings.

NATIONAL ECLECTIC MEDICAL ASSOCIATION. President, L. A. Perce, Long Beach, Cali.; Recording Secretary, William P. Best, 2218 East Tenth Street, Indianapolis, Ind. Meets at Kansas City, Mo., June 17–20, 1908.

ARKANSAS. President, W. C. Dallenbaugh, Pine Bluff; Secretary, T. J. Daniel, Magazine. Next meeting at Eureka Springs, June 12–13, 190S.

CALIFORNIA. President, F. J. Petersen, Lompoc; Secretary, J. Park Dougall, Douglass Bldg, Los Angeles. Meets at San Francisco, May 19–21, 1908.

CONNECTICUT. President, J. W. Fyfe, Saugatuck; Secretary, G. A. Faber, Waterbury. Next meeting at Hartford, May 12, 190S,

GEORGIA. President, J. F. Owens, Hahira; Secretary, George A. Doss, Atlanta. Next meeting at Atlanta, May, 1908.

ILLINOIS. President, C. H. Merritt, Alton; Secretary, W. E. Kinnett, Peoria. Next meeting at Chicago, May 20–22, 1908.

INDIANA. President, A. E. Teague, Indianapolis; Secretary, E. B. Shewman, Waymansville. Next meeting at Indianapolis, May 26-27, 1908.

IOWA. Secretary, E. H. Wiley, Des Moines. Next meeting at Muscatine, May, 1908.

KANSAS. President, E. B. Packer, Osage City; Secretary, F. P. Hatfield, Grenola. Next meeting at Kansas City, June 15, 1908.

KENTUCKY. President, J. J. Morrill, Otter Pond; Secretary, Lee Strouse, Covington. Meets at Louisville, May 13-14, 1908.

MASSACHUSETTS. Secretary, Pitts E. Howes, Boston. Next meeting at Boston, June 4-5, 1908.

MAINE. President, Sylvania A. Abbott, Taunton, Mass.; Secretary, H. Reny, Biddeford. Next meeting at Preble House, Portland, May 26, 1908.

MICHIGAN. President, J. E. G. Waddington, Detroit; Secretary, F. B. Crowell, Lawrence. Next meeting at Detroit, June 3-4, 1908.

MISSOURI. President, J. T. McClanahan, Boonville; Secretary, E. F. Cook, 710 Felix Street, St. Joseph. Next meeting at Kansas City, June 15-16, 1908.

NEBRASKA. President, E. J. Latta, Kenesaw; Secretary, S. J. Stewart, Beatrice. Next meeting at Lincoln, May 5-7, 1908.

NEW ENGLAND. President, G. A. Faber, Waterbury, Conn.; Secretary, S. A. Abbott, Taunton, Mass. Next meeting Keene, N. H., May 27-28, 1908.

NEW YORK. President, J. W. Thompson, New York City; Secretary, Earl H. King, Saratoga Springs. Next meeting at Albany, March 4-5, 1908.

OKLAHOMA. President, J. F. Son, Ardmore; Secretary, E. G. Sharp, Guthrie. Next meeting at Oklahoma City, May 14-15, 1908.

OHIO. President, A. S. McKitrick, Kenton; Secretary, W. N. Mundy, Forest. Next meeting at Dayton, May 5-7, 1908.

PENNSYLVANIA. President, C. J. Hemminger, Rockwood; Secretary, Kimmel Rauch, Johnstown. Next meeting at ———.

SOUTH DAKOTA. President, W. P. Collins, Howard; Secretary, W. E. Daniels, Madison. Next meeting at ———.

TENNESSEE. President, B. D. Austin, Rome; Secretary, B. L. Simmons, Granville. Next meeting at Nashville, May 19-20, 1908.

TEXAS. President, G. W. Johnson, San Antonio; Secretary, L. S. Downs, Galveston. Next meeting at Dallas, October, 1908.

VERMONT. President, J. B. H. Cushman, East Charleston, Secretary, P. L. Templeton, Monpelier. Next meeting at State House, Montpelier, June 3-4, 1908.

WEST VIRGINIA. President, George R. Miller, Amos; Secretary, J. A. Monroe, Wheeling. Next meeting at Clarksburg, May 5-6, 1908.

WISCONSIN. President, A. A. Duclos, Milwaukee; Secretary, J. V. Stevens, Jefferson. Next meeting at Devil's Lake, May 25-26, 1908.

National Association Bulletin for March.

The National Association Bulletin, which was mailed early in the year, was addressed to every Eclectic whose name and address could be obtained. We are more than satisfied with the good it did, which, according to all indications, more than justifies the effort and expense. We are pleased to note that many "take notice," and since have been giving evidence of arousing to action.

We are pleased to note the efforts being made by the Missouri Eclectics to insure the National Association not only a welcome to Kansas City, but to start the enthusiasm with a two-day meeting of the sister States in joint session on Monday and Tuesday, June 15-16.

They promise to make our meeting a rousing success, and to "shake the bushes" all over the West to bring out every available man. The National Executive Committee has arranged to waive the use of Tuesday, June 16, on which date our meeting should open, in favor of the joint meeting of Missouri and Kansas. The National Association will convene promptly at 9 : 30 A.M. on Wednesday, June 17, and continue in session until and including Saturday.

Our headquarters will be at the *Midland*, one of the best hostelries anywhere in the West. The rates will be such as to accommodate any and all. Dr. J. T. McClanahan, the hustling President of the Missouri Eclectic Medical Society, and now serving for his sixth term, writes : "Rates will be $1.00 and up, per day, European. Fine cafés in the hotel and near by. Rooms all over the house will be $1.00 ; single rooms with bath, $1.50 and $2.00 ; double rooms and bath, $2.50 and $3.00.

We regret to announce that the Transactions have been much delayed in appearing, and we trust you will pardon us for mentioning it, but this need not occur again if the members will remember that their MSS. should be in the hands of the Secretary not later than twenty days after the adjournment of the annual meeting.

We trust our people will awaken, and recollect that we stand for the only strictly original and truly American practice of medicine. To quote from the *Harbinger*, January, 1908, page 162 : "When we go into history and trace the evolution of medicine, we note that Regularism as well as Homeopathy, are of European origin, while Eclecticism is purely American, being endowed with American ideas of freedom and liberality, so characteristic of American principles, and as we ponder our wonder grows as to why American-born citizens should cultivate and foster a hatred to the advance of American therapeutics and medicine.'

The work being done by the Council of Education and the Committee on Organization and Legislation cannot but elicit praise and commendation when they make their reports at the coming meeting.

The President will soon announce the names of the section officers, and we trust all members will promptly reply to requests for essays for the next meeting. Do not forget the importance of an immediate reply, and of having your MSS. type-written and ready whether you attend the meeting or not.   Very fraternally,

WILLIAM P. BEST, Secretary, Indianapolis.

T. A. E. Notes.

The year 1908 sees the T. A. E. Fraternity rising in power. We have, with the aid of staunch Eclectics, succeeded in establishing chapters in the American Medical College of St. Louis, and in the Kansas City Eclectic University of Kansas City, Kas.

To Bro. D. E. Bronson, '06, is due the honor of establishing and installing Zeta Chapter in the Kansas City Eclectic University. This chapter begins with the following charter members: N. L. Johnson, T. B. Young, E. L. Hobson, J. F. Cave, S. G. Boyce, S. C. Hutton, W. S. Hord, D. B. Craig, H. E. Snyder, W. E. Hare, C. O. Hoover. This chapter was installed January 9, 1908, and is growing fast.

Bro. H. H. Helbing, Secretary of the National Eclectic Association, aided us very materially in establishing the Epsilon Chapter in the St. Louis American Medical College. This chapter, consisting of twenty charter members, was installed by Bro. C. C. Hamilton, January 24, 1908, with the following officers at their various stations: W. T. Burdick, E. A.; M. C. Kimball, D. E. A.; S. F. Freeman, Prel.; W. Kelley, M. of E.; G. C. Wallace, Scribe; E. C, Rohrbach, Chron.; W. E. Aubuchon, M. G.; G. O. Wilhite, C.T.; W. G.Wood, I. W.; and R. E. Scott, O. W.   Bro. Hamilton reports this chapter as very enthusiastic in its work, and speaks highly of his entertainment while in St. Louis: W. D. DYER, Chronicler.

E. P. Notes.

We have forty-five members in college at present. Twenty-four have been added to our number this year.

They are of unquestionable character and the kind of material that is needed to carry on the work you so well planned.

There never was a more brotherly feeling, interesting meetings, or higher average of attendance than this year.

The annual banquet of the E. P.'s will be held on or about March 27, and will be up to the usual standard.

Bro. William York, '07, is located at Williamson, W. Va.

Bro. Sponseller, '07, is located at Sycamore, O. He recently brought two patients to the hospital for operation.

Bro. Hartwig, '07, Anthem, W. Va., gives us a very vivid picture of a country doctor.

The Eclectic Phylomatheans are still alive and kicking.

Brothers, listen ! The work you left to be done has been most accomplished. The degree work (thanks to Bros. Rank, Swanson and others) has been perfected and the candidate who ventures to "ride" the E. P. "goat" in the future will surely be entertained by His Majesty in a most becoming manner. Our plans now are to establish chapters in other Eclectic colleges. The propaganda work will commence next year.   A. C. LAMBERT.

Sigma Theta Notes.

Old Father Time does not tarry, but constantly adds year after year to our ever-increasing age; therefore, let us improve present opportunities, for money can be replaced, but time never; let us not idle it away, our very existence depends upon it. When we look into the past we were basking in the sunshine of spring, while now with most of us the summer is nearly over and fall is approaching, and yonder, not very distant, we can discern grim old winter looming up, slowly, 'tis true, but with a step so firm that he cannot be denied. Our alma mater also soon will have added another to her many years of usefulness.

The fellows who are not engaged in life's battle deserve considerable credit for the success they have achieved in the cause of Eclecticism, and we have every reason to feel satisfied that the fellows at present being prepared in the old E. M. I. will with willing hands take up the share of work allotted to them and do credit to the cause. Let us ever be true to our precepts, and success must attend us in our various walks of life.

Fellows! it becomes our duty to inform you that Fellow D. E. Morgan, '08' recently surprised us by taking unto himself a wife. Congratulations are in order. We will add that a committee of '08 congratulated D. E. in due form.

With a feeling of pleasure we learned of the installation of a chapter at St. Louis by the T. A. E. Fraternity. We are always pleased to hear of progress along this line, and tender our hearty and sincere congratulations to Tau Alpha Epsilon.   SCHANTZ.

At the December meeting of the Cincinnati Homeopathic Lyceum Prof. Bloyer was an invited guest, and read a paper on "Materia Medica," which was highly commended, Dr. Geoghegan remarking that it "expressed a healthy, optimistic view as to the use of medicines."

The Board of Medical Registration and Examination of Ohio at its recent meeting elected the following officers : President, A. Ravogli, Cincinnati ; Vice-President, S. M. Sherman, Columbus ; Treasurer, E. J. Wilson, Columbus ; Secretary, George H. Matson, re-appointed. Twenty-three out of twenty-seven applicants passed the examination for regular practice, and one in three of Osteopaths failed to pass.

PERSONALS.

Location in Ohio town of 500, on Big Four Railroad ; modern nine-room house, four-room office, large barn ; designed for physician. For particulars address Forest B. Dowell, Prospect, O. (son of Dr. Dowell, E. M. I., 1894, deceased.

The *Chicago Medical Times* is now under the editorial management of Dr. J. S. Horovitz, and is published at 412 Fulton Street, Chicago. The subscription price has been increased from $1.00 to $1.50 per year. The size of the journal has also been enlarged and divided into various departments; that of medicine and therapeutics will be in charge of Drs. Graves and Pollock ; surgery and obstetrics under Drs. Robertson and Bushnell ; dermatology and genito-urinary under Drs. Latimer and Winne.

The physicians of Virginia are demanding that the license tax on physicians shall be repealed. There are some 2,700 doctors in the State, and they pay something like $10 each. They contend that no other State exacts a tax from physicians, and that they should not be required to pay the tax.

Good country location. Am retiring from practice. For particulars address, with stamp, Dr. W· H. Mahoney, Alhambra, Texas.

A good location ; practice worth $1,800 to $2,500 ; fifteen miles from Cincinnati ; will sell house and lot ; want to leave and go to California on account of family's health. Address Dr. C. W. Silver, Mt. Carmel, O.

Good country location in Kentucky. For particulars address Dr. L. J. Poe, Butler, Ky.

Two country locations in Southern Ohio. For particulars address Dr. W. E. Bloyer, Lancaster Building, Cincinnati, O.

The first commencement exercises of the new Seton Hospital Training School for Nurses took place February 14, with appropriate exercises. Miss M. E. Redmond received her diploma after the completion of a three years' course. She will locate at 220 Dorchester Avenue, Mt. Auburn. Tel. N 2441 L. THE JOURNAL wishes Miss Redmond every success in her chosen profession.

Dr. George M. Gould has resigned the editorship of *American Medicine*, which has been sold to New York parties. As a parting shot, he has lately written an extensive article on medical colleges, advocating the preservation of the small, independent colleges as against the university medical school wielded by politics. Incidentally, he advocates the reading of State medical journals as a remedy for *insomnia*.

OBITUARY.

Dr. Theodore F. Scott, E. M. I., '91, Lynchburg, Ohio, January 29. He was a member of the Ohio State Society.

Jos. G. Pierce, E. M. I., '83, at Sebastopol, Cal., December 21, aged seventy-three.

Peter Shaw, Philadelphia, '86, at Mt. Bethel, Pa., December 24, aged fifty-eight.

Edward D. Messenger, Bennett, '87, a veteran of the Civil War, at Chicago, January 8.

F. C. Semolroth, Bennet, '73, at Walnut Grove, Ill., January 8, aged seventy.

Robert G. Gahrer, New York, '70, at Brooklyn, January 13, aged sixty-three.

James B. Hayes, St. Louis, '78, at Carrollton, Ill., January 15, aged sixty-three.

J. W. Thomas, California, '81, at Weeping Water, Neb., January 16, aged sixty-five.

Ira F. Cameron, E. M. I., '76, at Keswick, Iowa, January 14, aged sixty.

B. F. Baird, Memphis Bot., '67, at Vildo, Tenn., January 22, aged seventy-one.

James B. Hudson, E. M. I., '70, at Lafayette, Ind., January 20, aged seventy-one.

Harvey D. Williams, Bennett, '80, at Kansas City, Kas., January 17, aged seventy-eight.

P. VonLackum was born in Germany, March 28, 1842, and died from cerebral hemorrhage, in Council Bluffs, Iowa, January 19. He graduated in medicine from the Physio-Medical College, in Cincinnati, Ohio, 1869. From this time he carried on a successful practice in Minnesota and Iowa until the fall of 1888, when he located in Omaha, Neb., where he enjoyed a large and successful practice until his death.

READING NOTICE.

Eliminative Treatment.

It cannot be denied that faulty elimination of the products of metabolism is a common predisposing cause of disease. Such cases, regardless of name, are promptly relieved by stimulating elimination through the kidneys. There is no better renal eliminant than Alkalithia.

THE ECLECTIC NEWS

A MONTHLY NEWSPAPER

| No. 4. | APRIL, 1908. | Vol. XIII. |

BOOK NOTICES.

The Eclectic Practice of Medicine. By Rolla L. Thomas, M.D., Professor of the Principles and Practice of Medicine in the Eclectic Medical Institute, Cincinnati, O.; Consulting Physician to the Seton Hospital. Second edition, 1908, Illustrated with two lithographs in in colors; six color prints and fifty-seven figures in black; 8vo., 1033 pages. Price, cloth. $6.00; sheep, $7,00. The Scudder Brothers Company, publishers, No. 1009 Plum Street, Cincinnati, O.

One of the standing needs of the Eclectic school is adequate representation in medical literature. We welcome the second edition of the Eclectic Practice of Medicine, by Dr. Rolla L. Thomas, of the Eclectic Medical Institute of Cincinnati, because it fills a real need, and because the thorough and scientific manner in which the book is written and the excellent workmanship it represents in typography reflects credit not only upon its author and publishers, but upon Eclecticism as a school.

This is a work that will even stand the test of those hypercritical judges who look with disdain upon Eclecticism for some reason or other. Physicians of all schools who are losing faith in the efficacy of medicinal therapy should purchase Thomas' text-book to correct their pessimism and increase their efficiency. Those who are prejudiced against Eclecticism as a school of medical practice will have their prejudices dispelled in two minutes by a perusal of the two-page preface to the work, and will thus be placed in the right mental attitude to profit by the wealth of information condensed in its thousand pages.

It has been said that the chapter on typhoid fever is characteristic of every text-book on practice, as it usually reflects the qualities and deficiences of such work. If that be so, and if practical features are what count in a text-book, the author of this Eclectic work should be proud of his accomplishment. The Scudder Brother Company is also to be congratulated for the excellent form in which they have gotten out the work.—Editorial *Chicago Medical Times*, February, 1908.

Essentials of Medical Gynecology. By A. F. Stephens, M.D., Professor of Medical Gynecology in the American Medical College, St. Louis, Mo. 12mo., 428 pp. Fully illustrated. Cloth, $3.00. The Scudder Brothers Company, Publishers, Cincinnati, Ohio.

It has been a privilege and an opportunity to have my attention drawn to this book. It is not large or expensive, but on account of its clear, concise and methodic presentation of subjects contained it is unusually comprehensive on medical gynecology. It is needless to say the text is correct. The first chapter treats of the remedies indicated, and of their specific medication. He who has not used the specific administration of medicines does not realize what he loses, and how much can be gained by their judicious selection. Medicines prepared from fresh, pure drugs, and in a concentrated form, in small doses, representing the active ingredients of the drug, free from inert useless constituents, are a great desideratum; unfortunately, not generally appreciated. Here they are referred to for medical gynecological use. We are pleased with this work, and can cheerfully recommend its purchase.   CHAUNCEY D. PALMER, M.D.,

Emeritus Professor of Obstetrics, Gynecology and Clinical Gynecology in Medical College of Ohio, Cincinnati.

_____

The Treatment of Fractures. With notes on a few common dislocations. By Charles L. Scudder, M.D., of Boston. Octavo, 600 pp. Illustrated. Cloth, $5.50. W. B. Saunders Co., Philadelphia, Pa.

This work has been standard for several years. Has been revised eight times and is probably in the libraries of a majority of the medical men of this country. It doubtless also has had a large sale abroad. The author is Surgeon to the Massachusetts General Hospital and Lecturer on Surgery in the Harvard College Medical School. With such sponsors it will hardly be expected that any one will have the· hardihood to say ought but praise in review of it.

Careful examination justifies in most respects the strong hold that it has on the good opinion of the profession. It is especially gratifying to note the importance assigned to massage in treatment, and the emphasis given to the necessity of frequent inspection and re-dressing, lest the soft tissues suffer from compression and impaired circulation. It seems to be taken for granted that every physician understands the effect of massage, and how to apply it. It is to be hoped this confidence is well founded. One is led to think that, in revising, too much of the old treatment is retained, with rather scant acknowledgement of newer and better methods.

A disposition to rely upon force in adjusting and maintaining adjustment, increasing the force to any extent in unyielding cases, which has always characterized bone surgery, is still manifest. This is shown in the author's treatment of Colles' fracture, to which he devotes no less than sixteen pages and twenty-six illustrations. We are told that "very great force is needed to accomplish satisfactory reduction of impacted fractures." Anesthesia is advised, and he claims "it is because of the use of too little force that often a slight bony deformity remains after union." It is easy to see that the method of adjusting advised must require very great force, and, at that, will often fail, even if supplemented by pads fore and aft.

On page 263 of the 1906 JOURNAL a treatment of this fracture is given that requires no anesthetic, only a moderate degree of force, no retentive pads, and with or without a single light pasteboard splint, results in recovery in three weeks, with no bony deformity.

The mechanism and pathology of fractures are very clearly presented, and it must be considered authoritative in most respects for a considerable time yet.　　　　——————　　　　w. b. c.

Transactions of the National Eclectic Medical Association. Volume xxxv, 8vo, 348 pp., cloth. Edited by the the Secretary, Dr. William P. Best, Indianapolis, Ind.

We are in receipt of the annual volume of the Transactions, which has been delayed owing to the late receipt of several papers and essays. This volume contains a frontispiece of ex-President Stevenson, and includes the proceedings of the thirty-seventh annual meeting, held at Los Angeles, Cal., June 18–21, 1907, together with the addresses, papers and reports. This volume is the equal of its predecessors in the character of its papers and discussions; but we do not believe it compares favorably with those of several of our State societies, owing to the fact that the various chairmen of sections do not have sufficient control of the papers presented. An improvement should be made in this direction, which would greatly increase the value of these annual volumes.

——————

Surgery: Its Principles and Practice. In five volumes. By sixty-six eminent surgeons. Edited by W. W. Keen, M.D. Volume III. Octavo of 1132 pages, with 562 text-illustations. Philadelphia: W. B. Saunders Company. Per volume, cloth, $7.00.

Close scrutiny will reveal new and important matter in each chapter of this third volume to fully justify the addition of this great work to the very numerous surgeries already in use.

The every-day physician will perhaps maintain that in some instances too ready resort is had to surgery, when non-surgical treatment might have been effective. For instance, one might well shrink from the extensive neurectomies advised for the treatment of spasmodic wry-neck, and continue to apply remedial and medical measures, which have proved effectual in many cases. In the chapter devoted to the nose and its accessory sinuses, timely and highly important consideration to the sinuses is given. It is notorious that in infectious diseases, especially influenza, a fatal issue is often dependent upon extension of infection and inflammation to the maxillary, ethmoidal and frontal sinuses, which fails to be appreciated and radically treated.

"Surgery of the Stomach," by A. W. Mayo Robson, of London, and Chapter L, "Surgery of the Liver, the Gall-Bladder, and the Biliary Ducts," by the Mayo Brothers, are beyond criticism.

On the whole. Volume III is of absorbing interest, and represents the very crest of the wave of surgical progress to date.

The completed work, in five volumes, will be in itself a very complete surgical library.   _____   W. B. C.

Thorndike's Orthopedic Surgery. Cloth, $2.50.   P. Blakiston's Son & Co., Philadelphia.

This is a most attractive little volume, as near perfection externally as internally.   It is a difficult work to review, if one is anxious to find something for adverse criticism.   The English is undefiled, and unusual pains has been taken to incorporate in the text all the latest and best ideas and methods.   It is evident that Dr. Thorndike is most fastidious and exacting, but this child of his brain ought to give him immense satisfaction.   W. B. C.

Practical Diagnosis. By H. A. Hare, M.D.   Octavo, 616 pp., illustrated.   Cloth, $4.50.   Lea Brothers & Co., Philadelphia.

The author has presented to the profession in this work a plain, intelligent, practical and strictly up-to-date method of diagnosis, one in which the general practitioner may find without loss of patience any information relative to diagnosis. The chapter on the urinary bladder and the urine, together with its microscopic and chemical examination, is very comprehensive and complete. The application of the pathological changes found in the urine and their significance in diagnosis is very instructive. The chapters on the blood and its diseases and the eye and its diseases, together with a complete and lucid explanation of the latest methods of examination, are arranged in a concise manner, and are well fitted for the use of the general practitioner. The chapter on the different varieties and the diagnostic significance and cause of cough and expectoration, and the examination of the sputum and its pathological significance, together with the chapter on vomiting and pain and their significance, are more than worth the price of the volume. The clearness with which the physiological and pathological facts are demonstrated, and the intelligent manner in which the symptoms are presented as they are met with at the bedside, make the work of especial value. In short, it is as its name implies—*a Practical Diagnosis.*   J. C. E.

Medical Diagnosis. By Charles L. Green, M.D. P. Blakiston's Son & Co., Philadelphia, Pa. Flexible leather, price, $3.50.

The subject is thoroughly covered without a redundancy of words. A commendable feature, and one that adds greatly to the value, is the system of marginal notes, by which one is able at a glance to get the important points on any subject.

One of the good things is the chapter treating of the nervous system and its diseases. Special mention is made of the necessity of examination of the eye, particularly with the ophthalmoscope, which the author says "every physician should be able to use, as it frequently proves the master-key in diagnosing obscure cerebral lesion, syphilis, tuberculosis, arterio-sclerosis and chronic nephritis." The text is here illustrated with several very fine plates, showing different conditions of the retina in the various diseases mentioned above.

Other valuable chapters are those treating of differential diagnosis, heart and blood-vessels, and urinary analysis.

The book ends with an appendix, treating of the different methods of preparing blood and bacterial specimens for microscopical examinations.   L. C. W.

The Principles and Practice of Modern Otology. By J. F. Barnhill, M.D., and E. W. Wales, M.D. Octavo of 575 pp., with 305 original illustrations. Philadelphia: W. B. Saunders Company. Cloth, $5.50 net.

This composite work on the ear, from its title, would lead one to infer that radical changes had been made in the methods of treatment, but a careful perusal does not support this idea. There is, of course, the individuality of the authors in their methods of treatment, but the general line is in the same rut that has been used for the last twenty years. In operative work, however, it is up to date, and is better in many respects than the works of a majority of the older writers.

A commendable feature of the volume is the excellence of the plates ; also the portion dealing with central or intracranial complications.

For any one wishing a comprehensive work on the ear, they will not be disappointed in this Modern Otology.   K. O. F.

Modern Medicine; Its Theory and Practice. In original contributions by American and foreign authors. Edited by William Osler, M.D. In seven octavo volumes of about 900 pages each, illustrated. Volume iii, just ready. Price per volume, cloth, $6.00 net. Lea Brothers & Co., publishers, Philadelphia.

In volume iii the grand division of Infectious Diseases is concluded and Diseases of the Respiratory Tract considered. This volume might almost be called the tuberculosis volume, since 300 of the 900 pages are devoted to this important subject. This disease, which is holding the attention of the laity as well as the medical world as no other, is treated in a most careful, interesting and exhaustive manner. The treatment may be said to be a résumé of all the best methods now in use by skilled physicians for this dreaded scourge. So valuable is this article that one will be repaid for the outlay of the entire work for this one volume.   R. L. T.

What to Do for the Stomach. By G. E. Dienst, M.D. 202 pages. Cloth, $1.00 net. Philadelphia : Boericke & Tafel.

Perhaps a thorough simon-pure homeopath may learn what to do for the stomach by a perusal of this little book, but we are willing to confess that it is too much for us. For example, "No appetite," sixty-one remedies are named, seventeen leading and forty-one lesser remedies, with no directions as to selection of the above-named remedies. The indications for the proper remedy are not specific enough for the average practitioner.   R. L. T.

Business Methods of Specialists. By J. D. Albright, M.D.; 12mo, 110 pp., cloth, $1.25. Published by the author, No. 3228 North Broad Street, Philadelphia, Pa.

This is a very interesting little book by the editor of *Albright's Office Practitioner*. It presumes to lay bare the inside workings of the advertising specialist, and shows how the advertising doctor is presumed to succeed. One lesson which the reader will soon learn from the perusal of the book is that a very great deal of their success is due to systematic business management, in which the so-called ethical physician is frequently lacking.

Elements of Homeopathy. By Dr. F. A. Boericke and E. P. Anshutz. Cloth, $1.00. Boericke & Tafel, publishers, Philadelphia.

This little work is full of meat, and will well repay the time spent in its perusal. The elements of homeopathy are clearly and concisely stated, and one may begin to test the efficacy of remedies as herein given. A book that can be of help to all careful prescribers.
                                                R. L. T.

COLLEGE AND SOCIETY NOTES.

National Association Bulletin.

Encouraging reports coming to hand from some of the section officers and the committees appointed by the Kansas City Eclectics insure the success of our coming meeting, in so far as it is possible for success to come from their efforts alone. It is now a good time to realize that your committees and officers, alone, cannot make a successful meeting, and that each individual Eclectic owes it to himself, the cause and to all concerned to be present.

The next meeting should be the best in attendance in the history of our organization, because matters of vital mportance will be up for consideration, and for this one reason the meeting will be the most important in our history.

Never in the seventy-five years of Eclecticism has the need of our system of practice been so accentuated, nor has the necessity for organized effort to meet the demands for more Eclectic practitionesr been so great. Never has the Executive Committee had to assume so much work, nor has there ever before been so much undertaken and accomplished in the interest of liberal medicine.

This is true of our cause and likewise true of the cause from the Homeopathic and Physio-Medical standpoint. The American Institute of Homeopathy meets at Kansas City, and through the President, R. S. Copeland, M.D., Ann Arbor, Michigan, has invited Dr. Perce to attend their meeting and address the members thereof on the subject of closer affiliation with them, in so far as our mutual interests are concerned. We are pleased to say, parenthetically, that this is in keeping with the policy outlined last year, and the place of meeting was selected with this in view, and the Councils of Education have worked jointly and harmoniously for the common good.

It is now only a short time until the meeting, and the officers and committees have much to accomplish before all is in readiness, and we have every reason to believe that our men will loyally support us with good attendance and active coöperation.

New and stronger State societies, new and stronger colleges, better and stronger organization, renewed interest and loyalty cannot but produce good results, and the National Association should be the general index of such.

A full list of the section officers was promised for this bulletin, but on account of unavoidable delay it will appear in the May bulletin.

Very fraternally,   WILLIAM P. BEST.

Railroad Rates to the National Association.

We were unable to obtain special reduced rates to our meeting at Kansas City on account of the two-cent law in various States. The two-cent per mile, however, is the same rate as we have heretofore obtained, and we will not be bothered with certificates. The law now, in many States, requires the payment of two cents per mile each way, while before we paid three cents one way and one cent returning.

Dr. Scudder informs me that parties of ten or more from his district can obtain a reduction of about 10 per cent. on their fares. We cannot obtain such concession from St. Louis, but you might from your district. Dr. Scudder says: The single fare from Cincinnati is $13.50, Columbus, $15.50, Pittsburg, $19.50, and Wheeling, $18.00. We can get a reduction of $1.00 each if we can get ten or more going through or from Cincinnati, and this will be my plan.'' Write him and prepare to go in a body, as this will be more enjoyable. Perhaps Dr. Howes, of Boston, can make the same arrangement. I havn't had time to obtain a reply from him since knowing of this.

H. H. HELBING, Corresponding Secretary,
1208 North Kingshighway, St. Louis, Mo.

T. A. E. Notes.

L. C. Wottring, M.D., and L. A. Hays were taken from the land of the barbarians and naturalized as Greeks, March 14. Afterward a smoker was given, and an altogether pleasant evening was spent.

The following officers were installed for the ensuing year March 28: L. W. Page, E. A.; F. C. Leeds, D. E. A.; M. C. Karr, Scribe; A. F. Burson, M. E., E. S. Haas, Prel.; H. F. Killen, Chron.; G. E. Black, C. T.; L. A. Hays, M. G.

Brother J. F. Wuist, Dayton, O., writes the fraternity, and expects to visit us soon.

Epsilon Chapter reports several new members, and among them several members of the faculty.

I wish to thank all brothers for the aid given me in my office during the past year, and ask your further continuance to our new Chronicler, H. F. Killen. W. K. DYER, Chronicler.

Notice.

The Arkansas Eclectic Medical Association will hold its annual meeting at Eureka Springs, Arkansas, June 13, 1908, at 10 A.M. Each Eclectic in the State is requested to be present at this meeting, for it promises to be one of the most interesting meetings in the history of the Association. A cordial invitation is extended to every Eclectic outside the State to be present.

W. C. DALLENBAUGH, M.D., President.
T. J. DANIEL, M.D., Secretary.

The Kentucky Society meets in the School Board Educational Rooms, 418 W. Walnut Street, Louisville, May 6 and 7, beginning at 10 A.M. Railroad tickets, one fare for round trip, can be secured on the 5th and 6th, returning on the 8th and 9th, on account of the Republican State Convention. Headquarters at Hotel Willard, $2.00 per day, American plan.

PERSONAL.

Dr. E. A. North, E. M. I., 1906, formerly of Kentucky, is now located in partnership with Dr. G. R. Cooper, at Childress, Texas.

Dr. Charles R. Campbell, E. M. I., '06, has been appointed surgeon for the Portsmouth division of the Norfolk and Western Railroad, and has also been appointed health officer of Newtown, Hamilton County, O.

Dr. Charles Camp, E. M. I., '65, died at his home in Camden, Indiana.

Lacation, at Prescott, Kan. For particulars, address Dr. J. W. Reynolds, Prescott, Kan.

Dr. J. A. Dungan has passed the Colorado Board and is now located at Greeley, Colo.

Good country location in Ohio. For particulars, address with stamp, Dr. X, care this journal.

Dr. Thomas F. Collins, E. M. I., ,04, has moved to 61 S. Jefferson Street, Newcastle, Pa. There are now two or three good locations in his neighborhood, about which he would be glad to furnish information if addressed with stamp.

Dr. Charles J. Otto, E. M. I., '05, has opened up offices at Room 294, Arcade Building, Dayton, O.

Good location in northeastern part of Ohio. Was compelled to leave on account of ill health, and offer my house and practice for sale at a bargain. Good references. For particulars, address with stamp, Dr. H. C. Spencer, Gainesville, Fla.

Wanted, a good, honest young Eclectic as assistant, one who is thoroughly familiar with specific medication. Have a good proposition for the right man as assistant, and will soon be retiring on account age. Good practice, in town of 12,500 inhabitants. For particulars, address with stamp, Lock Box 562, Bristol, Conn.

For sale—property and practice in a beautiful village of 1,200 inhabitants, in a rich farming and vineyard country. Good schools and churches. Wish to retire because of age. This is a most unusual opportunity to step into a lucrative business. To right man will sell at cost of property, and make it make it an object to purchaser, and on easy terms. For particulars, address Dr. W., care this journal.

Good country location; good business can be done from the start; nothing to sell. Am moving to a larger place. For particulars, address with stamp, Dr. G. W. Collins, Volant, Pa.

We regret to record the death of Dr. William Jean Krausi which occurred in New York City in February. Dr. Krausi was a graduate of the New York Eclectic, in 1890. He was born in Germany forty-nine years ago, and was a prominent member of the New York Eclectic Medical Society, of the College, and the New York Specific Medication Club. His funeral services were conducted by the Masonic lodge, of which he had been a member for a number of years. His wife survives him. THE JOURNAL extends sympathy to his New York friends.

READING NOTICES.

ARTERIOSCLEROSIS.—Auto-intoxication from faulty metabolism and imperfect elimination ranks with gout and lead as a cause of high blood pressure. This, in time, leads to arterio-sclerosis, cardiac hypertrophy and dilatation, mitral and aortic insufficiencies, cerebral apoplexy and retinal hemorrhage. Lowering the blood-pressure is at once a preventive and curative measure. This is best accomplished by renal eliminants, and we know of no better remedy of this class than Alkalithia.

EINHORN (*Therapeutic Gazette*, January, 1908) submits a method for investigating the functions of the intestinal tract, the principle of which is the administration of test substances with the food and observation of the effects of the digestive fluids upon these substances.
The author divides his cases of intestinal digestive disturbance into two groups :
1. Those of pure nervous intestinal dyspepsia. 2. Those of genuine intestinal dyspepsia.
In that great class of cases of intestinal dyspepsia in which the starch digestion alone is disturbed, Taka-Diastase (Takamine) has proved of especial value.

ANTIKAMNIA has also stood the test of exhaustive trial, both in clinical and regular practice, and has been proven free from the usual untoward after-effects which accompany, characterize and distinguish all other preparations of this class. Therefore antikamnia and codeine tablets afford a very desirable mode of exhibiting these two valuable drugs. The proportions are those most frequently indicated in the various neuroses of the larynx as well as the coughs incident to lung affections, grippal conditions, etc.—*The Laryngoscope*.

ANTIPHLOGISTINE AND PNEUMONIA.—In five cases of pneumonia where the acute trouble did not end in complete resolution, but left circumscribed and affected areas which, in my judgment, were doomed to caseous degeneration, the liberal and persistent use of Antiphlogistine slowly but surely caused the absorption of the abnormal patches within the lungs and left them as normal as they were prior to the pneumonitis.—H. ENTON, M.D., Brooklyn, N. Y.

CLINICAL POPULARITY.—Llewellyn Eliot, M.D., says : In irrigating these cases, we may use the solution of bichloride of mercury, carbolic acid or any other medication which individual preference may suggest ; for my part, I employ a solution of Tyree's Antiseptic Powder, which is non-poisonous.''

URETHRAL INFLAMMATION.—Usually the only treatment needed to cure urethritis is to administer Sanmetto and alkalies, with an occasional purge, and very mild injections of chloride of zinc.

Good country location, at Helena, O. Vacancy caused by death of Dr. J. M. Crismore. For particulars, address with stamp. Dr. W. E. Crismore, Helena, O.

The Eclectic News

A Monthly Newspaper

No. 5.　　　　　MAY, 1908.　　　　　Vol. XIII.

BOOK NOTICES.

Essentials of Medical Gynecology. By A. F. Stephens, M.D., Professor of Medical Gynecology in the American Medical College, St. Louis, Mo. 12mo, 428 pp. Fully illustrated. Cloth, $3. The Scudder Brothers Co., Publishers, Cincinnati, O.

The interest manifested in the non-surgical treatment of many supposedly surgical conditions indicates that the pendulum is swinging backward, for in practically every branch of medicine therapeutic measures are again given more than passing attention. In no special line of work is this tendency more noticeable than in gynecology, and the cutting age seems, for a time at least, to have passed.

Dr. Stephens' book on medical gynecology deserves the attention of the general practitioner, especially so if he makes any pretense of specializing in diseases of women.

The remedial means suggested in this work are largely taken from the Eclectic Materia Medica, although by no means exclusively so. This fact should not deter any practitioner from obtaining it, as there is nothing mysterious or difficult about it, but, on the other hand, the specific medication of the Eclectics, if properly studied and correctly applied, will be sure to prove something of a revelation to the physician unacquainted with it. We have never been therapeutic nihilists and never expect to be, but have long ago recognized the fact that accurate diagnosis of conditions (not necessarily diseases) is an essential to definite results, and that familiarity with the indications for and action of Eclectic and Homeopathic remedies is one of the best acquisitions of the old school physician.

In this work surgery is not decried when necessary, but it does much to instruct in the way of avoiding that same necessity by its sound, practical and dependable teaching on the medical side of this important subject.—Dr. J. D. Albright, in *Albright's Practitioner*.

Diseases of the Skin. By H. W. Stelwagon, M.D. Fifth revised edition. 267 illustrations. 8vo. 1135 pp. Cloth, $6.00. Saunders & Co., Philadelphia.

A thorough review of this latest edition of Stelwagon impresses one that it contains all that is new in treatment and only that which is of utility in cure. Special stress is laid on hygiene, diet and internal treatment of the various diseases, being more specific in directions and indications than in most of the works on the skin. It therefore becomes a very valuable book to the student and especially the practitioner, who will find illustrative cases to meet the types he may come in contact with. The illustrations, both in number and beauty, compare with the best atlases. There is a good deal of new material to be found in this book.   E. F.

Diseases of Genito-Urinary Organs and Kidneys. By R. H. Greene, M.D., and H. Brooks, M.D. 292 illustrations. 8 vo. 550 pp. Saunders & Co., Philadelphia. Cloth, $5.00.

This new work is very creditable to the authors and publishers. The style of the bok is attractive. A great deal of space is devoted to details of diagnosis and treatment, and the surgical as well as the medical side is considered. Illustration by clear line drawings are very helpful. Gonorrhea and its treatment are most satisfactorily presented and Bright's disease and uremia are exhibited in a manner highly instructive to the busy physician.   E. F.

Practical Fever Nursing. By Edward C. Register, M.D. Octavo, 352 pp. Philadelphia: W. B. Saunders Co. Cloth, $2.50 net.

An excellent text-book on practical fever nursing, written especially for nurses, it is a work which cannot fail to be of great value, the chapters devoted to treatment and diet being especially worthy of mention.

Sections on disease itself are important, as a nurse to intelligently care for a patient must have some knowledge of the disease.

The chapters on typhoid fever, spinal meningitis and scarlet fever are good, giving in detail the isolation, disinfection, etc.

The work as awhole is unusually clear and completely covers the field of fever nursing.   R. L. T.

The Battle Creek Sanitarium System: History, Organization and Methods. By J. H. Kellogg, M.D., Superintendent, Battle Creek, Mich.

In noticing this book we will want to say a few words concerning the work which Dr. Kellogg has been doing for the past twenty-five years. The two dominant features of the Battle Creek idea stand out in prominence. One can be covered for the sake of brevity under the word "diet;" the other under the heading "water," its uses in various ways. ' Many would call Dr. Kellogg a crank, but he is a man of many ideas. Many times you will have a patient who would do well there with its various methods, independent of medication.

Woman. A Treatise on the Normal and Pathological Emotions of Feminine Love. By Dr. Bernard S. Talmey. Cloth, 8vo., 258 pp., with 23 drawings in the text. Price, $3.00. Practitioners' Publishing Co., 55 W. 126th Street, New York.

A second edition of this somewhat unique book has been soon called for, and the author has taken the opportunity to revise and enlarge the text. The first edition received the endorsement of medical book reviewers generally, and the same can be predicted for the second. The only criticism is the rather large price for so small a book. J. K. S.

The Correction of Featural Imperfections. By C. C. Miller, M.D. Including the description of a variety of operations for improving the appearance of the face. 136 pages. 73 illustrations. $1.50. Published by the author, 70 State Street, Chicago, Ill.

In this little book the author has attempted to give the profession a concise volume on this subject. In many instances the conciseness will confuse the novice. There are many admirable features in the book, but the reviewer would suggest that the descriptive portion and illustrative portion be placed together, as often there is confusion in referring to the plates. However, for any one wishing to study this line of surgery the book will be of value. K. O. F.

Diseases of the Nose and Throat. By D. B. Kyle, M.D.; fourth edition, revised. Octavo of 725 pp., with 215 illustrations, 28 in colors. Philadelphia: W. B. Saunders Co. Cloth, $4.00 net.

This popular work on the nose and throat has been reviewed before in THE JOURNAL. Considerable of the present edition has been re-written and much new material added. The latest methods of operating are fully described, and nearly thirty new articles introduced, bringing the volume thoroughly up to date as a text-book on this subject. The author is too well known to need an introduction. It can be profitably studied by both the general practitioner and specialist. The new plates are artistic, and all the illustrations are of such a character as to make a study of the subject comparatively easy. K. O. F.

Home Practice of Medicine. By Dr. L. S. Downs, Galveston, Texas. 12mo, 80 pp. flexible leather. Price, $1.00.

This is a little manual written by Dr. Downs to instruct his patients in the use of the simpler forms of specific medication in domestic or family practice. The author will probably be open to the same criticisms that were made against Beach, King, Gunn and Scudder, in attempting to teach the simpler forms of medication direct to the laity. But he handles his subject well, and so far has given satisfaction to such of his clientèle as seem fitted for it.

--- ---

The Reward of Motherhood is Great. Julia Ward Howe tells young mothers not to undervalue it.

"I would not exaggerate even so great a blesing as that of maternity," says Julia Ward Howe in the May *Delineator*. "Every woman cannot be a mother; and many women in our days have gifts and callings which detain them far from the pains and pleasures of the nursery. Their lives may be replete with good to themselves and their community, nay, to the world at large. Heaven knows that of all women I should be the last to undervalue their labor and their reward."

Minor Surgery. E. M. Foote, M.D., D. Appleton & Co., New York.

Close study of Dr. Foote's new book shows it to be one that is abreast of the times. Every practitioner treats minor surgical cases, and many times they are the least scientifically cared for of any of his patients. Bad results often follow simply because he has neglected to inform himself as to the best methods of caring for these cases in use at the present time. For the sake of the "other fellow" he should possess a good text-book detailing the care of just such cases, and this is one of the good ones. B. V. H.

Bound JOURNALS.—Bound JOURNALS of 1907 are now ready for shipment. We can furnish nearly all the bound JOURNALS from 1890 to 1905 in half-sheep binding, prepaid, for $2.00 each. Where subscribers will send in unbound JOURNALS, we will return the bound JOURNAL for $1.00 postpaid. We have the years 1906 and 1907 bound in green buckram cloth, $2.00 postpaid, or in exchange for unbound JOURNALS, 75 cents each.

We are in receipt of the February issue of the *Bloodless Phlebotomist*, which is a little twenty-four page pamphlet gotten out in the interest of Antiphlogistine. It will be sent free on request to any of our readers by addressing The Denver Chemical Manufacturing Company. 57 Laight Street, New York City.

COLLEGE AND SOCIETY NOTES.

National Bulletin for May.

SECTION OFFICERS.

Section on Specific Diagnosis and Specific Medication—Chairman, J. P. Harvill, M.D., Nashville, Tenn.; Secretary, J. M. Keys, M.D., Omaha, Neb.

Section on Practice of Medicine—Chairman, C. E. Pace, M.D., Osawatomie, Kan.; Secretary, Pearl Hale-Tatman, M.D., Eureka Springs, Ark.

Section on Materia Medica and Therapeutics—Chairman, Finley Ellingwood, M.D., Chicago, Ill.; Secretary, Mary B. Morey, M.D., Gonzales, Tex.

Section on Pediatrics—Chairman, E. H. Stevenson, M.D., Fort Smith, Ark.; Secretary, Hanna Scott Turner, M.D., Pomona, Cal.

Section on Gynecology—Chairman, O. C. Welbourne, M.D., Los Angeles, Cal.; Secretary, A. F. Stephens, M. D., St. Louis, Mo.

Section on Dermatology and Syphilology—Chairman, J. V. Stevens, M.D., Jefferson, Wis.; Secretary, J. S. Stewart, M.D., Hastings, Neb.

Section on Electro-Therapeutics—Chairman, R. P. Rudd, M.D., Fulton, Ky.; Secretary, J. R. Spencer, M.D., Cincinnati, O.

Section on Ophthalmology, Rhinology, Otology and Laryngology—Chairman, J. P. Harbert, M.D., Bellefontaine, O.; Secretary, A. H. Reading, M.D., Chicago, Ill.

Section on Surgery—Chairman, H. H. Brockman, M.D., Eldon, Mo.; Secretary, C. E. Laws, M.D., Fort Smith, Ark.

Section on Obstetrics—Chairman, P. C. Clayberg, M.D., St. Louis, Mo.; Secretary, J. A. Archer, M.D., Grenola, Kan.

Section on Pathological and Bacteriological Research—Chairman, J. D. Robertson, M.D., Chicago, Ill.; Secretary, Lyman Watkins, M.D., Blanchester, O.

Section on Genito-Urinary Diseases—Chairman, A. P. Hauss, M.D., New Albany, Ind.; Secretary, G. Adolphus, M.D., Atlanta, Ga.

Section on Orthopedic Surgery—Chairman, Lee Strouse, M.D., Covington, Ky.; Secretary, J. C. Mitchell, M.D., Louisville, Ky.

Section on Neurology—Chairman, C. W. Brandenburg, M.D., New York, N. Y.; Secretary, S. B. Pratt, M.D., Boston, Mass.

Section on Sanitation and Hygiene—Chairman, Lee H. Smith, M.D., Buffalo, N. Y.; Secretary, G. A. Weeks, M.D., Richmond, Me.

Since the appearance of the last bulletin it has been learned that the Midland Hotel, at which it was intended to have held the meeting of the National at Kansas City, will have given up the building before the time set, therefore the place of meeting will of necessity be changed.

Dr. March informs me that he has arranged with the management of the Coates House, and that he has secured the session room and three large rooms adjacent for committee rooms, all free of charge to the Association.

The rates at the hotel are $1.00 a day and upward on the European plan, and $2.50 a day and upward, American plan; the latter includes bath.

We trust each member who intends to prepare an article for the National will not fail to have his article ready, and forward it if he finds it impossible to attend.

All reports from the section officers should be in the hands of the Secretary no later than May 1.

Let every man make it his business to do something toward making the coming meeting a success. We need every individual and the individual physician needs the organization.

We should not fail to do our part to make the attendance and the enthusiasm the best ever, especially when we consider how much the good Eclectics of Kansas City are doing to assure us a delightful time while their guests. Very fratrnally,

WM. P. BEST.

May Meetings.

Arkansas.—The twenty-eighth annual meeting of the Arkansas E. M. Association will be held at the Basin Park Hotel, Eureka Springs, June 13, 15 and 16. An interesting program has been arranged and a large attendance is looked for. Quite a delegation will go up to Kansas City following the meeting to attend the National.

Pennsylvania.—The Pennsylvania State Society will meet at Harrisburg, in the Capitol Building, May 21 and 22. Drs. Foltz and Russell have been invited to attend. Dr. Nannie M. S. Glenn, Recording Secretary, State College.

Kentucky.—The Kentucky Society will meet in the School Board Education Rooms, 418 W. Walnut Street, Louisville, May 6 and 7. Headquarters, Hotel Willard. Dr. Lee Strouse, Secretary, Covington.

West Virginia.—The West Virginia Society will meet at the Hotel Windsor, in Wheeling, May 5 and 6. Dr. G. R. Miller, President; Secretary, Dr. J. A. Monroe, Wheeling.

Indiana.—The Indiana Society will meet at Indianapolis May 26 and 27. Headquarters, Grand Hotel. A large attendance is anticipated. Dr. E. B. Shewman, Waymansville, Secretary.

Connecticut.—The Connecticut E. M. Association will be held at the Allyn House, Hartford, Tuesday, May 12. President, J. W. Fyfe, Saugatuck; Secretary, Geo. A. Fisher, Waterbury.

Iowa.—The Iowa Society will be held at Muscatine May 27 and 28. President, E. B. Fulliam, Muscatine.

Illinois.—At Chicago, May 21-22; headquarters, Sherman House. President, C. H. Merritt, Alton; Secretary, J. B. Standlee, Peoria.

The annual Commencement Exercises of the Georgia College of Eclectic Medicine and Surgery was held Tuesday, March 31, in the Grand Opera House at Atlanta. An interesting program was rendered. There were twenty-three graduates.

E. P. Notes.

Bro. H. E. Price, located at Weldon, Ill., reports prosperity, and says he has many times in his short professional life had reasons to be thankful that he cast his "lot" with the Eclectic school.

Bro. Chas. J. Shaffer, '07, is located at Noble, Ill.

Bro. J. W. Reynolds writes from Sager, Texas, that he expects to be back with us at the E. M. I. this coming session.

The fourth annual banquet of the Eclectic Philomatheans was held at the Palace Hotel, March 31. About eighty members and friends were present. During the evening a very appropriate program was rendered by members of the "frat." Hofer's orchestra furnished the music.

E. P. officers for the coming year are: N. M., John Swanson; M., E. J. Burnett; S., R. L. Alsaker; A., N. B. Baird; R. N., H. S. Monroe; L. N., G. D. Harris; R. G., R. M. Jean; L. G., G. C. Aurand; G. C., A. C. Lambert; Chap., C. F. Flannery; Cho. R. E. Hecock. Reporter for E. M. J., A. C. Lambert; Trustees, John Swanson, John Thiel, A. C Lambert, G. W. Martin, J. W. Bowers, E. J. Burnett, J. D. Estell, C. O. Bayless, H. R. Wynn.

We wish to introduce to the "fellows" Bros. G. W. Martin, Fred. Preston and J. D. McCaffery, of the E. M. I. '08.

We wish to thank the E. M. JOURNAL for its many courtesies during the year. We feel sure the members at large appreciate the space allotted to us. If you are not a subscriber or know of a brother who is not, get busy! A. C. LAMBERT.

Vacation address, 200 Twenty-ninth Street, Wheeling, W. Va.

Sigma Theta Notes.

Fellows! the finals are over, and the curtain has been rung down the session of '07 and '08.

Let us spend our short vacation in a manner both enjoyable and profitable to ourselves. Let it not be all pleasure, as idleness brooks no good; on the other hand, let it not be all work; let us say to ourselves, we will make it the well-balanced happy intermediate. By so doing we will all look longinly forward to the month of September, when our Alma Mater will call us hither.

Sigma Theta wishes well her own who have recently gone forth to enlist in the army of exponents of Specific Medication.

We recently had a very pleasant letter from Fellow O'Hara, of Lewisburg, O.; he is enjoying a constantly increasing practice.

Fellow Blough, '07, writes us that he expects to enlarge his present office at Pittsburg, Pa. This is very gratifying.

Some days ago a letter from Fellow Saxton, '07, of Tampa, Fla., informed us that the world continued to treat him very kindly.

A recent communication from California told us that Dame Fortune continued to smile upon Fellow Dickinson, '07. He was recently appointed resident physician in one of the leading hotels in Los Angeles.

Fellow Rausch, '07, continues to do nicely at Stone Creek, O.

One of the most pleasant events of the year was a recent visit paid us by Fellow Winter, '07, of Indianapolis, Ind. He informed us that

Specific Medication was doing for him what it ever has done and always will do for every well-trained Eclectic, keeping him busy.

The close of the session marks the appearance of new faces within our walls. These men have crossed the burning sands and have demonstrated to us that each and every one possesses all the characteristics necessary to become a Sigma Theta.

The past year, under the watchful eye of M. W. M. Finlaw, has been one of harmony, prosperity and fraternalism, and we feel satisfied that M. W. M. Jones will continue this good work. SCHANTZ.

T. A. E.

The following brothers are in this year's graduating class: W. K. Dyer, C. C. Hamilton, D. S. Strong, F. M. Wurtsbaugh, E. E. Watson and H. F. Pohlmeyer. T. A. E. wishes them all the success and happiness due a true T. A. E., and may they wear the red carnation with the same pride that they have in the past three years.

The wedding bells will soon be ringing in Johnstown, Pa. The T. A. E.'s extend congratulations to Dr. and Mrs. J. D. Keiper and wish them a happy and successful life.

The fifth annual banquet of the Pan-Hellenic Asociation, composed of forty fraternities in the United States, was held at Dayton, O., Friday, April 3. The T. A. E. is the only Eclectic Fraternity that is a member of this association. Our representative, J. F. Wuist, reports a fine large time and advises more of the brothers to take part in the festivities next year.

I wish to make an appeal to our brothers in practice to write to the fraternity often; we will be glad to hear from any of you. "Don't forget to hit the stride."

My address for the summer will be care of E. M. J.

H.F. KILLEN, *Chronicler.*

PERSONALS.

Locations—Several good locations in Oklahoma. For particulars address with stamp Dr. Geo. H. Stagner, Coyle, Logan County, Okla.

Wanted—An active young Eclectic as partner. For particulars address with stamp Dr. W. H. Devore, Canyonville, Oregon.

For Sale—Practice, office and furniture in small town with good surrounding country. For particulars address with stamp Dr. P. D. Gaunt, Gilman, Iowa.

Location.—Good opening for an Eclectic physician. For particulars address with stamp Willanna L. Hawk, 817 S. Clinton Street, Trenton, N. J.

Died—At Trenton, N. J., Dr. W. W. Wyckoff, Pa. '63.

Died—In Michigan, March 22, Cullen A. Battle, President of Battle & Co.. Chemists, St. Louis, Mo.

Died—At Huckabay, Texas, March 24, Dr. Claude E. Standlee. Dr. Standlee graduated from the American Medical College of St. Louis, in 1891, but after an active practice he was compelled to go to Arizona for his health. He was a brother of Dr. John B. Standlee, of Peoria, Ill., and the late Dr. E. Lee Standlee, of St. Louis.

READING NOTICES.

DYSMENORRHEA.—It should not be forgotten that simple, painful menstruation, in the absence of ovarian disease or uterine displacement, is often a pure neurosis, due to a faulty state of metabolism, and a dose of Alkalithia, night and morning during the month, will in many such cases insure a painless flow.

The following extract from a letter written recently to Dr. W. C. Abbott, Chicago, tells its own story:

"The skin on Paul's back was cut into sheds; Luther was turned out of church; Servetus was burned at the stake, and Columbus was sent to jail. Do you think you are better than they? Take courage. We are traveling to the beautiful City of the Ideal. We know that we shall never reach it—but the suburbs are very pleasant."

WE desire to reassure our friends in the medical profession that Cactina Pillets contain only the therapeutic principles of Cereus Grandiflorus. No other species of cactus is employed in their manufacture, nor does any other medicinal ingredient enter their composition.

SULTAN DRUG CO.

IMPORTANT FOR THE DOCTORS.—For the doctors' convenience in prescribing, the Dios Chemical Company have quite recently adopted abbreviations for their products, viz.: Dioviburnia (Dov.), Neurosine (Nuo.), and Germiletum (Glou.). The doctors can, if they desire, thus indicate in prescribing. We think this will be acceptable as many doctors dislike to do much writing.

WHILST the formula of Tyree's Antiseptic Powder is known to every practitioner, we deem this an opportune moment to submit, as additional evidence of its incomparable value, the views of those whose judgment of therapeutic agents of this class is universally accepted as authoritative in the highest degree. Literature and a trial package will be mailed free of charge to physicians if they will send their name and address to Mr. J. S. Tyree, Chemist, Washington, D. C.

VAGINITIS is treated first by douching the parts with a solution of Glyco-Thymoline, one ounce to a quart of hot water, applying strips of cotton or gauze saturated with the solution and left in place for twelve hours; even may be reeated more frequently than twice a day. This may be alternated with other antisetic and astringent solutions. In other and severe forms of vaginitis, douching and irrigation of the parts with Glyco-Thymoline may be practiced with advantage and after the application of a stronger caustic and other remedies.—J. W. HEROLD, New York City.

OKLAHOMA REGISTRATION.—The Oklahoma *Medical News-Journal* states that the present State Board of Health is too previous in asking for re-registration of physicians for a nominal fee. The new State has not passed any new law on the subject as yet. The Constitution distinctly provides that the legal practitioner under the old laws of Oklahoma and Indian Territory should not be disturbed.

SOCIETY CALENDAR

NATIONAL ECLECTIC MEDICAL ASSOCIATION. President, L. A. Perce, Long Beach, Cali.; Recording Secretary, William P. Best, 2218 East Tenth Street, Indianapolis, Ind. Meets at Kansas City, Mo., June 17–20, 1908.

ARKANSAS. President, W. C. Dallenbaugh, Pine Bluff; Secretary, T. J. Daniel, Magazine. Next meeting at Eureka Springs, June 12–13, 1905.

CALIFORNIA. President, F. J. Petersen, Lompoc; Secretary, J. Park Dougall, Douglass Bldg, Los Angeles. Meets at San Francisco, May 19–21, 1908.

COLORADO. At the office of Dr. B. F. Richards, June 6.

CONNECTICUT. President, J. W. Fyfe, Saugatuck ; Secretary, G. A. Faber, Waterbury. Next meeting at Hartford, May 12, 1905,'

ILLINOIS. President, C. H. Merritt, Alton; Secretary, W. E. Kinnett, Peoria. Next meeting at Chicago, May 20–22, 1908.

INDIANA. President, A. E. Teague, Indianapolis; Secretary, E. B. Shewman, Waymansville. Next meeting at Indianapolis, May 26-27, 1908.

IOWA. Secretary, E. H. Wiley, Des Moines. Next meeting at Muscatine, May, 1908.

KANSAS. President, E. B. Packer, Osage City; Secretary, F. P. Hatfield, Grenola. Next meeting at Kansas City, June 15, 1908.

KENTUCKY. President, J. J. Morrill, Otter Pond; Secretary, Lee Strouse, Covington. Meets at Louisville, May 13-14, 1908.

MASSACHUSETTS. Secretary, Pitts E. Howes, Boston. Next meeting at Boston, June 4-5, 1908.

MAINE. President, Sylvania A. Abbott, Taunton, Mass.; Secretary, H. Reny, Biddeford. Next meeting at Preble House, Portland, May 26, 1908.

MICHIGAN. President, J. E. G. Waddington, Detroit; Secretary, F. B. Crowell, Lawrence. Next meeting at Detroit, June 3-4, 1908.

MISSOURI. President, J. T. McClanahan, Boonville; Secretary, E. F. Cook, 710 Felix Street, St. Joseph. Next meeting at Kansas City, June 15-16, 1908.

NEBRASKA. President, E. J. Latta, Kenesaw; Secretary, S. J. Stewart, Beatrice. Next meeting at Lincoln, May 5-7, 1908.

NEW ENGLAND. President, G. A. Faber, Waterbury, Conn.; Secretary, S. A. Abbott, Taunton, Mass. Next meeting Keene, N. H., May 27-28, 1908.

NEW JERSEY. President, D. P. Borden. Patterson. Next meeting Thursday, May 21, at Newark.

OKLAHOMA. President, J. F. Son, Ardmore; Secretary, E. G. Sharp, Guthrie. Next meeting at Oklahoma City, May 14-15, 1908.

OHIO. President, A. S. McKitrick, Kenton; Secretary, W. N. Mundy, Forest. Next meeting at Dayton, May 5-7, 1908.

PENNSYLVANIA. President, C. J. Hemminger, Rockwood; Secretary, Nannie M. S. Glenn, State College. Next meeting State Capitol, Harrisburg, May 21-22.

SOUTH DAKOTA. President, W. P. Collins, Howard; Secretary, W. E. Daniels, Madison. Next meeting at ———.

TENNESSEE. President, B. D. Austin, Rome; Secretary, B. L. Simmons, Granville. Next meeting at Nashville, May 19-20, 1908.

TEXAS. President, G. W. Johnson, San Antonio; Secretary, L. S. Downs, Galveston. Next meeting at Dallas, October, 1908.

VERMONT. President, J. B. H. Cushman, East Charleston, Secretary, P. L. Templeton, Monpelier. Next meeting at State House, Montpelier, June 3-4, 1908.

WEST VIRGINIA. President, George R. Miller, Amos; Secretary, J. A. Monroe, Wheeling. Next meeting at Hotel Windsor, Wheeling, May 5-6, 1908.

WISCONSIN. President, A. A. Duclos, Milwaukee; Secretary, J. V. Stevens, Jefferson. Next meeting at Devil's Lake, May 25-26, 1908.

The Eclectic News

A Monthly Newspaper

No. 6.   JUNE, 1908.   Vol. XIII.

BOOK NOTICES.

Diseases of the Nose, Throat and Ear. By Kent O. Foltz, M.D. 117 illustrations. 12mo. 643 pages. Cloth, $3.50. The Scudder Brothers Co., Publishers, 1009 Plum Street, Cincinnati, O.

"The Eclectic School is generally known as being 'long' on medication, depending, perhaps, more on drug treatment than the others, and especially is this true when it comes to the treatment of conditions in which local applications are usually resorted to.

"This work on the treatment of diseases of the nose, throat and ear is intended to bring therapeutics more prominently before the profession, although by no means losing sight of the recognized value of purely local treatment.

"The author believes that many of the inflammatory diseases of the upper respiratory tract and ears can be cured by tne institution of the proper systemic measures, and makes a plea for their more general adoption.

"For students and practitioners this book is well adapted. It covers the subject, as expressed in its title, in a manner that is characterized by clearness and without unnecessary verbiage, giving special prominence to diagnostic points and indications for specific medication. Its many illustrations, both of pathological conditions and office equipment, will be appreciated by the practitioner wishing to become more proficient in this line of work."—*Albright's Office Practitioner.*

A Text-Book of Clinical Medicine—Treatment. By Clarence Bartlett, M.D. 1222 pages, cloth, $8.00. Philadelphia: Boericke & Tafel. 1908.

The fact that this book is from the pen of Dr. Clarence Bartlett, one of the foremost writers of the Homeopathic school of medicine, assures us of its value.

It is a work for the general practitioner, and is full of good, practical points. One refreshing feature is the belief in the value of medical treatment expressed by the author, which is contrary to the view taken by the medical nihilists.

Instructions as to the applications of the different therapeutic measures are clearly explained, and of great practical value. The treatment is along rational lines.

We quote the author's views on such remedies as control the active delirium of typhoid fever. Speaking of hyoscyamus, hydrobromate of hyoscine, stramonium and agaricus, he says: "Of these, hyoscyamus is the favorite remedy with the majority of physicians. It is successfully used in those cases of typhoid fever presenting an actively muttering delirium, associated with a generalized twitching of the tendons. Patient picks at the bed-clothing or his lips, or grasps at imaginary objects in the air. Associated symptoms are such as we find in most severe cases of typhoid fever."   L. C. W.

Diseases of the Heart. By PROF. TH. VON JURGENSEN, of Tubingen; PROF. DR. L. KREHL, of Greifswald; and PROF. L. VON SCHROTTER, of Vienna. Edited, with additions, by George Dock, M.D. Octavo of 848 pages, illustrated. Philadelphia: W. B. Saunders Co. Cloth, $5.00 net.

Volume 12, "Diseases of the Heart," completes the series of "Nothnagel's Encyclopedia of Practical Medicine." For carefulness of detail and thoroughness of investigation the Germans lead the world, and Vol. 12, on diseases of the heart, shows on every page the master hand. Endocarditis, by Jurgensen, is worth the price of the volume, while Krehl's article on the myocardium and its affections is equally valuable. Ably edited by Prof. George Dock, of Ann Arbor, Mich., important American and English contributions, which were not brought out at the time of the original articles, have been added. As a work on cardiac lesions it is almost invaluable.   THOMAS.

The Essentials of Medical Gynecology. By A. F. STEPHENS, M.D. Cloth, $3.00. The Scudder Bros. Co., Cincinnati.

I have just finished a careful examination of this book, and I am of the opinion that it is one of the best books on the subject that has come from the press for a long time. To the younger men in the ranks of medicine it will be invaluable; to those who know nothing of specific medication of any age, who will carefully study this book, and then faithfully carry out its therapeutics, it will be a revelation; it will lessen their drug bills, increase their success in their chosen vocation, and add much to the comfort of their patients.

There is little to be criticised. I think, however, cancer of the uterine cervix can be managed better than by either excision or strong caustics. I can treat syphilis without mercurials. But I believe I can treat them better by adding the judicious use of these agents, and I feel assured the author of this book could use mercurials without the frightful results of which he seems to be afraid, and which were so often seen years ago.

I could wish for this book a place in every medical library.

J. FEARN.

Nervous and Mental Diseases. By CHARLES S. POTTS, M.D. 12mo. 570 pages, with 133 engravings and 9 full-page plates. Cloth, $2.50 net. Lea & Febiger, Philadelphia.

The second edition of this very excellent manual is placed before the profession and a careful examination of the book shows much to commend.

It is well written, the illustrations are good. The descriptions of disease, etiology, pathology and diagnosis are clear and to the point.

The chapter on symptomatology and methods of examination is a useful part of the work, and gives much valuable information in regard to the importance and significance of symptoms and their proper classification, and is particularly instructive as to methods of examination.

The diseases of the nervous system are taken up systematically and each given a brief though careful description, and the diagnosis made as plain as may be.

The work is up to date in regard to pathology and classification. It is particularly suited to the needs of the general practitioner. It gives in a condensed and simple form the description and diagnosis of the different diseases, and one does not have to read through pages to find out what can be told in a few sentences. Yet it contains as much as most physicians care to study along these lines.

W. E. P.

An Aid to Materia Medica. By R. H. M. DAWBARN, M.D. Fourth edition, revised and enlarged by E. V. DELPHEY, M.D. The MacMillan Company.

This edition has been brought fully up to date to conform with recent changes in the latest edition of the pharmacopeia. All of the good things have been retained, many new ones added.

The author believes the book to be of special value to students, since examiners require much that the practitioner soon lays aside;

to graduates, as a ready reference to doses, new remedies, changes of dose, etc., etc.

The book, though not large, certainly contains a fund of knowledge in a most readily accessible form.   W. E. B.

Surgical Therapeutics. By Emory Lanphear, M.D.   Cloth, $1.00.
Clinic Publishing Co., Ravenswood, Chicago.

This little book of Professor Lanphear's covers very briefly and forcefully the practical suggestions for the management of surgical cases, "with tips" in regard to after-treatment. I am quite sure that a copy of this work will be well appreciated by the practitioner, and, as the author says, "while it is not exactly Eclectic, I hope you will find it—in the language of the druggist—'just as good.'"   L. E. R.

SAUNDERS' FORTHCOMING BOOKS.—Messrs. W. B. Saunders Company, medical publishers of Philadelphia and London, announce for publication before June 30 a list of books of unusual interest to the profession. We especially call the attention of our readers to the following:

Bandler's Medical Gynecology—treating exclusively of the medical side of this subject.

Bonney's Tuberculosis.

Volume II, Kelly and Noble's Gynecology and Abdominal Surgery.

Volume IV, Keen's Surgery.

Gant's Constipation and Intestinal Obstruction.

Schamberg's Diseases of the Skin and Eruptive Fevers.

John C. DaCosta, Jr.'s Physical Diagnosis.

Todd's Clinical Diagnosis.

Camac's Epoch-Making Contributions in Medicine and Surgery.

All these works will be profusely illustrated with original pictures.

COLLEGE AND SOCIETY NOTICES.

National Association Bulletin for June.

Coates House, Kansas City, Mo., June 17, 18, 19, 20, 1908.

Again our National Association meeting is but a few days away. Again we bring to your notice the need of every loyal Eclectic of the Association and its influence, and the duty of each to the National body.

Throughout the year we have tried to keep all in touch with the efforts of the officers and committees to serve your interests.

The N. E. M. A. exists for you, not for the officers and commit-

-tees. *We* desire *you* to be present, for it is to *you* that our reports should be read, it is for you to know the full year's work, our needs and the *true* situation.

Every officer and every committeeman has done a full share, and much is to be reported, considered and acted upon.

Not for many years have your officers and committees had so much to do and so much to report that is of interest and of *vital importance*, and that demands careful and thoughtful action.

While this meeting is primarily one for business, our brethren of Kansas City and Missouri and Kansas will not allow you to return without a taste of genuine Western hospitality.

Many good things await all who, in duty to themselves and loyalty to the cause, will be at the meeting.

The program will prove of unusual interest and contains many surprises which will prove entertaining and agreeable.

We hope to meet every Eclectic that can possibly spare the time to attend. Fraternally,

WILLIAM P. BEST, Indianapolis.

Rates to the National.

None but the Western Passenger Association has granted us special rates, and they are practically the same as the regular rates. The Southwestern Association, which includes Arkansas, Texas, Oklahoma, etc., have a summer excursion rate to Kansas City which is lower than any they could grant us specially. The round trip rate from North Pacific Coast points is $60. The dates of sale, however, are a little early for us, being June 5 and 6. The rate from California points is the same, viz., $60, the dates of sale being June 9, 10 and 11. There is also a round trip rate of $90 from Pacific Coast States to Kansas City. Tickets on sale daily. As stated before, the two-cent laws in the various States make the rates the same as has been granted us heretofore, so that the matter of rates should not deter anybody from attending this most important meeting. Remember the date, June 17-20. H. H. HELBING, *Corresponding Secretary*,

1208 N. Kingshighway, St. Louis, Mo.

At the annual meeting of the California Board, Dr. J. Park Dougall, the Eclectic member from Los Angeles, was chosen President for the ensuing year. We congratulate Dr. Dougall and the Eclectics of Southern California on this new honor.

Dr. C. W. Seeley, of Wileyville, W. Va., writes that the State Board of West Virginia has begun reciprocity and is now empowered to reciprocate with Illinois and Utah on examination, and with Iowa, Kansas, South Carolina and Wisconsin on either diploma or examination.

The Missouri State Eclectic Medical Association will be held in Kansas City, Monday, June 15 and 16. Headquarters at Midland Hotel. Dr. E. F. Cook, Recording Secretary, St. Joseph, Mo.

The tenth annual Commencement of the Eclectic Medical University was held in the Auditorium Hall, Kansas City, Kan., April 30. Nineteen students received the degree of Doctor of Medicine.

PERSONALS.

Dr. J. V. Athey, E. M. I., '99, has moved from Belpre, Ohio, to Bartelsville, Okla.

The *Charlotte Medical Journal* and the *Carolina Medical Journal* have been consolidated, and will hereafter be published under the former name at Charlotte, N. C., under the management of E. C. Register, M.D. This is one of the best Southern journals which comes to our editorial desk.

CONSOLIDATION.—The *California Medical Journal,* of San Francisco, and the Los Angeles *Eclectic Medical Journal* have been consolidated, and will hereafter be issued from Los Angeles under the name of the *California Eclectic Medical Journal,* subscription price $1.00 per year. It will be under the editorial management of Dr. O. C. Welbourn, of Los Angeles, who will have the assistance of the former editor, Dr. Daniel Maclean, of San Francisco.

WANTED—To exchange a good location in city of 7,000 or 8,000 for a good location in country. Address Doctor D, care ECLECTIC MEDICAL JOURNAL, 1009 Plum Street, Cincinnati, O.

FOR SALE—American Case and Register Company desk. New and in good condition. No bookkeeping required. Also Yale Operating-Chair, less than a year old. Apply to R. E. Harding, 408 Walnut Street, Elmwood Place, O.

Dr. J. S. Horovitz has retired as editor of the *Chicago Medical Times,* which will hereafter be published by the Medical Times Company, at 412 Fulton Street, under the management of the Editors' Board, consisting of Drs. Robertson, Francis, Graves, Pollock and other members of the Faculty of the Bennett Medical College. The subscription price has been raised to $1.50 per year. In the April issue the *Times* states that it will continue to be the exponent of

Eclectic medicine and surgery, and that its editors are all medical cptmists with the firm belief in the efficacy of direct medication.

FOR SALE—Back issues of THE ECLECTIC MEDICAL JOURNAL for twenty-six years, in good condition, for $5.00. Address J. O. Latimer, M.D., West Farmington, O.

Good location at Rushville, Ind. For particulars address with stamp, Dr. Bert Coffey, R. R. No. 1, Rushville, Ind.

Battle & Company, of St. Louis, have just issued the fifth of their series on Dislocations, which they will be glad to send free to readers of this journal on request.

OBITUARY.

At Pyrmont, Ohio, April 14, Dr. Orion W. Tobey. Dr. Tobey was born in 1849, studied medicine under Dr. G. W. Dickey, and graduated from the E. M. I. in 1873. He was a member of the Methodist Church. Dr. Tobey has been a prominent member of the State Society for several years. Two children survive him, a daughter and a son, Dr. Wilbur C. Tobey, of Dayton, O.

At Pasadena, Cal., January 9, 1908, Dr. Ira F. Cameron, E. M. I., '76, aged sixty years. Dr. Cameron practiced medicine at Keswick, Iowa, for nearly thirty years.

J. A. Elliott, New York, '74, at Northumberland, Pa., from paralysis, January 28, aged sixty-five.

Robert D. Unger, Philadelphia Ecl., '59, at Chicago, January 30, aged eighty-three.

H. P. Sharp, E. M. I., '76, at Arcade, N. Y., January 29, aged fifty-three.

George W. Roffey, E. M. I., '77, at Columbus, O., February 9, aged sixty.

Edward Walker, E. M. I., '49, at Delphi, Ind., February 17, aged seventy-eight.

O. Michaud, Bennett, '73, at Clifton, Ill., February 13.

J. C. Ball, E. M. U. of K. C., '04, at Kansas City, February 28.

T. B. Bartlett, E. M. I., '79, at Mount Clare, W. Va., February 25, from paralysis, aged seventy-two.

James J. Rowe, E. M. I., '58, at Abingdon, Ill., February 29, aged seventy-six.

D. D. Stevens, N. Y. Ec., '78, at New York City, November 19, 1907.

J. Surman, Cali., '82, at Portland, Ore., February 24, aged sixty-six.

W. S. Ross, E. M. I., '58, at Madisonville, Ky., February 26, aged seventy-eight.

D. J. Brannen, E. M. I., '81, at Washington, D. C., March 4, aged fifty.

C. W. Dunlop, N. Y. Ecl., '80, at New York City, March 6, aged sixty-three.

R. T. Hart, E. M. I., '67, at Pickens, Miss., aged seventy-five.

N. J. Barry, Georgia, '93, at Gainesville, Fla., November, 1907, aged forty-three.

C. B. Smith, Phila., '79, at E. Portland, Ore., March 14, aged sixty-one.

J. W. Owens, N. Y. Ecl., '75, at Carthage, N. Y., March 16, aged eighty.

READING NOTICES.

CYSTITIS.—It should not be forgotten how prominently a condition of hyperacidity of the urine figures as an etiological factor in the ordinary case of acute cystitis. Proof of this is found in the readiness with which such cases yield to Alkalithia. This is the alkaline treatment in a form which permits of the alkalies being pushed to the point of alkalinizing the secretions without disturbing the stomach as with the use of the plain alkalies.

During the spring months, especially if the weather has been of the varied sort, the profession has its hands full of cases recovering from respiratory ailments and which need particular care to steer them safely to normal health. To bridge this gap nothing is quite so serviceable as a palatable cod liver oil preparation. The representative of this class of remedies is Hagee's Cordial of the Extract of Cod Liver Oil Compound, and it is in constant use by the profession and with most gratifying results.

In taking a paragraph on "Cactus," the *American Journal of Clinical Medicine* says:

"The above paragraph is taken from Lloyd Brothers' 'Dose-Book of Specific Medicine,' just published by them. It is a fair illustration of the quiet, sensible, moderate tone used by Lloyd in speaking of the remedies which are put out by that firm. The 'Dose-Book' we find exceedingly interesting. We would suggest to our readers that they will find in it many a useful hint to try in their practice. We presume that the 'Dose-Book' would be sent to those requesting it of Lloyd Brothers, Cincinnati, O. We make one more significant quotation: 'Every jobber's stock in America is made up of fresh specific medicines. No bottle in any stock is older than 1907.' Now, doctor, when you send a prescription to your pharmacist, are you *always, invariably,* sure that the latter takes the precaution which so great a chemist as Lloyd finds necessary, that your prescription does not contain a single ingredient which is older than 1907? Possibly the reply to this question may enlighten you as to some of the disappointments you have experienced in the application of medicines."

NEW LABORATORY COMPLETED.

"No Dope for Quackery Made Here."

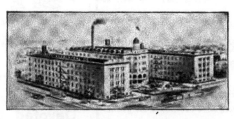

"Nothing succeeds like success." Another milestone in the progress of the Abbott Alkaloidal Company is marked by the completion of their new laboratory shown to the left in the picture above. This is the finest building of its kind in the country for supplying the needs of the doctor. It is absolutely fireproof, reinforced-concrete construction, with every modern improvement, and up-to-date equipment. The central building, to be used for executive offices, will be completed next year.

We suggest that our readers send to the Abbott Alkaloidal Company, Chicago, Ill., for their new therapeutic price list which is now ready for distribution. There is much of interest and value in this list for every progressive physician.

GOOD FAITH WITH THE MEDICAL PROFESSION.—It means much to the thoughtful practitioner to have remedies at his command in which he can place implicit confidence as to quality, uniformity, and therapeutic efficiency. The substantial success won by Gray's Glycerine Tonic Comp. during the past fifteen years is the strongest possible evidence of the good faith that has constantly been kept with the medical profession. To prescribe an original bottle of Gray's Glycerine Tonic Comp. is to insure a maximum of benefit to a patient, and a minimum of uncertainty as to the desired results. When other tonics fail to prevent bodily decline, Gray's Glycerine Tonic Comp. will prove a veritable sheet anchor.

Over sixty years ago, the Pond's Extract Company began the preparation of Pond's Extract, selecting therefor the best and most luxuriant growths of the shrub at the season of the year when richest in extractive material, and perfecting a process whereby an extract of uniform strength and efficiency was produced.

Nervous exhaustion and melancholic mania are relieved by Celerina in teaspoonful doses three times a day.

INDEX TO ADVERTISEMENTS.

ECLECTIC NEWS

THE

A MONTHLY NEWSPAPER

No. 7. JULY, 1908. Vol. XIII.

BOOK NOTICES.

Essentials of Medical Gynecology. By A. F. STEPHENS, M.D., Professor of Medical Gynecology in the American Medical College, St. Louis, Mo. 12mo, 428 pp. Fully illustrated. Cloth, $3.00. The Scudder Brothers Co., Publishers, Cincinnati, O.

WHAT OTHERS SAY.

"That the greater attention which now is being paid to medical gynecology is the natural reaction following the recent supremacy of gynecological surgery, is likewise a fact. Dr. Stephens has written a good book, whose title should have been medicinal gynecology instead of a medical gynecology."—OTTO JUETTNER, M.D.

"The arrangement of subjects is excellent, and the treatment by our own remedies will, I am sure, be very pleasing to our practitioners, enabling them to cure all cases that medicine will reach, and indicating those that need surgical attention. There is need of this work."—S. M. SHERMAN, M.D.

"In this work Professor Stephens has fully and graphically given the views of the gynecologist from the standpoint of a medical practitioner, and has very carefully described these lesions, with the best known remedies for betterment. The author says that where diseases can be cured by surgical measures only, he has frankly said so, and dismissed the subject. I think this manly statement of Professor Stephens will win for him the commendation of the practitioner."—L. E. RUSSELL, M.D.

The Eclectic Practice of Medicine. By ROLLA L. THOMAS, M.D. 8vo., 1033 pages. Price, cloth, $6.00; sheep, $7.00. The Scudder Brothers Company, publishers, 1009 Plum Street, Cincinnati, O.

Here is another of the splendid Eclectic works published by the Scudder Brothers. It is a complete treatise on general medicine and embraces the etiology, pathology, symptomatology, diagnosis, prognosis and treatment of the entire list of diseases usually classed as medical diseases.

Apart from its therapeutics it does not differ from other works of like character, except in so far as the personal observations of the author may modify the usual descriptive matter, but in the treatment a most important feature is the application of the specific Eclectic remedies which are held in such deserved esteem by all followers of that school, and a great many of the old and Homeopathic persuasion.

No one who has ever studied the specific indications and actions of the specific remedies used by the Eclectics ever gives them up.

For those who are unfamiliar with these indications a chapter is devoted. The various chapters are considered in alphabetical order and the information given is clear, brief and specific. It is a splendid addition, and a fitting ending for a work on this subject.—J. D. ALBRIGHT, in *Albright's Practitioner.*

Progressive Medicine. Vol. X, No. 1, Whole Number 37, 1908.

Lea & Febiger, Philadelphia. $6.00 per year.

This quarterly digest of advances, discoveries and improvements in the medical and surgical sciences comprises a valuable and comprehensive review and synopsis of the best articles appearing in periodical literature. The groups treated and their authors are the following: "Surgery of the Head, Neck and Thorax," by Charles H. Frazier, M.D.; "Infectious Diseases, Including Acute Rheumatism and Croupous Pneumonia," by Robert R. Preble, M.D.; "The Diseases of Children," by Floyd M. Crandall, M.D.; "Rhinology and Laryngology," by D. Braden Kyle, M.D.; "Otology," by Arthur R. Duel, M.D.; and index. One who would keep abreast with medical literature should have access to such compilations, and we know of none better than this quarterly digest.   FELTER.

COLLEGE AND SOCIETY NOTES.

Last month the Commencement Exercises of the Eclectic Medical College of the City of New York were held at the Carnegie Lyceum. Professor Gunning read the report of the faculty, and Dr. Boskowitz, the Dean, conferred the degrees. Mrs. Krausi has decided to donate an entirely new laboratory equipment for the college. The following graduates reveived degrees: J. F. A. Arnold, H. Fried, A. S. Gombar, Sarah K. Greenberg, J. A. Redi, Jr., O. J. Ruzicka and Stella Shaffer.

The twentieth annual session of the Kentucky Eclectic Medical Association was held in Louisville, May 6 and 7, 1908. It was the best meeting in our history, seven new members being taken in. Sixteen in attendance. Papers were good and discussions well timed. All seemed full of enthusiasm. Membership list thirty-six, with thirty-three in good standing. Motion carried that as a body we join the National, providing the combined cost of auxiliaries, State and National, do not exceed five dollars a year, and the Secretary ordered to act accordingly. The following visitors were in attendance: Drs. Coons, Ashabranner, Hauss, Best and Watkins; written communications from Drs. Wilder and Howes. Also greeting from the Ohio State Association, then in session at Dayton, Ohio, came by telegram, on the eve of adjournment. The following officers were elected for the ensuing year: President, J. A. Farabaugh, Clinton; Vice-President, T. A. E. Evans, Farmers; Secretary, Lee Strouse, Covington; Corresponding Secretary, Wm. Leming, Louisville; Treasurer, J. C. Mitchell, Louisville. Next meeting at Louisville, May, 1909.

The annual meeting of the Connecticut Eclectic Medical Association was held May 12, being presided over by Dr. Fyfe. The suggested plan of affiliation with the National was approved. Several excellent papers were read and discussed. A concise plan for better organization was adopted. The following officers were elected to serve for the ensuing year: President, John W. Fyfe, Saugatuck; Vice-President, Frank B. Converse, West Millington; Treasurer, Leroy A. Smith, Higganum; Secretary, Geo. A. Faber, Waterbury.

The twenty-ninth annual meeting of the Tennessee Eclectic Medical Association convened at the Maxwell House, May 19 and 20. The meeting was well attended and one of the best in many years. Prof. R. L. Thomas, of Cincinnati, was a welcome visitor. The society voted favorably upon the question of National affiliation. The following officers were elected for the ensuing year: President, R. O. Williams, Humboldt; First Vice-President, W. W. Phebus, Ridgely; Second Vice-President, A. S. Corbin, Tennessee City; Recording Secretary, B. L. Simmons, Granville; Corresponding Secretary, J. O. Cummings, Nashville; Treasurer, Geo. M. Hite, Nashville. Next meeting at Nashville, May 11 and 12, 1909.

The West Virginia Eclectic Medical Association was held at Wheeling, May 5 and 6, and the meeting was larger and more interesting than usual. The following resolutions were adopted:

"*Resolved,* That we, the members of the West Virginia State Eclectic Medical Association, in annual session assembled, do endorse the proposed action of the National Association whereby the State societies may be more closely allied with it in its interests and its work.

"*Resolved,* That we do most heartily commend the measures the Trustees of the Eclectic Medical Institute have taken towards improving the course of study, the teaching facilities and the new hospital."

The following officers were elected for the ensuing year: President, Allen Bush, Morgantown; First Vice-President, M. H. Waldron, Naugatuck; Second Vice-President, F. W. Vance; Secretary and Treasurer, W. B. Hartwig, Uniontown; Corresponding Secretary, C. W. Seely, Wileyville. Next meeting at Clarksburg, first Tuesday and Wednesday in May, 1909.

The fortieth annual meeting of the Illinois State Eclectic Medical Society was held at the Sherman House, Chicago, May 20, 21 and 22, 1908, with a full auditorium. About two hundred were in attendance, and this proved to be one of the most interesting and enthusiastic meetings ever held for a number of years.

We had the pleasure and honor of having with us Dr. L. E. Russell, of Ohio; Dr. J. D. McCann, of Indiana; Dr. H. Hugh Helbing, of Missouri; and many others of note from different States. The program was very interesting, and all responded to their papers, which made the work of more interest to every one. In the department of Medicine, Materia Medica and Therapeutics, an interesting paper was presented entitled "A Specific Vegetable Diphtheritic Antitoxin," by Dr. Ernst Jentzsch, of Chicago, in which he claims to have discovered a vegetable antitoxin in our well-known drug lobelia. In his paper, the doctor has readily shown a safe, immediate, potent and permanent relief by the injection method of this drug as an antitoxin in diphtheria. All who heard the paper were greatly interested. Twenty-six new applications were voted on, and added to our large list of membership.

The following officers were elected for the ensuing year: President, Charles H. Bushnell, Chicago; First Vice-President, G. O. Hulick, East St. Louis; Second Vice-President, John A. McDonell, Chicago; Secretary, William E. Kinnett, Peoria; Treasurer, John B. Matthew, Blue Mound; Corresponding Secretary, John B. Standlee, Peoria.

The next meeting will be held in East St. Louis, May 19, 20 and 21, 1909.   Fraternally,

> JOHN B. STANDLEE, M.D.,
> *Corresponding Secretary.*

The thirty-fifth annual meeting of the Pennsylvania Eclectic Medical Association was held at Harrisburg, May 21 and 22, 1908. The meeting was fairly well attended. A number of good papers were read and discussed at length. Prof. K. O. Foltz, of Cincinnati, was with us and gave several interesting and instructive talks. We also had Dr. C. C. McCormick, of Bowling Green, Ky., to address the society for a few minutes. Six new members were added to our membership. The following are the newly elected officers: President, W. S. Glenn, State College; Vice-President, R. E. Holmes, Harrisburg; Second Vice-President, L. A. Gardner, Columbia X-Roads; Corresponding Secretary, E. F. Shaulis, Indiana; Recording Secretary, R. Meek, Avis; Treasurer, S. J. H. Lowther, Somerset. Place of meeting next May, Harrisburg.   NANNIE M. SLOAN-GLENN.

PERSONALS.

Good country location in Oklahoma. For particulars address with stamp, Dr. Wm. Hall, Carter, Okla.

Good location for a young Eclectic. For particulars address with stamp, Dr. F. G. Wachtendorf, Fincastle, Ohio.

Dr. William Seitz, E. M. I., '08, has passed the Florida State Board, and is now located at 2407 Florida Avenue, Tampa, Florida.

Dr. D. M. Ulery, E. M. I., '03, formerly at 129 West Seventh Street, has removed to Flat 1, Sixth and Central Avenue, Cincinnati, Ohio.

Dr. R. O. Hoffman, E. M. I., '91, passed the California State Board, and is now located at the corner of Fifth and E Streets, San Diego, Cal.

Dr. H. H. Helbing, of St. Louis, will leave for Europe about July 6 for special study, and expects to return to St. Louis about September 15.

Location—Good location for an Eclectic physician in northwestern Ohio. An established Eclectic practice in a town of 400. Good surrounding country. No competition. Address with stamp, Dr. J. J. Sutter, Bluffton, Ohio.

OBITUARY.

C. R. Kobb, Bennett, '84, at Linesville, Pa., May 13.

Wm. C. Sweezey, E. M. I., '56, at Olivet, Kan., March 26.

C. E. Starrett, Bennett, '84, at Chicago, May 1, aged forty-three.

T. Conrad, St. L., '81, at San Francisco, May 10, aged fifty-two.

W. H. Davis, E. M. I., '65, at Chicago, May 19, aged sixty-five.

E. C. Guild, Bennett, '74, at Wheaton, Ill., April 25, aged seventy-six.

F. B. Brewer, Bennett, '72, at Evanston, Ill., May 12, aged seventy-six.

Sarah J. Hogan, Bennett, '86, at Chicago, April 23, aged eighty-three.

I. N. Hughey, St. L., '78, at Pomona, Cal., April 16, aged sixty-seven.

J. H. Mack, E. M. I., '63, at Madison, Iowa, March 16, aged seventy.

J. W. Jay, E. M. I., '55, at Richmond, Ind., December, 1907, aged eighty-two.

C. G. Crosse, E. M. I., '53, at Sun Prairie, Wis., April 21, aged seventy-nine.

J. H. Stebbins, Amer. Cin., '54, at Geneva, N. Y., April 8, aged seventy-four.

C. M. Maxfield, E. M. I., '70, at Chicago, March 31, of heart disease, aged sixty.

Willis L. Snyder, E. M. I., '93, at Muncie, Ind., April 2, from aneurism, aged thirty-nine.

Fred. W. Range, E. M. I., 96, at Monmouth, Ill., from cerebral hemorrhage, aged thirty-six.

READING NOTICES.

PROSTATIC IRRITATION.—The influence of residual urine in setting up prostatic inflammation is well known. When the urine is concentrated or unduly acid it becomes doubly irritating. To induce a bland, free, unirritating urine is to remove a common exciting cause of the trouble. For this purpose there is no better remedy than Alkalithia. Shut off the use of rhubarb, tomatoes and strawberries.

PUBERTY.—At this time the administration of a proper remedy can go a long way toward establishing normal functioning of the reproductive system of girls approaching maturity. Hayden's Viburnum Compound exerts a beneficial influence upon the nervous and reproductive system, and if administered just prior to the initial catamenia, its antispasmodic and tonic action will be found of particular advantage.

WHERE hysteria is the result of uterine troubles, Aletris Cordial Rio combined with Celerina is an excellent remedy.

IN studying the action of Pond's Extract, it is found to possess marked anodyne, antiphlogistic, astringent, antiseptic and styptic properties. It relieves pain, irritation and congestion by its soothing and cooling effect on the surface structures, and a coincident improvement in the local capillary circulation. It is astringent through its pronounced contractile influence on protoplasm and, while antiseptic, is not so much so because of its immediate destruction of bacteria, as by reason of its astringent and sedative action on inflamed areas, thus making the tissues attacked less favorable locations for the growth and propagation of germ life. Its styptic action, which is specially marked in capillary hemorrhage, or bleeding from small vessels, is accomplished by both contraction of the vascular coats and an increase in the coagulation of the blood.

THE ECLECTIC NEWS

A MONTHLY NEWSPAPER

No. 8.   AUGUST, 1908.   VOL. XIII.

BOOK NOTICES.

A Text-Book of Physiological Chemistry. For students and physicians. By CHARLES E. SIMON, M.D. New third edition, octavo, 490·pp. Cloth, $3.25 net. Lea & Febiger, Philadelphia, Pa.

In this edition the author considers the chemistry of the three classes of foodstuffs, their digestion, assimilation, metabolism and excretion, and of the products of the various glands and organs. His presentation adapts the work for use as a text-book, a laboratory manual, or for the office needs of the physician in active practice. The tendency of college curricula is distinctly towards requiring a knowledge of general chemistry for entrance, and the limitation of subsequent chemical study to its bearings on physiology and pathology. On the first of these two great divisions, Professor Simon's work has won recognition as a leading text-book.

Essentials of Medical Gynecology. By A. F. STEPHENS, M.D., Professor of Medical Gynecology in the American Medical College, St. Louis, Mo. 12mo, 428 pp., fully illustrated. Cloth, $3.00. The Scudder Brothers Company, Cincinnati, Ohio, Publishers.

I have thoroughly examined this publication, and believe it a most timely work. It contains a chapter on "Remedies Used in Gynecological Practice and Their Specific Indications," also a chapter on "Conditions and Symptoms and Indicated Remedies for Their Relief." These two chapters alone are worth the price of the book to any practitioner who has not familiarized himself with the Eclectic practice of medicine.

While it is a most valuable addition to any one's medical library, it is, however, most important to a practitioner who is called upon to treat diseased conditions of the female generative organs, and especially to such of our brothers in the medical profession who are not equipped to do anything in the way of surgical treatment. Indeed, it is a book for any general practitioner, especially at this age, when most of the works on gynecology give little space to the medical treatment. I can heartily recommend this book to my friends.—J. J. LINK, M.D., *Professor of Surgery, American Medical College, St. Louis, Mo.*

Bier's Hyperemic Treatment in Surgery, Medicine and the Specialties. By WILLY MEYER, M.D., and DR. V. SCHMIEDEN. Philadelphia: W. B. Saunders & Co. Cloth, $3.00.

The medical profession has been awaiting with interest the appearance of a practical text-book on this new and important therapeutic measure. Bier's teachings have been the chief subject of interest among German surgeons for the past two years, and no doubt they will be generally applied in America sooner or later. Their importance lies in the fact that they aim to prevent operative interference to a large extent, and passive hyperemia will frequently accomplish without danger or distress to the patient results that are impossible by operative methods. The application of the hyperemia treatment, however, is not as easy as it would seem at first thought, for much of our success depends upon the time and frequency of application, the selection of cases, etc.

Therapeutics of Vibration. By WM. LAWRENCE WOODRUFF, M.D. J. F. Elwell Publishing Co., Los Angeles, Cal. Price, $1.50.

This little volume of 144 pages represents, according to the author's statement, an attempt to reduce the therapeutics of vibration to an exact science. In the elaboration of his purpose the author resorts to the speculative reasoning and to the well-worn demonstration by analogy so popular with the natural philosophers of ages gone by. The theoretical part of the book is a confused and motley mixture of fragmentary and half-digested scientific matter. It is books of this character that have impeded the legitimate development of vibration and other forms of physical therapy because they prejudice the mind of the unbiased physician by unscientific methods of reasoning. The medical student would be hopelessly confused if he attempted to get any information on vibration out of this book.   JUETTNER.

Studies in the Psychology of Sex: Erotic Symbolism, the Mechanism of Detumescence, the Psychic State of Pregnancy. By HAVELOCK ELLIS. Cloth, 8vo, $2.00 net. F. A. Davis Company, Publishers, Philadelphia.

We have before us the fifth volume of this series by Professor Ellis. The preceding volumes were reviewed at some length by the late Dr. Foltz. The present volume is up to the usual standard of excellency. The work is only sold by subscription to physicians, lawyers and scientists, and is very valuable to those studying along these lines.

COLLEGE AND SOCIETY NOTES.

Faculty Changes.

The Trustees of the College have appointed J. P. Harbert, M.D., of Bellefontaine, Ohio, Professor of Ophthalmology, and Chas. S. Amidon, M.D., Professor and Clinical Instructor on Otology, Rhinology and Laryngology. Dr. Amidon will continue in the office of the late Dr. Foltz, at 105 Odd Fellows' Building, Seventh and Elm Streets.

Dr. H. E. Sloan has opened his office for the practice of general surgery at 808 Andrews Building, Fifth and Race Streets.

The Michigan State Eclectic Medical Society held its thirty-second annual meeting in the parlors of the Griswold House, Detroit, June 3-4, 1908. It was enthusiastic from start to finish, the papers were exceptionally good, and reflected much credit upon the writers. The discussions were lively and many valuable facts in therapeutics were brought out. On Wednesday evening the association was entertained at the home of the President, Dr. Waddington, the evening being passed in social chats, music, readings, and an elegant lunch was followed by toasts of high order. Four new members were taken into the society—Dr. Frank A. Howland, Adrian; Dr. Enoch Mather, Detroit; Dr. Mart Hammond, Adrian; Dr. C. H. Murphy, Perry. The following were the guests of the association: Dr. W. B. Church, of Cincinnati; Dr. W. J. Pollock, of Chicago, and Dr. R. M. Tafel, of Phoenix, Arizona. Dr. Best, of Indianapolis, Ind., was unavoidably detained. The following officers were elected for the ensuing year: President, C. S. Sackett, Charlotte; Vice-President, H. G. Palmer, Detroit; Treasurer, P. B. Wright, Grand Rapids; Secretary, E. B. Crowell, Lawrence. Next meeting will be held at Adrian, June, 1909.

The annual meeting of the Arkansas Eclectic Medical Association was held at Eureka Springs, June 15, 1908. Professor Katz opened the convention with music, to the pleasure of the delegates. In the absence of the President and Vice-President, Dr. Stevenson, of Ft. Smith, was chosen temporary chairman. Dr. Daniels, of Magazine, offered prayer. Dr. Wm. P. Best, of Indianapolis, Ind.; Dr. Ray, of

Kelly, Okla., and Dr. Mary A. Thomas, of Chicago, were guests of the Association. By unanimous consent, after most earnest discussions, the State Association voted to ally itself with the National Eclectic Association as a member of that body. The following officers were elected to serve for the ensuing year: President, G. A. Hinton, Hot Springs; First Vice-President, A. E. Tatman, Eureka Springs; Secretary, Claude E. Laws, Fort Smith; Treasurer, T. J. Daniels, Magazine.

The forty-third annual meeting of the Vermont Eclectic Medical Society was held in the Supreme Court Room of the State House, June, 1908. The annual address was given by Prof. J. W. Marsh, President. A number of interesting papers were read and discussed. The following officers were elected for the ensuing year: President, Joseph M. Moore, West Rupert; First Vice-President, J. B. H. Cushman, East Charleston; Secretary, P. L. Templeton, Montpelier; Treasurer, H. E. Templeton, Montpelier.

The forty-third annual meeting of the Maine Eclectic Medical Society was held at Portland May 26, 1908. Reports of the Secretary, Treasurer and various committees showed the society fairly prosperous. The following officers were elected for the ensuing year: President, E. Palmer, Ripley; Vice-President, Geo. A. Weeks, Richmond; Recording Secretary, S. A. Abbott, Taunton, Mass.; Corresponding Secretary, J. L. Wright, Durham; Treasurer, A. Fossett, Portland. The next meeting will be held at Portland, May 26, 1909.

The fourteenth annual meeting of the New England Eclectic Medical Association was held at Keene, N. H., May 27, 1908. A number of interesting papers were read, also letters and telegrams from absent members and friends. The Committee on "Standing of Eclecticism in New England" reported a great need of young Eclectics in the northeast, and the Secretary was instructed to invite, through the Eclectic journals, graduates to locate herein. The following officers were eleced to serve for the ensuing year: President, S. A. Abbott, Taunton, Mass.; First Vice-President, James T. Tonks, Westbrook, Conn.; Secretary, F. W. Abbott, Taunton, Mass.; Treasurer, Henry Reny, Biddeford, Maine. The next meeting will be held at Boston, Mass., June 2 and 3, 1909.

The annual meeting of the Missouri Eclectic Medical Association was held at Kansas City, Mo., June 15 and 16, 1908. A resolution was adopted in the form of a protest entered against the tendency to relegate therapeutics, the discovery and application of remedies for disease, to a secondary place in the curriculum of the profession. The cardinal principle of Eclectic medicine is declared to be the study and application of therapeutics. The following officers were elected for the ensuing year: President, H. H. Brockman, Eldon; First Vice-President, E. C. Hill, Smithville; Recording Secretary, E. F. Cook, St. Joseph; Corresponding Secretary, Geo. E. Krapft, St. Louis; Treasurer, A. W. Davidson, Poplar Bluff. Next meeting at St. Louis in May, 1909.

Sigma Theta.

The summer is moving slowly, and it is by supposition only that we know the whereabouts and occupations of our fellows, but in whatever they may be engaged, our thoughts are with them in hearty co-operation.

Fellows, let us bear in mind the fact that the short vacation we are now enjoying should not all be consumed by amusements, but that some of our time should be expended in a way to enlarge the mind on subjects with which the profession deals.

Fellow Watkins is in his father's office during the summer, acquainting himself with the many good traits of a loyal Eclectic.

Fellow Frederick sent us a letter telling us of his loneliness and solitude, but he concluded with a lengthy description of a banquet which he had attended, convincing us that he is not "faring bad" after all.

In a short communication from Fellow Lynch we learn that he is blending a little work with his vacation. He has been making elaborate preparations for a camping trip. Good work, "Dick," I would like to join you.

We are glad to note that Fellow Jones, who is pursuing the study of medicine in a practical way at Shepard Hospital, Shepard, O., is greatly enjoying his work. Owing to the fact that it is very quiet at times, he requests the boys to write him often.

Indirectly, we are able to report that success is following the efforts of Fellows Kinsey, Detrick and Yawn.   MARPLE.

Triadelphia, W .Va.

Good location at Frankfort, Ky. Small property to sell cheap. Address Dr. G. A. Budd, R. R. No. 1, Frankfort, Ky.

PERSONALS.

Dr. Daniel S. Strong, E. M. I., '08, also passed the Indiana board and is located at Hillsdale, Ind.

Dr. C. C. McCaffrey, E. M. I., '08, has passed the Ohio board, but is at present practicing at Huntington, W. Va.

Dr. Jesse W. Bowers, E. M. I., '08, has passed the Indiana board and is located at 918 Harmer Street, Ft. Wayne, Ind.

Several good locations for young Eclectics in West Virginia. Address with stamp, Dr. C. W. Seely, Wileyville, W. Va.

Dr. George W. Martin, E. M. I., '08, passed the Ohio board and will probably locate with his brother at Chillicothe, Ohio.

Dr. Fred H. Finlaw, E. M. I., '08, passed the Indiana board, and if he does not locate in Indiana he will locate in Pennsylvania.

Good location in Kansas for energetic young Eclectic. For particulars address with stamp, Dr. T. C. Burton, Hoisington, Kan.

Location—Good opening for an Eclectic physician in Idaho. For particulars address with stamp, Dr. Russell Truitt, Cottonwood, Idaho.

We are glad to learn that Dr. C. C. Hamilton, E. M. I., '08, has passed the Indiana board with an average of 94.2, which gives him an honor grade. He is located at Ewing, Ind.

Dr. H. L. Henderson, of Astoria, Ore., who is one of the special contributors to this journal, is now President of the City Council of Astoria, and represented the Mayor of Astoria at Seattle during the reception to the United States fleet.

Doctor, would you work to become rich? Dr. T. Ormsbee, of Woodstock, Oregon (a suburb of Portland), has a fine location (no other doctor and thousands of people nearest him), will turn over his practice to a thoroughly competent young Eclectic physician without pay. Reason: seventy-three years old. Has drug-store which he will sell at price no reasonable person will object to; part cash, balance easy terms.

The attention of our readers is called to the new announcements under the head of professional cards in the front portion of the JOURNAL. We have frequent inquiries for the names and addresses of various physicians, and it has been thought advisable to maintain and extend this new arrangement. One inch cards, including the JOURNAL one year, will cost $10. Half-inch and JOURNAL, $6. One-quarter inch and JOURNAL, $4.

HYSTERIA is the expression of one form of nervous debility. Celerina is thus peculiarly indicated because of its tonic effect on the whole nervous system.

GASTRALGIA.—Papine in teaspoonful doses, given every two or three hours, will promptly relieve the severe pain associated with gastralgia. The effect of one dose is often prolonged for five or six hours.

THE old and reliable house of Wm. R. Warner & Co. will be incorporated under the laws of Pennsylvania, with Mr. Wm. R. Warner, Jr., retaining his connection as President of the corporation. This move enables Mr. Warner, who has managed the entire business, to transfer to others many of the details of management, and at the same time assures his host of friends and patrons in the trade of a continuation of the safe and conservative policy which has proven the keynote of its success, and which has characterized it from its foundation in 1856.

CYSTITIS.—The treatment includes rest, administration of sanmetto, plenty of cold water or milk, bland and mild food, laxatives, hot sitz baths or vaginal douches, irrigation of the bladder with antiseptic solution followed by solution of nitrate of silver.

IN cases of intermitten fever it is best to prescribe doses of one or two antikamnia tablets when the first chill comes on. I also find them most valuable in controlling headaches of a neuralgic origin. Rarely more than two tablets are necessary; the pain is promptly dissipated and the patient can go about as usual. The tablets of antikamnia and codeine, I consider the best and most useful in controlling severe pain. I have used them after surgical operations as a substitute for morphine, and find them eminently satisfactory. In controlling the severer forms of neuralgia they rank next to morphine itself.— C. P. ROBBINS, M.D., Louisville, Ky., in *Medical Progress.*

IN regard to the therapeutics of hamamelis, of which Pond's Extract is admittedly the standard preparation, no better evidence can be brought forward than the statement of prominent medical authorities. For instance, Potter, in his well-known work on "Materia Medica, Pharmacy and Therapeutics," says: "Hamamelis is used with great benefit, both externally and internally, in cases of hemorrhoids (particularly those of the bleeding variety), varicose veins and ulcers, venous congestion and threatening local inflammations. It is highly recommended in hemorrhages from the nose, stomach, lungs, rectum and kidneys, and externally for sprains and bruises, foul ulcers, the pruritus of eczema, and catarrhal diseases generally."

INDEX TO ADVERTISEMENTS.

ᴛʜᴇ ᴇᴄʟᴇᴄᴛɪᴄ ɴᴇᴡs

A Monthly Newspaper

No. 9. SEPTEMBER, 1908. Vol. XIII.

BOOK NOTICES.

A Text-Book of Surgical Anatomy. By W. F. CAMPBELL, M.D. Octavo, 675 pages, with 316 original illustrations. W. B. Saunders & Co. Philadelphia. Cloth, $5.00.

As stated in the preface, "No teacher can impart, or student assimilate, all the details of anatomy. The facts must be sifted, their comparative values fixed, and the reason for their acquisition demonstrated by directing attention to the practical problems with which they are associated. The single purpose of the book is to aid the student and practitioner in mastering the essentials of practical anatomy."

With this purpose the author has produced a book in which regional anatomy is presented in a concise and simple manner, with emphasis laid upon the surgical considerations. Only those structures are mentioned which have a clinical interest, and about these only those facts that can be applied. The student will appreciate the simple style and the avoidance of technical terms, and the graduate of some years will thank the author for his adherence to the old nomenclature.

In this as in other books, mistakes are found and some portions are not clear. For example, the diploic veins are given as one division of the veins of the scalp; the great sciatic is called the great sacro-sciatic nerve; descriptions of the relations of the third portion of the common bile duct are contradictory; in hammer toe the third phalanx is said to be flexed upon the second; lymph nodes is certainly preferable to lymph glands or ganglia. In introducing sounds into the urethra we are admonished to use no force, "the sound's own weight is sufficient force." Such expressions have been found in our text-books for years, and have certainly served their day. It would require a vivid imagination to enable the student to accept that statement literally after making a few attempts. The description of the descent of the testicle and the formation of the inguinal canal is far from clear.

The illustrations as a whole are good, and aid the text in the presentation of the subject. In a few of them we are reminded that illustrators of medical books should learn their anatomy. In Fig. 72 the action of the palatal muscles in separating the edges of the cleft is not well shown. In Fig. 219 the longitudinal fissure of the liver is not properly designated. In Figs. 223, 224, 225, the common bile duct is represented as having no supra-duodenal portion. In Fig. 263 the round ligaments are shown posterior to the uterine tubes. In Fig. 266 an entirely wrong impression of the course of the external iliac vessels and round ligaments is given. These errors do not impair the usefulness of the book, and every physician, whether he does surgery or not, should be familiar with the facts it presents.   SLOAN.

Clinical Materia Medica. By E. A. FARRINGTON, M.D. 8vo.; 826 pp.; cloth, $6.40. Boericke & Tafel, Philadelphia.

This is a reprint of the course of lectures delivered at the Hahnemann College in Philadelphia by Professor Farrington, and was reported phonographically by Professor Bartlett. The lectures are very concise and comprehensive, and afford much valuable information to Homeopathic physicians when the clinical side of the study of materia medica is taken into consideration. It seems to one not so well versed in this line of study a more simple guide than some of the more complex works.

State Board Questions and Answers. By R. MAX GOEPP, M.D. 8vo; 684 pp.; cloth, $4.00. W. B. Saunders Company, Philadelphia.

Now that recent graduates must submit to a State board examination in every State but one, a demand for a work of this order has become imperative. This book is very full and explicit. The author has taken a varied assortment of questions and added the answers. The only criticism we might offer is that the questions and answers on Eclectic and Homeopathic materia medica and practice have been omitted. But as our men are quite well qualified in these directions, the omission will not prove serious.   J. K. S.

Modern Medicine: Its Theory and Practice. In Original Contributions by American and Foreign Authors. Edited by WILLIAM OSLER, M.D. Assisted by THOMAS McCRAE, M.D. Volume IV. Subscription only, $6.00 per volume. Lea & Febiger, Philadelphia, Pa.

Volume IV is devoted to diseases of the circulatory system, diseases of the blood, diseases of the spleen, and diseases of the thymus and lymph glands, lesions, unfortunately, that in most cases baffle the efforts of the medical man. Thus of the 830 pages devoted to the work, only 40 pages are given to treatment.

The contributors to this important volume have been selected with care, and each has contributed that which will make Volume IV take rank with the other volumes which have preceded this great work. The illustrations are unusually good, and the publishers are to be congratulated on Volume IV and the reader on the possession of the latest material on these important subjects.   R. L. T.

Gray's Anatomy has maintained its lead as one of the best publications on this subject for the last fifty years, and thousands of copies have been sold to various medical students, who have burned the midnight oil in perusing its pages. A new edition will appear soon under the personal supervision of Professors DaCosta and Spitzka. While the recent revised editions have been very elaborate, about the only criticism one could well make would be that a very great deal of new material has been added in the shape of notes in finer type, which can hardly be assimilated by the average medical student, but which are of more value to professors of materia medica, or to one doing research work in this direction. This edition will be reviewed at greater length as soon as it is issued by the publishers, Lea & Febiger, Philadelphia, Pa.

COLLEGE AND SOCIETY NOTES.

There are several fall society meetings. The Connecticut holds a semi-annual meeting at Allyn House, Hartford, October 13; New Jersey and Newark in October, and the Texas Society at Dallas.

The Missouri Valley Eclectic Medical Association has recently organized at Kansas City. It will unite and form a Mississippi Valley Association at St. Louis in September.

THE annual meeting of the Colorado Eclectic Medical Association was held in the Adams Hotel, in Denver, June 9, 1908. From the beginning to the close of the second session considerable enthusiasm was manifested, and after each paper was presented lively discussion followed. A banquet was given in a private dining-room in the hotel, at which each physician did his best in filling the measure of happiness to the overflowing point. Four new members were added to the society. This was most gratifying, for Colorado has room for many more enterprising, straightforward Eclectic physicians. The Association voted to ally itself with the National Eclectic Association. The delegates who were to attend the National meeting in Kansas City were instructed to make a pull for its next meeting in Denver, or pave the way for 1910. The following officers were elected: President, W. S. Bogart, Denver; Vice-President, Chas. W. House, Denver; Secretary and Treasurer, B. Franklin Richards, Denver. The next meeting will be held in Denver, June 8, 1909.

PERSONALS.

Dr. Julius E. Bach, E. M. I., '08, passed the Kentucky State Board and is located at Newport, Ky.

Dr. Louis L. Moench, E. M. I., '03, formerly of Lewis, Idaho, is now located at Kilkenny, Minn.

Dr. Frank P. Hatfield, of Olathe, Kan., has been elected President of the State Board of Medical Examiners.

Good opening for a young Eclectic in Ohio. For particulars address with stamp, Dr. P. E. Decatur, Marseilles, O.

Dr. Geo. W. Thompson has been elected President, and H. Harris, Registrar, of the New York Eclectic Medical College.

Frederic E. Elliott, M.D., E. M. I., '04, has passed the New York Board, and his present address is P. O. Box 201, New York City.

Dr. George T. Sauter, E. M. I., '08, successfully passed the Kentucky Board and is located at 908 Ann Street, Newport, Ky.

Dr. C. T. Saylor, E. M. I., '08, passed the Pennsylvania State Board, and is now located at Boswell, Pa., where he is doing nicely.

Dr. George E. Miller, E. M. I., '05, represents the Foreign Christian Missionary Society, and is located at Mangeli, Central Province, India.

WANTED—A bright up-to-date man to take half interest in $4,000 practice. Cash yearly business can be increased to $6,000. For particulars address Dr. J. M. Hamblin, Westboro, Mo.

Dr. E. H. Gregg, formerly of Yorktown, Ind., spent the winter at Talfurrias, Tex., which he reports is a delightful place to spend the winter. He is now pleasantly located in Sulphur Springs, Ind., where we wish him an abundance of success.

OBITUARY.

Z. P. Bradley, Kansas City, '06, at Kansas City, July 3, aged sixty years.

David M. Shoemaker, E. M. I., '81, at Chicago, July 19, aged sixty-three.

Bela St. John, N. Y., '82, at Torrington, Conn., July 16, aged eighty.

Filson Cooper, E. M. I., '69, at Villisca, Iowa, July 27, aged seventy-one.

Wesley Robbins, Indiana, '84, at Detroit, Mich., July 13, aged fifty-two.

Rody E. Warner, E. M. I., '75, at Pittsburg, Pa., July 15, aged fifty-seven.

Nathaniel J. Beachley, E. M. I., '54, at Lincoln, Neb., July 10, aged seventy-six.

William T. Williamson, St. Louis, '79, at Fort Branch, Ind., July 22, aged sixty-four.

READING NOTICES.

PSEUDOANEMIA.—Do not forget that not every anemic-looking patient has anemia, a lack of red blood corpuscles. The diathetic state known as lithemia very often induces such a contraction of the peripheral circulation as to produce a condition of pallor that may be mistaken for anemia. The condition, however, is one of ischemia instead of anemia, and does not call for iron. The therapeutic indications are to overcome the underlying lithemia, and for this purpose there is no remedy superior to Alkalithia, made by the Keasbey & Mattison Co., Ambler, Pa.

CARDIAC TONIC.—"I have prescribed Cactina Pillets in a number of cases of heart trouble and find them a reliable cardiac tonic, especially in weak heart with small, frequent intermittent pulse. They are a specific in functional heart trouble."—R. A. CLOPTON, M.D., Milan, Tenn.

A STERILE EYE BATH.—An eye bath fashioned from a single piece of aluminum has been introduced by the Kress & Owen Company (which will be sent free upon request). That this little device will be well received by the medical profession is not to be questioned when one considers the many points of advantage this metal cup has over the old style glass contrivance. It is cleanly, unbreakable and can be sterilized instantly by dropping into boiling water. The surgical bag in the future will hardly be complete without one of these cups, which will give happy results in many an emergency. It will be found invaluable for treating ophthalmia, conjunctivitis, eye strain, ulceration and all inflammatory conditions affecting the eye.

Directions.—Drop into the eye bath ten to thirty drops of Glyco-Thymoline; fill with warm water. Holding the head forward, place the filled eye bath over the eye, then open and close eye frequently in the Glyco-Thymoline solution. It is soothing, non-irritating and reduces the inflammation.

RATIONAL TREATMENT OF INFANTILE DIARRHEA.—For years the treatment of diarrhea in children, commonly known as summer complaint, has been a stumbling block for the practitioner mainly because the true nature of the disease never was thoroughly understood. As a matter of fact, the prevention of the disease is quite easy, but as it depends altogether upon the parent who has the children in charge, neglect is always accountable for the sickness. The result is that the physician is seldom called until mischief has been done. Under the circumstances, rapid treatment has to be resorted to if fatalities are to be avoided. The main point is to modify the diet, suppressing objectionable food, particularly milk not properly modified in strength and sterilized. Meanwhile the bowels should be kept in a thoroughly aseptic condition. An experience of ten years or more has demonstrated that this is better accomplished through the use of Tyree's Antiseptic Powder; one teaspoonful or less of this powder diluted in a pint of tepid water makes an ideal washing for the intestine as an enema. Sample with chemical and bacteriological analysis sent upon request to J. S. Tyree, Chemist, Washington, D. C.

THE VARIETIES OF DYSMENORRHEA.—In an article on Dysmenorrhea, Solomon Henry Secoy, M.D., of Jeffersonville, Ind., refers especially to its causes and treatment and offers some valuable suggestions as follows:

"The treatment of dysmenorrhea very naturally comprises such remedies and procedures as will correct the cause, and the administration of anodynes to relieve the pain. In the neuralgic form we must correct the cause. If that be malaria, quinine must be given. In most cases where the neuralgic form is presented there is anemia, and no relief will be secured till this factor is overcome. Iron in some available form must, therefore, be given. During the period of menstruation the administration of antikamnia and codeine tablets in doses of two tablets every two hours, will relieve the pain. If these tablets are given at the beginning of the attack, we can often entirely prevent pain."

THE ECLECTIC NEWS

A MONTHLY NEWSPAPER

No. 10.   OCTOBER, 1908.   Vol. XIII.

BOOK NOTICES.

Diseases of Children. By WILLIAM NELSON MUNDY, M.D., Professor of Pediatrics in the Eclectic Medical Institute, Cincinnati, O. Second edition, revised and rewritten. Illustrated, 8vo, 512 pp. Cloth, $3.00. The Scudder Brothers Company, Cincinnati, Ohio, 1908.

The second edition of Professor Mundy's "Diseases of Children" marks a distinct advance in Eclectic medical literature. In this edition many important changes have been made. A complete rearrangement of subjects, making the book more convenient of consultation, is one of the improvements. The introduction of excellent illustrations have greatly enhanced the value of the book, and we have never seen a better selection calculated for teaching value. These illustrations have not been selected for pictorial embellishment merely, but to forcibly impress the meaning of the text in specially required instances. The illustrations showing the marasmic child, the victim of adenoid vegetations, the desquamation of scarlatina, the variolous eruption, the cutaneous maculæ and conjunctival suffusion of measles and the vesicles of varicella cannot fail to be useful, as they vividly portray these diseases as ordinarily met with. We question if ever the beginner in practice could mistake his diagnosis after having seen these pictures.

In the description of diseases Dr. Mundy has rightly recognized, at stated periods, that there is a difference in anatomy and physiology of the child as compared with the adult, and that the symptoms and course of disease in the child does not always coincide with those of the adult. He brings out clearly the essential diagnostic points, and has not burdened his work with useless or questionable and lengthy descriptions. All through the work is the evidence of the sound common sense so strongly a part of the author. He is positive even to bluntness in some instances in recording his opinions. This gives an individuality to the work that greatly increases its worth as a guide.

There is no better field for the exhibition of specific medication than in diseases of children, and this the author seems never to have lost sight of. We question if any work on diseases of children now published contains so full and rich a therapy with reasons for the application of medicines and guides for the beginner in specific diagnosis. The work is supplemented by a section on the drugs most used in diseases of children, with full indications for their selection and form of administration and dosage. This is the only recent work in the Eclectic school on children's diseases. It originally incorporated the best of Scudder's "Diseases of Children." This the second edition, is, however, fully revised and rewritten, and presents the best that there is in Eclectic medicine to-day on the subject considered. It is well written, with better typography than the first edition, has a larger page, and makes a much larger book. No progressive Eclectic should fail to buy this book and buy it early.   FELTER.

Suggestion in the Cure of Diseases and the Correction of Vices. By GEORGE C. PITZER, M.D. Cloth, seventh edition, pp. 254. Published by the St. Louis School of Suggestive Therapeutics and Medical Electricity, Los Angeles, Cal. $1.00.

That suggestion is one of the most powerful factors in all human action will scarcely be denied by any one. That it should exercise great control over human feeling and bodily and mental processes is equally plausible. To the same extent it is admitted by many that it may be brought into requisition in the treatment of disease and the correction of vicious tendencies. At any rate, it is equally certain that much of the success of some physicians in practice may be accredited to their use of suggestion, perhaps unconsciously, on their part; but suggestion nevertheless. Pitzer's book upon this subject may be read with benefit by the physician and layman, particularly teachers, lawyers and clergymen, and may open up to them a better insight into crime and very often show to some extent the blamelessness of the perpetrator of crimes; and how crime may, in many instances, be averted.

This book embodies the principles upon which Professor Pitzer works in teaching and applying suggestion. Underlying the subject are the fundamental principles of Thomson Jay Hudson: That man has two minds—an "objective mind" and a "subjective mind." "The subjective mind is constantly amenable to control by the power of suggestion;" and that "the subjective mind has absolute control of the functions, conditions, and sensations of the body." The book shows how these forces under perverted action can excite and develop diseased conditions, and how under corrective action can be made to remove the conditions thus brought about by perverted action. If this book teaches us how to correct vice, break the liquor and tobacco habits, prevent functional diseases of a nervous type, and lend contentment to us in our daily work and life, it will have done a power of good for humanity and for the doctor in particular. The book is neat and well printed and written in the simple, direct, and understandable language characterizing all of Professor Pitzer's writings. It will be recalled by older practitioners that Dr. Pitzer was once an active Eclectic physician and editor of the *American Medical Journal* of St. Louis. Subsequently he became interested in medical electricity, making that a specialty. He is now engaged in teaching medical suggestion.   FELTER.

Progressive Medicine. A quarterly digest of advances, discoveries and improvements in the medical and surgical sciences. Edited by H. A. HARE, M.D. Vol. x, No. 2. June 1, 1908. Lea & Febiger, Philadelphia. $6.00 per annum.

This quarterly digest includes "Hernia," by W. B. Coley, M.D.; "Surgery of the Abdomen, Exclusive of Hernia," by E. M. Foote, M.D.; "Gynecology," by J. G. Clark, M.D.; "Diseases of the Blood," "Diathetic and Metabolic Diseases," "Diseases of the Spleen, Thyroid Gland and Lymphatic System," by A. Stengel, M.D.; and Ophthalmology," by E. Jackson, M.D. This number is of unusual value, and the general topics above given show but poorly the wealth of subjects noticed. This number gives a comprehensive view of the best thought and results in the special fields considered. There is no better method of keeping abreast of current views and work than by reading publications of this character, and of such works there has never been a more practical and useful series than Progressive Medicine.

                                              FELTER.

Medical Gynecology. By S. WYLLIS BANDLER, M.D. Octavo of 675 pages, with 135 original illustrations. Philadelphia: W. B. Saunders Co. Cloth, $5.00 net.

The pendulum that has long swung toward the surgical aspect of gynecology is slowly swinging back to the medical side of the subject, and it is well that it is so. Many have felt that surgery has been carried too far into gynecology, and that medical treatment is sufficient for many cases that have ben subjected to the knife. However, both the surgeon and the internist are finding their true places, and we are glad to see several works coming out on the medical treatment of diseases of women. The non-operative is the side that appeals most to the general practitioner, and he needs guides to direct him in the treatment of cases that may never need the knife, or at least will not need operation if properly cared for early and medically. The work of Bandler is, therefore, very welcome at this time, and can be commended for its comprehensiveness, its good illustrations, and its plain, direct and readable style. The student and practitioner who have both this book and Stephens' (to give Eclectic therapy) book on "Diseases of Women," have a useful working library at a moderate cost. We cheerfully recommend Bandler's Gynecology. FELTER.

Reference and Dose Book. By C. HENRI LEONARD. Cloth, 16mo., 145 pages; price, 75 cts. The Illustrated Medical Journal Company, Publishers, Detroit, Mich.

The changes in the new edition of the U. S. Pharmacopeia are given in this edition of "Leonard's Dose Book" in two groupings, one showing those of "Increased Strength," the other of "Decreased Strength," and the new doses for these changes. All the Dose List has been carefully "proof-read" by several different readers, so as to insure absolute accuracy in the (nearly) 4,000 remedies given. The U. S. Dispensatory has been followed for medium and maximum dosage. The common name (in small type) is given after the drug name and dose. Besides this complete Dose List, the book has numerous useful Tables and a therapeutic index.

Anatomy: Descriptive and Surgical. By HENRY GRAY. New American edition by J. C. DACOSTA and E. A. SPITZKA. Octavo, 1625 pp. and 1149 engravings. Price, sheep, with colored plates, $7.00. Lea & Febiger, Publishers, Philadelphia.

We are just in receipt of a copy of the new (seventeenth) edition of Gray's Anatomy. This work has held its own for the past fifty years, and thousands of students have received their knowledge of anatomy from this book. No expense has been spared on this new edition. Every page has been revised and improved, and the section on the nervous system has been entirely rewritten. Both revisers are well-known anatomists and surgeons, and are well prepared for this work. It has been stated that Gray's Anatomy reduces to a minimum the labors of both student and teacher, and the only criticism we might offer is that very much new material has been put into the later edition in the shape of foot notes in fine print, which could not very well be omitted, but which material adds to the work of the student. . J. K. S.

COLLEGE AND SOCIETY NOTES.

At a meeting of the Legislative Committee of the Eclectic Medical Association of Pennsylvania, held August 5 at Bethlehem, all of the bills on medical legislation as proposed by the dominant school were rejected, and it was resolved to ask the Legislature to continue the three State Medical Boards as at present. Dr. C. L. Johnstonbaugh was Chairman of the Committee.

RECIPROCITY.—In this State we have three examining boards, representing the three schools of medicine. The law gives each board the right to grant reciprocity, and the Eclectic board exercises that right in the case of all applicants who present a license based upon an examination *equal* to that required in this State.

JOHN WILLIAM FYFE,
President Connecticut Eclectic Examining Board....

PERSONALS.

Dr. M. A. Cooper, E. M. I., '06, formerly of Leakey, Texas, has moved to Sabinal, Texas.

Good location, with the prospect of succeeding me in practice. For particulars address with stamp, Dr. John A. Lanius, Bonham, Texas.

For Sale—My office furniture, and practice, to a good Eclectic physician. Correspondence solicited. DR. JACOB F. LEWIS, 700½ Main Street, Little Rock, Ark.

Dr. George H. Granau, E. M. I., '07, formerly of Milton, Florida, is now located at Bagdad, Florida, and is physician to the large lumber firm of Stearns & Culver.

Wanted—A good unopposed country practice, in Ohio. Will buy property if suited. Address "DOCTOR," care of the Scudder Bros. Co., 1009 Plum Street, Cincinnati, O.

Wanted—Assistantship, salaried position, or partnership, by a woman physician, Eclectic, seven years' experience. Address Dr. J. Miller, Des Moines, Iowa, General Delivery.

Although there were 40 per cent. of failures at the August examination of the Kentucky Board, D. Edward Morgan, E. M. I., '08, passed same with a general average of 84 per cent., and is now located at 17 E. Third Street, Maysville, Ky., where we feel sure he will do well.

Dr. Marquis E. Daniel, of Honey Grove, Texas, who served the new Texas board very creditably for over a year as President, has been chosen Secretary and Treasurer for the ensuing year. Dr. Daniel has given considerable time and labor as well as money in representing our branch of the profession on the new board and he should receive the thanks of all our men in the State of Texas. It takes just such broad-minded men, who are willing to sacrifice some of their business, to help us place our branch of the profession to the front.

We have just learned that the Antikamnia Chemical Company are about to erect a new building at the corner of Pine and Fourteenth Street, St. Louis, Mo., at an estimated cost of $75,000. Mr. Frank A. Ruf is President of the Company, and also a Director in the Mercantile Trust Company. We are glad to be able to congratulate the company on the growth of their business.

OBITUARY.

Jas. A. Lonsdale, St. Louis, '91, at Detroit, Mich.

Alva L. Snyder, E. M. I., '60, at Bryon, aged eighty.

Absolom B. Hostetler, E. M. I., '55, at Covina, Cal., aged eighty-two.

George W. Pangle, King Eclectic, '91, at Council Bluffs, Iowa, aged sixty-two.

Shelby L. Lenox, St. Louis, '94, at Eureka Springs, Ark., aged thirty-eight.

Cyrus Pickett, M.D., of Dunning, Neb., one of the oldest members of the National, who was made an honorary member at the Kansas City meeting at the advanced age of eighty years, passed away on August 7. He has been a subscriber to this journal for over forty years.

READING NOTICES.

CHOREA.—Omitting those cases due to organic changes in the brain or cord, chorea may, in the vast majority of cases, be considered a manifestation of the "rheumatic diathesis." In fact, it often precedes or follows an attack of rheumatism, and this explains why Alkalithia, which is an ideal remedy for rheumatism, so promptly overcomes choreic movements.—KEASBEY & MATTISON Co., Ambler, Pa.

IN an address delivered before the Danbury Medical Society on "The Practical Value of Old Remedies," John V. Shoemaker, M.D., of Philadelphia, Pa., spoke of Hamamelis in the following terms:

"Hamamelis Virginica, an excellent old-time remedy, has a well-defined range of usefulness within which it is without a rival. Externally and internally, it is sedative and astringent. It is used as a lotion and ointment in many diseases and injuries of the skin, in leg-ulcer and varicose veins. It is serviceable in acute and chronic diarrhea, internal hemorrhages, bronchorrhea, epistaxis (nose bleed) and varicose ulcers, etc."

"I AM well pleased with effects of Ecthol in severe cases of blood poisoning; as an external remedy in all painful affections, especially rheumatic, as was demonstrated in the case of my wife, who was laid up in bed with a painful rheumatic affection of one of her feet, which, after bathing and wrapping with Ecthol, to my surprise was about the house again the next day. I have also found it excellent in pruritus ani and erysipelas. I am now using it in a case of ulcer in an old man, on the bottom of his foot, which is healing."—G. A. GORSE, M.D., Meadowbrook, N. Y.

IN chronic diffuse interstitial nephritis the patient is generally anemic, and iron will agree with but few. Indeed, in many cases the nervous symptoms are aggravated by its use. Here is where Hagee's cordial of the extract of cod-liver oil compound is indicated. It should be given in tablespoonful doses four times a day.—*American Journal of Dermatology*.

H. V. C.—The success which attends the conjunctive employment of Viburnum Opulus, Dioscorea Villosa and Scutellaria Lateriflora as presented in Hayden's Viburnum Compound for the treatment of diseases of women, is due as much to the quality of each individual drug as it is to their proper proportioning; hence, it is seldom, if ever, possible to secure ideal results by the extemporaneous combining of such specimens as are procurable in the open market.

If it has once satisfactorily served you in your practice, it will do so again, provided you prescribe the original H. V. C. and see that a substitute is not administered.

SINCE Trousseau announced the great efficacy of belladonna in the "petit mal" it has held high rank as a valuable addition to the bromides. Of cannabis indica it is well said: "In morbid states of the system it has been found to cause sleep, allay spasms, compose nervous disquietude and relieve pain. In this respect it resembles opium, but it differs from that narcotic in not diminishing the appetite, checking the secretions, or constipating the bowels." (U. S. Disp., p. 351.) The literature upon this subject is so vast that volumes might be filled with quotations from standard authorities, but we make the briefest reference to these only with a view of calling attention to Neurosine (a most efficient neurotic, anodyne and hypnotic) an elegant preparation of the following ingredients: C. P. bromides of potassium, sodium and ammonium, bromide of zinc, pure extracts belladonna, henbane and cannabis indica, extract lupuli, fluid extract cascara sagrada, with aromatic elixirs.

INDEX TO ADVERTISEMENTS.

ECLECTIC NEWS

A MONTHLY NEWSPAPER

No. 11.   NOVEMBER, 1908.   Vol. XIII.

BOOK NOTICES.

What is Man?—Or Creationism vs. Evolution. By JUDSON D. BURNS, M.D. New York: Cochrane Publishing Co., 1908. Price, $2.00.

This is a serious, bold, plucky attempt to undo all that Darwin, Spencer, Huxley, *et al.*, did for the theory of evolution. A vast and daring undertaking, certainly, but not more so than would be the attempt to disestablish the law of gravity. The author's effort calls for our admiration, for who does not like a gamey man? The theory of evolution has its detail difficulties, especially those pertaining to the origin of species, and the author expands upon these with relentless pertinacity. He puts up the best anti-evolution argument I have seen. It must be conceded that he is an able, and very extensively read man, and that he is an earnest and vigorous writer. The astonishing thing is that a man of his intellectual measurement should be so far behind the scientific front. It startlingly illustrates the tenacity of the preteristic instinct, and especially it exemplifies the fixedness of religious conviction.

The idea of a nearly definite number of separate creations, commencing with the moneron and ending in man, merely substitutes the immanence of God for the immanence of natural law. It rules out the necessity of natural law, or else it rules out the necessity of God— you can take your choice. It makes a distinction where there is no difference. If we recognize the eternal immanence and assertiveness of natural law, there is no room or need of a God; if we recognize the eternal immanence and assertiveness of God, there is left no room nor need of natural law—God and natural law are one. This is pantheism, but all are pantheists—even the most devout religionists —for all believe in God's omnipresence, *i.e.*, his immanence. I know we cannot logically reconcile the idea of heredity to that of natural selection, and I know that the difficulty with reference to intermediate species is nearly as great, but I know that evolution is a fact, for I see it is going on right under my eyes. The pollywog evolves into the frog, whatever may have been the previous history of the tadpole. If evolution can be once a fact, it can be always a fact. The biontic evolution going on under our eyes should be conclusive, for biontic is, essentially, condensed phyletic evolution.

The book is necessarily retrogressive, for it makes for that ecclesiasticism which well-nigh wrecked the world, and which would have completely done so if increasing freethought had not come to the rescue. I take the liberty to give here my own definition of evolution as it occurs in my forthcoming booklet, "The Primitive Fundamental." Here it is: Evolution is natural law's immanent assertiveness in coincidence with the ceaseless stress of cosmic momentum. It is worth any one's while to buy this book, for it exhibits in brilliant phrase the nether side of modern thought, and it contains much valuable information which is merely collateral to the main subject.

COOPER.

Principles and Practice of Gynecology. By E. C. DUDLEY, M.D., of Chicago. Fifth edition, octavo, 806 pp., 421 illustrations. Cloth, $5.00 net. Lea & Febiger, Publishers, Philadelphia.

In this edition Professor Dudley has followed the plan of the previous ones and divided his subject along etiological and pathological rather than anatomical lines. This method is of decided advantage in giving the student a better understanding of the lesions from the same etiological factor in the various organs. Thus the infections of the vagina, uterus and tubes are grouped together and their relationship made clear in a way that would be impossible if vaginitis, metritis and salpingitis were found in different sections of the work.

This is essentially *Dudley's* Gynecology, his conception of gynecological diseases and his treatment being presented. The criticism that is so often made that too many methods have been described does not apply to this work. Its value as a book of reference would have been increased by descriptions of more of the standard operations.

The illustrations which were made especially for this work are numerous and accurate, many being in colors. The steps of the more important operations are illustrated so well that the technique is easily grasped.

The arrangement and clearness of the subject-matter presenting the views of such an able man, and the excellent illustrations make this a valuable book. SLOAN.

COLLEGE AND SOCIETY NOTES.

Ohio Society.

The Executive Committee met at the Grand Hotel and made arrangements for the meeting, April 27, 28 and 29, 1909.

The sections and section officers were arranged as follows:

Section I—Pediatrics. At 11 A.M. Tuesday. A. L. Schwartz-welder, Cleveland, Chairman; Ivadel Rogers, Delaware, Secretary.

Section II—Surgery. At 2:30 P.M., Tuesday. Herbert E. Sloan, Cincinnati, Chairman; A. S. McKitrick, Kenton, Secretary.

Section III—Materia Medica and Therapeutics. Tuesday, P.M. Guy J. Kent, West Liberty, Chairman; Jos. B. Barker, Piqua, Secretary.

Section IV—Pathology and Practice. At 10 A.M., Wednesday. A. N. Herring, DeGraff, Chairman; W. F. Weikal, Middletown, Secretary.

Section V—Eye, Ear, Nose and Throat. Wednesday, A.M. C. S. Amidon, Cincinnati, Chairman; S. W. Mattox, Marion, Secretary.

Section VI—Obstetrics and Gynecology. At 3 P.M., Wednesday. Edwin Scott, Toledo, Chairman; E. A. Ballmer, Columbus Grove, Secretary.

Section VII—Miscellaneous, including mental and nervous diseases, skin, electro-therapeutics, etc. W. E. Postle, Shepard, Chairman; E. M. Wright, Warsaw, Secretary.

The Committee decided to hold section officers responsible for the success of their respective sections, and urge them to fill their sections and report promptly to Dr. J. L. Payne, Cincinnati. The Grand Hotel has been selected as headquarters, and all meetings will be held at the hotel.

The Governor has appointed the new Oklahoma State Board of Medical Registration, which is composed of eight members, no school of medicine having a majority membership. Dr. Frank P. Davis, of Enid, is the Eclectic representative. He is a graduate of the Eclectic University of Kansas City in 1902. Further information in regard to the new board and their regulations will be given after its organization.

The Southwestern Ohio Eclectic Medical Association was organized at the Grand Hotel in Cincinnati, on Tuesday, October 13. Thirty-nine physicians were in attendance and considerable enthusiasm was shown. It is proposed that the new society shall meet on the first Wednesday of every other month, five times a year, in alternate counties. Annual dues will be fifty cents per year. The following officers were elected: President, Lyman Watkins, Blanchester; Vice-President, O. P. McHenry, Hamilton; Secretary, J. L. Payne, 918 W. Eighth Street, Cincinnati; Treasurer, E. R. Freeman, Seventh and John Streets, Cincinnati. The next meeting will be held at Blanchester, in Clinton County, Wednesday, December 2.

The President of the National has appointed the following general committees: Committee on the new "By-Law for State Societies affiliating with the National," Dr. E. H. Stevenson, Ft. Smith, Ark., Chairman; Dr. Finley Ellingwood, 100 State Street, Chicago, Ill.; Dr. M. M. Hamlin, 5255 Page Avenue, St. Louis, Mo. "Bok Committee," to formulate a reply to the editor of the *Ladies' Home Journal*, Dr. F. Ellingwood, Chairman, 100 State Street, Chicago, Ill.; Dr. P. E. Howes, 703 Washington Street, Dorchester District, Boston, Mass.; Dr. G. W. Boskowitz, 140 W. Seventy-first Street, New York. The Transactions for 1908 are now ready and will be mailed to members during October.

T. A. E. Notes.

The Tau Alpha Epsilon fraternity was organized in the Eclectic Medical College, at Cincinnati, O., in 1896, and the first regular meeting was held February 28, 1897, with Bro. Young, E. A., and Bro. Mumm, Scribe.

The gathering of that little band of loyal Eclectics was the start of the first Eclectic fraternity in the country, and T. A. E. has grown from one chapter with a handful of men to a fraternity that has a chapter in the six leading Eclectic colleges, and therefore a member of the Pan-Hellenic Association, which is composed of forty Greek letter fraternities and holds a meeting each year.

The past year has been a year of progress and advancement for T. A. E. We have added two new chapters to our list and organized our National Association, which will meet for the first time this year. To say that we have prospered and that harmony and good fellowship has prevailed the past year is putting it mildly. Any man that has ever entered the sacred precincts of our beloved fraternity knows what a spirit of fraternalism is always present in the T. A. E. hall, and the meetings the present year will not be an exception, because we are sure the E. A., Page, will keep up the good work that was started on the 28th of February, 1897, which standard has ever been maintained throughout the past year.

The following is the list of the chapters of the fraternity: Alpha Chapter, Cincinnati, O.; Beta, Chicago, Ill.; Gamma, Lincoln, Neb.;

Delta, New York City; Epsilon, St. Louis, Mo.; Zeta, Kansas City, Mo.

During the summer we have received letters from all the chapters stating that they are anxious for college to start so that they can get into the college and frat. work once again.

Bro. C. C. Hamilton, '08, writes us that he is nicely located at Ewing, Ind., and that specific medication is bringing him good results.

Bro. D. S. Strong, '08, is located at Hillsdale, Ind. Good luck to him.

A letter from Bro. E. G. McLaughlin, 07, informed us that he is "making lots of money." Mc. and Bro. Wood, '07, are thinking of forming a partnership.

Once again we are back in old E. M. I. and have entered with more enthusiasm and determination to do better college work. There is an old saying, "that you can't keep a good man down." Let each one show that he is a good man.   H. F. KILLEN, *Chronicler.*

PERSONALS.

Dr. Glenn E. Miller, E. M. I., '06, is located at White Oak, Okla., where he is doing well.

Dr. Herbert E. Truax and Dr. Florence E. Truax are making quite a success of their sanitarium at 474 Cherokee Avenue, in Atlanta. The latter is a graduate of the E. M. I., '01.

Prof. A. F. Stephens, author of the new work on "Medical Gynecology," has been elected as Dean of the American Medical College in St. Louis, and has been transferred to the chair of Principles and Practice of Medicine.

FOR SALE—ECLECTIC MEDICAL JOURNAL, Volume 24 to date. Volumes 24 to 30 are well bound in sheep. The remainder are unbound. Am getting old and will sell this set at a reasonable price. Address Dr. N. M. Carpenter, Ellington, N. Y.

The Chicago Medical Book Company has purchased the business of E. H. Colegrave & Company, and will continue that store at 67 Wabash Avenue as a branch house. The other West Side house will still be continued at Congress and Honore Streets.

Dr. H. Ford Scudder has moved from Long Beach to 125 Cajon Street, Redlands, Cal., where he will devote his attention to general medicine, making a specialty of diseases of the respiratory system. Any cases referred to him from the East will be given special attention.

OBITUARY.

Dr. Hiram E. Zimmerman, E. M. I., '54, Laurence County's oldest physician, died at Mt. Jackson, Pa., October 3, 1908, aged seventy-eight years, after more than half a century of active practice, in which he was unusually successful. He was a man of great determination and endurance, and died almost in the harness. He was highly esteemed by all who knew him.

READING NOTICES.

M. R. DINKELSPIEL, M.D. (Philadelphia).

In all the simple acute inflammations of the upper air passages, such as pharyngitis, laryngitis, rhinitis, etc., especially when they are due to exposure, to cold or to dampness, I have found the judicious employment of *Glyco-Thymoline* an excellent remedy and when the patient is seen at once, practically an abortive remedy.

WE have just read a very interesting paper on the new "Dietetic and Injection Method of Treating Typhoid Fever," by Dr. F. J. W. Maguire, which recently appeared in the *Michigan State Medical Society Journal*. He reported 138 consecutive cases successfully treated during the past ten years. A reprint of this article will be furnished on request by Parke, Davis & Company, Detroit, Mich.

PHARMACOLOGICAL INSURANCE.—The physician who prescribes Gray's Glycerine Tonic Comp., in original bottles, knows that he is getting a product representing quality, uniformity and therapeutic efficiency. The definite responsibility of a reputable firm always insures reliability, and the manufacturers of Gray's Glycerine Tonic Comp. are proud of the faith they have kept with the medical profession.

FOR twenty-six years Hayden's Viburnum Compound has remained standard both as to quantity and quality of its component parts as well as to the uniformly satisfactory results following its administration. Hayden's Viburnum Compound is prepared with that care, both as to the selection of drugs and in the proper combining, to make it a perfect and dependable product which is impossible where a substitute formula is extemporaneously prepared from the stock and with the limited facilities of the average drug store.

THE fall season brings cool weather and raw winds. This condition checks elimination through the skin. More work is thrown upon the kidneys. It is not always that they are equal to the extra task imposed. Imperfect elimination is the result. The auto-toxic state which soon develops is expressed in either so-called gouty bronchitis, with or without asthma, gouty eczema, recurrent tonsillitis, or rheumatism. To establish adequate elimination is to remove the cause and thus effect a rational cure. The ideal eliminant in such cases is Alkalithia, made by the Keasbey & Mattison Co., Ambler, Pa.

IN a very excellent article on "Various Forms of Headache" which appeared in *Medical Progress* a short time ago, Dr. J. U. Ray, of Blocton, Ala., states that "We must not only be particular to give a remedy intended to counteract the cause which produces headache, but we must also give an anodyne which will relieve the pain until the constitutional dyscrasia to which this trouble is due has been neutralized. To answer this purpose, two antikamnia tablets will be found a safe an convenient remedy. Usually they relieve the pain within twenty minutes. The remedy, having none of the drawbacks common to other agents of this class, it is eminently fitted to be applied in the treatment of the cases just described."

A POPULAR SALINE LAXATIVE.—Druggists doing a large prescription business report a phenomenal increase in the demand for granular effervescent aperients. There are any number of these upon the market of various grades of efficiency; but physicians seem to prefer the simple salts, prescriptions calling for sulphate of magnesia and sodium phosphate outnumbering materially those demanding compounds of known or partially secret character. Saline Laxative (Abbott) seems to be regarded as the representative preparation of magnesium sulphate, and as it is even stronger than the official magnesii sulphas effervescens and decidedly more pleasant to take, it is very generally given the preference.

ETHICAL ELEGANCE.—To obtain an antiseptic and germicide the equal of bichloride and carbolic without their dangerous features, has been a great study with the friends as well as the foes of these two corrosive agents. Dr. Tyree believes the problem is solved by the clinical and scientific tests made with Tyree's Antiseptic Powder. These tests, with the opinions of gentlemen eminently qualified to pass upon the therapeutic value of any chemical agent, are embodied in an interesting little booklet, which will be sent free. While Tyree's Powder has hitherto been largely confined to obstetrical and gynecological work, careful experiments in the hospitals of this country and London, indicate its equal value in general, rectal, laryngeal and oral surgery, whether of operative or mechanical application.

A prominent author says: "The distilled extract of Hamamelis is a valuable application to sprains and bruises. Hamamelis is very useful in checking epistaxis. bleeding sockets after the extraction of teeth, bleeding hemorrhoids, and many other forms of hemorrhage. An ointment containing Hamamelis is of service in burns, eczema, erysipelas, sunburn, seborrhea, acne, etc. When given internally, this remedy exerts an astringent and sedative action. It is also highly valued in the treatment of acute and chronic diarrhea, dysentery, hemorrhage from internal organs, purpura hemorrhagica, varicose veins and ulcers." This and other statements from reputable men concerning the usefulness of Hamamelis are well borne out in general clinical experience. provided always that a uniform, active product— such as is only found in Pond's Extract—be employed.

INDEX TO ADVERTISEMENTS.

ᴛʜᴇ Ᵽᴄʟᴇᴄᴛɪᴄ Ɲᴇᴡꜱ

A Ɱᴏɴᴛʜʟʏ Ɲᴇᴡꜱᴘᴀᴘᴇʀ

No. 12.   DECEMBER, 1908.   Vᴏʟ. XIII.

BOOK NOTICES.

Nervous and Mental Diseases. By A. CHURCH, M.D., and F.-PETER-SON, M.D. Octavo, 960 pp.; 350 ill. Cloth, $5.00. W. B. Saunders Co., Philadelphia.

The fact that this work has reached the sixth edition is presumptive evidence of its merit, and a careful examination of its contents shows that it well deserves the favor.

In the section on nervous diseases Dr. Church has endeavored to bring out all that is of practical value with reference to lesions of this nature, so that it contains the best that is known to-day both as to pathology and treatment of the diseases of the nervous system.

The chapter on psychasthenia is a new and valuable addition, and presents the more recent views as to the etiology and nature of lesions falling under this heading.

In the section on mental diseases Dr. Peterson has arranged the classification in accordance with the present-day views, and gives the terms and definitions in use by the alienists of America.

The treatment recommended is such as is being found most successful, and is in use in the best hospitals and sanitariums of the country.

The book as a whole leaves little to be desired. As a text-book for the student or the physician, or a work of reference for the specialist, it fills the place, and is one of the best works on these subjects before the profession.   W. E. P.

Pulmonary Tuberculosis. By SHERMAN G. BONNEY, M.D. Octavo, pp. 778. Illustrated. W. B. Saunders Co. Cloth, $7 net.

Among the *many* works on the subject of tuberculosis, this new book by Prof. Bonney is, to the mind of the writer, one of the best.

The subject is presented in a readable and interesting manner, greatly at variance with the bulk of such works. The book is exceedingly well illustrated. The methods of examination are the best, special attention being given to the detection of incipient phthisis. The best method being to have the patient cough, followed immediately by forced inspiration, which in cases of infection give a series of fine crackling râles in the affected area.

Fever is one of the most important early symptoms. The author insists that superficial examinations, or those made other than dictly to the skin over the thorax, are of no value whatever. In the more advanced cases the Roentgen ray is highly spoken of as a means of determining the extent of infiltration, an objection to this method being that an expert is required to conduct the examination.

In the treatment of the subject the author takes up in detail every phase of the life of the patient under observation, an essential being to secure the intelligent co-operation of the patient himself. Each case should be regarded as a law unto itself.

The treatment consists principally of outdoor life and hygienic means under careful observation, with such remedial agents as the physician thinks indicated, the object being to conserve and build up the patient's resisting power.

The book can be studied by student and practitioner alike with great benefit.   L. C. W.

The Cure of Rupture by Paraffin Injections. By CHARLES C. MILLER, M.D. Published by the author, 70 State Street, Chicago, Ill. Price, $1.

Without going into a discussion of the histological changes which follow the injection of paraffin into the tissues, it is certain that our present knowledge does not justify the teaching that this method is a safe and efficient treatment for hernia.

The cases recited by the author in which there was no recurrence within seven days to two months after treatment, do not warrant very definite conclusions. It is probable that had Dr. Miller waited for a few years before writing his book. the number of complications and recurrences would have deterred him. We await more conclusive evidence.   H. E. S.

Diseases of the Eye. By EDWARD JACKSON, M.D. Second edition, 615 pages. Illustrated. Cloth, $2.50. W. B. Saunders Co., Philadelphia.

While this new edition has been brought thoroughly up to date, yet a close examination of the work reveals the fact that it is strikingly free from the latest fads which so often permeate the present-day publications. Consequently one feels that whatever is suggested in the way of care and treatment in this book has back of it the author's personal experience. This healthy conservatism materially adds to the value of the book.

The work is practical throughout, and the chapter on "Remedies and Their Applications" is alone worth the price of the work to the student or practitioner.   HARBERT.

Pathological Technique. By F. B. MALLORY, M.D., and J. H. WRIGHT, M. D. Fourth revised edition, octavo, 480 pages. Illustrated. Philadelphia, W. B. Saunders Co. Cloth, $3 net.

This book is divided into three parts:

Part I.—Post-mortem examinations.

Part II.— Bacteriological methods, giving materials used and methods of preparing culture media, bacteriological examinations, methods of studying, and a description of and differential staining for the pathogenic bacteria.

Part III.—Histological methods. Pathological histology.

This is a valuable addition to the works on technique. The subjects are ably handled and well written, and any one doing postmortem, bacteriological or pathological research will find much of value in this book, and occasion to refer to same almost daily.

PAYNE.

Catechism of Hematology. By ROBERT LINCOLN WATKINS, Professor of Hematology, Eclectic Medical College of the City of New York.

The author devotes about twenty-five pages of the thirty-one in this essay to questions and answers upon the function of the blood. He gives a description of the microscopical appearence of blood in various pathological states, and claims to be proficient in diagnosis by this method. Some of the writer's statements are at variance with accepted theories. The essayist claims a new line of diagnosis for students and physicians. L. W.

Transactions of the National Eclectic Medical Association. Vol. XXXVI. Published by the Secretary, W. P. BEST, M.D., Indianapolis, Ind.

This embraces the proceedings of the thirty-eighth annual meeting held at Kansas City, June 17-20, 1908, together with addresses, papers, essays and reports; 340 pages are devoted to papers and 112 to other material, sufficient to make four quarterly *Bulletins* of about 80 pages each. It seems to us that the day of bound transactions is at an end, and most scientific societies are resorting to periodical form. This matter should be thoroughly discussed in Chicago next June.

Physician's Visiting List for 1909. Leather, $1. P. Blakiston's Son & Co., Philadelphia.

This very necessary little book should be in the possession of every physician. Its value is proven by the fact that this is the fifty-eighth year of its publication.

The book contains, in addition to the visiting list, a dose table revised according to the 1905 U. S. P., table of poisons and antidotes, incompatibility, metric system of weights and measures, etc.

The book is bound in leather and is a model of neatness and conciseness. L. C. W.

COLLEGE AND SOCIETY NOTES.

Texas Eclectics.

The twenty-fifth annual convention of the Texas Eclectic Medical Association convened in Dallas, October 28-29, 1908. While only forty-eight of the two hundred and fifty Eclectics of Texas were on hand, the meeting proved to be a very interesting one. The papers presented were exceptionally good, and elicited hearty discussions.

R. L. Thomas, M.D., of Cincinnati, O., R. O. Braswell, M.D., Physio-Medical member of the State Board of Medical Examiners, and Dr. W. M. Brumby, State Health Officer of Texas, were among the distinguished guests of the convention, and each was frequently heard to compliment the papers presented as some of the best ever heard at a State association.

The treasurer's report showed the association in a healthy financial condition, and all bills paid.

One hundred dollars each was voted to Drs. M. E. Daniel and J. P. Rice, Eclectic members of the State Board of Medical Examiners, as part payment for time sacrificed in behalf of the Eclectic cause in Texas.

The Credential Committee reported the names of five for membership as follows: R. O. Braswell, Ft. Worth; L. H. Freedman, Ft. Worth; M. W. Lowrey, Sanger; G. Yates, Sierra Blanca, and H. A. Kling, Reedville. Prof. R. L. Thomas, of Cincinnati, was elected an honorary member.

JOINED THE NATIONAL.—At the last session of the National at Kansas City, Texas was given the honor of being the first State association to vote favorably on the proposition to join the National. Their previous action was ratified by the following resolution, offered by Dr. H. H. Blankmeyer and unanimously adopted:

"*Be it resolved*, That the rules be suspended and our Advisory Committee be empowered to so amend our By-Laws as to provide for our State association becoming an auxiliary of the National, at the next June meeting to be held at Chicago, Ill.

"*Be it further resolved*, That our dues be changed to four ($4) dollars per annum, which shall cover both State and National cost, including initiation in the National; same to go into effect on and after its passage."

SPECIAL ADDRESSES.—Tuesday evening was specially designated for some fine talks that every one enjoyed. First was a rich, scholarly address by Dr. J. P. Rice, of Alpine, Tex., on "Premedical Education." Then Dr. R. L. Thomas, in his characteristic forceful way, made a good talk on "Co-operation and the Needs of the Eclectic Colleges." This was followed by an interesting annual address by President G. W. Johnson. Dr. R. O. Braswell, Physio-Medical member of the State Board of Medical Examiners, being present, was called upon for a few remarks. He made a very interesting talk on the "Advanced Schools of Medicine." He called upon the various advanced (or so-called minor) schools to co-operate for their own protection and interests, and suggested the appointment of a standing committee of two from each school in Texas. His suggestion was accepted, and, upon motion of Dr. L. S. Downs, he and Dr. J. P. Rice were appointed to represent the Eclectics.

On Wednesday, on account of the very excellent tuberculosis exhibit at the Dallas Fair, it was decided to abandon the afternoon session and commence promptly at 9 A.M. and remain in continuous session until all business was completed, and then go in a body to the exhibit. So, after completing the various sections and inviting the National to meet with us in grand old Texas, in 1910 or 1911, at Galveston or any Texas city they may choose, the election of officers was taken up and the following were elected: President, C. D. Hudson, Waco; First Vice-President, E. H. Cowan, Crowell; Second Vice-President, M. F. Bettencourt, Gladewater; Treasurer, M. E. Daniel, Honey Grove; Secretary, H. H. Blankmeyer, Honey Grove.

Next place of meeting, Dallas, October, 1909, when we expect to have the largest meeting in the history of Texas Eclecticism.

Watch for the program, then come and see.

Fraternally,

H. H. BLANKMEYER, *Secretary.*

T. A. E. Notes.

We take pleasure in introducing G. A. Smith, D. W. Richmond, A. L. Coffield, of the class of '11, and J. T. Lafferty, class of '10, our new brothers who successfully overcame the Dragons and Fiery-Eyed Demon.

Bro. W. R. Dyer, '08, visited and gave the fraternity a nice little talk filled with advice and encouragement. He is located at Winchester, Ill., and doing well.

Bro. H. E. Sloan, '98, a charter member of the fraternity, has the chair of didactic surgery in his alma mater.

Bro. Charles S. Amidon is our professor on the ear, nose and throat.

Bro. W. B. Cunningham, '06, is located at West Liberty, W. Va. Bro. A. R. Rhinehart, '06, is located at Grafton, W. Va.

Bro. A. A. Dewey, '06, formerly of South Bend, Ind., is now located at Bristol, Conn.

Bro. Pearl Bennett, '05, formerly of Farmersburg, Ind., is now located at Springfield, Ill.

Bro. A. C. Prichard is located at Diggs, Ark.

Bro. A. E. Rhien, '06, visited the fraternity last month. He is located at Brownsburg, Ind.

Bro. M. C. Karr, '09, is one of the internes for the first half of the college year. Bro. L. W. Page, '09, serves after the holidays.

Remember, brothers, that the fraternity would like to hear from you at any time. Get in touch with the fraternity by correspondence.

H. F. KILLEN, *Chronicler.*

E. P. Notes.

After a long and enjoyable vacation we are once more gathered together as brothers to listen to the teachings of our alma mater. It it well to bear in mind that it is not what we attain, but what we aim, which determines our worth; so let each one of us aim high, and we are sure to meet with success.

Bro. G. W. Martin, of Portsmouth, O., writes us he is comfortably located and doing well.

Bro. J. W. Bowers is located at Fort Wayne, Ind. We predict excellent results for this estimable brother.

Bro. A. M. Uphouse is serving as interne at the Seton Hospital.

Bro. C. T. Saylor, who is now located at Boswell, Pa., recently favored us with a long and very interesting letter. He is enjoying quite a large practice and speaks very highly of specific medication.

Bro. R. M. Jean has resumed his practice at Pottsville, Ark. He says he is too busy to attend E. M. I. this year, but will be with us next term.   T. L. FULLER.

Sigma Theta.

The winter session is well under way, and we are looking forward to the annual holiday vacations, which will permit most of us to visit home.

Our fraternity is in good shape and the characteristic *Sigma Theta* spirit and harmony ever prevails. Let it ever be uppermost in our minds to preserve this true fraternal feeling for all time.

The fellows who are engaged in active practice should not forget to turn their thoughts toward the home of their fraternity and alma mater. It is always a source of pleasure to hear from those who have gone from us.

Fellow Blough, '07, is doing well at Pittsburg, Pa. He says specific medication gives results first, last and all the time.

We recently had a very pleasant letter from Maysville, Ky., which informed us that Fellow Morgan, '08, has every reason to feel satisfied with his location.

Fellow Saxton, '07, is doing nicely at Tampa, Fla. He recently purchased an automobile, and from all accounts it is a beauty.

Fellow O'Hara, '07, reports progress at Lewisburg, O., going all the time, day and night.

Fellow Bowman, '07, of Garrett, Pa., recently spent a few days in the city. He is a firm believer in the old adage, "Follow your indications and success will surely be thine."   MARPLE.

PERSONALS.

Wm. H. H. Shrock, E. M. I., '08, passed the Pennsylvania board and is now located at Berlin, Pa.

Dr. G. A. Hinton is the only Eclectic located at Hot Springs, Ark. His address is Kempner Bldg. He will be glad to look after any case sent to him in consultation.

Locations.—Three good locations in New York State. For particulars, address with stamp, Mrs. F. Smith, 1 W. Walnut Street, Oneida, N. Y.

Dr. A. A. Dewey, E. M. I., '06, who was formerly located at South Bend, Ind., has moved to 108 High Street. Bristol, Conn, and entered into partnership with Dr. F. H. Williams, a practitioner of over forty years' experience. Together they are doing a large and lucrative practice, mostly office work.

The State Medical Board has received information that some medical students, having preliminary educational requirements less than demanded by the Ohio law, have been induced to attend medicall colleges in other States under the impression that after gradu-

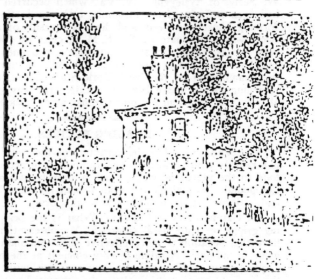

ation they can return to and obtain a license to practice in Ohio under reciprocity. This should be corrected. All medical students who have or who contemplate matriculating in colleges in other States with such impressions should understand that a license from another State is accepted in place of an examination only. The applicant in all other particulars must comply with the laws of Ohio and the rules of this Board. The preliminary educational attainments must be the same as required of students of Ohio colleges.

OBITUARY.

Elijah F. Davis, M.D., died in Lakewood, Cleveland, October 15, aged seventy-nine. He was born at Bazetta, O., August 9, 1829. He graduated at the Eclectic Medical Institute in 1857. He was a successful practitioner for over fifty-two years—forty-two spent in Cleveland. He was an active member of the Ohio Society for many years.

We regret to learn of the death of Dr. P. P. Outland, which occurred at Zanesfield, O., November 5. Dr. Outland had been suffering for some time from Bright's Disease, which was the cause of his death. He was a graduate of the E. M. I., '81' and had been a member of the State society for a number of years. He was a brother of Dr. W. H. Outland, who is located at Bellefontaine, O.

We regret very much to announce the sudden death of Dr. Charles W. Seely, of Wileyville, W. Va., which occurred October 29. He had been suffering from insomnia, and was in the habit of chloroforming himself to sleep, and died as a result of an overdose. Dr. Seely was a graduate of the E. M. I., class of 1903, and had been very successful in practice, and was a prominent member of his State society. About two weeks ago he was successful in passing the examination of the New York State Board, and had intended returning to his native State to locate. He was very well liked by all who met him, and his death comes as a shock to the community.

READING NOTICES.

MENORRHAGIA.—The desideratum for the relief of this condition is a remedy which will not only stimulate contraction, but will impart tone to the uterus as well. Such a remedy is Hayden's Viburnum Compound. Its action is superior to and far more lasting than Ergot and is devoid of the toxic effects of this drug.

LA GRIPPE—ACUTE CORYZA.—What is the best method of aborting grippe or acute nasal catarrh? My observation leads me to believe that sedation is more effective than stimulation. I can see no value in quinine. A saline is very efficient at the beginning. Glyco-Thymoline in a 25 to 50 per cent. solution with water, used with the K. &. O nasal douche, allays the congested mucous membrane of the nose and throat. It is alkaline, antiseptic and sedative, and always makes the patient feel comfortable. The patient should be instructed to keep the naso-pharyngeal mucous membrane in a clean aseptic condition, as it is doubtless during colds that many cases of tubercular infection occur.—W. T. MARRS, M.D., Jewett, Ill.

As THE cold, damp winds of fall chill the skin, more of the work of elimination is thrown upon the kidneys. It is not always that the function of the kidney can be adjusted to this increased demand, and imperfect elimination of waste products results. This auto-toxic state gives rise to such conditions as rheumatism, tonsillitis, neuralgia, catarrhal bronchitis, with or without asthma, winter eczema and pruritus, catarrhal rhinitis, and many other less distinctly defined conditions. The best results in treatment are to be had from establishing thorough renal elimination. Nothing accomplishes this so promptly and so effectually as Alkalithia in teaspoonful doses, in half a glass of water, every four hours, and a cure follows the removal of the cause.

IN the wasting diseases, as well as in rickets, scrofula and marasmus, it is of the greatest importance that a remedy be selected which will quickly check the pathological condition, and restore the organism to the normal without producing digestive or other functional disturbance. Cod liver oil has always stood first in the category of remedies calculated to bring about this desirable result, but unfortunately its peculiar odor and taste are features which are quite often objectionable to patients. Hagee's cord. ext. ol. morrhuæ comp. is an elegant preparation, containing all the essential therapeutic properties of cod liver oil combined with tissue-building chemicals (hypophosphites of lime and soda) and aromatics, which renders it agreeable to the palate.—*Am. Jour. Dermatology.*

THE FIRST SYMPTOMS OF MIGRAINE.—Dr. J. J. Caldwell, of Baltimore, Md., in *Medical Progress* writes as follows: "The treatment of migraine, to be correct, must be adjusted on the basis of the element of causation. Constipation, if present, should be treated by a proper dietary and regular habits, but purgatives should be avoided. Only mild laxatives should be employed, and they should be abandoned when diet regulates the bowels, as proper diet will do. During the premonitory stage we can generally abort or rather prevent the development of an attack by the administration of two antikamnia tablets. They should be given as soon as the first symptoms of the attack are manifest. If then, all symptoms are not speedily dissipated, another dose should be given in three-quarters of an hour or an hour. This means is a most effectual one to abort an attack, and when the attack is developed, antikamnia tablets will relieve the pain usually in about forty minutes."

Colden's Liquid Beef Tonic

Arouses the Gustatory Organs and Sharpens the Appetite.

Stimulates the Digestive Glands, Promotes Secretory Activity and Tones the Gastro-intestinal Tract.

Indications: Impaired Appetite, Gastro-intestinal Torpidity—and All Digestive Disorders in which the Secretory Activity of the Digestive Glands is Subnormal.

When Anæmia Complicates Colden's Liquid Beef Tonic with Iron is Indicated

Sold by Druggists

THE CHARLES N. CRITTENTON CO., 115 Fulton Street, New York

Sample with literature sent *gratis* to any physician on request.

INDEX TO ADVERTISEMENTS.

The Eclectic Medical Journal

1009 Plum Street, Cincinnati, Ohio.

JOHN K SCUDDER, M.D.,
EDITOR.

THE SCUDDER BROTHERS,
PUBLISHERS

Subscription Price, $2.00 per year in advance. Single Copies, 20 cents.

TABLE OF CONTENTS.

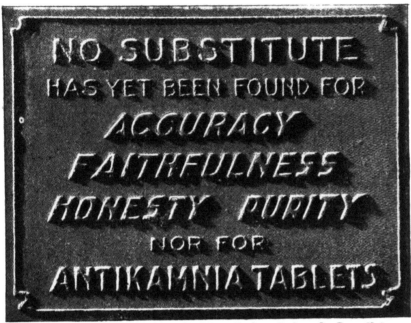
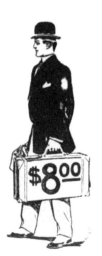

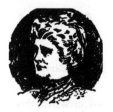
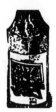

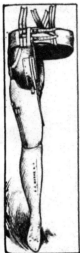
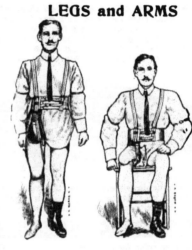

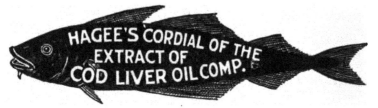

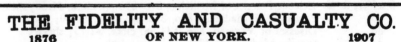

Eclectic Medical Books

All of the Books below are listed at strictly net prices.

Cooper, Wm. Colby. Tethered Truants, 12mo, 199 pages, cloth . . . $1
do   do   Immortality, 12mo, 173 pages, cloth 1
do   do   Preventive Medicine, 147 pages, cloth 1
Dodge. Social Purity, 16mo, cloth . . . .
Ellingwood. Materia Medica and Therap., 8vo, 811 pp. cloth, $5.00; sheep, 6
  do   Treatment of Disease, 2 vols, 8vo, 1100 pp. cloth . . . 6
Farnum. Orthopedic Surgery, 8vo, 554 pp. illustrated, cloth . . . 5
Felter-Lloyd. American Dispensatory, 2 vols, each 950 pp. cloth, $4.50; sheep, 5
Foltz. Diseases of the Eye, 12mo, 566 pp. cloth 2
  do Nose, Throat and Ear, illustrated, 12mo, 650 pages, cloth . . . 3
Fyfe. Materia Medica and Therapeutics, 12mo, 344 pp. cloth. . . 2
Howe. Fractures and Dislocations, 8vo, 426 pp. cloth, $1.50; sheep 2
  do Operative Gynecology, 8vo, 360 pp. sheep. 4
King. Family Physician, 8vo, 1042 pp. morocco 6
  do Chronic Diseases, 8vo, 1700 pp. sheep 8
  do Am. Dispensatory (Felter-Lloyd), 2 vols each, cloth, $4.50; sheep . 5
  do Eclectic Obstetrics, 8vo, 757 pp. sheep 5
  do Diseases of Women, 8vo, 366 pp. cloth, $1.50; sheep . . 2
Lloyd. Etidorhpa, 8vo, illustrated, 362 pp. cloth 1
  do The Right Side of the Car, paper . . . . .
  do Stringtown On the Pike. 12mo, cloth 1
  do Warwick of the Knobs, 12mo, 305 pp. cloth 1
  do Redhead, illustrated, 12mo, 208 pp. cloth. 1
  do Scroggins, 12mo, 110 pp. cloth 1
Locke-Felter. Materia Medica, 12mo, 500 pp. cloth 2
Mundy. Diseases of Children, 12mo, 600 pp. cloth 2
Munk. Arizona Sketches, 8vo, 230 pp. cloth 2
Neiderkorn. A Handy Reference Book to Specific Medication, 151 pp. leather . 1
Palmer. Digestive Organs, 8vo, 524 pp. cloth 3
Petersen. Materia Medica and Clinical Therap. 12mo, 400 pp. cloth . 3
Scudder, J. M. Eclectic Practice of Medicine, 8vo, 816 pp. cloth, $4.50; sheep 5
  do   Principles of. Medicine, 8vo, 350 pp. cloth, $1.50; sheep . . 2
  do   Diseases of Women, 8vo, 534 pp. cloth, $2.75; sheep . . 3
  do   Specific Medication, 12mo, 432 pp. cloth . . . 2
  do   Specific Diagnosis, 12mo, 388 pp. cloth 1
  do   Medication and Diagnosis, 1 vol, cloth 3
  do.   Materia Medica and Therap., 8vo, 748 pp. cloth, $4.00; sheep, 4
  do.   Eclectic Family Physician, 8vo, 900 pp. clo, $3; sh. $4; hf. mor. 5
Thomas. Eclectic Practice of Medicine, illus, 8vo, 1033 pp. cloth, $6; sheep, . 7
Stephens. Medical Gynecology, 12mo, 428 pp. illustrated, cloth . . . 3
Watkins. Compendium of the Practice of Medicine, 12mo, 460 pp. cloth . 2
Webster. Eclectic Medical Practice, 2 vols in one, 8vo, 1233 pp. clo, $6.50; sh. 7
Wintermute. King's Eclectic Obstetrics, 8vo, 757 pp. sheep . . . 5
Wilder. History of Medicine, 12mo, 946 pp. cloth 2
Woodward. Intra-Uterine Medication, 12mo, 208 pp. cloth . . . 2

Any Book on this list will be sent Post-paid on receipt of Price, by

THE SCUDDER BROTHERS COMPANY,

Medical Publishers,

1009 Plum Stree   Cincinna

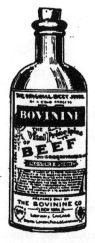
Post-Graduate Instruction in Cincinnati.

THE overtowering importance of the so-called physical or mechanical me_ thods (physiological therapeutics) in the modern treatment of disease is admitted on all sides. No physician can be considered an up-to-date practi- tioner who has not some knowledge of massage vibration, Swedish move- ments, hydro-therapy, thermo-therapy, electricity in its various forms, Fin sen-rays and other forms of light treatment, X-rays, and the fundamental branches of physiological therapy, to wit, hygiene and dietetics.

The Cincinnati Post-Graduate School of Physiological Therapeu- tics is a school of scientific medicine, and the only post-graduate school of its kind in the West. It is open to physicians only. The school has the most complete equipment to be found anywhere in the United States. The courses of instruction are short and practical. A two weeks general course, includ- ing instruction in static electricity, galvanism, faradism, high-frequency currents, Roentgen rays, hydro-therapy, thermo-therapy, Finsen rays, Minin rays, electric light baths, massage, Sweedish movements, etc., given from time to time for the benefit of busy practitioners who can not afford to spend much time away from home. The school has the unqualified endorsement of the profession. Every member of the graduating class of the Eclectic Med- ical Institute is given a course in drugless therapeutic methods at the Cin- cinnati Post-Graduate School of Physiological Therapeutics, the course being obligatory and a part of the curriculum of studies.

> The text-book of practice used at the school is "MODERN PHYSIO- THERAPY," a practical hand-book of Physical and Mechani- cal Therapeutic Methods, by Otto Juettner, M. D.

Illustrated prospectus of the School and specimen pages of "Modern Physio Therapy" sent upon application. Address

Cincinnati Post-Graduate School of Physiological Therapeutics,
No. 628 Elm Street. CINCINNATI O.

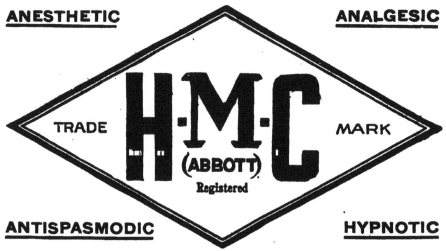

PROFESSIONAL.

WILLIAM B. CHURCH, M. D.

SURGEON
The Berkshire, 628 Elm St.
CINCINNATI.
Will visit any part of the country in consultation or to perform operations.

OWEN A. PALMER, M D.,
Gynecological and General Surgery,
CLEVELAND, - - - OHIO
New No. 1948 101st St., N. E.,
Sanitarium accommodations. Will visit any part of the country.

K. O. FOLTZ, M. D.
EYE, EAR, NOSE and THROAT,
105 Odd Fellows' Building,
7th and Elm sts. CINCINNATI.

J. STEWART HAGEN, M. D.
SURGEON
1506 Harrison ave. Cincinnati, O.

JOHN L. PAYNE, M.D.,
Microscopist,
918 W. Eighth St., CINCINNATI.
Tel. W. 1146.

Sputum urine-and tissues examined.

Dr. WILLIAM E. BLOYER,
THE LANCASTER,
22 West Seventh St. Cincinnati,
General Consultant.
Telephone, Canal 2248.

L. E. RUSSELL, M. D.
SURGEON
The Groton—Seventh & Race
CINCINNATI.

R. L. THOMAS, M. D.
Consulting Physician.
792 EAST MCMILLEN ST.
Walnut Hills, CINCINNATI.

H. C. BURSON, M. D.
SURGEON
115 Main St. TOLEDO, O.

JOHN R. SPENCER, M.D.,
General Consultant,
952 W. Eighth St.
Tel. W. ATL.

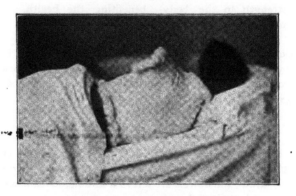

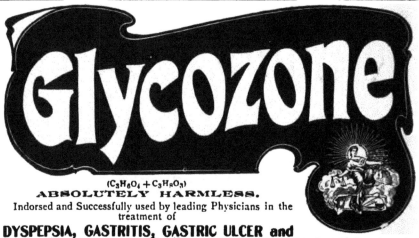

THE
ECLECTIC MEDICAL INSTITUTE

CHARTERED MARCH 10, 1845.
3,918 GRADUATES

The SIXTY-FIFTH SESSION will begin Monday, September 20, 1909, and continue thirty-two weeks. Hospital instruction in Cincinnati and Seton Hospitals. Clinical instruction in the daily *Dispensary* of Seton Hospital, conducted by the Sisters of Charity, at 625 Kenyon Avenue.

New students are urged to perfect their entrance qualifications and matriculate early. Fees are Ninety Dollars a year, no extras.

For announcement and further information address

JOHN K. SCUDDER, M.D., *Secretary*,
1009 Plum Street, Cincinnati, O.

FACULTY.

Professors

JOHN URI LLOYD, Phr. M.,....................*Chemistry and Pharmacy.*
BISHOP McMILLEN, M.D.................*Mental and Nervous Diseases.*
ROLLA L. THOMAS, M.D...................*Practice of Medicine; Dean.*
WILLIAM E. BLOYER, M.D...........*Materia Medica and Therapeutics.*
JOHN K. SCUDDER, M.D..............................*Secretary; Latin.*
LYMAN WATKINS, M.D...................*Pathology and Physiology.*
HARVEY W. FELTER, M.D............................*Medical History.*
L. E. RUSSELL, M.D....................*Clinical Surgery and Gynecology.*
JOHN R. SPENCER, M.D...................................*Obstetrics.*
JOHN P. HARBERT, M.D................................*Ophthalmology.*
CHARLES GREGORY SMITH, M.D..........................*Chemistry.*
HERBERT E. SLOAN, M.D............................*Didactic Surgery.*
WILLIAM N. MUNDY, M.D......................*Diseases of Children.*
THOMAS BOWLES, M.D............................*Diseases of Women.*
BYRON VAN HORN, M.D.....................................*Anatomy.*
CHARLES S. AMIDON, M.D.........*Otology, Rhinology and Laryngology.*

Lecturers

WILLIAM L. DICKSON, M.D.....................*Medical Jurisprudence.*
JOHN L. PAYNE, M.D.....*Hygiene, Histology, Pathology and Bacteriology.*
WILBUR E. POSTLE, M.D.................*Mental and Nervous Diseases.*
EDWIN R. FREEMAN, M.D..................*Skin and Venereal Diseases.*
J. STEWART HAGEN, M.D....................*Surgery and Gynecology.*
J. CORLISS EVANS, M.D...........................*Physical Diagnosis.*
OTTO JUETTNER, M.D............................*Electro-Therapeutics.*
LOUIS C. WOTTRING, M.D...........................*Clinical Medicine.*
VICTOR P. WILSON, M.D.................*Clinical Diseases of Women.*

Lightning Source UK Ltd.
Milton Keynes UK
UKHW020625120219
337137UK00005B/528/P